Textbooks in Contemporary Dentistry

This textbook series presents the most recent advances in all fields of dentistry, with the aim of bridging the gap between basic science and clinical practice. It will equip readers with an excellent knowledge of how to provide optimal care reflecting current understanding and utilizing the latest materials and techniques. Each volume is written by internationally respected experts in the field who ensure that information is conveyed in a concise, consistent, and readily intelligible manner with the aid of a wealth of informative illustrations. *Textbooks in Contemporary Dentistry* will be especially valuable for advanced students, practitioners in the early stages of their career, and university instructors.

More information about this series at https://link.springer.com/bookseries/14362

Tiril Willumsen • Jostein Paul Årøen Lein
Ronald C. Gorter • Lena Myran

Editors

Oral Health Psychology

Psychological Aspects Related to Dentistry

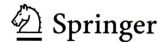 Springer

Editors
Tiril Willumsen
Institute of Clinical Dentistry
University of Oslo
Oslo, Norway

Ronald C. Gorter
Social Dentistry & Behavioural Sciences
Academic Center for Dentistry Amsterdam
Amsterdam, The Netherlands

Jostein Paul Årøen Lein
Levanger Hospital
Levanger, Norway

Lena Myran
Oral health center of expertice Mid-Norway
Trondheim, Norway

ISSN 2524-4612   ISSN 2524-4620   (electronic)
Textbooks in Contemporary Dentistry
ISBN 978-3-031-04247-8   ISBN 978-3-031-04248-5   (eBook)
https://doi.org/10.1007/978-3-031-04248-5

This Springer imprint is published by the registered company Springer Nature Switzerland AG
The registered company address is: Gewerbestrasse 11, 6330 Cham, Switzerland

Foreword

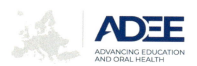

Association for Dental Education in Europe
International Office
Dublin Dental University Hospital
Lincoln Place, D02 F859, Ireland

To the authors of the book *Oral Health Psychology*

The book *Oral Health Psychology* should be a must for both current and future dentists and other oral health professionals. The authors define "oral health psychology" as a collection of scientific, pedagogical, and professional contributions from psychology to the promotion and maintenance of oral health. The book thus contributes to placing oral health as an integral part of general health and well-being. In order to understand and help all patients, dental professionals should have knowledge and skills in communication, disease prevention, and anxiety problems. Oral health psychology also deals with the professionalism in the role of oral health professionals and should therefore be set clearly and included in modern curricula for dental health professionals.

Registered in Ireland: Tax Reference Number 9624753K
Registered Charity Number 20058111

Charitable Tax Exemption Number CHY16249
EU transparency registry: 224420913440-79

Pål Barkvoll
Professor dr.odont. (Oral Surgery and Oral Medicine), President ADEE
(Association for Dental Education in Europe), Lincoln Place, Ireland

Preface

Dentistry aims to provide a dental patient the opportunity to experience good oral health throughout life. In order to achieve this aim, adequate attitudes, knowledge, and skills within the dental team are essential. Traditionally, (bio)medical knowledge and technical/manual skills have been the basis of dental care. The biopsychosocial model has informed us that these perspectives are not sufficient to provide optimal care for all patients. We know today that many patients are at risk of poor oral health due to reduced benefit from traditional dental care. They may not be able to take advice and instructions from dental personnel, they struggle to perform daily oral care, and when showing up in a dental clinic, they fight with anxiety, helplessness, or hopelessness.

In 2021, the World Health Organization (WHO) issued a World Health Assembly Resolution in which it paved the way for better oral healthcare. Together with emphasizing the need for accessibility to oral care for all, the WHO also stressed the fact that "oral health is a key indicator of overall health, well-being and quality of life." The WHO also recommends a shift from the traditional curative approach towards a preventive approach that includes promotion of oral health within the family, schools, and workplaces, and includes timely, comprehensive, and inclusive care within the primary healthcare system.

To help patients, dental staff need to include a psychological dimension in their professional field. Within a broader (medical) context, psychological understanding of healthcare-related issues is defined as health psychology. Therefore, following the American Psychological Association's definition of health psychology, we define *oral health psychology* as:

> "Oral health psychology is the aggregate of scientific, educational, and professional contributions from psychology to the promotion and maintenance of oral health. This includes the prevention and treatment of illness, the identification of etiologic and diagnostic correlates of diminished oral health, and the analysis and improvement of the oral healthcare system and oral health policy formation."

The field of dentistry is ever developing. Dentistry is no longer only about oral diseases. In 2016, the World Dental Federation (FDI) redefined oral health as "Oral health is multi-faceted and includes the ability to speak, smile, smell, taste, touch, chew, swallow and convey a range of emotions through facial expressions with confidence and without pain, discomfort and disease of the craniofacial complex (head, face, and oral cavity). Oral health means the health of the mouth. No matter what your age, oral health is vital to general health and well-being."

The purpose of this definition is to integrate oral health in the patient's overall health and well-being. The new definition represents a paradigm shift in dentistry. In this paradigm shift, understanding and implementing oral health psychology in daily dental practice is fundamental.

The dental health service has emphasized and will continue to place great emphasis on operational treatment of discomfort and/or disease in the craniofacial complex. But modern dentistry also includes seeing the patient as a whole, including psychological issues and challenges that affect oral health.

This book aims to give both oral health students and staff a comprehensive introduction and understanding in many aspects related to oral health psychology. It will also address many of the challenges faced by oral health staff when meeting patients with different degrees of psychological well-being associated with their oral health and treatment. Hopefully, these perspectives and increased understanding will contribute to fulfill the needs of every patient.

> ❯ Dental patients are not difficult, but they may be in a difficult situation.

As editors, we have chosen to refer in the text to other relevant chapters rather than writing the same thing several times, although there may be some overlap. For students, the chapters are presented in a carefully planned order, and it is recommended to read the entire book. For dental and other oral health professionals, or any interested reader, the chapters can often be read separately.

For reasons of readability, in the text the word dentist is regularly used just to refer to the dentist, whereas in many cases it is also used to refer to the dental staff in a broader sense.

We want this book to contribute to better oral health in patients of all ages, and to help improve collaboration among dental professionals, their patients, and the patients' caregivers. In addition, we hope that improved knowledge will increase job satisfaction and reduce risk of burnout among dental staff.

This book is a result of international collaboration, with authors from various countries and various continents. We would like to thank all authors for their contributions and dedication to help create this book.

Tiril Willumsen
Oslo, Norway

Ronald C. Gorter
Amsterdam, The Netherlands

Lena Myran
Trondheim, Norway

Jostein Paul Årøen Lein
Levanger, Norway
16. 02. 2022

Contents

Part III

IV   Patients with Complex Reactions and Co-morbidity

Part IV

V   Professionalism

     and Education 305
     Sandra Zijlstra-Shaw and Ronald C. Gorter

21   **Living in a Golden Cage? Work Stress, Burnout Risk, and Engagement in**
     Dental Practice: Background and Prevention 315
     Ronald C. Gorter, Lena Myran, and Tiril Willumsen

22   **Working in Partnership for Better Oral Health Care** 327
     Lena Myran, Jostein Paul Årøen Lein, Margrethe Elin Vika, Ulla Wide,
     and Wendy Knibbe

     Supplementary Information
     Index 345

Contributors

Maren Lillehaug Agdal   Oral Health Center of Expertise in Western Norway, Bergen, Norway
maren.gry.lillehaug.agdal@vlfk.no

Trine Anstorp   Private Practice, Oslo, Norway
ansfri@online.no

Koula Asimakopoulou   King's College London, London, UK
koula.asimakopoulou@kcl.ac.uk

Sarah R. Baker   University of Sheffield, School of Clinical Dentistry, Sheffield, UK
s.r.baker@sheffield.ac.uk

Jan Bergdahl   Department of Psychology, University of Umeå, Umeå, Sweden
jan.bergdahl@umu.se

Karin Goplerud Berge   Oral Health Center of Expertise, Bergen, Norway
Karin.Goplerud.Berge@vlfk.no

Anne Kristine Bergem   Oslo Metropolitan University, Oslo, Norway

Therese Varvin Fredriksen   Tannhelsetjenesten i Telemark og Vestfold, Tønsberg, Norway
therese.fredriksen@vtfk.no

Paula Frid   Department of ENT and Division of Oral and Maxillofacial Surgery, University Hospital North Norway & Public Dental Service Competence Centre of Northern Norway, Tromsø, Norway
Department of Clinical Dentistry, UIT The Arctic University of Norway, Tromsø, Norway
paula.frid@unn.no

Ronald C. Gorter   Department of Oral Radiology/Digital Dental Training and Assessment, Academic Centre for Dentistry Amsterdam (ACTA), University of Amsterdam/VU University Amsterdam, Amsterdam, The Netherlands
r.gorter@acta.nl

Marianne Hoås Gudmundsen   Oral Health Center of Expertise, Bergen, Norway
marianne.gudmundsen@vtfk.no

Anne Elisabeth Münster Halvari   Department of Dental Hygiene Science, University of Oslo, Oslo, Norway
ahalvari@odont.uio.no

Jenny Harris   Consultant in Community Paediatric Dentistry, Wheata Place Dental Clinic, Sheffield, UK
jenny.harris@nhs.net

Mariann Saanum Hauge   Faculty of Dentistry, University of Oslo, Oslo, Norway
mariann@tannsor.no

Ann Catrin Høyvik   Faculty of Dentistry, University of Oslo (UiO), Oslo, Norway
a.c.hoyvik@odont.uio.no

Ingrid Berg Johnsen   Karolinska Institute, Stockholm, Norway
ingjo@tkmidt.no

Jan-Are Kolset Johnsen   Department of Clinical Dentistry, UIT The Arctic University of Norway, Tromsø, Norway
jan.a.johnsen@uit.no

Wendy Knibbe   Department for Orofacial Pain and Dysfunction, Academic Centre for Dentistry Amsterdam (ACTA)/Centre for Special Dental Care (SBT), Amsterdam, The Netherlands
w.knibbe@acta.nl

Vibeke Kranstad   Oral Health Centre of Expertise in Eastern Norway, Oslo, Norway
vibekek@viken.no

Jostein Paul Årøen Lein   Trøndelag fylkeskommune and Helse Nord-Trøndelag, Norway
jostein.lein@gmail.com

Zoe Marshman   School of Clinical Dentistry, University of Sheffield, Sheffield, UK
z.marshman@sheffield.ac.uk

Lena Myran   Center for Oral Health Services and Research Mid-Norway (TkMidt), Trondheim, Norway
lenmy@tkmidt.no

Åshild Nupen   Oral Health Centre of Expertise in Eastern Norway, Oslo, Norway
ashildn@viken.no

Peter Prescott   Solli District Psychiatric Center, Oslo, Norway
Iprescottnorge@gmail.com

Helen Rodd   School of Clinical Dentistry, University of Sheffield, Sheffield, UK
h.d.rodd@sheffield.ac.uk

Adam Rogers   Department of Pediatric Dentistry and Behavioral Science, Faculty of Dentistry, University of Oslo, Oslo, Norway
a.a.rogers@odont.uio.no

Anne Rønneberg   Department of Paediatric Dentistry and Behvioural Science, Institute of Clinical Dentistry, Faculty of Dentistry, University of Oslo, Oslo, Norway
anne.ronneberg@odont.uio.no

Julie Satur   Melbourne Dental School, University of Melbourne, Melbourne, VIC, Australia
juliegs@unimelb.edu.au

Borrik Schjødt   Centre for Pain Management and Palliative Care, Haukeland University Hospital, Bergen, Norway
borrik@uib.no

Siri Søftestad   Kristiansand, Norway
siri.softestad@gmail.com

Linda Stein   Department of Clinical Dentistry, UiT The Arctic University of Norway, Tromsø, Norway
linda.stein@uit.no

Bent Storå   Agder Dental Health Service, Kristiansand, Norway
bent.stora@agderfk.no

Kjetil Strøm   Faculty of Dentistry, University of Oslo (UiO), Oslo, Norway
kjetil.strom@odont.uio.no

Jorun Torper   Oral Health Centre of Expertise in Eastern Norway (OHCE), Oslo, Norway
myrulljorun@gmail.com

Margrethe Elin Vika   Oral Health Center of Expertise in Western Norway, Bergen, Norway
margrethe.elin.vika@vlfk.no

Ulla Wide   University of Gothenburg, Gothenburg, Sweden
ulla.wide@gu.se

Tiril Willumsen   Dental Faculty, University of Oslo, Oslo, Norway
tiril.willumsen@odont.uio.no

Marit Irene Woldstad   Outpatient Clinic Adult Psychiatry, University Hospital of Northern Norway, Tromsoe, Norway
marit.woldstad@unn.no

Sandra Zijlstra-Shaw   Education Research, School of Clinical Dentistry, University of Sheffield, Sheffield, UK
s.zijlstra-shaw@sheffield.ac.uk

Basic Oral Health Psychology

Contents

Basic Oral Health-Related Psychology

Jan-Are K. Johnsen, Adam Rogers, Jan Bergdahl, and Tiril Willumsen

Contents

1.1 Introduction

This book addresses many different issues included in the field *oral health psychology* and examines the application of psychological knowledge within the oral health sciences. Psychology itself is a large subject area that can be defined as *the study of behaviour and mental processes*. Through the perspective of psychological science, one can find answers as to why people act, feel, and think as they do and obtain ideas for how to change or influence behaviours, thoughts, and feelings.

In recent years it has become more common for psychologists worldwide to work in, or be affiliated with, oral health care [1]. Furthermore, subjects focused on psychological and behavioural science have been increasingly recognized as important in the education of oral health professionals [2, 3]. Students training to be oral health clinicians appear to value behavioural science teaching [4–8], although negative attitudes or hidden curricula concerning behavioural science teaching might still exist among students and teaching staff [9, 10]. In this chapter we will look at some basic perspectives and theories that may have direct clinical applications for oral health professionals and also help to form a basic working knowledge of psychology that will be useful during continued learning about applications of psychology within the field of oral health.

⊜ Learning Goals
 — To establish a basic understanding of the relationship between thoughts, feelings, and behaviours.
 — To gain knowledge of psychological theories that may help interpret reactions from both clinicians and patients to stress, challenging clinical encounters, and other factors within the dental treatment environment.
 — To learn about the practical benefits of emotional competence and affective awareness within dental health care.

1.2 The Bio-psychosocial Model of Disease and Health

The evolution of oral health psychology can be seen as a result of the bio-psychosocial model [11] being introduced in health services, adding psychological and social relationships to the traditional biomedical model of disease and health. This traditional biomedical model is based on the premise that every disease has an underlying biological explanation, whereby an organism is affected by pathogens (i.e. bacteria, viruses), with the treatment of disease occurring when influence is exerted over such biological factors. Within this model, the absence of obvious pathogens or disease-related symptoms is taken as an indication that the individual is in good health. However, while such models have their values (e.g. in the treatment of infectious diseases), they have proved less suited to tackling modern health challenges related to complex individual lifestyles (lifestyle diseases). In these scenarios, treating only identifiable disease may have little lasting effect on the factors that led to the disease in the first place. Dental caries is one example of a disease in which a pure biomedical disease model falls short of explaining the phenomenon, namely because long-term disease control is largely connected to individual behaviour (i.e. diet, hygiene measures) rather than therapeutic measures (e.g. filling teeth, etc.). In other words, while the removal of biological plaque and caries is beneficial, it does little to influence the chronic disease processes that led to disease development. Therefore, for a clinician to attest that they have improved the health and well-being of their patient, efforts must be made to alter these root causes.

Identifying the causes of disease beyond proximal factors, however, is not an easy task. According to Engel's bio-psychosocial model [11], one may traverse the causal hierarchy all the way to the sub-atomic level in order to explain an emergent phenomenon. The bio-psychosocial model suggests that the determinants of any event can be ranked from large (e.g. the universe) to small (e.g. atoms, quarks), with a prerequisite that all parts of this system are interconnected and interact with each other. Thus, small changes in biological neural cells can elicit changes in thoughts, which can change behaviour, which can change social factors. Simultaneously, working down the hierarchy shows that the social context may limit the available behaviours, which can limit the associated thoughts or cognitive reactions. Essentially, each level acts as a framework for potential actions, while also being influenced by the infinite cumulative interactions occurring at the levels below. Understanding dental caries therefore necessitates more than identifying and treating the illness, one must look at the psychological factors that preceded risk behaviour and disease, as well as the social and environmental factors that may steer these psychological processes (◘ Fig. 1.1).

The basis for this shift towards bio-psychosocial models within medicine and health sciences is the growing acceptance that a close relationship exists between patients' individual lives and encounters and their experience with illness. This perspective has also contributed to the development of the fields of health psychology and psychosomatic medicine, disciplines that acknowledge the need to address both psychological and social factors, in addition to symptoms, during the treatment and prevention of disease. In recent years, both public health authorities and oral health professionals have

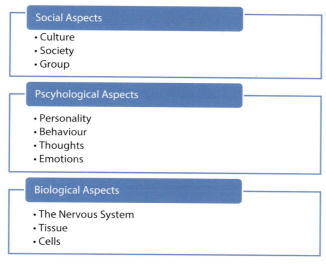

Fig. 1.1 Example of a hierarchical, bio-psychosocial model of health and disease; from social relationships to biological factors

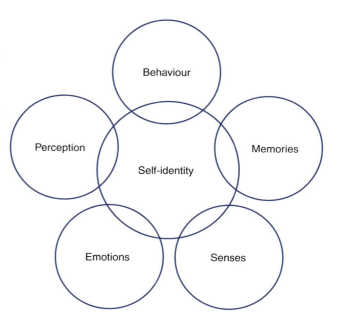

Fig. 1.2 The experience of self-identity as a result of the interaction of many factors

also started to appreciate the importance of this perspective, which includes the realization that some individuals might fall outside of established oral healthcare systems due to psychological and social factors. To understand why patients are unable to access existing care networks, even when there are real treatment needs, it is necessary to look for causal mechanisms beyond the dental clinic itself.

> For individuals that are unable to utilize the existing oral healthcare system, it is unlikely that this is caused by single factors (e.g. aversion to treatment). Instead, there could be an interaction of thoughts, emotions, behaviours, as well as cultural or social factors that contribute to their self-identity and well-being at any point in time. In other words, explaining the persistence of oral disease necessitates a broader understanding of how people think and act in the face of dental health concerns.

1.3 Self-Identity: Who Are We?

In order to recognize how psychological and biological elements may influence each other and disease development, it is important to look at the way they contribute to the stable set of characteristics that we carry during our daily lives – our self-identity. A fundamental part of being human is that we all have a defined self-identity and experience life as a unique individual ('I'). This experience, also called self-awareness, has been interesting for both philosophy and psychology. Early notions suggested that self-awareness originated outside the body, with ideas such as the existence of the *soul* creat-

ing a so-called mind–body dualism, as described, for example, by Rene Descartes [12]. Here, the body and soul are completely separate, with the soul constituting a metaphysical phenomenon. In contrast, there are also those who claim that consciousness is instead a pure physiological process ('monism'), suggesting that rather than being a separate entity, it should be possible to identify a specific source of self-awareness in the brain. However, research suggests that self-awareness, and our concept of self-identity, is not situated in a single place but is the result of an interaction between many different parts of the brain and many different brain functions [13] (**◻** Fig. 1.2).

Because self-identity deals with how individuals experience and understand themselves, exploring the concept of self-identity can explain how people relate to the world and others around them. Delving into psychological and social processes in the realms of dentistry may therefore increase the appreciation of how practitioners understand themselves and their roles – that is, a form of professional self-awareness – in addition to recognizing the uniqueness of each patient, with each individual guaranteed to have their own experiences and needs. This chapter aims to show how a wider bio-psychosocial and psychological perspective may assist in achieving this desired level of understanding. Through a review of some principles of basic psychology, with a partial focus on the functions and processes that underpin our self-identity, this chapter aims to demonstrate how important psychology is to our communication and interaction with others in an oral health setting.

1.4 Relationship Between Behaviour, Thoughts, and Feelings

To examine the theoretical links between elements of self-identity, there are many different directions and perspectives. One of the most well-known directions is cognitive psychology, with the term 'cognition' (adj. cognitive) referring to the mechanism involved in establishing comprehension; namely, the process of obtaining and piecing together information from memory and from the world around us. Cognitive psychology thus deals with underlying mental processes such as thought, perception, attention, and problem solving. In early philosophy, the cognitive perspective was often contrasted against the *emotional* perspective, where emotions were seen as obstacles to rational thinking. Today, however, more interest is placed on the connection and interaction between cognition and emotion [14], with both suggested to influence action simultaneously.

One reason to emphasize cognitive psychology in this context is that, from this perspective, it encourages a closer look at the constituent components of information processing and decision-making. This can be contrasted against alternative directions that may be more concerned with, for example, the development of mental illness (e.g. psychoanalytic psychology) or exploring specific mental processes and tasks (e.g. learning psychology). The cognitive perspective also prompts us to search for a definition of abstract concepts such as 'thinking' and 'thought', which were described as a partial focus within this chapter. Although humans are engaged in cognition almost all of the time, and are capable of identifying current thoughts, that does not necessarily make it easy to define what a thought *is* or explain how it has arisen. In cognitive psychology, a *thought* is talked about as a *mental representation*, with these representations coming from an interaction between the collection of information from the environment (*perception*), the selection of important information *(attention)*, and the processing and storage of this information *(memory)*. Thus, the construct of thinking can be simplified as the active and deliberate use of this information that is continuously being collected, stored, and recalled, with individual thoughts and ideas being the experience of this process and its content. Within an oral health setting, a cognitive perspective means exploring how clinicians and patients collect information from their environment, how they determine which information is important, and how this information is stored and used in future situations.

Through influencing and controlling how information is processed and interpreted, one can fundamentally intervene in the processes related to thinking. This is one of the main reasons why the cognitive perspective in psychology has been so popular, leading to the development

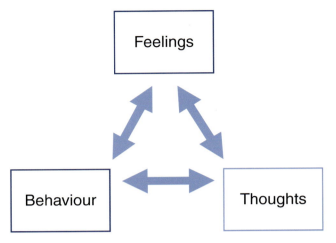

■ **Fig. 1.3** The relationship between feelings, thoughts, and behaviours

of therapeutic approaches to treating conditions such as depression, where it has been shown that thought content and emergent feelings are both interconnected and able to be manipulated. By changing or correcting the content of a depressed individual's thoughts, as well as coaching specific behaviours and self-reflection techniques, one has been able to remedy emotions such as chronically depressed mood. This also highlights the close relationship between behaviours, feelings, and thoughts and how they mutually affect each other (see ■ Fig. 1.3). The types of psychological therapies that explore and utilize the relationship between thoughts, emotions, and behaviours are commonly called cognitive therapy, or cognitive behavioural therapy (e.g. [15, 16]), where the distinction is that the latter form of therapy contains distinct behavioural components.

This simplified relationship between behaviours, thoughts, and feelings will be a general principle behind the theories addressed in this chapter, with these constructs having a conceivable influence on one another, on the self-identity of the individual, and on oral health.

1.5 Thoughts: Fast and Slow Thinking

As mentioned in the introduction, cognitive psychology is a field that attempts to explain abstract constructs, such as *thinking*, by looking acutely at how information is collected, processed, and stored. Although this handling of information may be incredibly complex, it is possible to distinguish between two key modes of processing: either it occurs in a deliberate and controlled manner or it can happen more or less automatically with little or no awareness. This duality between active and passive thinking is known as a 'dual-process' framework of information processing and is important for explaining many basic findings concerning the processing of information from our surroundings [17, 18]. There also seems to be agreement that the two pathways within a dual-process model operate in parallel, whereby the deliberate control pathway may serve as a kind of gate-keeper [19]; if deliberate control is not engaged, processing will occur via the automatic system. Such opportunities to exert deliberate control over thought processes are suggested to be limited by the capacity of working memory (short-term memory) and attention [18]. For many situations at work and in daily life, engaging in controlled and effortful thought processes can also be difficult. For example, in situations of high job-pressure and stress, where there are numerous pieces of information requiring processing and attention, it can be difficult to override automatic reactions or automated methods of thinking. In research on decision-making and problem solving, psychologists often talk about *heuristics* and *cognitive biases* to refer to these instances where individuals make decisions based on automated and learned strategies rather than controlled thinking. Terms like 'cognitive economy' are also used to describe this overall phenomenon where energy and time for processing are limited, meaning that there are considerable benefits associated with automated decision-making when the alternative is to carefully ruminate over all available choices. In these scenarios, past experience can serve as a useful guide for anticipating the result of future behaviour, meaning time and energy can be saved by using past experiences to direct automatic and instant decision-making processes.

Automated processes, however, do not always reflect an ideal method of processing information. In research literature, there are many examples that point to errors or biases that result from over-reliance on automated thinking. One of the most common 'errors' that results from automated reactions between thoughts, feelings, and behaviour is called *the fundamental attribution error* [20]. Attribution is a term used to refer to the process through which people try to explain the cause or outcome of their own or others' behaviour. Studies of the fundamental attribution error illustrate that when observing the behaviour of another person, the observer tends to systematically overestimate the importance of personal characteristics or traits as the cause of behaviour. The reason for this error may be related to the fact that a third-party observer in any situation might be most concerned with the subject or actor being observed, while situational and external factors remain secondary as part of the background. Conversely, actors themselves are often concerned primarily with the situational conditions that explain their behaviour, since their attention is most focused on their surroundings rather than their inner feelings or motives. This mismatch between actors and observers in attribution processes may be referred to as actor-observer asymmetry [21], and this implies that the ways in which oral health clinicians and patients attempt to explain their own and each other's behaviour (as 'actors' or 'observers') may be largely differentiated and can have implications for cooperation.

There is also another clinically relevant, and perhaps under-communicated, point regarding attribution that merits mentioning: patients' ideas about the root causes of their health status are likely to be dominated by their actor perspective, which highlights the influence of their life conditions. Likewise, there might be a tendency from oral health professionals', as observers, to evaluate patients in a more reductionist way, and to focus on patients' personal characteristics as a cause for health problems, or even focus solely on specific parts of patients, such as teeth and gums. Simultaneously, many patients may feel that it is irrelevant to talk about non-biological conditions with healthcare providers in the context of somatic medicine or oral health, and thus important factors contributing to health and disease can be overlooked. For example, patients may live in conditions that make it difficult to comply with recommendations or treatment measures; they may lead stressful lives that make it difficult to prioritize their health; or they may live where conditions are harmful and pathogenic. In many cases, these conditions are key determinants of oral health that needs to be addressed in the clinical setting, and oral health professionals need to be aware that acquiring insight into patients' life conditions requires adhering to a patient centred and individualized clinical perspective.

Another example of an automatic process that is of interest in decision-making is so-called *confirmation bias*, that is, a tendency to seek information confirming what one already knows [22, 23]. This process also exemplifies the strong interactions between attention, memory, and emotions in the context of behaviour. An example of confirmation bias is typically that people try to confirm their hypotheses rather than debunk them.

> ► **Example**
> The tendency in tasks like shown in ◨ Fig. 1.4 is to seek to confirm the rule, meaning that a participant typically will choose cards with even numbers and vowels (e.g. A or 2/4). However, since the task is essentially a logical problem, 'if X, then Y', the typical approach is incorrect. In this case, one must be able to test one card with vocals and one card with odd numbers (to check what happens if 'not Y') (see, e.g. [23]). The reason for this is that we get distracted by information that we already possess (the relationship between vowels and even numbers) and thus overlook important information (odd numbers). ◄

Confirmation bias has also been drawn into theories regarding the development and maintenance of mental disorders. For example, depressed people may have tendencies to automatically select information from the environment or their memory that confirms negative thoughts and beliefs, and people with health anxiety may associate random physical symptoms as evidence of a serious illness (for more examples, see [22]). Confirmation bias can ultimately help create *self-fulfilling prophecies* – experiencing a reality that conforms to an anticipated reality – in people with pre-held negative hypotheses about themselves and the world.

These types of problem-solving failures and thought patterns have been highlighted, along with a number of others (e.g. various forms of over-confidence), as among the most common sources of error in medical practice [24]. In health services, biases and heuristics create chal-

lenges in clinical decision-making. Preconceived ideas about what is wrong with a patient restrict the search for necessary information to debunk these ideas, which can lead to misdiagnosis [25]. In light of this, it has been argued that the teaching of health sciences should provide students with appropriate insight into decision-making processes and challenges related to automation, cognitive biases, and why suboptimal clinical choices occur [26].

> In addition to understanding the dual-process model and its consequences, several researchers also recommend that healthcare professionals should actively develop their *metacognitive skills* [27, 28] – that is, the ability to reflect on one's own thinking – to counteract the effects of errors in decision-making and automatic thought and action patterns.

Cognitive biases can also shape our expectations for the future. We often consider that the chance of negative things happening to us is lower than for the average population and that the chance of positive things happening is higher [29–31]. While it may seem trivial, many studies have looked at the challenges this can bring to risk behaviour and health problems if one is unable to assess risk in a correct manner.

Humans also seem to have considerable difficulty assessing their own skills. This phenomenon, called the *Dunning–Kruger effect* [32], shows that self-assessment bias (the difference between perceived and actual ability) is greatest for people who perform poorly, where the tendency is to overestimate their own achievement. In contrast, well-performing people tend to underestimate their own performance (see ◘ Fig. 1.5). In the original

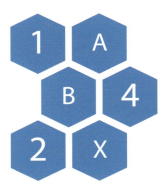

◘ **Fig. 1.4** Consider that the figures above are two-sided cards lying on the table. We want to find out if the rule 'if there is a vowel on one side of the card there is an even number on the other side of the card' applies. What two cards would you turn around to figure this out?

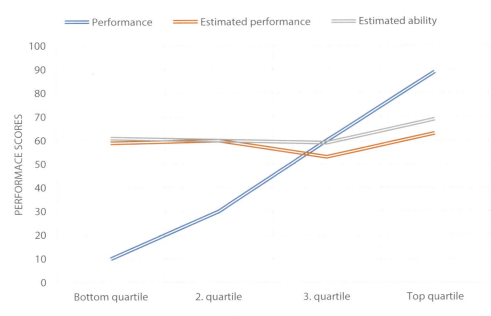

◘ **Fig. 1.5** Example of the Dunning–Kruger effect for a logical task. (Adapted from [32])

studies, the researchers showed that this applied to relatively academic exercises, such as grammar and logic; however, the findings have been subsequently applied to many other areas of human life including the ability to assess the feelings of others [33].

The reason for these findings seems to be slightly different for the two groups performing worst and best (◘ Fig. 1.5): for bottom quartile performers, overestimation of ability seems to concern an 'inner' illusion regarding one's own skills, accompanied by a failure to correct this error. This situation can be characterized as being 'twice cursed', as one's low capacity for thinking and reflecting about thought processes (in other words, metacognition) will impair both actual performance and the ability to recognize performance quality [34]. Low-performing individuals are also unable to use social comparison, the process of evaluating one's self relative to those around them, to assess their achievements [35].

In contrast, top-quartile performers tend to consider themselves as equal to others, employing ideas such as 'what is easy for me must also be easy for others' (also a form of social comparison) [32].

One way to avoid biased assessments and predictions regarding performance is to develop attitudes and mindsets aimed at understanding one's self, as well as reflecting on and analysing one's own thinking and problem solving. This can be particularly demanding within disciplines where there is no definitive solution to the set problems, such as fields of communication and relationship building. Here, it can be demanding to evaluate one's own performance in a situation where there are no exact right or wrong answers and when situations are inherently dynamic and unpredictable, such as an open conversation with a patient. Thus, metacognitive skills become even more important (as well as the requirements for educational skills of teachers/tutors) in order to imagine alternative scenarios and objectively compare one's current perceptions and performance against these hypothetical options. This may be particularly relevant to low-performers, who are also more likely to resist skill-training. Rather than giving directives regarding training requirements, the focus may instead be to help such individuals reflect and understand their own weaknesses as a means of motivating improvement.

> ► Example
> A young man has moderate gingivitis without pain. A young dental hygienist is very eager to give him the best possible oral health care. She is good at performing dental flossing herself and assumes it must be easy for others to floss every day as well. The patient experiences that he has no oral health problems and thinks he is performing 'well enough' and cannot see the need for learning proper use of dental flossing. For both parties, we can see that individual bias may influence perceptions regarding the best way to treat the moderate gingivitis, potentially creating difficulties in agreeing upon a treatment plan. ◄

> **Box**
> Imagine how a clinician might react when a person arrives late for dental treatment, potentially perceiving the patient to be 'unorganized' or 'uncaring'. However, there may be a valid explanation; for example, the bus was cancelled or the taxi did not arrive on time. Alternatively, in a treatment situation where something goes wrong, or where the clinician has trouble finding a specific instrument required for a particular treatment, the patient may perceive the clinician to be 'unorganized' or 'uncaring', when there might be valid reasons for the error or trouble.

1.6 Basic Information Collection and Processing

While cognitive biases demonstrate the susceptibility of the brain to rely on prior knowledge as a go-to guide for automated action, understanding when automated thinking is engaged involves looking more closely at how information is collected and processed. The idea of information processing is central to cognitive psychology and can be taken as a metaphor regarding the brain being a computer that continuously processes information collected from the environment through the senses, with different parts or modules of the brain working on different tasks and devoted to different information. Modules within the brain take care of visual impressions, language, motor skills, and many other tasks (◘ Fig. 1.6). These are fundamental processes that form the basis of human life including professional practice. Insight into how individuals process information from the environment is important for understanding how patients and clinicians make sense of the world and other people. For example, while understanding beliefs or motivations may help to explain visible behaviours, understanding the role of the senses can give us answers as to what patients notice in the treatment situation and what they remember from information given before, during and after treatment. Essentially, the environment, and how it is perceived, may have a formative role in shaping feelings, thoughts, and actions.

1.7 Perception

Perception is a process in which information from the surroundings (collected through the senses) is organized, interpreted, and understood. This fundamental capacity forms the basis for individuals to learn new skills, form

1

Motor and Sensory Regions of the Cerebral Cortex

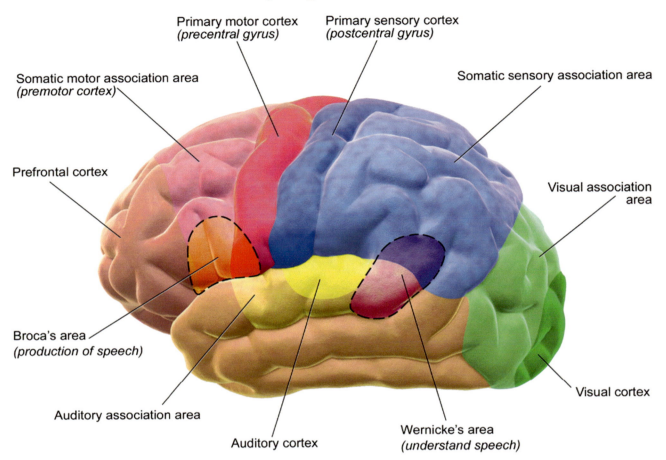

memories, and become active agents in their experience of life. The difference between perception and sensation is seen, for example, in apperceptive visual agnosia, a condition characterized by the inability to identify objects despite functioning vision. Here, the sense of vision works, but the information that enters the brain through the eyes cannot be properly assembled and interpreted by the brain. Individuals with apperceptive visual agnosia can often identify shapes or colours within an object but are unable to identify the whole object itself due to an inability to process sensory data (for an overview and case study, see [37]).

If the sensory apparatus is not faulty or compromised somehow it is reasonable to assume that the information gathered from the environment provides a correct and objective representation of the world. This notion of objectivity is skewed, however, during the perception phase, whereby the bottom-up collection of information is complimented by 'top-down' perceptive influences.

► Example

For example, observing that a patient is moving or trembling during treatment could be considered bottom-up information; however, concluding that the observed behaviour is caused by dental anxiety would be a top-down interpretation of this information. ◄

This is yet another example of interaction between thoughts, feelings, and behaviours. For instance, emotional responses can form the basis of how one interprets information from the world. Results from a study on arachnophobia demonstrated that those who were afraid of spiders considered spiders to be larger in size, and therefore potentially more dangerous and threatening, than people who were not afraid of spiders [38]. This may help explain why frightened patients may perceive instruments in the dental clinic to be very large and invasive, and why anxious patients expect injection syringes to be larger than they actually are. Although a clinician may assume that patients will interpret stimuli (e.g. the presence of a syringe on the table) in a rational manner, differences in expectations and predispositions may mean that the experienced reality of the patient is very different to that of the clinician.

Sensory impressions beyond the visual are also influenced by emotions. Negative emotions, or conditions such as depression, seem to lower pain tolerance [39] and people who are anxiety-sensitive (fear of anxiety-related emotions) have a tendency to experience pain in a more negative way [40]. Pain experiences are also altered through contextual conditions, such as negatively charged words or images, which can make pain feel more intense [41]. Modern pain theories (e.g. Gate-Control Theory) [42] describe pain as a multidimensional concept in which cognitive and emotional states can influence the experiences of pain stimuli [43]. In other words, similar stimuli, such as the sensation of a needle stick, can be interpreted differently by two individuals. Although, biologically, the same sensory neurons may detect the sensation of the needle, the addition of emotional reactions plus the content of any thoughts that are conjured up (e.g. positive or negative imagery) will create a unique pain experience for each person.

The interaction between top-down and bottom-up processes is often called *interactive perception,* and many studies have been designed with the intention of understanding how these processes complement one another [44]. Interesting examples are found in research on so-called Gestalt phenomena, where an individual is capable of filling in any gaps in objective bottom-up information using pre-held experiences and expectations.

► Example

The missing pieces in ◘ Fig. 1.7 are filled in using information from our experience-based knowledge of the world. In this way, it is possible to see the figures as a circle and a rectangle, respectively, despite the real image simply portraying a series of disconnected lines. ◄

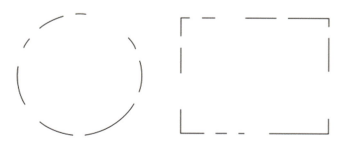

◘ **Fig. 1.7** 'The law of closure'. We fill in the missing information in the image based on our experiences. (Wikimedia Commons, public domain)

Bottom-up processes will be employed to obtain information whenever the situation is transparent, and the individual has the opportunity to focus on the task at hand. In situations where distractions are present, or when detailed information from the environment is not available, top-down processes are increasingly employed to interpret and understand our experiences. Thus, past experiences and expectations influence people's understanding of the current state of the world, simultaneously helping to facilitate a reliable understanding when limited information is available and reducing the likelihood of distress when information may be unavailable.

Box
When information is collected from the environment via the senses, without interference from other parts of the nervous system, this is referred to as 'bottom-up' processing.

Box
'Top-down' processing is constructed from the individual's expectations and thoughts regarding the world, as well as the values or meaning that are attached to events or collection of information.

1.8 Attention and Memory

While the shapes in ◘ Fig. 1.7 demonstrate an ability to automatically fill in the gaps, they also show how an individual's focus and memory play a role in perception. After all, most people will automatically perceive the broken lines as belonging to two distinct groups of lines rather than a combined melange of line segments, and most people will not have to think hard in order to identify the first shape as a circle or triangle. In other words, since people possess the circle shape in their memory, it will influence the ability to subsequently detect the shape in an abstract set of lines. Applied to people's daily lives, this means that when the brain is filling in the gaps, these gaps are likely dictated by which information is given attention, with the attention influenced by which patterns and knowledge we already possess.

Thus, people's understanding of the world depends heavily on where attention is directed. Attention can determine how stimuli are interpreted and stored in memory, and such memories may ultimately determine where attention is directed in the future. Attention itself represents a flexible resource that can be used in relation to most of the senses (e.g. to listen actively to a source, to feel a specific object, to look in a particular direction)

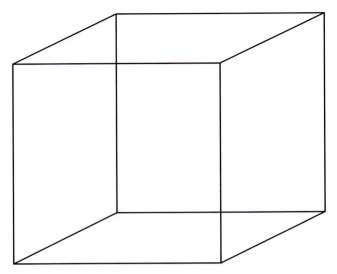

Fig. 1.8 A drawing of an ambiguous box, also known as a Necker cube: try and see if you can get the box to 'face' up to the right or down to the left (this work is licensed under a Creative Commons Attribution-ShareAlike 3.0 Unported License (CC BY-SA 3.0)) [46]. Notice that it requires effort to shift attention from one aspect/perspective to another

and relates to both the observation of external events and the designation of internal focus [44]. While a loud sound is capable of automatically capturing a person's attention, attention can also be used actively and deliberately, for example if someone wants to distinguish a friend's voice from other voices in a crowded public space. However, attentional resources are limited, and there are restrictions in place regarding how well someone can focus at any given time [45] (☐ Fig. 1.8).

Attentional resources can be regarded as a kind of filter that can prevent an overload of the cognitive information processing systems. If we had to attend to everything happening in our direct environment at all times, we would quickly become overwhelmed. Thus, attention is often given direction, and particular events or stimuli that are chosen as a focal point can be referred to as the targets of *selective attention*. This selection of information that can pass through the attention filter in such cases takes place not only on the basis of the quality of information ('bottom-up' aspects such as light, volume, or movement) but also through our own needs and conditions that serve as 'top-down' guides for attention.

> Laboratory experiments have shown that people suffering from social phobia, for example, direct their attention more towards angry faces than to neutral or happy faces [47], and the same applies to other types of anxiety [48]. Patients with dental anxiety may divert their attention towards factors they perceive as intimidating, such as characteristic smells ('dental odour') and instruments that are visible in the treat-

ment room. Just the same as the mental idea of a *circle* helped to fill in the gaps in the broken lines (☐ Fig. 1.7), the pre-held idea of an *intimidating scenario* can increase attention towards stimuli that fits this description, making it likely that the individual may fill in the gaps and perceive the clinic to be intimidating in the presence of just a few anxiety-provoking triggers. In other words, individuals' own need to protect themselves from potential threats, combined with pre-held schemas and ideas, can influence their attention to environmental stimuli in predictable ways.

What is attended to and perceived within our environment is naturally associated with the ability to remember. Put simply, one cannot remember things that have not been perceived and committed to memory. Because attention is also limited in terms of how many things one can monitor at any given time, this places additional limits on what can be captured and learnt from our surroundings as well. The selection of what is perceived may, as noted, be influenced by emotions (e.g. how important or threatening something appears) or the characteristics of the event itself (e.g. sounds, lights). In addition, information and past memories are utilized to guide the acquisition of new knowledge (see, e.g. [49]). Existing knowledge provides a framework that facilitates information collection and controls attention, which is linked to the existence of cognitive, automated schemas. Thus, there is a close relationship between pre-existing knowledge and the acquisition of new knowledge.

Memory is also a central part of the experience of being human, in terms of both its usefulness in storing knowledge about the world and its use as a means of understanding ourselves. Human memory consists of several different parts, with the simplest understanding of memory implying a division into *short-term* and *long-term* memory. Short-term memory is used to describe the process of holding finite elements of information in the memory for immediate applications. An example might be the process of learning the licence plate number of one's new car, where one may have to repeat the numbers several times before they can be remembered. As information in the short-term memory can be readily visualized and manipulated, it is often referred to as the working memory and represents the part of memory where information is processed before being understood and stored. Working memory capacity is limited in relation to the duration that information can be held and how many items are able to be processed (remembered) at a given time. If, after several years, one still remembers the licence plate number of an old car, it is reasonable to assume that it has been stored successfully in long-term memory and that it can be retrieved using voluntary control (when faced with cues such as 'what was the license plate number of my old Volvo?').

Long-term memory, as a separate entity, appears to be divided into several different parts, with a common differentiation between episodic, semantic, and procedural memory: episodic memory deals with events from our lives (e.g. a recent summer vacation in France), semantic memory refers to facts about things in the world (e.g. what is a zebra, Oslo is the capital of Norway), and procedural memory pertains to the performance of specific actions (e.g. how to ride a bike, how to drive a car). Together, these parts constitute what we require to be whole individuals with a life story and knowledge of the world around us.

Because memory is so central to human self-awareness, it is appropriate to query how accurate memories are: how well do people recall their life-journey and experiences? For example, how correct is our episodic memory of our trip to France? Intuitively, when answering such questions, one might be tempted to think of memory as a type of video camera that records what is actually happening and assume that later recollections are an objective and true representation of what took place. At the same time, though, we have seen that attention has limitations regarding what can be monitored and that our expectations and our existing knowledge of the world appear to influence both focus and observational capacity.

Many studies support a notion that memory does not function as objectively as playing back footage from a camcorder. The clearest examples of this are found in studies of bystander accounts and witness psychology, where one is interested in the degree to which one can rely on witness accounts retold in connection with criminal investigations and legal settlements. In a series of experiments, Loftus and colleagues illustrated that it is relatively easy to influence people's memories and that retrieving memories is not as simple as mentally 'replaying' the events in order to recount what actually happened. Even the questions used to elicit the recall of events may influence what is actually remembered and perceptions of facts pertaining to the incident. In a study by Loftus, subjects observed video of two cars that collided and were subsequently asked to assess the speed at which the car was driving [50]. The researchers manipulated the question composition so that some of the participants made the assessment based on the phrase 'how fast were the cars going when they smashed into each other?', while other participants received the same sentence with alternative verbs (e.g. collided, hit each other, contacted each other). The results showed that the phrase 'smashed' gave higher speed ratings than sentences with other verbs, even though the participants had watched the same film. A week after this assessment, the subjects were asked to assess whether they had seen any broken glass on the video footage (yes/no), which did not exist, and people who had assessed the speed on the basis of 'smashed' answered to a greater extent 'yes' than people who rated the speed after hearing alternate verbs. These and other similar results [51] show that people's memories seem to be the results of reconstructive processes, where available information in working memory is utilized to reconstruct and interpret an episodic event. As the results show, this can lead both to fallacies regarding the facts surrounding the event (such as speed), and also potential recall of things that did not actually happen (broken glass). This has led to changes in the recommended conduct of interviews with witnesses in criminal investigations [52, 53] and the increased use of open-ended questions to follow-up regarding specific information that appears within more freely recalled stories. The real-life consequences of violating these principles could be that people risk recalling things that have not happened, and even making false confessions [54].

These principles are important to think about when interacting with other people (and patients), even if we are not working with criminal investigations. Basic elements of conversation such as the way questions are formulated can have a profound impact on what answers are provided. For some topics, this can be absolutely crucial. For example, asking 'so I gather you are not using any medications at the moment?' or 'you're not sick at the moment, right?' as part of recording a patient's medical history violates information collection principles, because the way the questions are formulated is based on the assumption that the patient is healthy. This can lead to several problems. First, the patient will be put in a situation where he/she must actively dispute this assumption or assertion made by a professional (who is often in a position of authority). Second, it can activate linguistic concepts and schemas related to wellness and absence of disease, which can make it harder to recall chronic diseases or conditions and can change the likelihood of reporting ongoing medicine use. For these reasons, health professionals should strive to ask open questions to their patients and follow up on the information provided freely by the patients (see ▶ Chap. 6 for more on this).

This example points to another feature of information processing, namely that the brain, in addition to being module-based (different parts do different tasks), is also characterized by being a *network* with many connections where activation in one region can influence other seemingly unrelated regions simultaneously [55]. This may explain, for example, findings that physical temperature in the environment can affect subsequent social behaviour and decision-making. It turns out that moderate heat in the environment increases our motivation to establish relationships with others [56, 57] and that something as simple as holding a container of hot drink can increase motivation for social proximity [57], while cold drinks may have the opposite effect [58]. People who report being lonely, a form of social isolation, also report a higher frequency of taking hot baths or showers, as cold sensations may increase the experience of loneliness [59]. An explanation for the findings related to temperature may be that the parts of the brain that record physical temperature, for instance heat, are also involved in the emotional assessment of 'social warmth' (i.e. the experience of feeling connected to other people) [60]. Thus, studies have shown that the experience of heat triggers positive emotions [61] and increases the likelihood of behaviours associated with this. In addition, the network structure implies that there will be associative connections between, for example, language areas and sensory areas of the brain, meaning that language may influence how sensory information is interpreted (e.g. exposure to negative words increases pain perception) [41]. Such an understanding of the brain as a coherent neural network can make it easier to understand the close relationship between thoughts, emotions, and behaviours, and also observations of seemingly inseparable association between these entities. If activation of emotions is simultaneously activating areas of the brain associated with thoughts, it is logical that it becomes impossible to distinguish whether emotions triggered the thoughts or vice versa.

1.9 Emotions

Emotions or *feelings* are the lay terms for what is referred to in research literature as affective states. The development of affective states can perhaps best be explained from evolutionary and functional perspectives. People are born with the capacity to express their needs through emotions (we talk often about infants' temperament) and certain affective states are *basic* and *universal*. The latter is evidenced through the observation that connections between specific facial expressions and certain emotions seem to be culturally independent; that is, they are interpreted equally by people from vastly different parts of the world and cultural contexts [62, 63]. It is commonly suggested that there are six basic emotions: disgust, joy, surprise, fear, anger, and sadness (see, e.g. [64]). The physical facial expressions associated with these emotions have probably also been useful (and perhaps absolutely necessary) for the survival of early mankind. Especially in pre-lingual societies, the expression of emotions would have been a central part of communication, and this is still seen today in our closest relatives: primates. Emotional expressions can signal, for example, what kind of food should be avoided in order to avoid becoming sick (disgust), who to enter into relationships with (joy), the onset of a sudden change (sur-

prise), what situations should be avoided (fear), which individuals to avoid (anger), and that other people might need support in light of difficult events (sadness). Emotions can thus be described as a basic social language between human beings.

The term emotion is also used to describe aspects of emotional life beyond pure subjective experience. Although there is a lack of a unified definition of emotions [65], it is uncontroversial to suggest that emotions consist of four key components: (1) subjective feeling, (2) behaviour/action patterns, (3) physiological activation, and (4) motivation. The following example looks at how these components work together with regards to fear.

► Example

The subjective feeling of fear is a person's private experience of being afraid in the face of something threatening. Alongside this feeling there could also be associated behaviours; for example, it will occasionally be possible to see that a person is afraid by observing their facial expressions (cf. *basic emotions*) and fear might trigger behaviour, or the potential for behaviour, aimed at fighting the threat or initiating retreat. The feeling of fear is also associated with physiological processes and activation. In the brain, neural circuits related to the experience of emotion are activated including parts of the amygdala (basal nucleus), which in turn leads to activation of neuroendocrine processes. This will then influence blood pressure, heart rate, and the excretion of hormones (such as norepinephrine and testosterone) in the bloodstream. In addition, emotions are often used to understand motivation to initiate behaviour. Negative emotions can motivate us to initiate measures to reduce these emotions, whereby a frightened person will seek to become less afraid by removing themselves (i.e. escape, avoidance) from what is perceived as threatening or dangerous. Similarly, positive emotions can motivate a person to do more of what provides positive feelings. These four components of emotions therefore provide an entry point to understanding many sides to human behaviour. ◄

As previously mentioned, there is often a distinction made between cognitive processes and emotional processes, although there is little evidence to suggest that it is practically possible to distinguish these from each other [66, 67]. In other words, within the neural network of the brain, feelings and thoughts go hand in hand. This might be best understood by visualizing that all incoming sensory information is screened by structures within the brain that concern emotions (the limbic system), meaning that incoming sensory information is *always* given an emotional value. This value may then determine whether or not a person diverts attention towards the information [68, 69]. From an evolutionary perspective, this makes sense, as it could be argued that it is logical to notice events that have some emotional value (good or bad) to increase the chance of survival. In this way, emotional influence is central to our lives, even though we may not be aware of it at all times.

A number of studies have also shed light on how thoughts and feelings affect each other. According to early theories, it should be possible to understand emotions based on physiological activation, and each emotion should be accompanied by specific physiological activation (the so-called James–Lange theory) [70]. This was tested in a series of experiments by, among others, Schachter and Singer [71]. However, contrary to the James–Lange theory, Schachter and Singer found that study participants interpreted non-specific physiological activation (which was applied through adrenaline injections) based on the situational conditions. When the participants lacked a good explanation of why they felt physiologically activated, they behaved in line with a research assistant, who was placed in the same room as the subjects and either acted excited or angry. Participants who learned that they had been given adrenaline, and therefore had an adequate explanation for their physiological activation, did not do this. Such results led the researchers to formulate a theory of emotions, in which the experience of emotion consists of arousal (physiological activation; the autonomic nervous system) and a cognitive-emotional label (in which we seek an explanation for activation).

This distinction between physiological activation and the cognitive explanation model for activation has provided fertile ground for some interesting 'flaws' in how we assess our own emotions. This is often called the transfer of arousal and is about people occasionally choosing the wrong explanation model for why they are activated. In a much-cited study, it was revealed that male subjects who experienced emotional arousal from walking across a not-so-secure suspension bridge were more attracted to a female research coordinator whom they encountered on the other side than male subjects who crossed a regular bridge [72]. The authors of the study concluded that the fear experienced by the subjects was being misinterpreted as sexual attraction. Although both the two-factor theory and the transmission of arousal have been criticized in recent research (see, e.g. [73]), these experiments show the importance of the interaction between mental processes and the available environmental stimuli during the assignment, assessment, and development of emotions. Other studies also show how purposeful behaviour can affect the experience of our own emotions. For example, activating the facial muscles involved in smiling can elicit the experience of emotional stimuli (the so-called facial feedback hypothesis); in this state, individuals are more likely to find funny cartoons amusing and likely to react with stronger positive emotions to positive images than subjects who do not activate the same facial musculature [74, 75]. This has been shown to also apply to negative emotions (e.g. sadness) through the activation of the facial muscles used to express negative mood (see, e.g. [76]). In other words, it appears that muscular activity can influence the value of existing emotions. Adding further support to this hypothesis, studies of people who have received Botox injections (which paralyse the facial muscles) have also shown that emotional sensations become less intense after such injections, potentially due to the inability to enact the behavioural component of an emotional reaction [77, 78].

It may be useful for healthcare professionals to understand this interaction between internal and external factors in emotional experience. In other words, experiences of emotions within clinical situations are subject to influential forces that may be difficult to fully appreciate. Accepting emotional reactions in the clinical setting and working with patients to try and find explanations for such reactions may be useful. Understanding how emotions work may also help to sympathize with the experience of the patient, reducing the likelihood that a clinician will respond in unhelpful ways to negative emotions, such as fear or anger, in the dental clinic.

Emotions, in many cases, can also become strong motivating forces. As we have seen, information gathering and processing can be affected by the attention being directed towards objects and situations that have value for the individual [68, 69], and emotions can influence how objects or situations are perceived [38, 79]. On a more overarching level, these valuations tend to ascribe to the 'hedonistic principle', which suggests that a fundamental impetus in people's lives is to seek out positive emotions and avoid negative emotions. This is easy to understand when it comes to painful sensations: one will avoid contact with items or situations that are painful and prefer to seek out situations that elicit feelings of comfort.

This means that the emotional impact of behaviour is relatively controlling in regard to the choices an actor makes, and it is possible to imagine that some health behaviours are, to some extent, guided by such conditions. Thus, it may be that emotions tied to oral health can have a substantial impact on oral health behaviour. Specifically, people that are ashamed of their oral health status and their teeth are likely to actively avoid associated negative emotions by avoiding situations where such topics are discussed (e.g. dental treatment) or situations that may divert attention towards their teeth (e.g. own brushing, reading/hearing/watching information about oral health in various settings). There is also evidence that information that is emotionally aversive (i.e.

1

negative) influences people in a stronger way than positive information, which can be explained by the fact that negative information and threat-avoidance is more closely related to human survival [80]. Consequently, negative emotional states play an important role in shaping behaviour.

1.10 Emotions and Stress

Although threat-avoidance behaviours are understandable and to some extent functional, chronic states of worry about impending threats can be hazardous for health. Thus, in addition to sympathizing with worry, clinicians should also aim to understand the origins of threat arousal and how to potentially help individuals to cope with over-activation of threat detection mechanisms. Typically, this state of longer-term emotional arousal, due to concern regarding various impending threats, is known as the experience of *stress*.

Stress itself can be defined in several ways. Early definitions described stress as a non-specific biological response to pressure (the so-called general adaptation syndrome) [81], while a more recent definition by Folkman states that stress is a person–situation relationship that indicates deficiencies in a person's available coping resources and puts his or her well-being at risk [82]. Stress is associated with acute physiological activation where the purpose is to mobilize resources to deal with the current troubling event. This activation is therefore appropriate because activating resources, such as increasing blood flow to the muscles and focussing attention, enables the individual to meet the challenge it faces. Stress enables acceptance of testing situations and challenges, for example when learning a new skill. The vast majority will have some sort of stress activation connected with their first jump from a diving board, but with several successful jumps, this activation will go down (and something new has been learned). Stress activation is therefore essential for human development, and this scenario of activating resources to meet a challenge can be referred to as positive stress.

However, as suggested by Folkman's definition, it is also possible that stress can be problematic when the available resources for the individual are not sufficient to meet the anticipated challenge. In such cases, the situation itself may either be so chaotic and demanding that coping is not possible (typically in case of accidents or other traumatic events; see also ▶ Chap. 2) or entail a prolonged demand over time whereby the individual maintains a constant feeling of emergency preparedness. Studies show that such prolonged demand and maintenance of a state of high-arousal (chronic stress),

also referred to as 'allostatic overload' [83], is associated with the deregulation of inflammation-regulating mechanisms and disease development (see, e.g. [84, 85]). Stressful influences also relate to specific findings within the oral cavity, for example, that psychological stress can be detected in salivary biomarkers (e.g. alpha amylase and cortisol) [86, 87]. At the same time, higher levels of salivary cortisol, as a marker of chronic stress, is associated with development of periodontal disease [88, 89]. Furthermore, more overt consequences of stress activation on oral health also exist, such as negative consequences for the bite and jaw related to stress responses such as muscle tension and tooth grinding.

In addition, since stress can be considered closely associated with other states involving heightened emotional arousal, such as anxiety and fear, these states are likely to share many of the same behavioural, physiological, and psychological consequences [90]. Several studies point to the experience of stress as common in the development of depression and anxiety [90, 91]. Studies of stress management may focus therefore on the interpretation of situations (i.e. the cognitive processes or emotive states that are guiding attention and influencing how the current situation is interpreted) and the importance of accessing positive emotions to support coping with stress. This act of attaching positive emotions to stress arousal is often called 'positive reappraisal' and is an approach to stress management where one tries to see positive opportunities in challenging situations or to reinterpret a stressful situation so that the experience may not be dominated by negative rumination or attention to negative stimuli. Other approaches may be problem-focused coping, a technique focused on solving the problem – or those parts of the problem – that are under personal control (see, e.g. [92]).

As shown in the model in ▫ Fig. 1.9, both stress activation and performance are low in sleep and in very relaxed states. Similarly, in high stress activation, for example during the experience of panic, performance is also low. It is interesting to note however that performance capacity reaches its maximum during moderate stress activation. In this area the individual is attentive and possesses enough resources to meet challenges, resulting in a higher likelihood of experiencing adequate performance. This span from relatively low to relatively high stress activation, and the relationship with high performance, can perhaps be interpreted as a person's individual tolerance range for stress (dotted line). When the stress exceeds the tolerance range, performance suffers, with prolonged exposure to stress outside of our tolerance range becoming harmful over time. This will be elaborated when describing the 'Window of tolerance' later in the book (see ▶ Chap. 2).

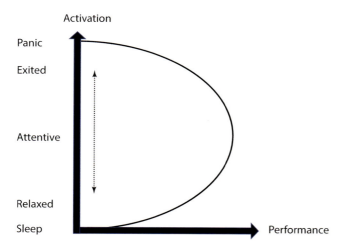

○ **Fig. 1.9** The relationship between performance and stress activation

1.11 Information Processing in the Clinical Context

The theories related to information processing, emotions, and stress are directly applicable in both private and professional situations. For example, consider the following scenario:

► Example

One of your colleagues at the dental clinic observes one of your patients in the waiting room. You have never met this person, but your colleague reaches out to you and warns you that this patient is considered 'difficult'. How can this expectation of a 'difficult patient' affect the relationship and interaction between you and the patient? What are you likely to remember in the aftermath of this consultation? ◄

This example focuses on the fact that health professionals' expectations for interaction, based on the theories and findings highlighted in this chapter, might well have a significant impact on the quality of their clinical work. It could be argued that ambiguous information or misunderstandings that arise in such cases, like in the given example, may be interpreted through a lens of top-down expectations regarding the stereotypical 'difficult patient', and attention may be drawn to aspects of the clinical situation that will confirm this expectation (an example of the automatic tendency to confirm things we already think we know, so-called confirmation bias). This may prevent this particular patient from receiving the same quality of treatment as another patient with similar problems but where these expectations and attentional biases did not exist.

An overarching point in the context of this discussion is the understanding that emotions are potent influ-

ences for interpreting and framing human behaviour and relationships between people, including interactions relevant to the provision of health services. Overall, the dimension that contains health and disease – as a singular topic – involves several complex emotions. These emotions may concern contentment, happiness, and wellness, on the one hand, and concern discomfort, pain, and death, on the other.

For example, *shame* is a negative and painful emotion that can frame how one interacts with oral healthcare systems. Shame is frequently associated with people who refrain from accessing dental care, potentially due to struggles with dental problems or anxiety about dental treatment. As argued previously, emotions can be regarded as a social language, and in expressions of shame lies a form of social submission that presumably has value for the individual's survival and that may explain the origins of the emotion itself. A person who is ashamed will withdraw from, or avoid, potential conflicts that may be detrimental to their well-being [93]. Arguably, for some people attending a dental clinic could elicit the experience of shame and the need to protect oneself from, or avoid, this emotional experience. The elicitation of shame in this context could both be based on current experiences (i.e. the real-time interaction between the patient and the oral health professionals), but also based on previous experiences with treatment or generalized expectations or impressions of oral health professionals. People who are experiencing impaired oral health because of their avoidance of the clinic may also experience 'internal shame', where they experience negative self-evaluation regarding the results of their actions. This may take the form of thoughts such as 'Why can't I address my teeth like everyone else? I'm completely useless!' Additionally, people can experience 'external shame', which implies focusing on others' evaluations of them and leading to thoughts such as 'What would others say if they discovered the state of my teeth?' (for a discussion of internal versus external shame, see [94]). Oral health professionals must be ready to meet and recognize negative emotions in dental patients and understand that patients can respond emotionally in the face of dental treatment. Although people working as health professionals tend to strive, or have been trained to strive for, a form of neutral professionalism when interacting with patients, there is little evidence to suggest that anyone is capable of completely detaching themselves from the influence of their own emotional life.

► Example

Consider the following situation: One of your patients behaves in a way that makes you feel uncomfortable and insecure. You cannot figure out what this is about, but you are experiencing the situation as quite uncomfortable.

1

During work, you feel nervous and notice that your hands are shaking, and you feel in a bad mood when you see the patient's name in the time schedule. How could these experiences impact the interaction with this patient and ultimately the quality of the work? Also see ◘ Fig. 1.10. ◄

1.12 Application of Psychological Theory in Oral Health Care

As this chapter shows, there are many challenges related to interpreting and understanding the environment and interacting with other individuals. These challenges place high demands on healthcare professionals whose task it is to obtain information from patients and make optimal decisions on the basis of this information. The challenges lie partly in the complexity of the surroundings, which may provide incomplete information or exposure to triggers that influence professional thinking and decision-making. Challenges can, alternatively, also originate from within. Predispositions to certain responses are likely to develop during a person's lifetime, which are likely to exert considerable influence over their actions. Solutions to such challenges may be realized partly by establishing systematic and pre-planned approaches to certain tasks or situations and partly through working on developing skills that may help overcome challenges as they occur. Lifelong learning and adaptation of systematic approaches and skill-developing measures should be part of a professional life for all health workers, including those in oral health. Through self-reflection around private and professional life and a focus on developing positive relationships with co-workers and patients, healthcare professionals will be able to increase the quality of their own life and the lives of others in the work environment.

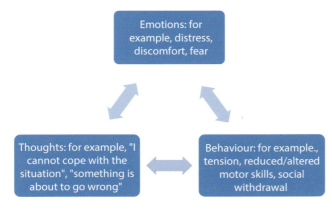

◘ **Fig. 1.10** The interaction between thoughts, emotions, and behaviour in an oral healthcare setting

1.13 Practical Approaches

As seen in this chapter, however, there are challenges regarding our capacity to collect and process information (i.e. selective attention, working memory) that can influence our ability to avoid stress and unwanted reactions. These limitations have long been suggested to play a role in performance in the workplace, and may be central to determining how an employee organizes their daily tasks, the degree to which they operate efficiently/productively, and their subjective experience of work as being positive or negative. Practical approaches are often aimed, therefore, at achieving stress reduction among workers. This can be done by ensuring an optimal balance between the strict work requirements set for employees and the degree to which they are given autonomy in the workplace [95]. Even solutions such as considering the aesthetic of the working environment may offset stress accumulation, with plants in office environments or healthcare settings shown to lower stress levels and increase attention [96, 97]. In health care, employees face several complex work situations, with numerous actors and interaction partners, and with potentially serious consequences when suboptimal choices are made. Similar concerns are also found in fields such as the airline industry, where pilots often operate in stressful conditions. Interestingly, in an industry characterized by technological development and modern solutions, paper-based checklists are still used frequently. These are primarily used for something called 'challenge response', where pilots first make settings based on memory and then use the list to verify their choices [98]. In the health care context, health professionals often deal with similarly complex issues and situations where errors can have major consequences both for patients and clinicians [99, 100]. In order to manage complex and congested work situations in oral health care and clinical practice, one possible solution is the design of checklists related to different situations and procedures.

Oral health professionals have a long tradition of remembering all their routines such as where and how long to apply dentine conditioner, how to apply bonding agents, and how to place a restorative material and initiate the curing process. This assumes, to some extent, that these procedures are automated in the process of repeating these actions each day. In today's dentistry, however, there is a constant development of new methods and materials that clinicians must deal with. The introduction of checklists for procedures can thus contribute to a greater level of quality assurance for the treatments. The same can also apply to communication with and follow-up of patients. When stressed, it is often easy to forget, for example, to take the patient's perspective in a conversation, but also to provide them with technical details.

1.14 Development of Metacognitive Skills: Mindware

In addition to developing practical checklists and tools to help us in complex situations, we can also work on improving our mental capacity to manage situational complexity. As previously mentioned, one of the challenges of being human is that our capacity to control our attention and reactions is limited, meaning that many of our actions are automated and beyond conscious control. These automatic actions and strategies can be seen as our 'personality' and represent our basis for conduct and relationships with other people. Intervening in these automatic action patterns and altering our tendencies therefore requires motivation, time, and cognitive capacity. Even with the aid of checklists, health workers may still be particularly vulnerable to stress that comes from working with people and the emotionality of continual inter-personal discussion with patients. Occasionally referred to as 'emotional labour' in the research literature, being constantly exposed to emotional surroundings can have a bearing on job stress, job satisfaction, and overall quality of life [101, 102]. The strong connection between working in emotionally charged situations and negative consequences related to

the work performed under such conditions may come from the fact that humans tend to automatically react with stress and discomfort when they detect discomfort and negative emotions in others (e.g. the idea concerning 'mirror neurons') [103]. At the same time, there is also evidence that some characteristics and skills in humans can likewise protect against these effects, such as the ability to engage in spontaneous self-reflection with the purpose of better understanding our emotional reactions [104, 105].

1.15 Emotional Competence

Several researchers have proposed models and programmes detailing how we can work to develop our own capacity to both manage and communicate our emotional states. Such methods are often described as programmes that target the development of affective, or emotional, awareness (i.e. recognizing how we feel and the influence of emotion on our current actions) and/or *Emotional Competence* (EC), which expands from basic emotional awareness to also understanding the cause and purpose of these emotions.

> In this context, EC can be described as how effectively individuals deal with both emotions and emotionally charged scenarios (see, e.g. [106]). EC can further be broken down into different sub-skills, with the literature describing five areas covered by this term: (1) identifying one's own and others' emotions, (2) understanding emotions, the origins of emotions, and consequences of emotions, (3) the capacity to express emotions in socially adequate ways and to attend to the emotional expression of others, (4) to regulate their own and others' emotions, and (5) using emotions to improve interactions and behaviours. In many ways, the final point emerges as an overarching purpose of working to develop emotional competence.

The purpose of working with the core competences involved in EC is that people who have good skills in these areas also appear to perform well elsewhere in life. This applies to both health status and to job/education performance, where high EC is associated with higher self-reported quality of life, less somatic and mental ailments, and increased ability to procure employment [107, 108]. The results also suggest that EC training appears to affect participants' personality traits, with participants reporting increased emotional stability and coping ability. This could lead to the assumption that the positive consequences of high EC may be due to emotional stability and emotional coping ability which protects the individual from negative effects of stress

45. Wickens CD, McCarley JS. Applied attention theory. Boca Raton: CRC Press; 2008.
46. Dale BF. A Necker cube. Wikimedia Commons: Creative Commons; 2007.
47. Mogg K, Philippot P, Bradley BP. Selective attention to angry faces in clinical social phobia. J Abnorm Psychol. 2004;113(1):160–5.
48. Bradley BP, Mogg K, Falla SJ, Hamilton LR. Attentional bias for threatening facial expressions in anxiety: manipulation of stimulus duration. Cognit Emot. 1998;12:737–53.
49. Chun MM, Turk-Brown NB. Interactions between attention and memory. Curr Opin Neurobiol. 2007;17:177–84.
50. Loftus EF, Palmer JC. Reconstruction of automobile destruction: an example of the interaction between language and memory. J Verbal Learn Verbal Behav. 1974;13(5):585–9.
51. Loftus EF. Leading questions and the eyewitness report. Cogn Psychol. 1975;7:560–72.
52. Hilgard ER, Loftus EF. Effective interrogation of the eyewitness. Int J Clin Exp Hypn. 1979;27(4):342–57.
53. Wells GL, Olson EA. Eyewitness testimony. Annu Rev Psychol. 2003;54:277–95.
54. Kassin SM. False confessions. WIREs. Cogn Sci. 2017:e1439.
55. Buckner RL, Andrews-Hanna JR, Schachter DL. The brain's default network. Ann N Y Acad Sci. 2008;1124:1–38.
56. Steinmetz J, Posten A-C. Physical temperature affects response behavior. J Exp Soc Psychol. 2017;70:294–300.
57. Ijzerman H, Semin GR. The thermometer of social relations: mapping social proximity on temperature. Psychol Sci. 2009;20(10):1214–20.
58. Chen Z, Poon K-T, DeWall CN. Cold thermal temperature threatens belonging: the moderating role of perceived social support. Soc Psychol Personal Sci. 2015;6(4):439–46.
59. Bargh JA, Shalev I. The substitutability of physical and social warmth in daily life. Emotion. 2012;12(1):154–62.
60. Inagaki TK, Eisenberger NI. Shared neural mechanisms underlying social warmth and physical warmth. Psychol Sci. 2013;24(11):2272–80.
61. Williams LE, Bargh JA. Experiencing physical warmth promotes interpersonal warmth. Science. 2008;322(5901):606–7.
62. Izard CE. Innate and universal facial expressions: evidence from developmental and cross-cultural research. Psychol Bull. 1994;115(2):288–99.
63. Ekman P. Facial expression and emotion. Am Psychol. 1993;48(4):384–92.
64. Ekman P, Friesen WV. Constants across cultures in the face and emotion. J Pers Soc Psychol. 1971;17(2):124–9.
65. Izard CE. Emotion theory and research: highlights, unanswered questions, and emerging issues. Annu Rev Psychol. 2009;60:1–25.
66. Ochsner KN, Phelps E. Emerging perspectives on emotion-cognition interactions. Trends Cogn Sci. 2007;11(8):317–8.
67. Storbeck J, Clore GL. On the interdependence of cognition and emotion. Cognit Emot. 2007;21(6):1212–37.
68. Damasio AR. Descartes' error: emotion, reason, and the human brain. New York: Avon Books; 1994.
69. Vuilleumier P. How brains beware: neural mechanisms of emotional attention. Trends Cogn Sci. 2005;9(12):585–94.
70. Cannon WB. The James-Lange theory of emotions: a critical examination and an alternative theory. Am J Psychol. 1927;39(1/4):106–24.
71. Schachter S, Singer J. Cognitive, social, and physiological determinants of emotional state. Psychol Rev. 1962;69:379–99.
72. Dutton DG, Aron AP. Some evidence for heightened sexual attraction under conditions of high anxiety. J Pers Soc Psychol. 1974;30:510–7.
73. Manstead ASR, Wagner HL. Arousal, cognition and emotion: an appraisal of two-factor theory. Curr Psychol Rev. 1981;1:35–54.
74. Soussignan R. Duchenne smile, emotional experience, and autonomic reactivity: a test of the facial feedback hypothesis. Emotion. 2002;2(1):52–74.
75. Strack F, Martin LL, Stepper S. Inhibiting and facilitating conditions of the human smile: a nonobtrusive test of the facial feedback hypothesis. J Pers Soc Psychol. 1988;54(5):768–77.
76. Larsen RJ, Kasimatis M, Frey K. Facilitating the furrowed brow: an unobtrusive test of the facial feedback hypothesis applied to unpleasant affect. Cognit Emot. 1992;6(5):321–38.
77. Davis JI, Senghas A, Brandt F, Ochsner KN. The effects of botox injections on emotional experience. Emotion. 2010;10(3):433–40.
78. Baumeister JC, Papa G, Foroni F. Deeper than skin deep - the effect of botulinum toxin-a on emotion processing. Toxicon. 2016;118:86–90.
79. van Ulzen NR, Semin RRD, Oudejans PJB. Affective stimulius properties influence size perception and the Ebbinghaus illusion. Psychol Res. 2008;72(3):304–10.
80. Baumeister RF, Bratslavsky E, Finkenauer C, Vohs KD. Bad is stronger than good. Rev Gen Psychol. 2001;5(4):323–70.
81. Selye H. Perspectives in stress research. Perspect Biol Med. 1959;2(4):403–16.
82. Folkman S. Personal control and stress and coping processes: a theoretical analysis. J Pers Soc Psychol. 1984;46(4):839–52.
83. McEwen BS. Stressed or stressed out: what is the difference? J Psychiatry Neurosci. 2005;30(5):315–8.
84. Danese A, McEwen BS. Adverse childhood experiences, allostatis, allostatic load, and age-related disease. Physiol Behav. 2012;106:29–39.
85. Kirkengen AL, Lygre H. Exploring the relationship between childhood adversity and oral health: an anecdotal approach and integrative view. Med Hypotheses. 2015;85(2):134–40.
86. Ali N, Pruessner JC. The salivary alpha amylase over cortisol ratio as a marker to assess dysregulations of the stress systems. Physiol Behav. 2012;106(1):65–72.
87. Nater UM, Rohleder N, Gaab J, Berger S, Jud A, Kirschbaum C, et al. Human salivary alpha-amylase reactivity in a psychosocial stress paradigm. Int J Psychophysiol. 2005;55(3):333–42.
88. Reners M, Brecx M. Stress and periodontal disease. Int J Dent Hyg. 2007;5(4):199–204.
89. Sabbah W, Gomaa N, Gireesh A. Stress, allostatic load and periodontal diseases. Periodontology. 2000;78(1):154–61.
90. Bystritsky A, Kronemeyer D. Stress and anxiety. Psychiatr Clin N Am. 2014;37(4):489–518.
91. Hammen C. Stress and depression. Annu Rev Clin Psychol. 2005;1:293–319.
92. Folkman S, Moskowitz JT. Stress, positive emotion, and coping. Curr Dir Psychol Sci. 2000;9(4):115–8.
93. Gilbert P. The relationship of shame, social anxiety and depression: the role of the evaluation of social rank. Clin Psychol Psychother. 2000;7:174–89.
94. Ferreira C, Moura-Ramos M, Matos M, Galhardo A. A new measure to assess external and internal shame: development, factor structure and psychometric properties of the external and internal shame scale. Curr Psychol. 2020;
95. Bakker AB, Demerouti E. The job demands-resources model: state of the art. J Manag Psychol. 2007;22(3):309–28.
96. Raanaas RK, Evensen KH, Rich D, Sjøstrøm G, Patil G. Benefits of indoor plants on attention capacity in an office setting. J Environ Psychol. 2011;31(1):99–105.
97. Dijkstra K, Pieterse ME, Pruyn A. Stress-reducing effects of indoor plants in the built healthcare environment: the mediat-

ing role of perceived attractiveness. Prev Med. 2008;47(3):279–83.

98. Degani A, Wiener EL. Cockpit checklists: concepts, design, and use. Hum Factors. 1993;35(2):345–59.

99. Gawande A. The checklist manifesto: how to get things right. New York: Metropolitan Books; 2009.

100. Provonost P, Needham D, Berenholtz S, Sinopoli D, Chu H, Cosgrove S, et al. An intervention to decrease catheter-related bloodstream infections in the ICU. N Engl J Med. 2006;355:2725–32.

101. Pugliesi K. The consequences of emotional labor: effects on work stress, job satisfaction, and well-being. Motiv Emot. 1999;23(2):125–54.

102. Nylander P-Å, Lindberg O, Bruhn A. Emotional labour and emotional strain among Swedish prison officers. Eur J Criminol. 2011;8(6):469–83.

103. Gallese V, Keysers C, Rizzolatti G. A unifying view of the basis of social cognition. Trends Cogn Sci. 2004;8(9):396–403.

104. Linville PW. Self-complexity as a cognitive buffer against stress-related illness and depression. J Personal Soc Psychl. 1987;52(4):663–76.

105. Jackson D, Firtko A, Edenborough M. Personal resilience as a strategy for surviving and thriving in the face of workplace adversity: a literature review. J Adv Nurs. 2007;60(1):1–9.

106. Ciarrochi J, Scott G. The link between emotional competence and Well-being: a longitudinal study. Br J Guid Counsel. 2006;34:231–43.

107. Kotsou I, Nelis D, Grégorie J, Mikolajczek M. Emotional plasticity: conditions and effects of improving emotional competence in adulthood. J Appl Psychol. 2011;96:827–39.

108. Nelis D, Kotsou I, Quoidbach J, Hansenne M, Weytens F, Dupuis P, et al. Increasing emotional competence improves psychological and physical well-being, social relationships, and employability. Emotion. 2011;11(2):354–66.

109. Victoroff KZ, Boyatzis RE. What is the relationship between emotional intelligence and dental student clinical performance? J Dent Educ. 2013;77(4):416–26.

110. Partido BB, Stafford R. Association between emotional intelligence and academic performance among dental hygiene students. J Dent Educ. 2018;82(9):974–9.

111. Kumar A, Puranik MP, Sowmyra KR. Association between dental students' emotional intelligence and academic performance: a study at six dental colleges in India. J Dent Educ. 2016;80(5):526–32.

112. Partido BB, Stefanik D, Forsythe A. Association between emotional intelligence and professionalism among dental hygiene students. J Dent Educ. 2020;84(12):1341–7.

113. Partido BB, Owen J. Relationship between emotional intelligence, stress, and burnout among dental hygiene students. J Dent Educ. 2020;84(18):864–70.

114. Pau A, Sabri BA. Relationship between emotional intelligence and job satisfaction in newly qualified Malayan dentists. Asia Pacific. J Public Health. 2015;27(2):NP1733–NP41.

The Importance of Trauma-Sensitive Care

Trine Anstorp, Åshild Nupen, and Tiril Willumsen

Contents

2.1 Introduction

This chapter aims to set new standards for dental treatment based on a psychological trauma-sensitive perspective. To incorporate this perspective in attitude, communication, and actions, certain educational objectives will be necessary to understand.

Each day dentists and hygienists strive to offer the best possible treatment for each individual patient. There are many challenges, however, that arise in the everyday running of a clinic. Despite the best of intentions, both patients and clinicians may feel confused and frustrated if something unexpected occurs. For instance, how can the dentist understand patients who suddenly leap out of the chair, faint, or behave as though they were in a completely different reality than the one shared with the dentist? How is it even possible to offer any dental treatment to patients who behave in this way?

To understand such complex reactions, knowledge of trauma and trauma-sensitive care is not only useful, but quite necessary in dental practice. Most dentists are unaware of what overwhelming life events their patients may suffer from. In consequence, the dentist unintentionally risks treating the patient so that uncomfortable memories from the past are triggered, and thus make the patient act in ways that are confusing to both patients and professionals as well. Hence, understanding trauma and knowledge of how to meet trauma reactions, will prevent many challenges in dental practice. In fact, the proper use of trauma theory and principles in trauma-sensitive care certainly will increase the quality of dental treatment, not only for those who are traumatized but for all patients.

🗨 Learning Goals
- How traumatic life experiences may impact on dental treatment and dental health in general.
- What is a psychological trauma.
- How does dissociation appear in the dentist's office.
- What is "The triune brain".
- Why "The window of tolerance" is a useful model for regulating emotions.

2.2 Why Is Trauma-Sensitive Dentistry Important?

Traditionally, a patient's problems and adverse reactions during dental treatment have been dismissed by labeling the patient as "difficult." Today, however, it is expected that the dental health practitioner has specific knowledge and enough expertise to make adequate treatment possible no matter how "difficult" the patient

may be. However, we know today that many "regular" dental patients carry with them unresolved traumatic experiences of a kind that certainly may challenge the treatment in different ways. Individuals who have a history of traumatic life events often experience heightened feelings of vulnerability and unsafety in new interactions. Physical closeness, as between dentist and patient during a treatment session, typically will trigger flashbacks of other situations where the person felt trapped or was unable to leave. In other words, it can be extra challenging for traumatized patients simply to sit in the dentist chair. Since most victims of traumatic life events do not inform dental practitioners what they struggle with, there will be only a small chance that the practitioner meets the traumatized patient in adequate ways. Whose fault is this? Is perhaps the patient to blame – for not informing the dentist? The answer is clear-cut: It is the professional responsibility of the dentist and hygienist to find applicable solutions when the situation gets difficult. Certainly, it is of little use telling the patient to "pull yourself together." So, how can we, as dental professionals, give the best of help?

Neither dentist nor hygienist should conduct psychological therapy or aim to process the patients' trauma history, if they have one. However, the entire dental health team must have knowledge of trauma and traumatic reactions to be able to give the appropriate professional dental care.

This chapter will discuss what dental professionals need to know to work successfully with patients with trauma-related problems. It will describe what dental professionals can do to support vulnerable patients in taking care of their own dental health in general, and more specifically in being able to receive professional care when necessary. Keeping this in mind, all dental care should be trauma-sensitive dental care.

> » Frida is 27 years old. She has not been to the dentist since she was 20. She feels intensely uncomfortable in just thinking about the dentist. Now she has had murmuring pain in a wisdom tooth for 3 months. When she enters the dentist's office, she proclaims that she "doesn't recognize herself", she loses control of her body, cries and just wants to run away. Eventually, Frida is examined and diagnosed with pericoronitis. Following simple measures will resolve the situation, but a tooth should be extracted within reasonable time. A treatment plan is made. After two hours of conversation around her anxiety, she sits quietly and thinks for a while, then she says; "Now I understand. When I was 17, I went to a party with friends, I drank too much, fell asleep and then I was raped. I get the same terrible feeling of helplessness and pain now, just thinking about sitting in the dental chair with the dentist so close to my body."

Frida's reactions were not a result of bad experiences from earlier dental treatment. Her anxiety and intense feelings of discomfort had an entirely different source.

It came as a big surprise to Frida when she realized that the incomprehensible, baffling, and frightening reactions she now experienced (in the dental office) were connected to a painful incident that she had tried to forget, but which still lived within her. She had unraveled an old mental wound, a trauma that occurred 10 years ago but still disrupted her life and limited her everyday functions even today. Something about the circumstances during dental treatment had brought to life memories from the rape many years earlier. How come Frida now managed to cope with the old trauma history, and thus finally could receive necessary dental treatment? In short, a dentist with skills described in this book seemed to be the key. That is, a dentist who focuses upon building a good relation and also has enough knowledge about oral health psychology, in general, in combination with good technical skills, to give the patient the quality of dental care that she needs.

2.3 Trauma-Sensitive Dentists Treat More Than Just Teeth

Dental health practitioners are in a position to contribute to the healing of old psychological wounds. Fundamentally, it is about not ignoring unexpected reactions and dismissing them as "strange" and incomprehensible, but quite on the contrary—to understand and accept the patient's reactions and what they may be signaling. By adopting such a proactive position, the dentist can help the patient through the necessary dental procedure. In this way the dental health practitioners are contributing to the creation of new experiences in the patient. Having previously been dismissed as "difficult," a traumatized patient can now experience that it is possible to be understood, helped to master new tasks and collaborate well. This may also contribute to the developing of generalized faith and belief in other people, which in return may increase the opportunities to receive support and master new situations.

Frida is one of many patients in the everyday life of a dental clinic. Like many victims of abuse, Frida does not perceive the connection between her previous traumatic experiences and her current problems during dentistry. While Frida's trauma was being raped, it is well known today that a variety of traumatic life experiences may lead to problems during dental treatment [1, 2]. Long-lasting and serious stressors such as bullying, physical and psychological violence, sexual abuse, or experiences of being neglected will all have serious consequences for those exposed to it. However, stressors of shorter duration and seriousness may also have an impact. Even when patients are aware of their trauma history, this it is not necessarily information that is shared with the dentist. This can be illustrated by examining Frida's case. Does Frida believe that the dentist can understand, without her saying anything herself? Does she wonder what others would think of her if she was open about the rape? Typically, she and other victims would be ashamed, afraid to reveal her own story, and worried about making a fool of herself to this kind dentist. Instead, she does not say anything, at least not in the first place. Altogether, this makes it easy to understand why not only Frida herself, but also the dentist, may get uncomfortable, feel irritated or helpless—which makes the treatment all the more difficult.

> When old traumatic experiences are triggered during dentistry, it is often expressed as anxiety. Traumatized people, however, are not necessarily afraid of either the dental instruments or the anesthetic or the white coat. They are probably more afraid of being close to, or under the authority of, another person. Sitting in the dentist's chair may trigger feelings of helplessness, being trapped or being at the mercy of another person connected to experiences from past traumatic events. In addition, patients may fear their own unpredictable reactions that even for them may seem incomprehensible or unmanageable. For dental professionals, and perhaps for the patients themselves, it can be difficult to distinguish between trauma-driven anxiety and more traditional oral phobia. Nevertheless, it is important to try to investigate what one is dealing with. Are anxiety reactions linked only to past experiences at a dentist's office or is it a consequence of more general adverse life experiences? At worst, a patient with trauma-driven anxiety may experience being re-traumatized if not properly understood and met by the dentist. As many people with traumatic experiences either are not conscious about the connection to problems with oral health, or camouflage it as dental anxiety, it is important to have an open and investigative attitude toward *all* patients. Consequently, what we call *a trauma-sensitive approach* should be implemented as a basic attitude for all professionals working with all kinds of oral health information, as well as in all dental treatment.

2.4   Trauma-Sensitive Approach: Responsiveness to an Unspoken Life Story

» John was born into a family with domestic violence. His father would beat his mother, and sometimes he hit John and his little sister as well. As a child his "bad teeth" gave John a lot of pain from infections. Dental treatment gradually became a true nightmare. At the age of 15, John ran away from home and started using heroin. Tooth infections regularly gave him a lot of pain. Only under the influence of heroin did he experience some pain relief. His dental care, however, was ignored when his time was focused on how and where to get his next hit. At the age of 40, John eventually was included in a treatment program that helped him believe that he too belonged in society. After 25 years on the streets, he now wants a life as a normal citizen. He wants a job, but says "It's hard, everyone just sees 'drug addict' when they see my teeth."

Many people live with wounds from violent experiences. These may have been caused by natural disasters, accidents, war, torture, disease, and not least—as the examples here show, various forms of violence in close relationships. Such overwhelming experiences will affect people's lives in many ways. When dental professionals ignore a patient's unexpected reactions during treatment, without stopping and finding out what is happening, it will reinforce the experience that John and others have: that no one really cares about what has happened. Ever again, traumatized individuals will be left all alone, not being able to count on the support of others and having to manage everything all by themselves.

It should not be too difficult, however, to use a trauma-sensitive approach in dental practice, also as a healing factor to reduce feelings of discomfort and stress [3–5]. The dentist may ask "Does your reaction today (… describe) have something to do with experiences from the past?" As a health professional you do not ask for any details but concentrates upon observing the patient's behavior here-and-now as important signals. For example, specific reactions of intense discomfort when being put backward in the chair or having instruments in the mouth may tell a story that has been difficult or even impossible to put into words. When simply having the toothbrush in the mouth causes re-enactments or intense discomfort, the patients need a dentist who does not criticize them for having poor dental care but understands that the lack of toothbrushing can actually be about avoiding painful memories. Without such understanding, the consequences turn out disastrous for oral health. Too many people have suffered from this lack of basic understanding from dental professionals.

❯ In sum, it is not important to know details of the traumatic event(s). What is required from the dentist is first and foremost to be able to show that you understand that something has happened in the past that makes it difficult for the patient to cope adequately here-and-now. This way of acknowledging the past without exploring it conveys "I see you, I know you have struggled, now someone knows something about how it was" in a matter-of-fact way that often calms the patient rather than activating traumatic memories. Secondly, of course, successful treatment requires skills and knowledge of how to make the situation more manageable to the patient.

2.5   The Theoretical Basis for a Trauma-Sensitive Approach

What tools and approaches do dental health professionals need to develop, to be able to offer traumatized patients the best of help? This chapter is centered around these issues. This next section, however, will specifically address the theoretical basis for *trauma-sensitive* dentistry. First a brief introduction into the development of the trauma-focused field in general.

2.5.1   Development of the Trauma Field: In Short

Understanding psychological trauma is in a way both a new and an old discipline in the field of mental health. At times, the recognition of what toxic stress can do to humans has been forgotten and neglected, and at other times it has been the subject of great attention. In the late nineteenth century, the French psychiatrist Pierre Janet, along with Sigmund Freud, Jean-Martin Charcot, and Gustav Jung, became one of the first to see a link between external stress and mental reactions [6]. A few years later this understanding was heavily criticized, not in the least by Freud, who then argued that libido, fantasies, and inner conflicts were the reason for various mental disorders. However, during the First and Second World Wars, Janet's early theory was again actualized in meetings with soldiers suffering from so-called shell shock in the aftermath of war. These soldiers had symptoms and disorders such as nightmares, re-enactments, intrusive thoughts, intense emotional outbursts, and a constant state of alertness/vigilance (hypervigilance). However, at the time there was little understanding that these were normal reactions to abnormal events. The psychological problems many soldiers came home with were most often dismissed as personal weakness or intolerance to enduring warfare.

It was not until the 1970s and early 1980s that a group of Vietnam War veterans had the American Psychiatric Association (APA) create a new diagnosis: Post-traumatic stress disorder (PTSD). PTSD was included in the association's Mental Disorders Diagnostic Manual (ICD) as the first diagnosis in which external stressors were described as a direct cause of disease [7]. It was a specific event that triggered the reactions that, in turn, developed into mental illness. The essence of PTSD is intrusive memories (flashbacks), increased alertness, and avoidance of anything reminiscent of the stressors in question. In other words, this new diagnosis described symptoms that were more or less common for many veterans with mental health problems as a result of experiences during war. Although they did not have physical injuries, they had been psychologically injured—traumatized—by the war.

Today it is well documented that a number of adverse life experiences including violence and sexual abuse can cause the development of a whole range of psychological reactions and disorders. Not only PTSD but also psychosis, anxiety and depression, obsessive compulsive disorder, eating disorders, self-harm, suicidal problems, substance abuse, and personality disorders can be trauma related.

2.5.2 Comorbidity

An American study from the 1990s has been of great importance to the trauma field. "The Adverse Childhood Experiences Study" (ACE) addressed a random sample of adults with questions concerning the occurrence of adverse experiences during childhood, such as physical and sexual abuse, family dysfunctionality, violence, threats, emotional abuse, etc. [8]. Of the nearly 17,000 participants, a third reported no adverse childhood experiences. Of the remaining two-thirds, 87% reported experiencing *more than one* adverse incident. With this comprehensive study, it was scientifically documented that adverse childhood experiences increased the risk of developing severe mental and physical illness in adult life.

The ACE study has been followed by a large number of new studies confirming the original findings—that the consequences of adverse child experiences are severe. It is consistently found that being exposed to abuse, violence, systematic threats, and general dysfunctionality in the family carries a significant risk of inadequate neurobiological development in children and adolescents. Deteriorating neurobiological function leads to a tendency to make poor choices in relation to health behaviors, which in turn again can lead to the development of serious illness and increase the likelihood of early death

(see ◘ Fig. 2.1). The explanation models are complex, and, among other things, are related to the fact that adverse childhood experiences lead to changes in the body's immune system.

The ACE Pyramid illustrates how childhood experiences shape attachment and health in adult age. Recently two more factors have been added to the Pyramid.

Social conditions/local context and Generational Embodiment/ Historical Trauma (see ◘ Fig. 2.1).

The ACE Pyramid has been used for decades, illustrating the implications of adverse childhood experiences in different ways—and in the end how such experiences may cause a risk of early death. Interestingly enough, a figure has also been developed that points out more precisely to the effects on dental health (see ► Chap. 17).

No one *wants* poor oral health. From a dental health perspective, the results of the ACE study provide important knowledge in order to understand the development of health-related risky behavior in vulnerable populations. According to the model, traumatic childhood experiences lead to poor health habits in general, and we know that poor health habits with poor oral hygiene and an unhealthy diet lead to dental caries and in a biopsychosocial development including economic resources lead to poor oral health. Increased incidence of caries will also increase the risk of dental anxiety [10], which in turn further increases the risk of poor oral health.

Even more specifically, being discussed currently is how periodontitis via diseases such as diabetes, depression, and autoimmune diseases can be affected by complex traumatic experiences [11]. It is argued that adverse childhood experiences, which we know can lead to both mental and physical stress disorders, again seem to increase the risk of chronic inflammatory conditions in the body. In this context, the necessity of cooperation across the various health professions is highlighted, for a better understanding and treatment of a wide range of trauma-related problems and diseases (see ◘ Fig. 2.2).

Along with poor economic resources, dental anxiety has been considered the main reason for poor oral-related quality of life [12]. This needs to be known and taken seriously. Modern dentistry with a biopsychosocial approach should always assess the complexity of poor dental care. It is essential to understand this complexity when patients avoid seeking necessary dental care or show poor dietary habits. When dental professionals have a deeper understanding of conditions that can lead to inadequate oral health, the possibilities for giving patients better guiding on self-treatment and prevention increases (see ► Chap. 5 Oral Health Literacy) and ► Chap. 7 (Habits, Motivation, and Change of Behavior).

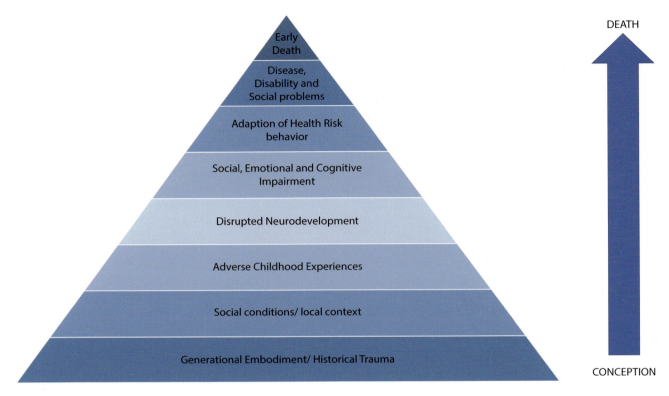

Fig. 2.1 The ACE pyramid [9]

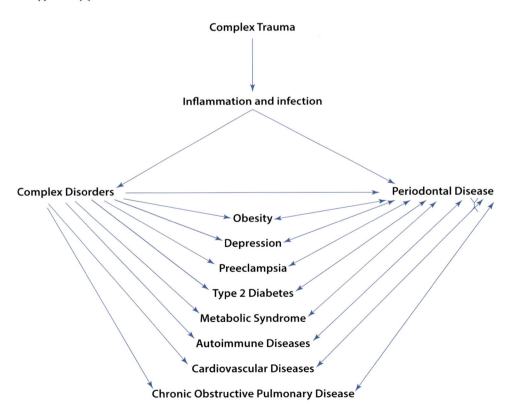

Fig. 2.2 By promoting inflammation and infections complex trauma causes and amplifies diseases, which in turn are correlated with periodontal disease. (Reproduced with permission [11])

The next part of this chapter will explore some of the *core elements* in understanding trauma. Here the knowledge is presented in a rather short version, but still aims to offer dental professionals a sufficient background for giving adequate treatment to traumatized patients. However, today there is currently a wide range of trauma-related literature available, which is recommended for further in-depth reading.

2.6 What Is a Trauma?

The word trauma comes from Ancient Greek and means wound or injury. A trauma is not the actual incident(s) that have occurred, but the *damage* inflicted by the incident(s). Physical traumas are wounds or injuries directly to the body, while psychological trauma injuries are emotional and mental. In this chapter, trauma is used in the sense of psychological damage. However, the trauma-focused academic community today is most concerned with how the body and psyche *play together* in the development of traumatic disorders [6]. Anxiety can be a psychological injury, but it is also a physiologically driven reflex. We say that "the anxiety is in the body." Humans are *both* body and mind, in an interaction.

Exposure to an event that involves intense fear, threat, or experience of complete helplessness may lead to the development of trauma or injury, but not automatically. Almost everybody experiences one or more dramatic events during their lives, but as humans we have developed resources to cope with it. However, when the extent and degree of the overwhelming situation exceeds a person's maximum coping strategies, one cannot deal properly with what has happened [13]. Depending on age, life history, personal resilience and, to a greater degree, access to support and comfort from others, we have different prerequisites to cope with stressful events. It is normal to be affected. In the aftermath of serious events, such as a car accident, rape, natural disaster, or experiences of war or torture, strong emotional, mental, physical, and cognitive reactions are to be expected.

Often, a person can feel oppressed, uneasy, distracted, and can experience for example disturbed sleep or eating problems. Others more typically may react with a sense of being stuck or frozen. We understand all these as normal reactions to abnormal events. Most often the wounds will heal after a while, provided the individual gets to safety and the opportunity to recover.

However, approximately 10% of those exposed to extreme stress will develop more lasting psychological injuries [6]. The nature of the events is crucial to the course of the healing. The greater the degree of guilt and responsibility one imposes on oneself for what has happened, the more the likelihood of persistent stress-related symptoms increases. Research shows that of rape victims, almost 90% will have post-traumatic stress reactions, and around 50% of those subjected to rape develop lasting psychological problems [14].

Typically, traumatized patients in medical (and dental) care are men and women who have been exposed to *a whole range of* adverse experiences, that is, far more than a single dramatic event. They have been exposed to different kinds of repeated adverse experiences (i.e., physical, psychological, and sexual violence) from an early age. In cases of repeated or recurrent trauma, a complex picture of symptoms and diseases is seen, involving difficulties with regulation, relational issues, and somatization [15]. Similar symptomatology may be seen in individuals with experiences related to *the absence* of events, that is, psychological wounds developed from neglect and lack of adult presence and support throughout childhood and adolescence [16]. The majority of those who develop more complex trauma problems have a long history over many years of violence, abuse, and neglect all together.

» Examples of children's experience of their own upbringing (from exhibitions and posters under the auspices of "Save the little ones"):

— Maria 10 years: I tried to keep away from the sound of mum and dad quarreling, but it didn't help.
— Lars 6 years: I tried to protect my mom, but I couldn't do it.
— Unknown child: I was so terribly scared at home. But when I read, I sort of forgot what was happening in the room next to me [17].

The children above share stories about adults who should provide safety and support, but instead behave erratically and make the children afraid. These children grow into adults and will be patients in dentistry. How does this kind of experience affect the situation at the dentist's office many years later?

» Ruth arrives at the dentist's office together with a friend. She is 47 years old and has suffered from major mental health problems throughout her whole life. In recent years, she has developed severe social anxiety. She also has dental anxiety and has only sought out dental services when she has been in great pain. Twice she has received dental treatment under general anesthesia. Ruth now attends psychological group sessions once a week, focusing upon trauma management. In one group session someone talked about a connection between having experienced childhood neglect and physical abuse and difficulty receiving dental treatment. Then at last Ruth understands the connection.

In Ruth's example, it took many years to find explanations that could shed light on her reactions that until then had been quite incomprehensible to her. Does it help Ruth, however, to understand her problems today in a context of early violence and abuse? For most people, it will be important to know that they are not crazy or stupid, but on the contrary, that their reactions—for example, in the dental setting—are normal reactions to abnormal events. The fact that Ruth found this connection gives her the opportunity to discuss the "strange" reactions of fear and helplessness when in the dental office and makes the dentist able to facilitate the treatment in a different way than before. This means, for example, simply to regulate the chair in a more comfortable position for the patient (i.e., not too much backward), stop and pause, talk in a friendly voice, inform the patient of what is going to happen in the treatment, how long time it will take, etc. Thus, Ruth is feeling a bit more in control of the situation. As a result, the possibility to find a way of treatment that suits Ruth's needs may be present for the first time. When the dentist or dental hygienist understand that Ruth is struggling with trauma-related problems, listen to the part of Ruth's story she wishes to share (no need for details) and show an understanding of the issues that are perceived as threatening, the chances increase significantly for a better treatment situation. This is a win-win situation for both Ruth and the dentist. On the one hand, the patient can receive high quality dental care, and on the other, the dental practitioner can provide care that will be as effective as possible.

2.7 How Does Dissociation Appear in the Dentist's Office?

So far, we have described how traumatic experiences in the past may affect daily life activities many years after, emphasizing that the dentist needs to understand trauma reactions to be able to offer adequate dental treatment. In addition, some knowledge of trauma-related dissociation is important.

Dissociation means a shift in the state of consciousness. All people can experience such shifts. One may not be 100% present but is still aware that it is "I" who act, feel, think, or talk. This form of flexibility in attention actually is one of the hallmarks of good mental health. Accordingly, for those who slightly dread visiting the dentist's office, it is a positive resource to disconnect a bit from the situation and think about something positive during the treatment. However, this capacity is understood as a selected shift in attention that is conscious and desired, while dissociation in the pathological sense occurs automatically. The patient who "floats away," faints, or perhaps jumps out of the dental chair, suddenly leaves the room, gets an anxiety attack, or otherwise behaves in unexpected ways during treatment is more likely to dissociate in the pathological meaning of the term. In trauma-sensitive dental care, dental professionals must therefore be able to distinguish between what are the degrees of a normal attention phenomenon, and what is more about splitting consciousness as a result of traumatizing.

Dissociative reactions can be associated with several different psychiatric disorders. According to ICD-11 WHO's diagnostic manual, in order to pose dissociation as a separate diagnosis, criteria such as amnesia, depersonalization, derealization, identity confusion and identity switching must be present [18]. The most severe dissociative disorder is the one that previously was known as Multiple Personality Disorder, but which is now called Dissociative Identity Disorder (DID). In the trauma field, the theory of structural dissociation of personality [19] has received a lot of attention. This theory explains how dissociation revolves around a form of different degrees of division at *the personality level*. In cases of such severe dissociation disorder, the dissociative structure is formed early. Structural dissociation with several "daily life awareness" (Apparently Normal parts of the Personality [ANP]) and several developed emotional parts (Emotional parts of the Personality [EP]) is the result of overwhelming stresses and disturbed patterns of interaction during critical periods of development [14, 20]. There is still one personality, but with several split parts of consciousness. Studies show that approximately 1% of a normal sample may have this serious diagnosis [21].

Dissociation in a pathological sense is not willful. In traumatized patients, dissociation has the character of an automatic way of disconnecting earlier overwhelming experiences from the here-and-now. It can happen during the actual event, described as "It was like I saw my body from the outside, from where I was somehow up under the roof." In retrospect, dissociation develops as a defense that helps the person to avoid relating to whatever triggers might come, that is, to avoid remembering. In this way, dissociation can be understood as an attempt to master the consequences of traumatic stress. In the long run, however, this solution develops several challenges. When not present here-and-now, one is also prevented from experiencing that the world is no longer as dangerous as before. The energy goes into some kind of re-living the trauma or in a state of protecting oneself from whatever might trigger flashbacks. Dissociative problems, therefore, will tend to tear down the person and hamper daily life functioning.

» When Anne walked into the dentist's office she stood with her coat on, against the wall, as far from the dentist and dental chair as possible. She looked down, made little eye contact, answered little, often with one-syllable words and evasive on questions. When she eventually sat in the dentist's chair, she seemed lethargic and distant but compassionate. It was like she was not quite herself anymore.

However, people struggling with dissociation can act completely "normal" until they are triggered. The patient who appears healthy and upright can suddenly become numb and lose sensation in different parts of the body. Or she/he can become very quiet and not contactable or get very angry. Some patients may also have convulsions reminiscent of epileptic seizure, or sudden paralysis. Sometimes the dentist may even notice that the person in the chair changes both expression and manner. A common feature of people in dissociation is that the adult patient in front of us somehow gets lost. When painful memories are triggered, we can meet the little scared child who had to flee into him/herself or an angry voice asking the dentist to go away. The person is no longer "here-and-now" but relates to a reality that she/ he experienced in the past.

» Beth has experienced many years of bullying, both physical and psychological, from her school mates. Her overbite was one of the topics regularly in focus of the classmates who harassed her. Some years later, at the dentist's, she is told "Please sit still and let me have a look at your teeth". Hearing this Beth mentally disappears. The sentence itself triggers her, and the physical reactions she gets are similar to those her body learned to use at the time when she just had to endure the bullying. That is, she literally "fled away". Today her body needs to unlearn this. In fact, the body needs to experience that in the dentist situation right now she is safe.

Dissociative reactions are confusing and perhaps also frightening to most professionals who are not trained in trauma therapy. Therefore, as a dentist it is important to remind yourself that what happens is not dangerous. What can be "dangerous" is to ignore the signals that the patient has switched off and continue treatment while the patient is not mentally present. This is challenging, because the signals of dissociation can be difficult to catch. It takes an attentive and trained look to observe what happens. For example, for the dentist, a person in a dissociative state can be perceived as a patient who simply is very silent and does not protest. It is therefore important in advance to talk to patients about dissociation. One might like to ask directly "Some patients are disconnecting or dissociate during dental treatment, is this something you think may happen to you?" If the patient responds that this could become a problem, then you can say "Is there anything special we should look for as a sign that you are about to unwind?"

In such an open-minded and straight-forward way, the dentist will communicate understanding, professionalism, and safety.

2.8 The Triune Brain and Reactions to Danger

Knowledge of neurobiological processes in the face of danger may be very useful for dental professionals when explaining to patients why they react as they do. An explanation of reactions presented in very simplified form may be beneficial when helping the patient to cope with dental treatment and to adopt good oral care.

From an evolutionarily perspective the body is designed for survival, and the brain controls the automatic reactions that provide protection when we are in dangerous situations. These are vital responses, but they become problematic if the brain is activated even when the danger is over. A core concept in the field of trauma is that in traumatized individuals, physical impressions, feelings, and thoughts have not been adequately processed after the harmful events. It is precisely because of this lack of processing that lasting psychological damage (trauma disorders) occurs.

> When subsequently exposed to situations that bare similarities to the original traumatic event, one reacts again by being afraid, unsettled and distracted. The alarm system has completely broken down. It "turns on" too easily and does not find the "shutoff button" again. Thus, the person is unable to distinguish appropriately between what is dangerous and what is not. The brain's ability to regulate affect has been disrupted after prolonged activation during danger, and the individual remains in survival mode where little or "nothing" is needed to trigger danger signals.

The term "the triune brain" is widely used in the trauma field. The brain is understood as it develops from the bottom-up [22]. ("Bottom-up," see ▶ Chap. 1). In short, this model divides the brain into three parts that are easily communicated to patients; the survival brain, the emotional brain, and the logic brain (see ▪ Fig. 2.3).

The brain stem *(latin truncus encephali)* and the lower parts of the brain are fully developed at birth. From here, all functions associated with survival are controlled: sleeping, eating, being awake, crying, breathing, noticing temperature changes, feeling hunger, feeling bodily sensations, feeling pain, and getting rid of waste substances through urine and feces.

Just above and around the brain stem (survival brain), we find the basic parts of the limbic system, here

2

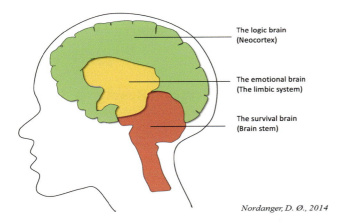

The logic brain
(Neocortex)

The emotional brain
(The limbic system)

The survival brain
(Brain stem)

Nordanger, D. Ø., 2014

▣ **Fig. 2.3**   The triune brain [23]

called *the emotional brain.* From the emotional brain, emotions, memory functions, and hormones involved in the instinctive defense mechanisms are controlled to fight, flight, freeze, and submission. Neurological development of this part of the brain takes place after birth and is completely dependent on interaction with other people. The emotional brain contains the lower part of the limbic system with the amygdala, also known as the body's smoke-detector or alarm system.

When a situation is perceived as dangerous (a potential risk to life), the alarm system is activated. The more dangerous the situation, the higher the alert level. When in extreme danger, this process is entirely automatic in order to rescue us. The amygdala picks up on perceived threats from somatosensory senses: sound, vision, smell, and touch (skin sensations) and sends signals directly to the brain stem (survival brain). The survival brain then triggers the sympathetic part of the autonomic nervous system, with the adrenal glands, which produce stress hormones such as adrenaline and cortisol that are then sent via the bloodstream to the heart, lungs, and muscles, to prepare for a battle. The ability to think rationally and reflect is now inhibited, as the cortex is disconnected in order not to delay life-saving responses. The amygdala part of the limbic system in the emotional brain also has a memory function. It stores sensations in the form of implicit memories/body experiences in order to make us able to quickly recognize the danger signals without having to think about it. For instance: *Lisa once got burned on a hot hob. Later, without giving it any thought, she automatically avoids touching the hob.* The hippocampus, also in the limbic system, is the library of the brain and stores experiences to make us link new experiences to those experienced in the past. This may be understood as the body *remembers*, with both good and bad consequences. An example:

» When he was three years old Peter had an experience at the dentist's that was both very painful and unpleasant.

The drill itself felt strange and scary, but even worse was the strict authority of the dentist, and the fact that Peter was held back in the chair as he tried to escape the situation. When he later at the age of 10 hears the sound of the drill, his body goes into total submission. Peter himself really does not remember the earlier experience. The bodily reactions he experiences, however, are so unpleasant that they frighten him. In this way, Peter develops an "anxiety of his own anxiety."

The logic brain consists of the cortex (neocortex) and the most advanced parts of the limbic system. This part of the brain matures throughout adolescence, until the pre-frontal cortex (front part of the neocortex) is fully developed in the early 20s [24]. The logic brain is the center of language and abstract thinking. It makes us able to integrate large amounts of information and understand it in a context. Activity in the pre-frontal cortex is absolutely necessary for skills like reflection, reasoning, and planning. If the emotional brain is the body's alarm system, then the logic brain is the regulation system. A well-developed logic brain acts as a regulating authority when processing somatosensory input or emotional arousal. When the alarm goes off as danger is detected, the logic brain will be able to connect and regulate the reactions: "Yes, this looks like something dangerous that has happened to me in the past. But it's not happening now. I am in another situation now, I am an adult, I am in control."

The brain's automated alarm system is highly effective when in danger. However, in traumatized individuals, the alarm system often does not work adequately. The access to the logic brain is often limited; the body's alarm system (emotional brain) fires too quickly or too slowly and makes it very challenging to function well in everyday life. The bodily reactions are perceived as incomprehensible and very troublesome. The patient who suddenly cancels dental treatment can despair "I do not understand what is happening to me. I am just so scared, and I just want to run away. But I know there's nothing dangerous going on here. I think I'm going crazy." The adequate response from dental professionals would be: "I am sure there is a good reason why you feel this way." Hearing this will make the patient able to calm down a bit. By calming down, access to the logical brain can be retrieved and thereby the possibility to ask oneself "What am I reacting to here?" The dentist has established a good start for a dialogue about how to make the situation less frightening for the patient.

The traumatized brain struggles to regulate emotions. A useful tool to help assist dentists in explaining to patients why frightening reactions come again and again, why they get the reactions they do and to help teach them to regulate themselves better, is that of "The window of tolerance."

2.9 Why "The Window of Tolerance" Is a Useful Model for Regulation of Emotions

The window of tolerance [24, 25] is a simple tool to use in psychoeducation when patients face stress-related problems. The model is easily understandable and shows how bodily and emotional activation occur during the experience of danger. Everyone has a zone of optimal arousal (activation) where there is neither too little nor too much going on inside the body. Emotions are experienced as tolerable and experiences can be integrated. This is the zone where we function at our best, we have access to our brain, we can learn new things and we are not overwhelmed with anxiety. The alarm is not on. This is where we want to be if attending an exam or doing something technically difficult. This zone is what we call our "window of tolerance."

In the face of stressors that are too much to cope with, our body reacts by going outside of the window, above or below. Going above the window gives reactions of increased activation (hyperactivation) in the body, and the sympathetic nervous system makes the body ready to fight, flight, or freeze. In this state it is normal to be agitated, panicky, angry, or experience flashbacks. Reactions if one goes below the window are associated with too little activation in the body (hypoactivation). Here physiological responses are inhibited, and the body becomes numb. Consciousness is influenced, the person becomes distant and partially disconnects from reality. This happens in situations where the danger is overwhelming with no benefit from fleeing or fighting back. In dentistry we see it as the patient suddenly becomes distant, lethargic, and acts almost as if he or she is unconscious.

❯ "The window of tolerance simply means the individual 'zone' of bodily activation, where we manage to relate attentively to others and can concentrate and learn" [25]. That does not mean that we are doing our very best, but rather that we can tolerate, cope with, and integrate stress activation (see also ▶ Chap. 1 on stress).

❯ The size of the window of tolerance will differ from day to day or hour by hour and may change quickly. If a person's window is small, activation is easily done—the alarm is on almost all the time. Traumatized individuals will typically have a very small window of tolerance and may swing quickly between hyper- and hypo-arousal (◻ Fig. 2.4).

As a rule, dentists should have a professional responsibility to make sure that the patient is within their window of tolerance during the entire dental treatment. Sometimes, the patient may be in a hyper-activated or hypo-activated state, but with the help of coping strategies, the dentist can help the patient to relax and "re-enter into the window."

» Eva comes to the dentist's office after avoiding dental treatment for 20 years. She was sexually abused as a young teenager. In the dental treatment room, she seems very uneasy, shifting the weight from one foot to another. She cannot control her breathing and her heart is beating way too fast. She feels terribly nervous and anxious.

The dentist notices that Eva is hyperventilating, she is clearly "above her window of tolerance." Eventually, the dentist can ask her to calm down, but it is unlikely to have any effect. Based on the model described above, it

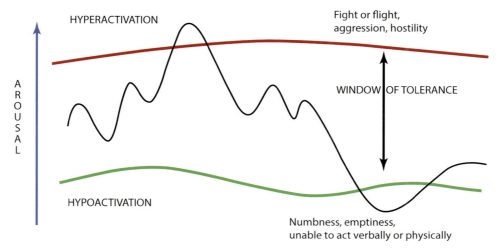

◻ **Fig. 2.4** Window of tolerance. (Adapted from Ogden, Minton & Pain, 2006 [26])

will be much more beneficial to sit down with Eva and get her to describe what happens when she is experiencing these reactions. Is there something that triggers the reaction? Maybe it is about something that happened a long time ago, or is it something in the situation right now that stresses her? This kind of approach will make Eva able to talk about why and how the dental situation is challenging. She may answer with statements like "I get scared of having someone so close to me." The dentist may then explain a little about the function of her triune brain and how her "window" has become narrow. And the two of them may begin to discuss what can be done to expand the window (see ▶ Chap. 15). Precisely what would make it more possible for Eva to be present in the room and carry out the treatment?

An opposite to over-activation, when reacting to perceived danger, is *under-activation* (hypoactivation). Physiological responses now are inhibited, and the body becomes numb. Consciousness is influenced so that one becomes distant, indifferent, and partially disconnected from reality. This happens in situations where the danger is overwhelming and when protecting oneself by fleeing or fighting back feels impossible. In dentistry this can be observed as the patient suddenly becomes distant and almost acts as being unconscious. He or she may dissociate as well. According to our model, this will be typical reactions when "under the window."

» Eric, an ex-solider suffering from posttraumatic stress symptoms after war experiences, seems in good spirits and tells a funny story as he settles in the dentist's chair. A few minutes into the examination, something suddenly happens. His body becomes rigid, he disappears mentally, and his breathing is almost unnoticeable. It may look like Eric is going into some kind of under-activation, he is hypo-activated.

When the dentist notices this, she stops the examination and says calmly and in a friendly, yet determined, voice: "You are here with me, the dentist, now. Please come back here." Eric may shake a bit and look surprised. He is offered some water and recovers quickly. Again, the dentist may comment on what just happened, and ask "Is this a reaction you can recognize from other situations as well? Did you notice the feeling right before you disappeared? What can we do to help you not fade away, but to stay more present here with me?"

If the patients remain "outside their window of tolerance" and do not get help to regulate back into the window again, they will experience strong negative reactions that later on probably will be linked to the dental treatment. Based on the window of tolerance model and knowledge of how the brain works during the experience of danger, dental professionals can counteract development of these negative reactions. In order to increase coping with dental situations that patients find uncomfortable, the aim will be to expand the window, which means increasing tolerance to their own reactions.

Today the "Window of Tolerance" model is used in many different health professional contexts, as well as in the general population such as the educational systems. The model has proved useful for dental professionals when explaining to traumatized patients why dentistry can be challenging but may be used to explain reactions and facilitate treatment for all patients as well.

Summary

"You won't see it until you believe it."

As clinicians the authors of this chapter have met patients with personal histories that include traumatic experiences, sometimes of a severity difficult to understand. Too often these patients have expressed a lack of empathy and respect of their reactions from former dental personnel. "The dentist just did his job and did not see how I was struggling." As a result, the patient typically will leave the dental office even more in risk of oral health problems than before. The dentist, on the other hand, would be ignorant of the patient's struggle as well as of the increased risk of developing future dental problems. It seems that if a dentist (or any other person) does not *believe* that being exposed to traumatic episodes may be something that might have happened to patients, he or she often does not *see* the patient's needs or struggles. Hence, interest in how trauma may affect personal health, together with knowledge of at least a few principles of trauma-sensitive techniques, should be a part of all ordinary health practice.

Trauma-sensitive care may be considered as a method. Even more relevant from the authors point of view, however, is to implement the basic understanding described in this chapter into every dental professional's attitude, professionality, and personal style. No patients are "difficult," they have difficulties. Dental personnel do not need to examine exactly why things are difficult, but must respect, tolerate, and be empathic toward all patients. Thus, in short, trauma-sensitive care means high quality dental care.

References

1. Bright MA, Alford SM, Hinojosa MS, Knapp C, Fernandez-Baca DE. Adverse childhood experiences and dental health in children and adolescents. Commun Dent Oral Epidemiol. 2015;43(3):193–9. https://doi.org/10.1111/cdoe.12137.
2. Leeners B, Stiller R, Block E, Görres G, Imthurn B, Rath W. Consequences of childhood sexual abuse experiences on dental care. J Psychosom Res. 2007;62:581–8.

3. Bath H. The three pillars of TraumaWise care: healing in the other 23 hours. Reclaim Child Youth J. 2015;23:6–11.
4. Raja S, Hoersch M, Rajagopalan CF, Chang P. Treating patients with traumatic life experiences: providing trauma-informed care. J Am Dent Assoc. 2014;145:238–45.
5. Kranstad V, Søftestad S, Fredriksen TV, Willumsen T. Being considerate every step of the way – a qualitative study analysing trauma-sensitive dental treatment for childhood sexual abuse survivors. Eur J Oral Sci. 2019;127:539–46.
6. van der Kolk B, McFarlane AC, Weisæth L. Traumatic stress. In: The effects of overwhelming experience on mind, body, and society. New York: Guilford Press; 1996.
7. American Psychiatric Association DSM-III. Diagnosis and statistical manual of mental disorders. Washington, D.C.: American Psychiatric Press; 1980.
8. Felitti VJ, Anda RF, Nordenberg D, Williamson DF, Spitz AM, Edward V, Koss MP, Marks JS. Relationship of childhood abuse and household dysfunction to many of the leading causes of death in adults. The Adverse Childhood (ACE) study. Am J Prev Med. 1998;14:245–58.
9. Centers for disease, control and prevention, About the CDC-Kaiser ACE Study, (updated April 6. 2021, cited May 17. 2021). Available from https://www.cdc.gov/violenceprevention/aces/about.html.
10. Raadal M, Strand GV, Amarante EC, Kvale G. Relationship between caries prevalence at 5 years of age and dental anxiety at 10. Eur J Paediatr Dent. 2002;3:22–6.
11. Kirkengen AL, Lygre H. Exploring the relationship between childhood adversity and oral health: an anecdotal approach and integrative view. Med Hypotheses. 2015;85:134–40.
12. Boman UW, Wennström A, Stenman U, Hakeberg M. Oral health-related quality of life, sense of coherence and dental anxiety. An epidemiological cross-sectional study of middle-aged women. BMC Oral Health. 2012;12:14.
13. Saakvitne KW, Gamble S, Pearlman LA, Lev B. Risking connection. A training curriculum for working with survivors of childhood abuse. Lutherville: Sidran Press; 2000.
14. Anstorp T, Benum K. Traumebehandling. Komplekse traumelidelser og dissosiasjon. Oslo: Universitetsforlaget; 2014. (in Norwegian)
15. Herman J. Trauma and recovery. New York: Basic Books; 1992.
16. Nordanger DØ, Braarud HC. Utviklingstraumer. Regulering som nøkkelbegrep i en ny traumepsykologi. Bergen: Fagbokforlaget; 2017. (in Norwegian)
17. "Redde små", a Norwegian network to support efforts to combat violence, abuse and neglect against children. (cited Nov 10th 2021). Available from https://reddesmå.no/ressurser/utstillinger.
18. World health organization (WHO) International Statistical Classification of Diseases and Related Health Problems (ICD). (cited May 17th 2021). Available from https://www.who.int/standards/classifications/classification-of-diseases.
19. Nijenhuis E, van der Hart O, Steele K. Traumerelatert strukturell dissosiasjon av personligheten. Teoretisk forståelse og begrepsavklaring. In: Anstorp T, Benum K, Jakobsen M, editors. Dissosiasjon og relasjonstraumer. Integrering av det splittede jeg. Oslo: Universitetsforlaget; 2006. (in Norwegian).
20. Anstorp T, Benum K, Jakobsen M. Dissosiasjon og relasjonstraumer. In: Integrering av det splittede jeg. Oslo: Universitetsforlaget; 2006. (in Norwegian).
21. Putnam F. Dissociative disorders. A clinical review. In: Siegel ID, editor. Dissociative phenomena. Lutherville: Sidran Press; 1993.
22. Holden C. Paul MacLean and the triune brain. Science. 1979;204(4397):1066–8.
23. Nordanger DØ. Nevrobiologi som veiviser for traumearbeid. In: Anstorp T, Benum K, editors. Traumebehandling. Komplekse traumelidelser og dissosiasjon. Oslo: Universitetsforlaget; 2014. (in Norwegian).
24. Siegel DJ. The developing mind. 2nd ed. New York: Guilford Press; 2012.
25. Ogden P, Minton K. Sensorimotor psychotherapy. One method for processing traumatic memory. Traumatology. 2000;6:1–20.
26. Ogden P, Minton K, Pain C. Trauma and the body. A sensorimotor approach to psychotherapy. New York: Norton; 2006.

Pain

Borrik Schjødt, Maren Lillehaug Agdal, and Margrethe Elin Vika

Contents

🅑 **Learning Goals**

To have knowledge about:
- Pain in a biological perspective.
- Mechanisms for pain transmission and pain perception.
- Personal and environmental factors in association with pain.
- Psychological interventions to ameliorate pain.

3.1 Introduction

Pain is an important topic in all somatic and psychologic health care. Pain can be transient or persistent, weak or overwhelming, understandable or diffuse. While most people feel pain from time to time, some have persistent pain and others lack the ability to feel pain. Pain is always personal and cannot be questioned by others. Dental procedures elicit pain and previous painful experiences may for some be the reason for their dental fear. Others may have conditions with persistent pain which influence their daily lives and make them vulnerable for new painful experiences. Pain may be the reason why the patient doesn't sleep at night, have problems in social interactions, and may be a barrier for the patient to seek regular dental care. Knowledge about pain is important to understand the person in pain. Knowledge about pain, pain conditions, and awareness of our attitudes towards persons in pain are essential in dentistry and for the professional care we give the patient.

Everyone – with a few exceptions - has experience with pain. Dental treatment is often associated with pain as many procedures can be painful, such as probing the teeth, pain when injecting the anaesthesia, drilling into the teeth and periodontal treatment with cleaning calculus. It can be argued that pain during dental treatment is less common now than in earlier days. The equipment has improved, medications to reduce the pain experience is routinely used and has become more effective. Altered perspectives, improved methods, together with increased knowledge about pain, means that patients should be treated in a way that both prevents pain, and when present reduces pain to a minimum. At the same time, there are conditions such as myalgia and neuropathy where pain in the jaw and face is not directly linked to the teeth, although the pain can be experienced as if the pain origins from one or more teeth. How to approach and treat the various pain conditions may thus be somewhat different.

Pain has a clear function – it is a warning signal – a warning that something is wrong, and that one must initiate an action that stops or reduces the pain. Pain is something we all have a relationship with, and everyone has an idea of what pain is. Despite this, it is difficult to both describe and define pain. Pain is a complex and compound experience.

The International Association for the Study of Pain's (IASP) definition of pain [1] has stood as the best definition until the IASP, after 2 years of discussions and hearings, came up with a new definition in 2020: Pain is 'An unpleasant sensory and emotional experience associated with, or resembling that associated with, actual or potential tissue damage' [2]. The definition is specified through six sub-items (see ▶ Box).

A study that included 46,394 people in 15 European countries as well as Israel shows how frequent the experience of pain is: As many as 19% reported that they had moderate to severe pain that had lasted for at least 6 months [3]. Other studies show about the same figures. The incidence of reported persistent pain varies from country to country, and both gender and age differences have been found for pain. Prevalence and incidence studies in children and adolescents are not consistent to which degree children experience pain in their daily lives. There is however a tendency that pain is an increasing problem in the younger population [4, 5]. In the adult population we see an increased incidence of pain with increasing age. Current data also indicate a predominance of women experiencing persistent pain. Incidence of pain is also related to socioeconomic status: the lower the status, the greater the incidence of pain [6].

3.2 Pain: A Complex Phenomenon

Pain is most often felt as something concrete that happens in the body. In early pain theories, it was assumed that an impulse from the periphery (e.g. a sting in the fingertip) followed a nerve thread to the spinal cord and further up to the brain, where it caused activity in a specific place in the brain. The intensity of the pain was thought to be related to the intensity of peripheral stimulation, while some assumed that pain intensity was the result of the sum of nerve impulses (◘ Fig. 3.1).

Later we have learned that it is far more complex. Pain has great personal variations and is influenced by previous learning, the person's state of mind, and the very perception of the cause of the pain. The complex interaction in the brain that leads to the concrete perception of pain is referred to as a neuromatrix/brain network.

IASP's definition emphasizes that pain is an experience, with both sensory and emotional qualities. Through many years of pain research, the research

3

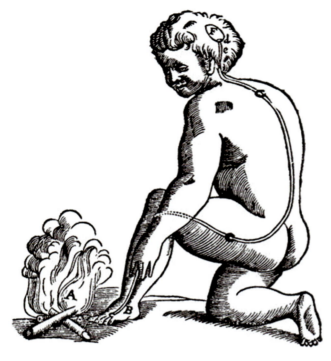

◘ Fig. 3.1 Pain transferred from peripheral tissues to the brain where it was perceived [7] (Descartes, 1664)

communities agree on the understanding that pain cannot be measured by describing activity in nerves that transmit pain impulses. There is no direct link between nerve activity and perceived pain. Pain is a subjective experience, and one must respect the person's expression of discomfort, regardless of whether one can explain the pain or not. Therefore, we should always respect the person's report of pain, whether we understand the origin of the pain or not.

Reasons for the large variation in pain experience will be discussed in more detail later in the chapter.

■ **Pain: Necessary for Development and Survival**

Pain is a warning signal that helps us to avoid dangerous situations that may involve injury or situations that challenge and strain body parts that need rest and relaxation. Pain is necessary to survive.

Everyone is born with the ability to feel pain — with a few exceptions. There are a few people with a genetic defect that makes them insensitive to pain (Congenital insensitivity to Pain or CIP). They have trouble recognizing and paying attention to injury or illness, and many die at an early age from sequela due to this disease. In children with this condition, burns, bitten or damaged fingertips, and bitten tongue tips are common. In older people with congenital insensitivity to pain, it is not uncommon with joint injuries and deformities as a result of previous bone fractures [8].

Pain

An unpleasant sensory and emotional experience associated with, or resembling that associated with, actual or potential tissue damage.

Notes

— Pain is always a personal experience that is influenced to varying degrees by biological, psychological, and social factors.

— Pain and nociception are different phenomena. Pain cannot be inferred solely from activity in sensory neurons.

— Through their life experiences, individuals learn the concept of pain.

— A person's report of an experience as pain should be respected. *

— Although pain usually serves an adaptive role, it may have adverse effects on function and social and psychological well-being.

— Verbal description is only one of several behaviours to express pain; inability to communicate does not negate the possibility that a human or a nonhuman animal experiences pain [2]

3.2.1 Nociceptive, Neuropathic, and Nociplastic Pain

A distinction has been made between different types of pain based on presumed underlying pathophysiology – with three different groups: nociceptive, neuropathic, and nociplastic [9].

Nociceptive pain: Pain that arises from actual or threatened damage to non-neural tissue and is due to the activation of nociceptors.

Neuropathic pain: Pain caused by a lesion or disease of the somatosensory nervous system.

Nociplastic pain: Pain that arises from altered nociception despite no clear evidence of actual or threatened tissue damage causing the activation of peripheral nociceptors or evidence for disease or lesion of the somatosensory system causing the pain.

Nociceptive pain is the most common category of pain, and it is this type of pain that is most often encountered. Pain is caused by the influence of peripheral nerve cells that transmit pain impulses, the so-called nociceptors (see section below). Nerve activity may be due to mechanical influence, temperature (heat / cold), or chemical influence. Examples of nociceptive pain are inflammation, stings or hard pressure on a body part, frostbite or burns. In other words, this is the type of pain found in a person with a normally functioning somatosensory nervous system. The nociceptive pain is the pain one normally expects in a dental treatment situation.

The patient feels pain at the sting of the syringe because the needle hits nerve endings as the skin is damaged when the needle is inserted. During drilling of a tooth, there is a corresponding cutting of nerve fibres in the dentine.

Neuropathic pain is defined as 'Pain caused by a lesion or disease of the somatosensory nervous system' [10]. Conditions of neuropathic pain may be present when nerves are damaged or cut or an underlying disease affects the nervous system. A well-known situation is that any surgical procedure which involves the probability that nerves will be cut, there is a chance that the cut nerves will in turn cause pain without external influence. In trigeminal neuralgia, the diagnosis is typically diagnosed by mapping clinical signs that may be the cause of the pain. Teeth can become hypersensitive in inflammatory processes due to damaged or hypomineralized teeth as in Molar Incisor Hypomineralization. In case of inflammation, there is an upregulation of inflammatory factors in close relation to the nerves in the teeth [11]. Accordingly, there is an increase in free nerve endings which over time reduces the threshold for pain, and pain is experienced at a lower degree of stimulus. Imaging, biopsies, and various clinical tests can be used to diagnose neuropathic pain. The presence of neuropathic pain is quite common and recognized with consensus as post effect for different diseases – for example postherpetic neuralgia. In the case of neuropathic pain, one may experience that a gentle touch causes intense pain, pain can occur without a clear external cause, and influences that were not previously painful cause intense pain.

Neuropathic pain is divided into central and peripheral neuropathies. Examples of central neuropathic pain are pain after stroke and brain injury. Peripheral neuropathies can be caused by pinched nerves or other forms of damage to peripheral nerves, such as polyneuropathy in diabetes, or canalis-carpi syndrome where there is a narrowing of the carpal tunnel and a compression of nerves in the wrist. Patients may develop neuropathies in the jaw after tooth extraction or tooth injury. Dental professionals must be aware that painful treatments can cause long-term pain experiences. This also applies to patients who cannot express pain during the dental procedure, such as patients who are being treated under general anaesthesia or who are on sedative medication. Therefore, dentists must always provide adequate local anaesthesia to achieve pain relief during procedures which are suspected to be painful. Some patients report pain in a tooth that has been extracted, other patients experience that the pain disappears when one tooth is extracted, but then moves to the next tooth. It is uncertain how common this is, but it is a considerable challenge when it occurs and underlines that treatment should never be performed without local anaesthesia solely on the basis of the patient's subjective pain experience and pain report during the treatment.

The third category, nociplastic pain, was proposed by Kosek et al. in 2016 and is endorsed by the IASP [12]. This is a type of pain defined as 'Pain that arises from altered nociception despite no clear evidence of actual or threatened tissue damage causing the activation of peripheral nociceptors or evidence of disease or lesion of the somatosensory system causing the pain' [12, p. 1383]. This definition is based on the premise that pain can occur without damaged nerve tissue, or that a threatening tissue damage can be detected, but where there is activity in the peripheral nerves that transmit pain impulses. In other words, the key is to change the function of pain-related sensory nerve pathways, centrally and/or peripherally. One example is fibromyalgia, where we know that there is increased sensation of pain, without damage to nerves or tissues. The mechanisms are uncertain, but it is assumed that there is both a central and peripheral sensitization of pain (that less stimulation is required before pain impulses are transmitted), which can be explained by changed activity in central and peripheral networks.

In the clinic, the most important message is that a person may experience intense pain, even if we cannot see or understand the cause of the pain. The pain is not imaginary, it is a result of activity in the part of the nervous system that transmits pain impulses and contributes to the experience of pain.

3.2.2 Acute vs. Persistent Pain

It is common to distinguish between acute and persistent pain. The thinking is that the acute pain – which serves as a warning signal – at one time or another no longer serves any function and turns into a troublesome, persistent pain. The question is how to define the difference between acute and persistent or when the pain changes from being acute to becoming persistent. In early studies, when the pain endures beyond natural healing time, the pain is defined as chronic [13]. When a bone fracture or wound after surgery has healed or the pain after an inflamed tooth has healed, the pain is expected to disappear. This definition is problematic in relation to a number of different pain conditions – for example, migraine. Can one talk about healing in connection with migraines? What about fibromyalgia or muscular pain associated with the jaw or neck muscles?

Another approach has been to set a fixed time – 3 or 6 months. Most injuries or painful conditions will heal after 3–6 months. From a research point of view, it is important to have a common reference, and there seems to be agreement that pain that lasts over 3 months is defined as persistent. In a clinical context, 3 months is often experienced as a short time, and most pain clinics or rehabilitation institutions set 6 months as a practical distinction between acute and persistent pain.

An important reason for distinguishing between acute and persistent pain is that the conditions should be treated differently. Acute pain should be relieved – for several reasons. An obvious reason is that it is troublesome, and we want to provide relief if we can. Another important reason is that pain which is left untreated can cause lasting changes in the nervous system [14]. In other words, the acute pain becomes unnecessarily persistent. Therefore, one should be largely liberal when it comes to drug relief of acute pain. For persistent pain, on the other hand, other treatment principles apply, as we will see later in the chapter. There are many indications that a one-sided focus on drug treatment of long-term pain over time can cause additional problems, without alleviating the actual problems contributing to the pain. Many patients report that after discontinuation of long-term opioid treatment of pain, they achieve better function in daily performance, increased quality of life, and almost unnoticeable changes in the pain problem compared with when they are on drugs. Well-designed studies on this area are sparse. Huffmann et al. collected data of approximately 1500 patients over a period of 12 months, patients who discontinued treatment with high doses of opioids, achieved significant reduction of pain, anxiety, and depression, and achieved better function [15]. It has also been shown that the use of opioids can lower the pain threshold, even after short-term use. At the same time, there is a small group that has a good effect and insignificant problems associated with long-term opioid use [16].

3.2.3 Chronic or Persistent Pain?

Pain that lasts longer than 3 or 6 months is described as persistent by some researchers and clinicians, whereas others describe the pain as chronic. Whether the word chronic is a good word for describing persistent pain has been debated for many years and is still debated. Chronic sounds like something that lasts forever. As pain treatment has progressed, new approaches have been developed and success has been experienced, and more people are getting rid of their pain problems. Therefore, it was proposed to replace chronic with persistent. Prolonged pain or persistent pain sounds more time limited or temporary. A chronic disorder sounds like a condition that will last a lifetime, while a persistent disorder sounds like something that can be altered and go away. Today chronic and persistent are used interchangeably. We prefer that people in the healthcare system talk about persistent pain, because we know that for most pain conditions there are approaches that can either make the suffering less troublesome or do something about all the unwanted consequences of the conditions.

3.3 The Physiology of Pain

3.3.1 Basic Neurophysiology

Research shows that there are large individual differences in how pain stimuli are experienced and reported [17]. It has also been documented that those who are highly sensitive to pain have higher activity in brain areas that process pain, compared to those who report low pain on the same stimulus [18]. Today it is known that pain signals that occur peripherally in, for example, the skin or in the tooth, can be amplified or reduced both in the peripheral and in the central nervous system. The peripheral nervous system is all the nerves in the body except the nerves in the spinal cord and brain. The nerves in the spinal cord and brain make up the central nervous system. Locally, for example in the mucosa, nociceptors that are thin C-fibres (unmyelinated) with free nerve endings can be stimulated, for example, by a small sting. The pain signal is transmitted as an electric impulse to the posterior horn of the spinal cord, where it in a synapse transmits the signal to a new neuron (secondary neuron) which carries the pain impulse to the brainstem. If A-delta (Aδ) fibres (myelinated) are stimulated in the same periphery area as the pain stimuli, small inhibitory nerve fibres in the posterior horn are activated. These inhibitory nerve fibres may reduce the pain impulse transmitted from the periphery C-fibre to the secondary neuron in the spine. Hence, the pain signal sent to the brainstem has a lower intensity than if Aδ fibres were not stimulated. The pain impulse in the C-fibres has a low speed of approx. 0.5–1 m/s, while Aδ fibres conduct the impulse significantly faster at a speed of 5–30 m/s. This understanding of possible alteration of a specific peripheral pain signal on its journey to the brain was launched by Meltzak and Wall in 1965 [19] and is called the gate control theory. In daily life, we use the opportunity to change the pain impulse both consciously and unconsciously. The gate control theory was the beginning of an extensive new understanding of the plasticity of nerves working together before the pain is subjectively felt and interpret.

3.3.2 Light Stimulation May Relieve Pain

If a child falls and is bruised, we blow on the wound. If we burn ourselves, it feels soothing to gently run our hand over the area that has been burned. In both cases, both by blowing and touching, nerves are stimulated which inhibit the transmission of pain impulses in the posterior horn of the spinal cord, as described in the gate control theory. Conversely, local factors can amplify the pain impulse. Inflammation of the mucous membrane intensifies the pain impulse in a sting due to various molecules in the tissue (see ◘ Fig. 3.2) [20].

The pain signals in the dorsal horn of the spine can also be amplified or reduced by descending impulses from the brain. With the same mechanisms as are seen in the gate control theory, descending nerves release noradrenaline, serotonin, and endogenous opioids into the dorsal horn [21]. According to the gate control theory, how the person perceives the situation, the person's emotional state, and previous experiences affect the transmission of pain in the dorsal horn. In dental clini-

cal practice, there are daily examples of how painful procedure produce different levels of pain.

3.3.3 Central Regulation of Pain

In addition to changing the intensity of the pain signal in the dorsal horn of the spinal cord, pain signals can be amplified or reduced in the brainstem. The changes that take place in the brainstem originate in activity from other brain areas. Central to pain modulation at this level is activation from the amygdala. This is seen in the fact that patients with high anxiety about pain will often experience more intense pain stimuli than patients who are not afraid. There is a modulation of pain where psychological processes are strongly involved. The pain signal is amplified and the activation in the sensory cortex is higher. This complex interaction is neither visible nor measurable [22]. It is such connections that contribute to us having to believe the patient's own subjective pain report. One no longer

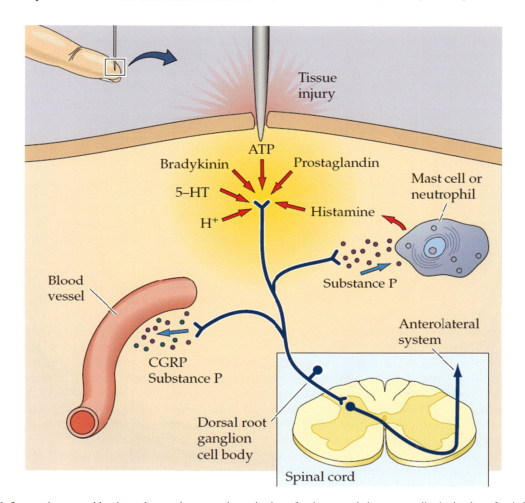

◘ **Fig. 3.2**   Inflammation caused by tissue damage increases the excitation of pain transmitting nerve cells. Activation of painful nerve cells also leads to the release of molecules that contribute to increased inflammation [20]. (Published with permission)

talks about an unreal or mental pain. In the brain, there are many areas that work together to shape a pain signal. The outcome – the pain the person is experiencing – should be taken seriously.

To describe how the different areas of the brain work together, the brain is referred to as a neural network where impulses from peripheral tissue (all tissues except the spinal cord and the brain) can be amplified or reduced. Melzack [23] believed that the theory of a neuromatrix could explain this. This network integrates a large amount of input, where the result is an experience of pain. The network includes sensory input, interpretation of what is happening, cognitive and emotional input from other parts of the brain (e.g., increased preparedness due to perceived danger), various inhibiting factors in the brain network, and activity in the body's stress-regulating system. Recent research on pain suggests that this is a fruitful way to go about understanding pain. Brodal [24] describes pain as activity in a complex central network, characterized by numerous connections and nodes, and which involves a number of brain structures (cortical and subcortical structures, amygdala, thalamus, PAG, etc.). An important point is that the network is fluctuating, and it is different from person to person and situation to situation. In other words, there is no pain centre, and it is unrealistic to imagine an objective measure of pain, even with the finest instruments.

This explains why people who are very afraid of pain may describe a certain exposure as terribly painful while others may describe the same exposure as pressure or mild pain. One should never dismiss the patient's experience of pain with the claim that the stimulation was 'just' pressure. As mentioned above, the bodily reaction to pain is unique for the person experiencing the pain. In some persons we can observe an overwhelming sympaticus activation during needle penetration or suddenly pain in a tooth under caries treatment. The startle reflex is also very prominent in some people. Afterward the patient may evaluate the actual pain experience as 'not so bad' and the duration 'a couple of seconds', and they feel the bodily reaction is exaggerated related to the actual pain they have felt. The problem is that it may be the bodily reaction they want to avoid in the future and not the pain per se. For many patients who are anxious of procedural pain, gradual and repeated exposure to pressure in the area where the syringe is to be inserted or the tooth is to be drilled will make the patient feel calmer in the situation, and gradually both the bodily reaction and the pain experience will decrease. With repetitive training the patient becomes able to perceive pressure as pressure, and not as pain due to changes in the brain that contribute to altered pain impulse in the CNS.

3.3.4 Referred Pain

Pain can be perceived as coming from one place in the body, while the origin is from another place. Some examples are what feels like toothache, but the pain comes from sinusitis, pain in the left arm that in fact comes from the heart, or pain in the jaw and temple that in fact originates from the neck muscles. When the pain is experienced as if it comes from a place other than the area where the nerves are stimulated, we call it referred pain.

Referred pain can have several explanations. The most common is that nerves from internal organs coincide with nerves from the skin and muscles in the dorsal horn of the spinal cord. When the internal organ is stimulated, it feels as if it comes from other areas, for example, as pain in the left arm by angina pectoris or under the right shoulder blade by gallstones. It is also likely that the nervous system becomes more sensitive when the pain persists over time, so that the pain can be felt even after the origin of the symptoms is gone.

Referred pain can also come from the muscles. We have trigger points all over the body which are hyperirritable points in the muscles that can be very painful when activated. Among other things, we have trigger points in the neck muscles, which when activated feel like pain in the temple or jaw. If you have activated trigger points in the large chewing muscle (masseter), it can be perceived as toothache, jaw pain, or earache.

3.4 Orofacial Pain

Disease in both the teeth and oral tissues, as well as pain during dental treatment, can involve unbearable pain. Pain is a significant etiological factor in the development of dental anxiety. Therefore, we will shed light on some common pain conditions related to the oral cavity and explain how the pain can lead to an increased degree of dental treatment anxiety.

Orofacial pain can be difficult to manage for the patient and for the dentist. Pain from the oral cavity can be acute, intense, throbbing, and persistent or more diffuse. Where does the pain come from? How can the pain be managed? The patients' sensation of the pain quality, duration, and alterations are valuable information and well-known diagnostic clues, but it is often not possible to conclude on the basis of pain report alone. The patient does not always know the origin and cause of the pain. The teeth and oral cavity are often difficult to access for inspection by the patient. Lack of information about the injury and lack of knowledge about oral diseases can make it difficult to judge whether the pain signals a malign condition or whether the pain is something the patient must live with.

3.4.1 Pain from Teeth and Surrounding Tissues

The innervation of teeth and surrounding tissues is a large research field. In this text we will only present a heading of the profound knowledge which is available on the issue.

Pain associated with teeth has different qualities depending on the cause of the pain. There are mainly two different types of pain-conducting nerve types from teeth and other oral tissues, such as the tongue, mucous membranes, and jaw joint. The thin and myelinated Aδ fibres that give the first acute and sharp pain, while the unmyelinated C-fibres with lower conduction velocity give the more diffuse and dull pain [25]. Verbally the quality of the feeling from Aδ fibres is 'pricking' while 'dull' and 'pressing' correspond to the innervation of C-fibres [26].

The equivalent to dorsal horn for orofacial pain is the Trigeminal Ganglion (TG). In the TG the first-order neuron transmits their signal to second-order neurons, which transfer the pain signal to the sensory cortex. The pain may be modulated at all levels in the transmission prom the periphery to the brain. As described above, the person's thoughts about the pain or feelings and anxiety associated with the pain have an impact on the duration and intensity of the nerve impulse.

■ **Pain from Healthy Teeth or Small Tooth Damages**
Centrally in the teeth there is a cavity called the pulp chamber. In the pulp chamber, there are soft tissues as nerves, both different A-fibres and C-fibres, blood vessels, and lymph tissue. All together the soft tissue is called the pulp. Between the pulp chamber and the surface of the tooth, the tooth is formed by dentin near to the pulp, and the outermost layer is called the enamel. On a weight basis, dentin is less mineralized than enamel (96% in weight), but more than bone or cementum (about 65% in weight) [27]. The organic part of the dentin is mainly collagen-rich tissue that surrounds the tubules, or small ducts. The dentin develops in an interaction between odontoblasts and free nerve endings, and these are in the dentin tubules. Nerve ends in the dentin are mainly Aδ fibres. The nerves mainly respond to changes in temperature and mechanical pressure that cause movement in the fluid around the odontoblasts. The enamel, a highly mineralized tissue, protects the dentine and the free nerve fibres. If the enamel is incompletely mineralized for various reasons, has cracks or there are caries and the enamel is weak or damaged, pain will occur due to stimulation of nerves in the dentine (■ Fig. 3.3).

Pain associated with dentinal pain is often referred to in everyday speech as 'icing pain' and can be characterized as sudden intense and severe pain due to an external influence on the tooth. For patients with dental

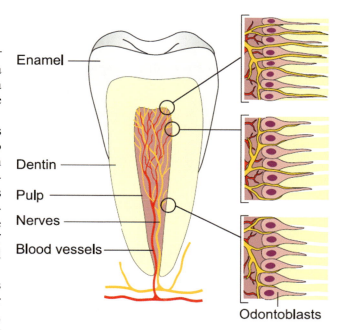

■ **Fig. 3.3** Figure showing innervation in the pulp and in the dentin in different parts of the tooth. (Figure from Nähri et al. [28] by permission)

anxiety and poor dental health, icing pain often makes it difficult to begin to perform good dental hygiene because major caries attacks will be painful when the toothbrush meets the dentine. At the same time, the tooth will be more sensitive to external changes in temperature and pressure when the bacterial coating is removed [28]. A person may experience comparable pain if you drill in a tooth with vital pulp tissue.

■ **Pain Associated with Caries**
It is common knowledge that bacteria cause infections in the teeth and gums if they are not removed regularly. The problem with bacterial infections in the teeth is that they are not immediately associated with pain. If pain was induced in early stages of caries, the person would be alerted, and the bacteria could be removed without considerable tissue damage. However, pain may be present without an obvious reason. When the patient is affected by pain in the face and jaw, without a clear explanation it may be a significant challenge for the patient – dentist relationship. Searching for underlying mechanisms can easily lead to scepticism and distrust towards the dentist. In order to meet the patient's problems interventions may be performed without clear indication. From our own practice, we have met patients who have had several teeth extracted, in search of the origin of the pain - but without getting better function or rid of the pain. Again, it is crucial not to perform irreversible interventions solely on pain indication, and at the same time to trusts the patient's description of the pain. In case of infection,

the blood supply to the tooth is changed to fight the infection. This creates increased pressure in the closed pulp chamber which is felt as pain upon innervation of C-fibres. Patients will feel this pain as more throbbing pain. The pain can also be triggered by external heat. At the same time, inflammatory signalling molecules secrete cytokines, growth factors and peptides [29]. These contribute to the increased sensitivity of the nerve fibres.

Pain Associated with Pulp Infection

When bacteria are in the pulp chamber, they move toward the root tip where there is a foramen. The bacteria spread to the tissue outside the tooth, there is however not much place for the bacteria to grow and multiply. In the narrow periodontal space where periodontal ligaments attach the tooth to the surrounding alveolar bone, the large pressure created by bacteria and inflammation elicits pressure and pain. The tooth will often feel like it is pushed up from its alveolar bone socket. All forms of pressure or force on the tooth which increase the pressure in the surrounding tissue will be very painful for the patient. Eventually, the infection may spread to the bone and adjacent tissues and form a swelling. Swelling is also normally very painful due to pressure in the tissue and the impact on surrounding tissues. An example is bacterial abscess around the crown of a not completely erupted wisdom tooth where swelling in the gingiva and surrounding tissues can make it difficult and painful to yawn and swallow.

Pain from Oral Mucosa

The soft tissues of the oral cavity can also be areas where pain occurs. Reasons for pain may be ulcerations such as aphthae, herpes outbreaks or chafing after dentures and sharp edges on teeth. Our experience is that patients with severe dental anxiety do not seek treatment due to pain associated with oral soft tissue.

Persistent Pain in Teeth

Inflammation and tissue destruction in teeth and surrounding tissues can lead to a sensitization of the pain. Locally, this may be a result of changes in the nerves. Inflammation in the tooth may induce sprouting of free nerve endings so that the tissue becomes more innervated [28]. Nerve endings may be excited or inhibited by local factors in the tissue or anatomic changes within the nerves or on the nerves cell membrane. Changes may also occur in the CNS with increase excitability or by inhibitory factors. And it is known that persistent inflammatory conditions in peripheral tissues can lead to permanent changes in the central nervous system and chronic hypersensitivity. After dental infections and inflammation, there are changes in the interaction between the neurons and glial cells in the Trigeminus

Ganglion resulting in increased nociceptive transmission. The interaction between nerve cells and glia cells after inflammation in orofacial tissues may result in persistent pain [30].

Case Study

The patient is a 31-year-old man. He says that for a long time he has had pain in one of the posterior molars in the lower jaw. The pain started approx. 2 years ago. He went to the dentist, but when the tooth had to be fixed, it was not anesthetized enough. Since he really wanted to have his tooth fixed, he tried to 'pull himself together' to get the treatment done. The pain during the treatment became so intense that he was unable to complete the treatment. The dentist said that he had received adequate anaesthesia and that he did not know how to help the patient.

The patient was then referred to a dentist with nitrous oxide. Unluckily the treatment was painful also this time. The patient experienced that he was not taken seriously when he expressed that the tooth was painful, but the nitrous oxide sedation made it difficult for him to stop the dentist and a permanent filling was placed.

Still, 2 years after treatment, his tooth is aching. According to dentists who have examined the tooth, it 'looks nice'. He is in pain when he eats, and he can only chew on the opposite side. He is now afraid that he will not dare to have dental treatment due to pain, even though the toothache still bothers him significantly in everyday life.

Treatment:

It is of outmost importance that the patient feels that he is met with respect and understanding. His pain should not be questioned as exaggerated nor mental. However, if there are no diagnostic signs which indicate need for treatment, the tooth should not be treated solely based on the patient's pain. Thorough information should be given about how peripheral and central sensitization may have occurred so that the tooth is painful without a diagnosis is valuable to alter the patient's cognitions regarding the pain. The sensitization may be in the tooth and surrounding tissues, in the Trigeminus Ganglion or in central parts of the brain.

If the tooth at any point is treated, pain-free treatment is crucial. Based on knowledge about peripheral nerves and reduced affinity for anaesthetics in case of inflammation, the patient should be given two to three times the dose that is normally given. Then there must be enough time for the anaesthetics to get in contact with the nerves. In addition, anaesthetic should be given in the PDL directly prior to the treatment. At any signs of pain, treatment must be stopped and additional anaesthetics must be supplied.

3.4.2 Pain from Other Locations

There are several pain conditions from other structures than the teeth. The International Classification of Headache Disorders third edition (ICHD-3) [31] describes 'Painful lesions of the cranial nerves and other facial pain' where most of the conditions are due to lesion or disease of nerves, that is, neuropathic pain. Some conditions are difficult to explain or linked to other structures or mechanisms. Atypical facial pain and burning mouth syndrome are the two most prevalent of these. Temporomandibular disorders (TMD), which originate from muscles or joints in the facial area, can present itself as orofacial pain.

- ■ **Pain Related to the Temporomandibular Joint and Mastication Muscles, or TMD**

Pain associated with the jaw joint/masticatory muscles and surrounding structures is defined as Temporomandibular Dysfunction (TMD). There are several tissues involved in TMD and pain associated with the condition can have different etiological factors and be experienced differently from person to person. The most common diagnoses associated with TMD are muscle pain (myalgia) and joint pain (arthralgia). In addition, the patient may experience headaches without this being linked to a special diagnostic code. Pain associated with the jawbone, jaw joint, and muscles may have a multifactorial ethology. There may be physical causes, such as injuries and inflammatory conditions, related to trauma and parafunctions. For many patients with TMD, the ethology is unknown with no obvious signs of injury or inflammation. As there is a predominance of women with TMD, it has been seen that oestrogen is important for the development of pain [32]. In addition, it is known that the pain may have a psychosocial origin. Today it is known that the chronic inflammatory condition and tissue damage in the masticatory muscles leads to local changes in the tissue so that a sensitization to pain occurs.

- ■ **Persistent Idiopathic Facial Pain**

Persistent idiopathic facial pain (PIFP), or atypical facial pain, is: 'persistent facial and/or oral pain, with varying presentations but recurring daily for more than 2 hours per day over more than 3 months, in the absence of clinical neurological deficit' [31]. PIFP may co-occur with chronic widespread pain or other pain conditions. According to ICHD-3 it may originate from a minor operation or injury. The pain typically starts on one side of the face and can spread to other parts of the jaw and face.

- ■ **Burning Mouth Syndrome**

Burning mouth syndrome (BMS) is well known among specialists, but uncommon in dental practice. The condition is described as an intraoral burning pain, without a causal explanation. The condition is most prevalent among women and higher age. Some studies show comorbid psychological problems [31]. As with most pain conditions, it is unclear whether psychological problems appear as a consequence of the pain or contribute to the appearance of the pain.

It is a significant challenge for many to be affected by pain in the face and jaw, without a clear explanation. Searching for underlying mechanisms can easily lead to the person experiencing scepticism and distrust, and that interventions are performed without clear indication. From our own practice, we have met patients who have had several teeth extracted, in search of the origin of the pain - but without getting better function or rid of the pain. Again, it is crucial not to perform irreversible interventions solely on pain indication, and at the same time to trusts the patient's description of the pain.

3.4.3 Dental Treatment and Pain

Dental treatment is intended to remove pathology. This can involve anything from drilling a tooth and filling or cleaning the teeth of calculus. Many people find dental treatment painful. Previously experienced pain together with subsequent fear and anxiety for new experiences of pain increases the risk of pain during later similar experiences [25]. Therefore, it is important to provide pain relief before dental treatment.

The most common method to prevent or relieve pain during dental treatment is local anaesthesia. Local anaesthesia is injected into the tissue where it binds to the nerve threads and the electric nerve impulses are stopped. Due to a large number of factors locally in the tissue, there is great variation in the amount of anaesthesia needed to achieve painless treatment. In cases where adequate anaesthesia is not achieved, care should be taken to continue treatment. Many patients with high dental anxiety have not had enough anaesthesia. Pain and the sense of lack of control during dental treatment is a high-risk factor for developing high dental anxiety [33]. Therefore, it is reasonable to believe that many patients who develop dental anxiety may have anatomical and/or physiological conditions that make them more difficult to anesthetize. With negative experiences of pain during dental treatment, patients develop a lack of confidence in the effect of the anaesthetic, high dental anxiety, as well as feelings of not having control in the dental situation. Together with poor dental health with painful infectious conditions and inflammation these conditions may result in central sensitization that reduces the chance of achieving painless dental treatment. It is therefore very important that dental health professionals meet the patient's need for pain relief. Sometimes it can be very time consuming to achieve and even difficult to obtain a good and pain-free dental situation and may also require good planning. Dental professionals must have 'in the spine' that pain-free treatment is an absolute necessity to help the patient out of the vicious circle of dental anxiety.

3.5 Psychosocial Factors

Psychosocial factors affect pain experience, and psychosocial factors are of great importance for the development of pain. There is a general over-representation of depression, catastrophizing or worst-case scenario thinking and abuse or neglect in childhood in people with persistent pain. This does not mean that it is these factors that induce or cause the pain, but they contribute to the development of the problems which in turn increase pain. We will provide an overview of some psychosocial factors which may be important to assess in order to gain an understanding of the patient's total burden of disease - especially in contexts where the pain has lasted over time.

3.5.1 Anamnestic Issues

As human beings, we are shaped by what happens around us and how we interact with the environment. How we develop as individuals affects how we cope with or face problems and challenges. Negative influences in early childhood can have significant consequences for later adjustment and problems. A large study in California conducted from 1995 to 1997 showed that the number of adverse events exposed to the first years of life correlated highly with health problems (both mental and somatic) later in life [34].

There is generally a higher incidence of sexual abuse in people with persistent pain than in the general population. Overall, one can get the impression that sexual abuse predisposes to later somatic or mental disorders, but it is not possible to predict which disorders or problems the person will experience [35]. Many explanatory models may be suggested, but the dynamics of the development of disease probably differ from person to person. A history of abuse can be stored as a trauma, or it may have given the victim an experience that "no matter what I do, I cannot influence what happens to me". The traumatic experience may lead to insecurity and reduced trust in others leading to continuous muscular activa-

tion to protect oneself from new abuse, shame can contribute to a poor self-image and lack of faith in one's own ability to cope with adversity, etc. In dentistry we know that sexual abuse can give rise to odontophobia, bothersome associations when someone operates in their oral cavity, and major reactions associated with having to sit passively in a dental chair. Naturally, pain in an area that has been traumatized also can give associations to the traumatic experience. Pain in the jaw or in a tooth may trigger nausea, fear and pain in persons who have experienced abuse in the mouth or face earlier in life.

3.5.2 Social Context

Some people have had a childhood and upbringing where it was important to have control. If the father is emotionally unstable, and may become quarrelsome, unreasonable, or angry seemingly without warning, it is important for the child to be watchful, looking for signs of anger. If the mother has a depressive disorder, and the child experiences that it is important to protect her so that her condition will not get worse, we can understand that the child develops his own ability to be attentive to incidents that could reinforce her mother's difficulties. If one of the parents is violent and the child wants to protect a little brother, the child will probably develop an alertness and try to be on guard continuously. Attempts to be in control, and constantly on guard, lead to increased stress levels, with a continuous stress-like condition. Prolonged, continuous readiness can contribute to increased muscular tension (which can be pain-provoking in itself) and generally contribute to increased incidence of long-term pain [36].

Social support is always important when a person is in pain. When people close to the person who suffers show support, understanding, and validates the person's experience, it is obvious that it contributes to feeling of safety and relaxation. During dental treatment, it is important that dental health professionals support the patient when the patient feels pain. The choice of words is important in this sense. Dental health professionals may in some cases define the acute pain experience with words that are intended to change the patient's experience of pain. Apparently supportive expressions such as 'It's probably just icing' or 'Yes, it can be uncomfortable' may give the patient the impression that it is not accepted to express feelings of pain during the dental treatment. Lack of social support during painful treatment may increase post-treatment rumination and fear of future pain.

3.5.3 Interaction with Family

The way you interact with other people and how they relate to the person's pain, affect pain. Bill Fordyce was one of the pioneers in modern pain management. He stated that 'people are complicated' and tried to use behavioural psychology to understand and influence pain. A basic principle in behavioural psychology is that the behaviour that receives attention will be reinforced. Fordyce showed how attention to pain behaviour resulted in more pain, while ignoring pain behaviour and increased attention to coping behaviours resulted in less pain. His book came in a new edition in 2015, with comments from invited key researchers and clinicians in the field of pain [37].

Many studies have been done on social interaction and pain behaviour. For example, Herta Flor [38] showed that patients with persistent pain, and who had solicitous spouses who gave them a lot of attention, tolerated far less pain when the spouse was present. If the spouse ignored pain behaviours, and instead paid attention to coping behaviours (focus on activity, use of relaxation and distraction, etc.), they tolerated more pain.

Social interaction and pain is a complicated area. In the clinic, the approach should be to give attention to coping behaviours, while you to a greater extent overlook pain behaviour. At the same time, it is important to show that you take care of the patient, provide support and understanding for the patient who is experiencing pain.

3.5.4 Pain and Cognitions

The way one perceives and relates to pain also affects the pain. One obvious example is attention. What we focus on or give increased attention to is reinforced. These are automatic processes that probably have to do with both cognitive or mental, and neurological conditions. If you have a small baby, you are extra aware of babies crying. Parents of young children hear children crying more easily than others - and they are also quick to identify whether it is their own children or not. The same also applies to pain: if you are aware of pain in your body, the processing of pain signals is intensified, and the pain feels more intense [39].

During procedural pain, pain is a natural result of the treatment that is given. Many patients are fearful and have negative thoughts about procedural pain. A calm patient who feels a little pain and who knows that it is transitory without creating other bodily discomfort may have thoughts such as 'The sting is only a little painful and only lasts for seconds. I need the anaesthetic.

It's important for me'. A person who has high anxiety in connection with the pain of the sting may have negative thoughts related to the pain that increases the perceived intensity of the pain. This person may have thoughts like 'The pain is so intense that I cannot cope. The syringe tip can hit something and damage the nerves and blood vessels and I will be injured'. Treatment should focus on both the pain associated with the actual procedure and the bodily reactions the patient feels in the situation. A question like 'Have you ever thought about how lucky you are having a skin that makes you aware if something penetrates?' may be an introduction to alter the patient's thoughts concerning the pain of the needle penetrating the skin. Another question addressing the startle reflex may be 'The whole body wants you to be alerted that something crossed the barrier of your skin. It is probably not a good feeling for you, but it is safe, and it will not affect how the infiltration is done'. Also, information about where and how the injection will be set, how the infiltration will be done, and why something will hurt can change the cognitions. Altered thoughts can reduce anxiety, which in turn reduces excitation of the afferent pain signal in the CNS and thereby reduces the pain sensation.

▪ Appraisals and Beliefs

The appraisals and beliefs one have towards the pain plays an essential role to how the pain is experienced. Assumptions about pain affect the interpretation of what we experience. If the pain is perceived as dangerous, it is experienced as more intense and unpleasant. One patient described the pain he knew was due to osteosarcoma or bone cancer as intolerable. He was born with clubfoot and had to undergo many operations. Because of this, he never got relief from pain in his foot. The pain in the foot had always been intense, but it did not bother him so much. He understood the reason for the pain, and it had become a natural part of him. The new pain, however, was a consequence of cancer. Although it had comparable quality and intensity, it became unbearable.

A pain that arouses fear will probably be experienced as more intense than a pain with a reasonable explanation without a serious outcome [40]. What beliefs we have of the pain also affect how we relate to it. If a patient fears that something is wrong with the jaw joint, and that it must be handled with care, it is likely that she will develop significant muscular tensions in the jaw, tongue, and neck muscles, which in turn will cause more pain.

▪ Catastrophizing

The term catastrophizing was introduced by Albert Ellis [41] and then adapted by Aaron Beck [42]. It describes a maladaptive cognitive style used by patients with anxiety and depressive disorders. Pain catastrophizing is characterized by a tendency to exaggerate what threat a pain represents. As a consequence, the person may feel helpless in connection with pain, and not be able to inhibit pain-related thoughts in anticipation of, during, or after a painful encounter. It is known as the most consistent psychosocial factor for predicting adjustment to persistent pain [43]. Catastrophizing has been shown to contribute to the development and maintenance of persistent pain and has better prediction for TMD than other variables [44].

■ **Fear Avoidance**

Vlaeyen et al. describe a model in which they showed that fear of pain can cause increased pain. The model is called a fear avoidance model [45]. They based the model on musculoskeletal pain and used it specifically for low back pain. The model can be used for all types of pain and describes how pain of different origins should be confronted. When the pain does not signal imminent injury or danger, it is generally best to confront the pain by for example stretching or lifting using the back in a way that the person fears could hurt. The principle is exposure, the same way we treat phobias. If the pain causes fear, they assume that the pain triggers worst-case scenario thinking, avoidance, increased pain-related fear, passivity, and depression. These conditions contribute to an increased experience of pain both in duration and intensity, triggers fear of pain, and lead to avoidance of situations they fear can affect the pain (◘ Fig. 3.4).

These are the same mechanisms we see in phobias, which is the reason why this is also called kinesophobia – or fear of movement. As with all phobias, the most effective treatment is systematic and gradual exposure together with cognitive restructuring of the patient's catastrophic thoughts or beliefs.

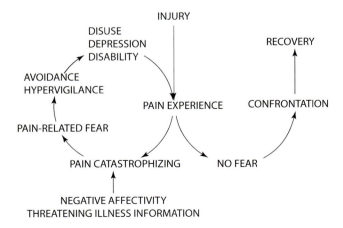

◘ **Fig. 3.4**   The fear avoidance model [45, p 329]

3.5.5 Emotional Factors, Psychological Problems, and Comorbidity

There is a high prevalence of psychological problems like catastrophizing, anxiety, depression, and PTSD among people with persistent pain. The numbers vary between studies, partly because of how they define persistent pain, depression or anxiety, and partly because of different sampling methods.

According to a national survey in the United States, 35.1% of the respondents reported anxiety and 20.2% reported depression among people with persistent pain, contrasted with 18.1% and 9.3% reported anxiety and depression, respectively, in the general population [46]. In a Canadian survey, they reported 19.8% depression among persistent pain sufferers, contrasted with 5.9% in the general population [47]. Most studies report a pooled odds ratio between 2 and 3 for anxiety and depression among pain sufferers, which indicate that emotional problems are at least twice as prevalent among people in pain, and probably even more prevalent among people with more serious pain problems.

It is also well known that people with depression have an extensively higher risk for pain, than the normal population. In a European survey, it was reported that 43.4% of persons with major depressive disorders suffered from persistent pain [48].

Anxiety and depression, together with pain, affects function and quality of life. According to Yu and McCracken [49], people with combined depression and pain have more days absent from work, higher degree of unemployment and lower quality of life, than people with one or none of the conditions.

There are different theories and explanations of the associations between anxiety, depression, and pain. Does depression predispose for development of persistent pain, or is depression a consequence of pain? The interaction is complicated, and probably varies from situation to situation. There is probably a mutual connection. Pain affects function, vitality, ability to participate in working life and social contexts, etc. Reduced participation and function probably affect the person's mood. To lose the opportunity for an ordinary life can result in grief, despair, and reduced self-esteem. All of these are factors that, of course, are reflected in fluctuations of mood and can result in increased depression scores.

From a clinical perspective, it is important to be aware of the associations. When dealing with persons with depression, one should ask for pain. When treating persistent pain, one should consider if the person suffers from depression. The knowledge that pain, together with emotional problems, is associated with lower quality of life and general function indicates that this is something we as clinicians should relate to.

Turk [50] describes anxiety sensitivity (AS) as a possible predisposing factor for persistent pain. AS is defined as the fear of anxiety-related sensations. Individuals with high AS tend to interpret unpleasant physical sensations, like feeling faint, increased heart rate, rapid breathing, as a sign of danger. We have described pain as a warning signal earlier in this chapter. The response to a warning is normally heightened alertness that might resemble an anxiety response. The combination of persistent pain and high AS probably contributes to increased muscular tension and more intensive pain, as described earlier [36].

Dentists and dental hygienists are trained to help patients achieve good dental health. Prophylactic treatment is the gold standard for preventing tooth decay and pain. Nevertheless, when illness is present there is often a considerable focus on helping the patient and eliciting pain and decay. Therefore, when a patient comes to the clinic and expresses despair over toothache, there is a potential dilemma where the dentist wants to relieve the pain with treatment. The urge to help the patient may in some cases cause initiation of dental treatment without carefully considering the indication for the treatment. In such situations, it is important to remain calm despite the patient's pain. A diagnosis of the dental or oral condition is a prerequisite before treatment is planned and performed. The dental professional must always have in mind that the pain experience alone is not a diagnostic criterion for operative treatment. Because the wish to help is very strong among healthcare professionals, it is important to have strategies for how to deal with the patients' pain when there are no diagnostic findings that provide a basis for dental treatment.

3.6 Treatment and Relief of Pain

Pain has a vital function as it signals tissue damage. If we did not become aware of the tissue damage, we would not respond adequately to avoid future damage. The skin is a wonderful organ that distinguishes man from the outside world. A painful stimulus from the skin notifies that the barrier is threatened. In view of an evolutionary perspective, the skin can ultimately become a gateway for bacteria and thus inflict an infection on the individual. However, most people endure the pain of minor injuries, such as cutting themselves on paper or a cat claw. Therefore, it may seem illogical to become phobic of dental and medical injections. The sting is not, viewed from the outside, a real threat or danger. The physiological, emotional, cognitive and behavioural anxiety reaction associated with the phobic stimulus

(sting) is therefore irrational and exaggerated. The anxiety reaction is intended to prevent the patient from entering the situation that triggers the pain. At the same time, anxiety creates negative thoughts about the situation and bodily activation that raises attention to the painful stimuli. Physiologically, activating of the amygdala will intensify the pain signal in the brainstem towards the sensory cerebral cortex. At the same time, the amygdala will reduce the patient's ability to think rationally about the pain. Statements like 'This is going to be okay!' or 'It's just a little sting!' won't matter when the amygdala and anxiety maintain negative thoughts like 'This is getting too bad, I can't do it!' At the same time, attention to the pain (reviewed more later in the chapter) will increase as long as the pain is considered a threat to health. Furthermore, people with high anxiety about pain during dental treatment tend to exaggerate previously experienced pain [51]. The memory of pain helps to avoid new pain, which is functional from an evolutionary perspective. However, therapists must be aware that dental treatment combined with a high anxiety response frequently leads to feelings of loss of control and thoughts that the pain can be harmful. In these situations, the pain stimulus is reported to be stronger than the peripheral physiological stimulation implies. Therefore, we should be careful to anticipate how the pain will be experienced for the patient. It is recommended to focus on reducing the anxiety before pain is inflicted and hopefully to achieve an experience that the pain is weaker and/or more tolerable than what the patient thought initially. Otherwise, some individuals may fall into a painful circle where they are sensitized to pain. That is, increasingly weaker stimuli can cause increased pain sensations. Accordingly, the sensitization process can cause some people to find that the syringe sting becomes more painful every time they try.

The pain experience is the result of an interaction between feelings and thoughts, bodily reactions, and social relationships [52]. To have an opportunity to influence the anxious patient's experience of pain, we need information about the patient's thoughts about the syringe, how the patient experiences the pain of the sting, how is the feeling when the anaesthetic is injected, and what are the patient's thoughts about being sedated.

3.7 Psychological Strategies for Relieving Pain

Pain is an experience – experienced as physical discomfort and associated with actual or potential tissue damage. The experience can be influenced by attention, expectations, what perception one has about the pain, experience of control, degree of anxiety and worst-case thinking. There are also many ways to influence pain – regardless of their origin.

The strategies we propose in this chapter are all based on good communication. Mastering basic rules of good communication is essential for all actions intended to reduce pain and anxiety.

3.7.1 Expectations

Expectations affect pain. We know this after many decades of studying placebo. Placebo involves a change in symptoms or a condition after the person has received an initially non-effective treatment. When testing analgesics, it is always seen that some people who are given a non-active medicine report a decrease in pain. How many of the population would experience such an effect, and the magnitude of the analgesic effect varies. Häuser [53] showed in a meta-analysis that 18.6% of subjects reported a 50% or greater reduction in pain after receiving a non-effective medicine.

Expectations are probably the most important factor in placebo. When you get a medicine that may have an effect, many people expect it to work. This expectation has several consequences, among which it can affect the excretion of various biochemical substances - such as endogenous opioids, endocannabinoids, and cholecystokinin, all of which can have a pain-relieving effect [54]. Endogenous opioids and cannabinoids are the body's own analgesic mechanisms. While the endogenous opioids (endorphins), act in the same way as morphine or other opioids, the effect of the endocannabinoids is more uncertain. Conversely, cholecystokinin decreases the effect of opioids. The interesting thing is that expectations seem to influence the secretion of these substances in such a way that expectations of pain relief contribute to pain relief, while fear of pain can cause greater pain problems.

In clinical practice, this means that if one can stimulate a person's expectations that the pain will be relieved, there are chances that it will also affect the excretion of biochemical substances that can relieve pain. In dental practice, we have many opportunities to increase the placebo effect to relief pain. Application of surface anaesthesia before an anaesthetic injection could be a golden possibility. When the patient feels that the mucous membrane is sedated, we can respond with 'So nice that the anaesthetic cream works for you! Then you're more likely to feel less about the sting, even if I can't promise you won't feel anything'. During dental treatment, information about the effect one wants to achieve may contribute to reduced pain. For instance, in fluoride brushing, one can tell the patient about how fluoride binds to phosphate in the saliva and again covers all pits and free nerve endings in the tooth and that this is how we will reduce ice pain.

The opposite of placebo is nocebo. Nocebo implies an undesirable effect of a treatment that basically has no effect. One example of this is in a meta-study on medications for headaches. It emerged that 10% of those given a non-effective drug developed such strong side effects that they had to withdraw from the study [55]. In clinical practice, this means that we must be careful about how we tell the patient about the possible unfortunate consequences of a treatment. Even the slightest obscurity can have major negative consequences in some. A statement such as 'this does not look good' may cause some people to react by developing ailments. To give the patient a detailed list of possible side effects of an anaesthetic may contribute to a person developing some of these side effects. An example from dental practice was a patient who had begun root canal treatment. Between the treatment consultation, the dentist puts a drug in the tooth to kill the bacteria (calcium hydroxide). The dentist told the patient that he put poison in his tooth without giving more detail about what he meant by this. The patient subsequently experienced extreme pain in his tooth and high anxiety about 'having poison in his body', which resulted in avoidance of dental treatment for 13 years.

Summarized, through good communication, one can facilitate positive expectations and also pain relief. Through unfortunate communication, one may increase doubt or uncertainty, and produce genuine side effects.

3.7.2 Control vs. Catastrophizing

Catastrophizing is well studied as an important cognitive factor in relation to pain. Several studies find that catastrophizing is a good predictor related to the development of jaw pain [56], the degree of pain after knee operations [57], the likelihood that one will develop low back pain [58], and the likelihood of the development of prolonged pain after surgery [59].

The relationship between catastrophizing and pain is probably complex. However, catastrophizing has common features with anxiety and implies a likelihood of increased attention directed to pain. Furthermore, avoidance behaviours may also contribute to the development of pain [60]. It probably contributes to a lack of experience of control and contributes to less security.

Catastrophizing implies a loss of control. In the clinic, it is important to give the patient a sense of control. The strategy may vary according to what kind of catastrophizer the patient is, but in most cases, the following should be considered:

Principles from congnitve behavioural therapy should be used. This implies 'an intervention with systematic, structured, and didactic knowledge transfer for an illness and its treatment, integrating emotional and motivational aspects to enable patients to copePainpsychological strategiescontrol vs. catastrophizingPsychological strategiescontrol vs. catastrophizing with the illness and to improve its treatment adherence and efficacy' [61]. Inform the patient of what is going to happen and why. Be sure that the patient understands what you are telling them.

Give the patient a tool to pause the interventions. A Norwegian psychologist has developed a procedure for children, where they are equipped with a stop sign. The deal is that when the child tells the health care worker to stop, they are obliged to do so, whatever procedure they carry out. Their experience is that the children are more secure, feel comfortable, and the procedures are easier to complete [62].

Ask the patient for earlier experiences. What worked in similar situations, may also work this time.

3.7.3 Relaxation

Pain causes many of the same responses that we see in anxiety. A natural reaction to pain is to be prepared for fight, flight, or freeze with tightening musculature, and also be ready for action. This response pattern may also occur when you fear that you will experience pain. We have some, but modest evidence [63, 64] that relaxation can be a helpful strategy, both against pain and anxiety. In clinical practice, relaxation is widely used.

One relaxation technique is not suitable for everyone, and what can be effective for one doesn't have to work for another. Hence, it is important to master a larger arsenal of strategies. The simplest strategy is to focus on breathing, while perhaps the most advanced is the use of hypnosis.

■ Breath

Calm, deep breathing contributes to relaxation for most people. It's hard to breathe deeply and calmly when you're anxious. The easiest thing is to ask the person to take a deep breath and breathe out calmly, preferably with their lips slightly facing each other. Alternatively, one can teach the person to 'breathe in square': Imagine a square. Start in one corner, such as the upper-left corner. Take a deep breath by raising your shoulders, chest forward and out with your stomach while following the line from left to right corner. Hold your breath while following the line from the top right to the lower right corner. Breathe out calmly – stomach, chest, shoulders – while following the bottom line from right to left. Hold

your breath while following the line from the bottom to the upper-left corner. And then you start breathing again. If you need visual support, there's almost always an accessible square — a window, a door, a house, or an imaginary square in the palm of your hand.

■ Imagery

Imagine a safe and quiet place, whether something you have experienced and have positive memories associated with, or a place you dream of coming to. The memory or image may be characterized by rest and stillness or movements if it fits better. Enter memory or image – use four different channels. (i) Visually – how it looks. Nature, people, sky, the chequered curtains in Grandma's kitchen. (ii) Auditory – what you hear. Grandma's voice, clattering glass from the sidewalk restaurant, the seagulls, the salt from the sea. (iii) Smell – how does it smell. Salty sea, moss, dark earth, grandmother's freshly baked bread. (iv) Tactile – contact with the surface. The rock you sit on, lying in the sand, walking across moss, flying off on skis.

One can also apply the principles of the imagery in a good conversation by asking the person about a good holiday memory or about a description of a place they like to be. Ask what it looks like, about sounds, smells and where they like to sit, lie down, or walk when they are there. For most people, it will help the other become calmer, lowering their shoulders and make them breathe more deeply and regularly – signs that they are entering a calm, tense state.

■ Body Scan

Body scans are used in various relaxation strategies, possibly in combination with progressive muscle relaxation or deep breathing. After breathing in square/breathing deeply, or otherwise achieving some relaxation, one must focus on body part by body part. Imagine loosening the tension in your musculature. Similarly, in the case of procedural pain, it can be helpful to explore with the patient what bodily reactions the patient experiences when pain occurs. Some patients experience the sudden pain, for example, of a sting or when the dentist is blowing air on their teeth as an extreme bodily activation.

Some patients experience the bodily alertness as so uncomfortable that they will do everything to avoid this bodily sensation, and consequently stay away from the pain experience. However, if the patient can express these bodily reactions, one can help the patient accept that the bodily reactions are only a signal to let the person decide whether the situation is safe or not.

■ Mindfulness

Those who teach mindfulness will, as a rule, not denounce it as relaxation. Nevertheless, we would argue that mindfulness frequently has a significant element of relaxation in it. The central thing about mindfulness is to be present in what is happening here and now, without thinking about the future or the past. These are strategies that have taken inspiration from Buddhist meditation and are used alone or in combination with other approaches. It is common to combine mindfulness with ACT (Acceptance and Commitment Therapy) and separate strategies have been developed against stress-based mindfulness, such as Mindfulness-Based Stress Reduction (MBSR) [65].

■ **Hypnosis**

Hypnosis is a more demanding form of concentration, relaxation, and influence of senses, thoughts, feelings, and actions. Hypnosis requires a more active therapist who has experience in using this type of approach. Hypnosis means that one person guides another into a state where one is focused, concentrated, and experiences good control.

Hypnosis is used in surgical procedures, in psychotherapy and in invasive medical procedures [66], and is shown to have good effect in various pain conditions [67]. Not everyone can be hypnotized. There are several tests to measure hypnotisability or susceptibility or to which extent the person is able to be hypnotized, of which the Stanford Hypnotic Susceptibility Scale [68] is probably the most widely used.

There are various phenomena that are active during trance. Some describe that the pain obtains other qualities – which are not necessarily painful, or that the pain disappears. Others may describe a more distanced relationship with the pain, as if entering a dissociative state. This type of strategy can be used systematically – as we see in some studies – or as an adaptation between the patient and the person who hypnotizes. The approaches typically include elements from both performance images and breathing techniques.

3.7.4 Distraction

Distraction has had a central place in pain management based on a cognitive approach. By shifting attention from pain, and over to more light-hearted or rewarding stimuli, it is believed that the pain decreases. Stimuli can be external (look at a landscape, listening to music, listen to a dentist's claims while drilling) or inner (imagine safe or relaxing places, being preoccupied with a mental task). There is clearer evidence for better effect on children and adolescents compared to adults [69].

It is very important that the dental health personnel are conscious of the importance of giving the patients a feeling of control. Patients who lack confidence in the dental staff and are anxious both for what the pain may lead to and the bodily activation of feeling pain, it will be more difficult to divert their attention. If distraction is used and the patient experiences that the pain suddenly occurs, the anxiety in the situation may increase and result in less confidence to the therapist. On a later occasion, such an experience may contribute to the deterioration of the pain experience with future exposures of the same character. Thus, it is very important to meet the patient's need for information and control before introducing distraction techniques.

Based on clinical experiences and knowledge of the nervous system, we have good explanations for why distraction works. We know that what we focus on is given priority. If you're looking for red hats in a crowd, you ignore other colours. A mother with infants is more attentive and notices a crying infant more quickly than others.

Likewise, we must assume that if you focus on pain, then the processing of pain signals in the central nervous system is amplified. Therefore, we can assume that distraction — drawing attention to conditions other than pain — has both a cognitive and neurological explanation.

What is most effective, comfort or distraction? A group of children underwent procedures that caused abdominal pain. The parents were either asked to distract the children or to comfort them. The children who were distracted found this to be better than children who were comforted. For the parents, the assessment was the opposite: they felt that they were the best support for the children when comforting them and that distraction was not good for the children [70].

This is interesting – the approach parents think is best for their children is the approach their children experience as the least supportive and vice versa. Distraction has a reassuring and pain-relieving effect, while comfort and attention can contribute to increased torment.

Similar results are reported in relation to adults.

3.8 Case Study

Woman, 43 years old

The patient is a 43-year-old woman. She is a trained nurse and has 2 children, but she is now out of work due to both physical and mental health conditions. Approximately 10 years ago she was diagnosed with depression. Periodically, she is admitted to the district psychiatric centre. She experiences that her mental illness is due to traumatic experiences with, among other things, sexual abuse in childhood.

She receives medication for depression, pain, anxiety, medication to relieve stomach ulcers, allergies, and hypothyroidism.

After a diagnostic interview with psychologist, she is diagnosed with odontophobia. She has problems brushing her teeth, and she brushes her teeth a couple of times every month. Her dental health is poor, and she has pain related to teeth and gums. Shameful for the condition she is in, she anticipates that dental professionals will belittle her. Being health educated she feels even more shame not addressing her own health issues better.

Her anxiety symptoms during dental treatment (scale 0–10):

Heartbeat: 10
Tremors: 10
Pressure over the chest/chest pain: 8
Dizziness: 10
Numbness: 10
Difficulty breathing: 8
Stomach pain/nausea: 8–10
Afraid of doing something uncontrolled (screaming/hitting): 6
Afraid to die: YES

The patient's dental anxiety is mainly related to her poor experience with anaesthesia. She has repeatedly experienced that she is not adequately anesthetized, and she has therefore undergone painful dental treatment. Dentists have repeatedly said that she has had more than enough anaesthesia and that they cannot give her additional doses.

Five years ago, two molars in the lower jaw were extracted. One tooth was extracted during nitrous oxide sedation and the other tooth was extracted under anaesthesia. On both occasions, the patient was in great pain after the procedure. The pain persisted long after healing. During this period, she was given several prescriptions for paracetamol/codeine medication which had only very limited effect. Today she has pain in large parts of her mouth, also in teeth with small damage without pulp involvement.

In addition to oral pain and poor dental health, she reports pain in the abdomen and pain related to fibromyalgia. The cause of the abdominal pain has not been diagnosed, and she is constantly very worried that the pain will increase.

Summary of the patient's health issues: The patient is very exhausted due to constant pain, both general and oral. She has lost confidence that she can be pain free. Her experience is that she needs significant number of painkillers for it to work. The last time she was hospitalized, her intense abdominal pain could not be treated, and she experienced the situation as completely unbearable. During a conversation with a psychologist

before treatment, she does not believe that the dentist will be able to help her with the oral-related pain problem.

3.8.1 Overall Treatment Goals

(a) Provide knowledge about pain that may occur in the oral cavity.
(b) Ensure that the patient experiences adequate pain relief both during and after dental treatment.
(c) Ensure that the patient experiences trust in her abilities to undergo dental treatment and has lasting confidence that she can have sufficient anaesthetic for pain relief during dental treatment.

Treatment Approach
(a) Establish a good relationship using basic communication techniques that increase her confidence and trust in the therapist and the treatment and motivate her to gradually try dental treatment.
(b) Psychoeducation – Thorough and customized explanations of the connections between anxiety, pain, and control.
(c) Increase the patient's understanding of the connection between being sexually abused and increased sensitivity to pain in the mouth.
(d) Always ensure the feeling of control in the situation.
(e) Give her dignity, by highlighting what she is able to do.
(f) Relaxation, with calm conversation and increased self-confidence.

I In the first dental consultation all the patient's anxiety symptoms are reviewed and thorough psychoeducation is given to normalize the anxiety reactions in order to increase the patient's understanding of what happens in the body. Then the patient's pain problems are discussed in a non-judgemental manner. Giving knowledge about pain is intended to give her hope for the opportunity to deal with pain during dental treatment and provide an increased understanding of her daily toothache. The importance of anxiety, cognitions, and knowledge are underlined as central in the pain modulation in the CNS.

She was reassured and encouraged to report any painful stimuli so that the dentist can give more anaesthesia. In addition, emphasis was put on securing her that she would never be pushed or forced to undergo painful dental treatment.

This was formulated as follows: 'I do not know your pain, therefore you must tell me when you feel any pain!' The patient was informed that previous doses of anaesthesia were not close to the maximum dose she can have. She was positively met on her wish to have more than the 'usual dose'. Reassuring her that her pain experience would never be questioned and that she would be offered more anaesthesia if she needed helped to reduce the anxiety about pain and the fear of not getting enough anaesthesia. Reduced anxiety and a feeling of being able to influence her own situation were important. By building a positive expectation of help and pain relief, previously negative expectation about the anaesthetic effect were altered.

Furthermore, it was emphasized that the pain she felt was real and would never be suspected to be thought or psychologic, or in other words, stigmatized as imaginary, both for the relationship and for the patient's self-esteem.

As the patient had a lot of pain in the teeth, it was important that the patient gained more knowledge about anatomical structures of teeth and reasons for pain related to teeth. She needed information described in the chapter on pain in the teeth related to vitality and pain that characterizes infection. Her experiences related to extractions turned out to cause pain from teeth with small injuries and made her very anxious that the teeth had to be extracted. The information about pain from the teeth was given very concretely in relation to each tooth from which the patient felt pain. Furthermore, X-rays of her teeth were shown to her and the conditions of her teeth and surrounding tissues were explained. Information was provided in a manner to give meaning to her experiences and to make it easier to understand different types of pain related to the oral cavity.

3.8.2 Dental Treatment

Prior to dental treatment, the patient received three times regular dose of xylocain/adrenaline buccal infiltration for tooth 16 (3×1.8 ml lidocaine). During test drilling, the patient still felt some pain. Without commenting on how much anaesthesia that had already been given, the therapist expressed joy that she gave notice of how she felt. A total of 1.7 ml of articaine was then given in the buccal and palatal intraligament. The patient now experienced to be pain free during drilling. However, she felt pain when the filling was put. She was offered more anaesthesia but chose to finish the filling without having more. Her choice was discussed after completing the filling, and she gave signs of being pleased with the situation and having been able to give sign of how she felt. Increased pain toward the end of the treatment gave the dentist the opportunity to support her in the experience that her body probably metabolizes anaesthesia faster than average patients and that she therefore needs more anaesthesia during treatment. For the relationship, it is important that the patient experiences that she is heard and believed, and this gives her faith that she will be taken seriously the next time she experiences pain.

How to Understand and Meet the Patient

A person with a lot of ailments caused by a basic feeling of lack of control. She has little experience that she can decide, and that she is generally characterized by a lot of preparedness (be on guard).

Low self-esteem and confidence of one's own abilities to influence the environment. Dissatisfied with oneself and with life. General feelings of shame and being ashamed of poor dental hygiene. These thoughts may also increase depression and the feeling of lack of good feelings in relation to how the life is lived.

Worst case scenario thinking - interprets signals in the worst sense. A little pain in the tooth means that something serious is wrong (while it may be the result of focused attention and interpretation of pain).

Painful sensation in the shoulder and neck may be interpreted as inflammation, while the actual reason may be that she is tense and on guard, and therefore have muscles in full tension. Numbness in the arms can mean that there is something with the nervous system, but it can also be due to tense muscles that affect the space conditions for the nerves.

Example: Pressure in the breast may indicate that she has high-costal breathing. In other words she is breathing tensely, with a tight stomach and using only the upper part of the lungs.

Psychosocial factors can aggravate pain

The pain can be generalized by, among other things, anxiety, alertness, difficulty sleeping and lead to sore muscles in completely different places than in the mouth.

History of abuse can be a cause of bad associations in the mouth, and increase discomfort in the oral area.

Dental professionals must be very clear that they believe the patient's evaluation of pain experience. "You are certainly one of those who need more anesthesia! Together we must make sure you get enough anesthesia!".

Complicating factor:

If the patient has grown up in a family where she has had to take care of others or be on guard. It can be especially important with good information to ensure that all elements of the treatment are predictable.

Also, have in mind that she may be sensible for being blamed for not taking her part, which make her vulnerable for enduring treatment that is really too difficult for her.

Box

by Beth Guildford, a consultant clinical psychologist in the Dental Psychology Service at Guy's Hospital. She works closely with the Departments of Oral Medicine and Oral Surgery, working with patients with various orofacial conditions (primarily persistent pain).

I work in an Oral Medicine department in a busy hospital in central London. We use a 'matched care' model, in which there are different intensities of psychologically informed interventions offered according to patient need. This helps the responsibility for psychological care of the patient to be held by all members of the team, rather than this being considered separate and only for the psychologist to deal with. The less intensive interventions, such as recognition of psychological distress and signposting to sources of support, are the remit of any clinician. The psychology team have developed leaflets that non-psychologists can share with patients, as well as training to help them feel confident to use questionnaires to screen for distress. If the need for more intensive input from a psychologist is identified, patients can either see a psychologist at the same time that they are attending their pain clinic appointment, or can be referred for an appointment on another day.

We have found it helpful if the whole team, including the psychologists, use similar terms and ways of explaining persistent pain. We achieve this through regular discussion between team members and training. The psychologists and Oral Medicine consultants have also jointly developed some written guidelines which are particularly useful for new members of the team and contribute to a consistent approach.

Finally, another important feature of how psychologists in our department work is through having regular informal liaison with our dental and medical colleagues. This helps us collaborate and share ideas about service improvements, as well as enhancing our work with individual patients.

References

1. Merskey H, Bonica J, Carmon A, Dubner R, Kerr FWL, Lindblom U, Mumford JM, Nathan PW, Noordenbos W, Pagni CA, Renaer MJ, Sternbach RA, Sunderland S. Pain terms: a list with definitions and notes on usage. Recommended by the IASP Subcommittee on taxonomy. Pain. 1979;6:249–52.

2. Raja SN, Carr DB, Cohen M, Finnerup NB, Flor H, Gibson S, Keefe FJ, Mogil JS, Ringkamp M, Sluka KA, Song XJ, Stevens B, Sullivan MD, Tutelman PR, Ushida T, Vader K. The revised International Association for the Study of Pain definition of pain: concepts, challenges, and compromises. Pain. 2020;161:1976–82. https://doi.org/10.1097/j.pain.0000000000001939.

3. Breivik H, Collett B, Ventafridda V, Cohen R, Gallacher D. Survey of chronic pain in Europe: prevalence, impact on daily life, and treatment. Eur J Pain. 2006;10:287–333.

4. Haraldstad K, Sørum R, Eide H, Natvig GK, Helseth S. Pain in children and adolescents: prevalence, impact on daily life, and parents' perception, a school survey. Scand J Caring Sci. 2011;25:27–36. https://doi.org/10.1111/j.1471-6712.2010.00785.x.

5. Fuglkjær S, Vach W, Hartvigsen J, Dissing KB, Junge T, Hestbæk L. Musculoskeletal pain distribution in 1,000 Danish schoolchildren aged 8-16 years. Chiropr Man Therap. 2020;2020:28. https://doi.org/10.1186/s12998-020-00330-9.

6. Mills SEE, Nicolson KP, Smith BH. Chronic pain: a review of its epidemiology and associated factors in population-based studies. Br J Anaesth. 2019;123:e273–83. https://doi.org/10.1016/j.bja.2019.03.023.

7. Descartes R. Traité de l'homme. Tratado do Homem. 1664.

8. Schon KR, Parker APJ, Woods CG. Congenital insensitivity to pain overview. 2018;[updated 2020 Jun 11]. In: Adam MP, Ardinger HH, Pagon RA, et al., editors. GeneReviews® [internet]. Seattle (WA): University of Washington, Seattle; 1993–2021. Available from: https://www.ncbi.nlm.nih.gov/books/NBK481553/.

9. https://www.iasp-pain.org/resources/terminology/.

10. Jensen TS, Baron R, Haanpaa M, Kalso E, Loeser JD, Rice AS, Treede RD. A new definition of neuropathic pain. Pain. 2011;152:2204–5. https://doi.org/10.1016/j.pain.2011.06.017.

11. Byers MR, Schatteman GC, Bothwell M. Multiple functions for NGF receptor in developing, aging and injured rat teeth are suggested by epithelial, mesenchymal and neural immunoreactivity. Development. 1990;109:461–71.

12. Kosek E, Cohen M, Baron R, Gebhart GF, Mico JA, Rice AS, Rief W, Sluka AK. Do we need a third mechanistic descriptor for chronic pain states? Pain. 2016;157:1382–6. https://doi.org/10.1097/j.pain.0000000000000507.

13. Bonica J. The management of pain. Philadelphia: Lea & Febiger; 1953.

14. Glare P, Aubrey KR, Myles PS. Transition from acute to chronic pain after surgery. Lancet. 2019;393:1537–46. https://doi.org/10.1016/S0140-6736(19)30352-6.

15. Huffman KL, Rush TE, Fan Y, Sweis GW, Vij B, Covington EC, Scheman J, Mathews M. Sustained improvements in pain, mood, function and opioid use post interdisciplinary pain rehabilitation in patients weaned from high and low dose chronic opioid therapy. Pain. 2017;158:1380–94. https://doi.org/10.1097/j.pain.0000000000000907.

16. Comelon M, Raeder J, Stubhaug A, et al. Gradual withdrawal of remifentanil infusion may prevent opioid-induced hyperalgesia. Br J Anaesth. 2016;116:524–30. https://doi.org/10.1093/bja/aev547.

17. Nielsen CS, Stubhaug A, Price DD, Vassend O, Czajkowski N, Harris JR. Individual differences in pain sensitivity: genetic and environmental contributions. Pain. 2008;136:21–9. https://doi.org/10.1016/j.pain.2007.06.008.

18. Coghill RC, McHaffie JG, Yen YF. Neural correlates of interindividual differences in the subjective experience of pain. Proc Natl Acad Sci U S A. 2003;100:8538–42. https://doi.org/10.1073/pnas.1430684100.

19. Melzack R, Wall PD. Pain mechanisms: a new theory. Science. 1965;150:971–9. https://doi.org/10.1126/science.150.3699.971.

20. Purves D. Pain. In: Purves D, Augustine GJ, Fitzpatrick D, Hall WC, Lamantia A-S, JO MN, Williams SM, editors. Neuroscience. 3rd ed. Sunderland: Sinauer Associates, Inc.; 2011. p. 209–28.

21. Swift A. Understanding pain and the human body's response to it. Nursing Times [online]. 2018;114(3): 22–26. https://www.nursingtimes.net/clinical-archive/pain-management/understanding-the-effect-of-pain-and-how-the-human-body-responds/7023422.article?search=https%3a%2f%2fwww.nursingtimes.net%2fsearcharticles%3fqsearch%3d1%26keywords%3damelia+swift. Accessed 31 July 2022.

22. Ness TJ, Randich A, Deberry JJ. Modulation of spinal nociceptive processing. In: Ballantyne JC, Fishman SM, Rathmell JP, editors. Bonica's management of pain. 5th ed. Philadelphia: Wolters-Kluwer; 2019. p. 52–61.

23. Melzack R. From the gate to the neuromatrix. Pain. 1999;199(Suppl 6):121–6. https://doi.org/10.1016/s0304-3959(99)00145-1.

24. Brodal P. The central nervous system. 5th edn. Oxford: Oxford University Press Inc; 2016.

25. Merrill RL. Central mechanisms of orofacial pain. Dent Clin N Am. 2007;51:45–59. https://doi.org/10.1016/j.cden.2006.09.010.

26. Beissner F, Brandau A, Henke C, Felden L, Baumgärtner U, Treede RD, Oertel BG, Lötsch J. Quick discrimination of adelta and C fiber mediated pain based on three verbal descriptors. PloS One. 2010;5(9):12944. https://www.ncbi.nlm.nih.gov/pmc/articles/PMC2944851/#.

27. Goldberg M, Kulkarni AB, Young M, Boskey A. Dentin: structure, composition and mineralization: the role of dentin ECM in dentin formation and mineralization. Front Biosci (Elite Ed). 2011;3:711–35. https://doi.org/10.2741/e281.

28. Närhi M, Bjørndal L, Pigg M, Fristad I, Haug SR. Acute dental pain I: pulpal and dentinal pain. Nor Tannlegeforen Tid. 2016;126:10–8.

29. Zhang J-M, An J. Cytokines, inflammation and pain. Int Anesthesiol Clin. 2007;45(2):27–37. https://doi.org/10.1097/AIA.0b013e318034194e.

30. Iwata K, Katagiri A, Shinoda M. Neuron-glia interaction is a key mechanism underlying persistent orofacial pain. J Oral Sci. 2017;59(2):173–5. https://doi.org/10.2334/josnusd.16-0858.

31. Headache Classification Committee of the International Headache Society (IHS). The international classification of headache disorders, 3rd edition. Cephalalgia. 2018;38:1–211. https://doi.org/10.1177/0333102417738202.

32. Bereiter D, Okamoto K. Neurobiology of estrogen status in deep craniofacial pain. Int Rev Neurobiol. 2011;97:251–84. https://doi.org/10.1016/B978-0-12-385198-7.00010-2.

33. Skaret E, Kvale G, Raadal M. General self-efficacy, dental anxiety and multiple fears among 20-year-olds in Norway. Scnad J Psychol. 2003;44:331–7. https://doi.org/10.1111/1467-9450.00352.

34. Felitti VJ, Anda RF, Nordenberg D, Williamson DF, Spitz AM, Edwards V, Koss MP, Marks JS. Relationship of childhood abuse and household dysfunction to many of the leading causes of death in adults. The Adverse Childhood Experiences (ACE) study. Am J Prev Med. 1998;14(4):245–58. https://doi.org/10.1016/s0749-3797(98)00017-8.

35. Dworkin ER, Menon SV, Bystrynski J, Allen NE. Sexual assault victimization and psychopathology: a review and meta-analysis. Clin Psychol Rev. 2017;56:65–81. https://doi.org/10.1016/j.cpr.2017.06.002.

36. Munk A, Reme SE, Jacobsen HB. What does CATS have to do with cancer? The Cognitive Activation Theory of Stress (CATS) forms the SURGE model of chronic post-surgical pain in women with breast cancer. Front Psychol. 2021;12:630422. https://doi.org/10.3389/fpsyg.2021.630422.

37. Fordyce B. Behavioral methods for chronic pain and illness. Mosby Company: St Louis; 1976.

38. Flor H, Breitenstein C, Birbaumer N, Füerst M. A psychophysiological analysis of spouse solicitousness towards pain behaviors, spouse interaction, and pain perception. Behav Ther. 1995;26:255–72. https://doi.org/10.1016/S0005-7894(05)80105-4.

39. Hauck M, Lorenz J. Supraspinal mechanisms of pain and nociception. In: Ballantyne JC, Fishman SM, Rathmell JP, editors. Bonica's management of pain. 5th ed. Philadelphia: Wolters-Kluwer; 2019.

40. Moore PJ, Chrabaszcz JS, Peterson RA. The cognitive processing of somatic anxiety: using functional measurement to understand and address the fear of pain. Psicológica. 2010;31:605–27.

41. Ellis A. Reason and emotion in psychotherapy. New York: Lyle Stuart; 1962.

42. Beck AT, Rush AJ, Shaw BF, Emery G. Cognitive therapy of depression. New York: Guilford Press; 1979.

43. Martinez-Calderon J, Jensen MP, Morales-Asencio JM, Luque-Suarez A. Pain catastrophizing and function in individuals with chronic musculoskeletal pain. Clin J Pain. 2019;35(3):279–93. https://doi.org/10.1097/AJP.0000000000000676.

44. Willassen L, Johansson AA, Kvinnsland S, Staniszewski K, Berge T, Rosén A. Catastrophizing has a better prediction for TMD than other psychometric and experimental pain variables. Pain Res Manag. 2020. https://doi.org/10.1155/2020/7893023.

45. Vlaeyen JW, Linton SJ. Fear-avoidance and its consequences in chronic musculoskeletal pain: a state of the art. Pain. 2000;85:317–32. https://doi.org/10.1016/s0304-3959(99)00242-0.

46. McWilliams LA, Cox BJ, Enns MW. Mood and anxiety disorders associated with chronic pain: an examination in a nationally representative sample. Pain. 2003;106:127–33. https://doi.org/10.1016/s0304-3959(03)00301-4.

47. Currie SR, Wang J. Chronic back pain and major depression in the general Canadian population. Pain. 2004;107(1–2):54–60. https://doi.org/10.1016/j.pain.2003.09.015.

48. Ohayon MM, Schatzberg AF. Using chronic pain to predict depressive morbidity in the general population. Arch Gen Psychiatry. 2003;60:39–47. https://doi.org/10.1001/archpsyc.60.1.39.

49. Yu L, McCracken LM. Pain and anxiety and depression. In: Ballantyne JC, Fishman SM, Rathmell JP, editors. Bonica's management of pain. 5th ed. Philadelphia: Wolters-Kluwer; 2019. p. 1414–20.

50. Turk DC, Swanson KS, Wilson HD. Psychological aspects of pain. In: Ballantyne JC, Fishman SM, Rathmell JP, editors. Bonica's management of pain. 5th ed. Philadelphia: Wolters-Kluwer; 2019. p. 76–89.

51. Kent G. Memory of dental pain. Pain. 1985;21:187–94. https://doi.org/10.1016/0304-3959(85)90288-X.

52. Grønseth R, Markestad T. Pediatri og pediatrisk sykepleie. 2nd ed. Bergen: Fagbokforlaget; 2005. p. 343.

53. Häuser W, Sarzi-Puttini P, Tölle TR, Wolfe F. Placebo and nocebo responses in randomised controlled trials of drugs applying for approval for fibromyalgia syndrome treatment: systematic review and meta-analysis. Clin Exp Rheumatol. 2012;30(Suppl 74):78–87.

54. Benedetti F, Frisaldi E. Neurochemistry of placebo analgesia: opioids, cannabinoids and cholecystokinin. In: Colloca L, Flaten MA, Meissner K, editors. Placebo and pain. San Diego: Academic Press; 2013. p. 9–14.

55. Mitsikostas DD. Nocebo in headaches: implications for clinical practice and trial design. Curr Neurol Neurosci Rep. 2012;12(2):132–7. https://doi.org/10.1007/s11910-011-0245-4.

56. Velly AM, Look JO, Carlson C, Lenton PA, Kang W, Holcroft CA, Fricton JR. The effect of catastrophizing and depression on chronic pain–a prospective cohort study of temporomandibular

muscle and joint pain disorders. Pain. 2011;152:2377–83. https:// doi.org/10.1016/j.pain.2011.07.004.

57. Burns LC, Ritvo SE, Ferguson MK, Clarke H, Seltzer Z, Katz J. Pain catastrophizing as a risk factor for chronic pain after total knee arthroplasty: a systematic review. J Pain Res. 2015;8:21,32. https://doi.org/10.2147/jpr.S64730.

58. Wertli MM, Eugster R, Held U, Steurer J, Kofmehl R, Weiser S. Catastrophizing-a prognostic factor for outcome in patients with low back pain: a systematic review. Spine J. 2014;14:2639–57. https://doi.org/10.1016/j.spinee.2014.03.003.

59. Theunissen M, Peters ML, Bruce J, Gramke HF, Marcus MA. Preoperative anxiety and catastrophizing: a systematic review and meta-analysis of the association with chronic post-surgical pain. Clin J Pain. 2012;28:819–41. https://doi. org/10.1097/AJP.0b013e31824549d6.

60. Linton SJ, Flink IK, Vlaeyen JWS. Understanding the etiology of chronic pain from a psychological perspective. Phys Ther. 2018;98:315–24. https://doi.org/10.1093/ptj/pzy027.

61. Ekhtiari H, Rezapour T, Aupperle RL, Paulus MP. Neuroscience-informed psychoeducation for addiction medicine: a neurocog-nitive perspective. Prog Brain Res. 2017;235:239–64. https://doi. org/10.1016/bs.pbr.2017.08.013.

62. Lindheim MØ. Når barn på sykehus trenger stoppskilt. Hel-sepsykologibloggen 2017. Available at https://www. psykologforeningen.no/publikum/blogger/helsepsykologibloggen/ naar-barn-paa-sykehus-trenger-stoppskilt

63. Jafari H, Courtois I, Van den Bergh O, Vlaeyen JWS, Van Diest I. Pain and respiration: a systematic review. Pain. 2017;158:995–1006.

64. Kwekkeboom KL, Gretarsdottir E. Systematic review of relax-ation interventions for pain. J Nurs Scholarsh. 2006;38:269–77. https://doi.org/10.1111/j.1547-5069.2006.00113.x.

65. Kabat-Zinn J. Too early to tell: the potential impact and challenges-ethical and otherwise-inherent in the mainstream-ing of dharma in an increasingly dystopian world. Mindfulness (N Y). 2017;8:1125–35. https://doi.org/10.1007/s12671-017-0758-2.

66. Lang EV, Benotsch EG, Fick LJ, Lutgendorf S, Berbaum ML, Berbaum KS, Logan H, Spiegel D. Adjunctive non-pharmacological analgesia for invasive medical procedures: a randomised trial. Lancet. 2000;355:1486–90. https://doi. org/10.1016/s0140-6736(00)02162-0.

67. Montgomery GH, DuHamel KN, Redd WH. A meta-analysis of hypnotically induced analgesia: how effective is hypnosis? Int J Clin Exp Hypn. 2000;48:138–53. https://doi. org/10.1080/00207140008410045.

68. Weitzenhoffer AM, Hilgard ER. Stanford hypnotic susceptibil-ity scale, form C. Standford: Consulting Psychologists Press; 1962.

69. Birnie KA, Chambers CT, Spellman CM. Mechanisms of distrac-tion in acute pain perception and modulation. Pain. 2017;158:1012–3. https://doi.org/10.1097/j. pain.0000000000000913.

70. Walker LS, Williams SE, Smith CA, Garber J, Van Slyke DA, Lipani TA. Parent attention versus distraction: impact on symp-tom complaints by children with and without chronic functional abdominal pain. Pain. 2006;122(1–2):43–52. https://doi. org/10.1016/j.pain.2005.12.020.

The Importance of a Safe Relationship with Dental Patients

Lena Myran and Tiril Willumsen

Contents

4

- Understanding the concept of relationship
- Knowing the key elements of professional relationship building
- Knowing the psychological concepts of attachment and transference, understanding how these concepts interact in dentistry
- Recognizing ruptures in alliances and knowing how to repair them

4.1   What Is a Relationship?

The concept of patient–care relations is over 100 years old, dating back to psychoanalyst Sigmund Freud's early works [1].

The relationship between dental professionals and patients involves a framework of conditions at two levels: external conditions and internal conditions.

External conditions involve practical matters like the legislation you must deal with, finances, as well as cancellations and holidays that intervene with treatment progress. Working conditions, like a clean and tidy dental clinic, and a schedule that allows for a calm atmosphere, will improve the consistency and predictability of the clinic environment and create a safe experience for both parties [2].

Internal framework conditions, on the other hand, concerns the treatment process that unfolds between the dentist and the patient. The foundation of the treatment process is the relationship. A good relationship is developed and strengthened through cooperation over time and relies on security, credibility, and trust. Therapeutic alliance is a term often used to illustrate the quality and strength of the relationship between the practitioner and the patient. The concepts of relationship and alliance are used interchangeably in psychological literature. The most commonly used definition of alliance today is a model consisting of three aspects: an emotional bond between the professional and the client, an agreement between the professional and the client on therapeutic tasks, as well as agreement on treatment goals [3].

4.2   The Importance of the Relationship in Patient Care

Several studies show that a good relationship has a positive impact on treatment outcomes [4]. A good therapeutic alliance is considered a prerequisite for success in treatment [5]. All patients need safety and predictability in the dental clinic. Almost everyone needs to experience a certain degree of control, although how much varies from individual to individual. A confidential relationship characterized by mutual trust is necessary for the patient to experience control during dental treatment. If the patient does not trust the dentist, the probability for increased anxiety, dissatisfaction, and increased risk of dropping out of dental treatment is high. In a Swedish study among patients with dental treatment anxiety, having a "safe relationship with the dentist" and "sense of control" were rated as the most important aspects in order to be able to go through with the treatment [6].

Establishing a safe relationship with the patient is also important to enhance the effect of preventive advice. Oral hygiene is a very sensitive issue and patients can easily feel ashamed when discussing their poor oral hygiene or bad breath. There are many examples where patients have felt guilt while discussing these issues with their dentist. If patients experience a safe relationship with a dentist who "wishes me well," the effect of oral hygiene instructions improves.

In addition, for dental professionals, having the knowledge and skills to build a trusting relationship can improve the confidence in their professional role. In the long run, relationship skills can help reduce the risk of professional burnout.

4.3   What Is a Good Relationship?

> In a psychological sense, a good relationship is a safe emotional relationship between the patient and the practitioner who have agreed on a treatment goal and on how to solve the tasks along the way.

In a psychological sense, a good relationship is a safe emotional relationship between the patient and the practitioner who have agreed on a treatment goal and on how to solve the tasks along the way. The ability of the healthcare professional to integrate these factors in their practice will contribute to achieving successful treatment [7]. The statement can be broken into the following three factors:

ℹ️ **The Golden Standard for a Good Relationship:**

A good relationship is a safe emotional relationship between people	The dental professional sees the patient as a person, not as a case, mouth, or a set of teeth. Dental professionals must work on themselves in order to be seen as trustworthy enough for a safe emotional relationship.
… who have agreed on the goal of treatment	The dental professional has a responsibility to facilitate a joint understanding of the treatment goal. This requires communication skills from the professional, including taking the patient's perspective.
…and on how to solve the tasks along the way	Lastly, the dentist and patient should agree on how to solve the tasks along the way, including all relevant elements of the treatment, e.g., practical issues (what should be done first, the time between appointments, etc.), emotional issues (for instance, making a coping plan, see ▶ Chap. 10), and financial issues or other relevant matters.

A good therapeutic attitude should signal safety; safety for the patient to speak up when something is problematic, safety to talk about their needs, and safety to talk about what is shameful. This understanding of a good therapeutic attitude is transferable to dentistry and other patient-oriented relationships.

American psychologist Carl Rogers was one of the first to describe the aspects of a good patient–professional relationship. Favorable characteristics of the therapist are described as authenticity, unconditional positive attention, and empathy [8]. These aspects are firmly rooted in psychological literature and have been shown to have a good effect on treatment results [9].

4.3.1 Authenticity

First, the professional must be authentic in contact with the patient. It is important to try to be yourself in the conversation and not build up an artificial professional façade. There should be a correlation between what you think or experience and what you say to the patient. Being authentic means that what you experience in the moment, comes out in ~~the~~ immediate communication. Being transparent with the patient provides safety. If negative feelings arise toward the patient, it is better to admit the negative feeling to yourself, reflect on how to deal with it, and act accordingly. (*"This patient makes me irritated, his aggression towards me is probably due to problems in his life (maybe anxiety), I will be extra calm and informative"* or *"This patient triggers something in me, I must find out why, but first I will take best possible care of him during treatment today"*) Authenticity is one of the most important core elements of the relationship because it signals, "I have no hidden agenda," "You can have confidence in me."

4.3.2 Unconditional Positive Acceptance

By meeting the patient's feelings and experiences in an accepting, empathetic, and honest way, the dental professional shows unconditional positive acceptance. The professional does not consider whether the patient is right or not but accepts the patient's experience. The patient needs to know that you respect the situation they are in, their emotional response to the situation, their dental health, and how they handle it. This does not mean that you must always agree. Unconditional positive acceptance signals, "I see you," "I have time for

you, just as you are." This can be conveyed by saying something like "We know that every life has its challenges and there are many reasons why people get poor oral health." You can also say, "I respect the way you deal with this very difficult situation." "I have great humility that you are in this process." "We recognize your fears." "We see you and see that this is very difficult for you."

If a patient corrects your actions or statements, you have a golden opportunity to establish an emotional climate where there is room for mistakes. By saying, "I heard that came out wrong." or "I thought about this and I realize I was wrong" you express authenticity, and the patient will know you do not have a hidden agenda. This is important when talking to patients who have had bad experiences with dental professionals.

4.3.3 Empathy

» If One Is Truly to Succeed in Leading a Person to a Specific Place, One Must First and Foremost Take Care to Find Him Where He is and Begin There. This is the secret in the entire art of helping
  S Kierkegaard.

Empathy can be described as finding the other where they are and from this perspective, take part in their experience. A professional is curious and interested in the patient's feelings and experiences and in conveying back to the patient that you listen to and take part in what the patient is recounting. To be empathetic is to try seeing the world through the patient's eyes, while being yourself. You don't get overwhelmed but manage to contain and hold the patient's feelings. This is not a simple matter in a work environment too often characterized by time pressure. Nevertheless, it is essential.

4.3.4 "NURSE"

❯ "The three core elements; authenticity, unconditional positive acceptance and empathy can be expressed and put into practice through the rule of thumb NURSE"

The three core elements – authenticity, unconditional positive acceptance, and empathy – can be expressed and put into practice through the rule of thumb NURSE: Name it, Understand it, Respect it, Support it, Explore it. This acronym is based on a model for relationship building [10] and is elaborated in ► Chap. 6. The NURSE mnemonic is also often used without the E; NURS (see ► Chap. 6).

4.3.4.1 Name It

Naming or identifying the patient's feelings is absolutely necessary and is the start of being able to communicate in a good way if the patient shows feelings such as insecurity, fear, or shame. You might say, "I perceive you as tense or anxious now" or "I get the impression that there is something that's not okay here/with you." By naming the patient's feelings, you signal that it is common and legitimate to feel the way the patient does, and that the dental clinic is a place where we can talk about difficult topics and show difficult emotions.

If you have misinterpreted the patient, the patient can guide you, and you are still in a constructive dialogue. Keep in mind that in this context the patient's criticism or correction implies that they have confidence in your ability to tolerate correction and that you are able to accommodate them.

4.3.4.2 Understand It

It is essential for the patient that you make it clear that you can not only name the feeling but also show that you understand that the situation is difficult. You could say, "I understand that it is difficult for you to be here today" or "I understand that this situation must be very upsetting for you." This way, you manifest that you empathically understand the emotional status of the patient even though you have probably never been in the same situation yourself. By saying this, you show the patient that you acknowledge the emotional cost of coming to the dental clinic, regardless of their personal experience (e.g., having been close to canceling appointments, not showing up at all or sleeping badly last night, dreading the waiting room).

> ❯ Beware of falling into the trap of telling the patient that you know how they are doing, because you do not know. "I understand how you feel" or "I know just how hard this is for you" can be well-meaning statements, but they often fail. If you do this, the patient thinks "How on earth are you going to be able to understand what it's like to be afraid of people like yourself?" Your authenticity is threatened, and the patient may have difficulty trusting you. It is difficult to establish trust with the patient if they don't think you are able to understand how they are doing.

4.3.4.3 Respect It

Perhaps the most important part of the interaction in an emphatic response is to convey respect for the patient. The patient needs to know that you respect the situation they are in, their emotional response to the situation, their dental health, and how they handle it. Examples of statements to express respect: "From what you have told me, it is natural that you feel and act like this" and "In light of your previous experiences, it is very obvious that this is a difficult situation."

4.3.4.4 Support It

To emphasize your emotional and practical support, you may say "Is there anything else I can do to help you through this situation?" Alternatively, you might say, "Don't hesitate to tell me if there's anything I can do to help you."

4.3.4.5 Explore It

Providing good support also involves exploring the patient's perspective to signal that you have an open mind and that you recognize that there are many ways to think. Explore both what lies behind the negative feeling the patient has and the thoughts of the patient on how to master the situation they experience as difficult.

> ❯ **Therapeutic Query Words**
> The words "how" and "what" work well. "How" opens doors, "How do you think that what we can do this in the best way possible?" "How can we in the office best help you with your problem of cancelling when you get scared." "What" encourages patients' stories. "What was it like for you to come here today?" "What did you think would happen?" "What do you need to make this situation better for you?"
>
> "Why" is a problematic word, as it can be perceived as accusatory. Too many patients have experiences with professional care givers they have not trusted. These patients are therefore extra "vigilant" of accusations or disappointments. The word "why" can be tolerated more easily by robust and safe individuals. The main rule is to avoid "why" until the relationship is established, and it feels natural to use the word spontaneously.

4.4 Challenges in Relationship Building

It may sound as if the relationship between the patient and the dentist will develop well and painlessly as long as the patient is met with authenticity, acceptance, and empathy. Unfortunately, it is not that simple. Patients may come from a childhood with economic or social difficulties. They may previously have been subjected to neglect or abuse, resulting in psychological problems in adulthood leading to difficulties collaborating with the dentist.

The challenge with Rogers' definition is that it does not address the patient's inability and motivation to utilize the therapist's empathy, authenticity, and emotional availability [11]. Some patients will always be challenging to ally with and difficult to commit to a collaboration. In order to understand why many patients are unable to utilize the dentist's attentiveness, it may be useful to enter psychological literature. Child abuse and neglect as a cause of the patients' problem attending dental treatment will be thoroughly discussed in ▶ Chap. 10. Other mental issues, the cause of a restrained alliance, will be discussed in ▶ Chap. 15. In this chapter, we will explore the concept of attachment, a key concept to understanding why we do as we do.

4.5 The Attachment Perspective in Patient Treatment

Attachment theory is an area of psychology essential to know for dental personnel. Dentists and dental hygienists meet people with different attitudes and personalities, and all patients have their unique history. Dentists meet people who express strong and unreasonable feelings during treatment, feelings such as anger, contempt, or fear. This section aims to make such feelings more understandable and easier to deal with.

Attachment is an innate system of action that develops over time, matures from experiences, and act as the foundation for our thoughts, feelings, and actions. The concept derives from John Bowlby's attachment theory and refers to a person's characteristic way of relating to other people [12]. Human life starts with attachment, the lifelong bond of love that the child forms to the primary caregiver. The attachment system primes children to seek "stronger and wiser" guides who both ensure physical and emotional survival and facilitate exploration and discovery [13]. This bond ensures that the child seeks closeness to his caregivers, using the caregiver as a secure base from which the child can explore the world, as well as a safe haven from which they can seek support, protection, or comfort in times of distress [12].

How the child's attachment approach is met by the caregiver, affects the child's development of self-esteem and personality, and follows us from the cradle to the grave [14]. A child who has hurt their knee and cries for their mummy can be met with comfort, ignorance, or yelling. A child meeting an angry dog and seeking parental support might be met with help, ridicule, or parental fear. A child sharing their enthusiasm for a newly discovered treasure might be met with rejection, shared enthusiasm, or be ignored. The relational experiences that we acquire from childhood form a set of expectations about how people will respond to you. The child might form expectations that they will be rejected, acknowledged, or ignored. This is known as a working

model. A working model is a mental representation of our relational experiences, which lay the foundation for how we perceive ourselves in the face of other people and influence how we meet others throughout life. The working model hence affects the individual's future relationships, including how well they will be able to ally themselves with their future dentist.

Canadian American psychologist Mary Ainsworth examined variations in attachment. By observing mother and child in various situations, she found three characteristic attachment patterns: secure attachment, anxious-ambivalent attachment, and avoidant attachment. A fourth category, disorganized attachment, was added later. This is explored further in ▶ Chap. 8. The attachment is not fixed, but once it is established, it is relatively difficult to change [15]. The attachment styles are thought to be stable and self-preserving over time, and it is important to emphasize that attachment patterns developed during childhood may be a prominent characteristic in the adult personality [14]. Thus, to be able to be empathic toward adults, attachment patterns need to be acknowledged and understood.

4.5.1 Secure Attachment

Seventy percent of children belong to this group. If the attachment to the child's caregiver is characterized by security, the parents have been secure, protective, and predictable. These people develop the ability to trust other people and to seek comfort and protection when they are afraid. A "secure attachment" style provides the basis for meeting others with an open mind, "knowing" that you are well taken care of, that others wish you well, that it helps to speak up when something is wrong, and that there is comfort available when discomfort or pain arises. People with secure attachment are often described as adaptable, capable, trusting, and understanding [15].

4.5.2 Anxious-Ambivalent Attachment

10% of all children have an anxious-ambivalent attachment. An anxious-ambivalent style can develop if the caregiver is unpredictable and more concerned with their own emotional needs rather than the needs of the child. The emotional instability of the caregiver can make the child unsafe and result in the child not knowing how to deal with the caregiver. As an adolescent and adult, people who develop attachments under this style can bear the mark of fear and skepticism towards approaching other people. They can pretend to need closeness and support when they really want to explore their surroundings, thus giving misleading signals to their surroundings. People with this form of attachment can also send very complex signals by appearing to be both dependent and independent.

4.5.3 Avoidant Attachment

Twenty percent of children fall into this category. Children who have developed under the avoidant attachment style seek little closeness and comfort and look seemingly unaffected even if they experience discomfort. A child with avoidant attachment is incurious and appears calm or uninterested. They pretend to be fine when they are really upset inside. The style is characterized by a caregiver who is predictable but emotionally unavailable or dismissive. The child has learned that they must deal with difficult emotions on their own and have thus become accustomed to fending for themselves early in life. In other words, there is no point in speaking out or seeking support as they expect not to be heard.

4.5.4 Disorganized Attachment

Children who have experienced neglect and abuse from their loved ones have learned that the caregiver poses a threat. Throughout life they may appear confused, frightened, and difficult to understand. This attachment style is characterized by caregivers who are a threat while being the only source of comfort and safety at the same time, resulting in fear without the possibility of resolution.

4.6 Meeting Attachment Styles in Adult Dentistry

> ❯ "When you meet a new patient, you will meet a person with expectations about the dental situation, assumptions about you as a human being and what your intentions are, as well as biases regarding the outcome of dental treatment."

The working models we carry through life, secure or insecure, are relatively stable and activate in attachment-related situations. Dental treatment is one of those situations. Every dental patient attends treatment with expectations about the dental situation, assumptions about you as a human being, and what your intentions are.

For individuals with a secure attachment style, their experience allows the individual to trust themselves and others, believing in the goodness of the self, and even

desire for interpersonal connection. In working together with their therapists, these individuals are more likely to be able to form an emotional bond, to agree on goals for treatment, and to agree on tasks to achieve those goals [3, 16]. The securely attached patient will therefore find it easier to establish a safe alliance with the dentist than those who have experienced other attachment styles. A secure attachment orientation predicts a positive working alliance and greater engagement in treatment [13]. A pattern of attachment characterized by security also proves important for children who have painful experiences at the dentist. Children with a secure attachment pattern are more likely to regulate and reduce fear of dental procedures after having a positive experience at the dentist [15].

People with any of the insecure attachment styles may have greater difficulty letting you get close to them, trusting you enough to establishing a safe relationship. A meta-analysis of connections between attachment style and outcome indicates that anxious attachment predicts a weaker alliance, a more difficult and potentially less helpful course of treatment [12, 13]. For individuals with an insecure attachment style, the assumptions connected to their attachment experiences reflect a distrust of the motives of others. They may have more negative self-representation or a pressing need to be reassured of the love of others [16]. Therefore, while working together with their dentist, these individuals have a more difficult time establishing a safe emotional bond, agreeing with their dentist on goals for treatment and on tasks to achieve those goals.

Be aware that the attachment style goes both ways. Both you and your patient bring an attachment style into the collaboration. A recent study suggests that the insecure attachment style of the professional affects the alliance between the professional and the client, especially in more symptomatic clients [17].

Knowing that many patients will struggle to commit to a collaboration with you, it is useful to understand that this can be caused by the patient's past experiences with close relationships. At the same time, we find in literature that the therapist's way of managing the patient's expectations, by being sensitive and responsive when the patient expresses a need for closeness and support, can strengthen the patient's sense of security, alleviate the patient's symptoms, and strengthen the patient's positive assumptions about themself and others [18].

> ❯ *Tom, a 35-year-old man with a history of insecure attachment and a problem trusting health personnel. He has a toothache. The dentist examines him and diagnoses an acute pulpitis in 26. Tom agrees to have local anesthesia. The dentist explains the procedure and injects local anesthesia.*

Tom (in an aggressive voice): This was more painful than you said it would be!

(The dentist admits the negative feelings the patient raises in her, reflects on how to deal with it and how to act according to this "This patient makes me irritated, his aggression towards me is probably due to problems in his life (maybe anxiety), I will be extra calm and informative")

Dentist: I am sorry about that

(The dentist raises the back of the dental chair to be at the same eye level as Tom, making sure that the interpersonal distance feels comfortable and focuses on presenting a very calm attitude)

Dentist: – I have injected once but I need to give you one more dose. This will probably be less painful, but it is important that you make a stop signal if you feel pain. It may also help if I inject slowly. In addition, it can be helpful if you try to relax your oral muscles. What do you think of that?

Tom: – I don't know

Dentist: – Do you have any suggestions on how to make it easier for you?

Tom: – Maybe it is worth a try to do what you suggest, but you must promise to be careful

Dentist: – I promise to be careful and to stop immediately if you give me a signal

Tom: – Okay

Dentist: – Fine, Now I am going to lower the back of the chair and we'll give it another try, Okay?

Tom: – Okay

4.7 Transference and Countertransference

The working model brought with you from the parent–child relationship is self-preserving and robust. It functions like tunnel vision; you see what you are looking for, and therefore give affirmative feedback on what you assume. From a health worker's perspective, it also means that the patient's behavior triggers something in your history and working model. It triggers reactions that neither you nor the patient is necessarily aware of, but which are unintentionally expressed. This section aims to make you aware of these reactions.

In order to understand some of the problems that arise in the cooperation between dentist and patient, it is essential to get acquainted with the concepts of transference and countertransference. Transference as a term originates from the psychodynamic model of understanding and describes the attitudes and feelings a patient develops in relation to a therapist. Transference is seen as a common phenomenon that colors and characterizes many of our relationships, probably most. In the face of other people, especially where strong emo-

tions are involved, we use previously central, emotionally important relationships as a starting point and template for attitudes and expectations. In that sense, we can say that transference refers to a way of remembering the past, to make use of what we have experienced [2].

If the patient is calm and without pain or fear, as most people are, it may be easy to establish a safe relationship. However, if the patient has a high level of stress and psychological pain, it may be challenging. When the patient expresses anger, contempt or despair, unreasonable feelings, or unrealistic expectations – health workers may experience the phenomenon of transference. The feelings and attitudes a patient may express toward the dentist may stem from their earlier relational experiences. The patient redirects their feelings toward others (such as their authoritarian mother or abuser) on to you.

Countertransference denotes the feelings and behavior the patient's behavior arouses in you as a dentist. It can initiate feelings of emptiness, irritation, or anxiety and will involuntarily affect your attitudes toward the patient. This may result in a dentist with a propensity for being a little too accommodating toward a patient, who does not properly adhere to framework and agreements, who stretches the appointment to avoid hurting or annoying the patient. The situation may, sometimes quite surprisingly, trigger thoughts, fantasies, or images in the dentist [19]. It can be about changing moods, variations in alertness and interest in what the patient says, boredom or drowsiness that act as signs of unconscious reactions in the therapist. There is a large spectrum of reactions that we can classify as countertransference [2].

▶ Example

Below you can find some examples of transference and countertransference.

A patient has scheduled a consultation for help with indistinct pain and sensitivity toward hot and cold drinks in her upper jaw. It is difficult to find a specific diagnosis. You try to explain this to the patient. The patient pours out all her frustrations and criticism. She talks about how angry she is at the world and how badly she has been treated by dentists. "No one has the competence to help me." She accuses you of not helping her. She has been rejected by health professionals many times before. This is the patient's typical behavior when she is afraid and feels that no one can help her (transference). As a dentist, you might feel a sense of inadequacy: "I'll never be able to fully help this patient." You might get annoyed, thinking "with that attitude, it's no wonder that no one is helping you." Maybe you get defensive "I doubt that everyone has been that useless?" (transference) or you feel a sense of weakness and inadequacy and even give up treatment. "This patient becomes too time consuming and complicated; "I'll leave it to someone who is more experienced" (coun-

4

tertransference). The patient thus receives a confirmation of her original assumption that no one is able to help.

A patient appears uninterested or even dismissive during dental treatment. He does not look at you (transference) and only answers in brief sentences to your questions. Treatment is slow going. Your attempts to chat fail and you feel helpless "I can't have a conversation with this patient, he dislikes the way I work or the way I talk to him" (countertransference). There may also be a feeling of inadequacy. You find that the patient apparently chooses not to try and improve the situation, and this in a situation where you are set to perform treatment that should be in the best interests of the patient. This provokes you and you may respond with anger (countertransference).

A patient talks nonstop, and you are unable to start treatment. The patient is actually very afraid. Constant chatter keeps you at a safe distance (transference). The stories are many and good, but as the dentist, you want to get started with treatment. You don't want to interrupt as you don't want to disappoint the patient and be a killjoy. Your frustration builds up. Finally, at the end of the appointment, you feel dissatisfied and stressed. You are delayed for your next appointment (countertransference). It is not fun anymore and has become a tricky situation that both parties are unhappy with. If the situation ends up this way, the dentist is, in addition to being annoyed with the patient, often mostly annoyed with himself for not being able to conclude the conversation and direct the patient toward treatment.

The "important patient" comes trotting into the office. He does not look at you, he doesn't say hello, he's well-dressed. He signals that he is an important person and must get the best treatment (transference). He awakens a feeling in you. You are afraid of making mistakes or of seeming less competent than what he expects of you. You are afraid of being exposed as ~~not~~ inadequate and may pretend that you know more than you do or are more competent than you actually are (concordant countertransference). ◀

These reactions are human and normal and happen to all of us regularly. At the same time, it is also very inappropriate in a professional setting. We handle some expressions worse than others and faced with those with which we have the greatest difficulty, we can almost instinctively react inappropriately, irrationally, and destructively. Should the patient dare to enter into a partnership with you as their dentist, they must be able to trust that you will meet them in a safe way. If the patient is to gain confidence in you and choose you as a confidential dental care professional, it requires you to avoid reacting in a destructive manner. This implies learning to reflect before acting on your emotions, reflecting on your own patterns of reaction, and becoming aware of your own vulnerabilities.

4.8 Developing Professionalism

Reacting emotionally to transference is inappropriate, but also very human. Common reactions are getting upset, becoming insecure, yelling, slandering the patient at lunch, rejecting, or caring too deeply about the patient. Patients who express emotions, like fear, anxiety, or grief, tug at our heartstrings.

Research suggests that therapists who report that they more often feel angry and annoyed with patients and who struggle to withstand their emotional needs form less constructive alliances with their patients [20]. Becoming aware of the emotions that may be triggered in yourself when treating patients is therefore an important part of developing professionalism.

Lack of reflection and awareness related to countertransference can also cause increased vulnerability to emotional strain. The less conscious the professional is of their own feelings and attitudes, the more empathetic mistakes will be made. This can make treatment more difficult. The professional will be less able to take care of themself, has reduced tolerance for strong feelings, and will more easily experience identity – and role conflicts. A professional who sees themself as tough and resilient can feel ashamed of constantly being overwhelmed by emotion. A professional who sees themself as warm and committed can be torn up by feeling fury directed at the client. A professional who sees themself as an optimist may fear taking on his client's sense of hopelessness [21].

The first step in developing professionalism is therefore to become aware of the feelings and thoughts that arise and become aware of the transferences from the patient. "Now I feel frustrated about not getting started with the treatment" or "I feel like I'm annoyed that he didn't come in before." You should accommodate and accept these feelings that emerge within yourself and address them as transference/countertransference. "The scolding I just got from the patient is probably not really about me" "The fact that I get scared doesn't say anything about me as a dentist/person."

It is possible to practice coping strategies for situations where a patient evokes your emotions. One technique is to take a break for a few seconds, so that the reflexive reaction can subside. This can be to count to three, to roll the ball of your foot against the sole of the shoe, or to use breathing techniques. This gives us time to connect to a suitable professional reaction.

When we endure and accept the emotions that emerge, we can look past them and look for the causes of the behavior. In the dentist–patient relationship, the dentist becomes someone who should strive to use the theoretical and practical competence to try to be empathic, to understand that the situation is difficult and to respect the patient's emotions and reactions. Questions you can ask yourself when meeting patients who evoke strong feelings in you can be "Can neglect or abuse (sexual, violent, or emotional) explain this behavior?" "Has the patient experienced something that scared them at the dentist's before?" "Is there a lot going on in the patient's life these days?" "Does the patient have concerns about finances?" "Is it shame or guilt that is expressed, is he afraid of what I will say about his teeth (condemnation)?"

Few people, including well-trained psychologists, are immune from countertransference, that is, to respond humanly and emotionally to the transferences from the patient. Nevertheless, it is a requirement that all health-care professionals, including dentists, strive to be aware of what is happening in the relationship with the patient.

❯ "A good professional relationship is one human being trying to help another human being."

Marsha Linehan, the originator of a psychological approach called dialectical behavior therapy, was once asked if she had any advice for novice clinical psychologists. She suggested that they be themselves and stop trying to act like therapists, reminding them that this entire venture is nothing more than "one human being trying to help another human being» [22]. The same advice also works for dental personnel. You will come a long way by being an authentic, accepting, and empathic human using your knowledge to help another human being.

4.9 Rupture and Repair: How to Repair When the Alliance Is Ruptured

❯ "While breaking alliances is possible, so is fixing them."

A rupture is a deterioration in the therapeutic alliance, manifested by a disagreement between the patient and dentist on treatment goals, a lack of collaboration on therapeutic tasks, or a strain on their emotional bond [23]. Alliances and relationships can be fleeting and are subject to change throughout life. All humans will most likely have many relationships, both professional and private, ruptured and broken. The dental situation is a situation that triggers our relational assumptions and, thus is vulnerable to rupture. Common ruptures in dentistry are absence from treatment, postponing of appointments or reduced compliance. While breaking alliances is possible, so is fixing them. Research implies that experiencing resolution of ruptures in the therapist–client relationship promotes client welfare even more than alliances with no ruptures (Eubanks, 2018). But how do you repair when the therapeutic alliance is broken or you feel that the relationship is tearing apart?

Listed below are research-supported suggestions on how practitioners can address and repair ruptures in the alliance.

> **Tip**
>
> Empathize with patients' expressions of negative feelings about the therapist or the therapy. Validate them for broaching a difficult and potentially divisive topic in the session. As a dentist you may say: "I appreciate your honesty, it gives me a chance to explain."

– Be attuned to indications of rupture, including confrontation ruptures marked by expressions of dissatisfaction or hostility, and more subtle markers of withdrawal such as patients evading or appeasing the therapist to distance themselves from the therapist or from the therapy. In dentistry, you should be aware of changes in the patient's reactions and attitudes, examples: suddenly being silent, aggressive, or not showing up for treatment.
– Preferably acknowledge the rupture directly and openly and non-defensively invite patients to explore their experience of the rupture. If the therapist–client bond is not strong enough for direct exploration or if this would divert from a priority therapeutic task, then address ruptures in an indirect, immediate manner, by changing the tasks or goals of therapy to satisfy the patient's concerns. As a dentist you may say: "I think we should try to make the situation more comfortable for you. I suggest we try to find a position which is more comfortable for you" or "It seems that the local anesthetic is not working the way I want it to, so my suggestion is to give you one more injection."
– Empathize with patients' expressions of negative feelings about the therapist or the therapy. Validate them for broaching a difficult and potentially divisive topic in the session. As a dentist you may say: "I appreciate your honesty, it gives me a chance to explain."
– Accept responsibility for your own part in the rupture; do not blame patients for misunderstanding or failing to comply with your wishes. As a dentist you may say: "I think maybe I was not precise enough in my description of the treatment plan and therefore it was easy to misunderstand."
– Anticipate that for some therapists, ruptures can evoke feelings of confusion, ambivalence, incompetence, and guilt. Develop your abilities to recognize, tolerate, validate, and empathically explore your own negative feelings, so that you can do the same for your patients. In dentistry, this may be relevant when the patient's behavior (not keeping the mouth open) interferes with the dental work and you feel that you are unable to perform according to your regular professional high standard.

You might recognize elements from NURSE, previously elaborated in this chapter. We will present a clinical example of a typical rupture in dental treatment. Then we will exemplify a dialog to back it up.

4

Case Study

The patient appears uninterested or even dismissive during dental treatment. He does not look at you and only answers in brief sentences to your questions. Your attempts to chat fail and you feel helpless and inadequate. You think: "I can't have a conversation with this patient, he dislikes the way I work or the way I talk to him." You find that the patient apparently chooses not to contribute, to try, and to improve the situation, and this in a situation where you are set to perform treatment that should be in his best interests. This provokes you and you respond with anger. The patient senses your frustration, the relationship ruptures, and he stops showing up for appointments. He only seeks treatment when in need of acute dental treatment. This is actually a relief to you as the appointments have been emotionally draining and you do not have to deal with the rupture. Still, it's not a good situation. The dental work is not finished, and you feel professionally responsible for the patient. The next time the patient makes an appointment, you decide to have a conversation about the rupture in the alliance.

Dentist: – Before we start the acute treatment, I would like to talk about our original treatment plan. I have noticed that you have cancelled several scheduled appointments *(acknowledge the rupture)*. I have been thinking, and I am wondering if maybe we got off on the wrong foot or if anything happened that made you feel uncomfortable coming back *(naming the feeling)*.

Patient: – (Silence) Mm-hmm

Dentist: – I understand if this seems weird to you *(being attuned)*. I just want you to know that undergoing dental treatment can be very demanding for many patients. It's important that you feel safe talking to me. So far, I have not done a good enough job making this a safe place for you to talk freely *(accept responsibility)*. I was hoping that I could change that.

Patient: – Ok, I think I know what you mean but... It is hard to explain... Hmm.

Dentist: – It's my responsibility to explain, and to make sure we understand each other *(accepting responsibility)*, and I suspect that some of our previous meetings didn't go too well. I would like for us to get a fresh start.

Patient: – Okay. You see, I often feel stupid coming in, fearing dental treatment. I am afraid I am taking up your time every time I come in late. Maybe feeling that it annoyed you a little?

Dentist: – Thank you for telling me how you feel *(empathizing with patients' expressions of negative feelings)*. You might be on to something too. When dental treatment doesn't go as planned, I can get frustrated. That is my responsibility, not being professional enough. I am working on that. I know that no one wants to be afraid of dental treatment and I do have great respect for the way you handle this difficult situation.

Patient: – Nice of you to say that. It's awful to have such terrible teeth. It scares me just to open my mouth to you.

Dentist: – Let's start over? I can tell you about dental anxiety, and maybe you will recognize some elements.

If therapists and clients process their therapeutic relationship (i.e., directly address in the here and now feelings about each other and about the inevitable problems that emerge in the therapy relationship), feelings will be expressed and accepted, problems will be resolved, the relationship will be enhanced, and clients will transfer their learning to other relationships outside of therapy [24].

Summary

A safe relationship between patient and dentist is crucial in dental treatment and is the foundation for successful treatment. Even if the dentist offers a safe space, building a relationship with the patient might not go as planned. There may be many reasons for this; in this chapter, we have elaborated on the patient's attachment experiences and have discussed how the dynamic between dentist and patient might develop. We further discussed ruptures in alliances and how to repair when a therapeutic bond is broken.

References

1. Horvath AO, Del Re AC, Flückiger C, Symonds D. Alliance in individual psychotherapy. Psychotherapy (Chic). 2011;48(1): 9–16.
2. Zachrisson A. Motoverføring og endringer i synet på den psykoanalytiske relasjonen. Tidsskrift for Norsk psykologforening. 2008;45(8):939–48.
3. Bordin ES. The generalizability of the psychoanalytic concept of the working alliance. Psychother Theory Res Pract. 1979;16(3):252–60.
4. Horvath AO. The alliance in context. Accomplishments, challenges, and future directions. Psychotherapy (Chic). 2006;43(3):258–63.
5. Friedberg RD, Gorman AA. Integrating psychotherapeutic processes with cognitive behavioural procedures. J Contemp Psychother. 2007;37:185–93.
6. Bernson JM, Elfström ML, Hakeberg M. Dental coping strategies, general anxiety, and depression among adult patients with dental anxiety but with different dental-attendance patterns. Eur J Oral Sci. 2013;121(3):270–6.
7. Elvins R, Green J. The conceptualization and measurement of therapeutic alliance. An empirical review. Clin Psychol Rev. 2008;28(7):1167–87.
8. Rogers CR. The necessary and sufficient conditions of therapeutic personality change. J Consult Psychol. 1957;21:95–103.
9. Nienhuis JB, Owen J, Valentine JC, Winkeljohn Black S, Halford TC, Parazak SE, Budge S, Hilsenroth M. Therapeutic alliance, empathy, and genuineness in individual adult psychotherapy: a meta-analytic review. Psychother Res. 2018;4: 593–605.
10. Smith RC. The patient's story. Integrated patient – doctor interviewing. Boston: Little, Brown and Company; 1996.
11. Horvath AO, Luborsky L. The role of the therapeutic alliance in psychotherapy. J Consult Clin Psychol. 1993;61(4):561–73.
12. Levy KN, Ellison WD, Scott LN, Bernecker SL. Attachment style. J Clin Psychol. 2011;67(2):193–203.
13. Slade A, Holmes J. Attachment and psychotherapy. Curr Opin Psychol. 2019;25:152–6. https://doi.org/10.1016/j.copsyc.2018.06.008. Epub 2018 Jul 5. PMID: 30099208.
14. Bowlby J. Attachment and loss, vol. 2. Anxiety and anger. New York: Basic books; 1973.
15. Eli I, Uziel N, Blumensohn R, Baht R. Modulation of dental anxiety – the role of past experiences, psychopathologic traits and individual attachment patterns. Br Dent J. 2004;196:689–94.
16. Diener MJ, Monroe JM. The relationship between adult attachment style and therapeutic alliance in individual psychotherapy: a meta-analytic review. Psychotherapy (Chic). 2011;48(3):237–48.
17. Bucci S, Seymour-Hyde A, Harris A, Berry K. Client and therapist attachment styles and working Alliance. Clin Psychol Psychother. 2016;23(2):155–65.
18. Mikulincer M, Shaver PR. An attachment perspective on psychopathology. World Psychiatry. 2012;11:11–5.
19. Zachrisson A. Analytic work with adolescents. Reflections on the combination of strict method and creative intuition in psychoanalysis. Scand Psychoanal Rev. 2006;29(2):106–14.
20. Moltu C, Binder PE. The voices of fellow travellers. Experienced therapist's strategies when facing difficult therapeutic impasses. Br J Clin Psychol. 2011;50(3):250–67.
21. Pearlman LA, Saakvitne KW. Trauma and the therapist: countertransference and vicarious traumatization in psychotherapy with incest survivors. WW Norton & Co; 1995.
22. Efran J, Fauber, R. Are Specialization and Clinical Complexity Really Necessary? [Internett]. Wisconsin: Psychotherapy Networker; April 2015. Available from https://www.psychotherapynetworker.org/blog/details/998/conversational-skill-the-common-denominator-in-good.
23. Eubanks CF, Muran JC, Safran JD. Alliance rupture repair: a meta-analysis. Psychotherapy. 2018;55(4):508–19.
24. Hill CE, Knox S. Processing the therapeutic relationship. Psychother Res. 2009;19:13–29.

Oral Health Literacy

Linda Stein, Jan-Are Kolset Johnsen, and Julie Satur

Contents

5

🎓 **Learning Goals**
- To understand the concept of health literacy
- To acknowledge the prevalence of low health literacy
- To learn how to identify groups at high risk of having low health literacy
- To know how to apply strategies aimed at low oral health literacy patients

5.1   Oral Health Information

Proper and appropriate use of reliable information is essential in health care where the consequences of invalid or misunderstood health information might be highly unfavourable for patients. In clinical dental practice, most dental professionals, at some point, will experience situations where some patients do not follow the given recommendations regarding their own or their child's oral health. Even though one thinks that information and recommendations were appropriately communicated, one can be left to wonder why patients show up to the next appointment as if nothing was explained at the previous visit, and you must explain the same thing all over again. Many questions may arise: *Why do parents think bottle-feeding the three-year-old during the night is ok, even after being told it is not? Why do the periodontic patient fail to start utilising the interdental brushes we agreed on? Why did the patient not complete the prescribed antibiotic treatment?* When facing these questions and the failures related to patient adherence, it might seem like information has gone in one ear and out the other. However, the problem may be that the information failed to go in the ear in the first place. A significant amount of information is often relayed to patients, but providers seldom evaluate patient comprehension. On the one hand, the patient may lack motivation or think dental health is not important enough to change behaviour. On the other hand, perhaps the patient did not understand the information presented by the dental professional because the information did not correspond to the patient's preconditions for understanding.

In today's information-rich society, health information is available to the public from various sources. Hence, oral health professionals have numerous competitors in providing relevant information to their patients. In addition to the more traditional sources like television, newspapers, and magazines, information from the Internet is a considerable challenge. Although more information and easier access is advantageous, it places heavy demands on some people with regard to retrieving and understanding health information. By utilising the Internet, an answer to a health-related question might be just a few clicks away. However, simply knowing how to obtain the information is not enough. The ability to judge the quality of information requires skills that not all people possess – many simply rely on the number of hits that can be hundreds or thousands, or even millions for some sites on the Internet. As a result, patients might trust misleading information and make important health decisions based on sensationalised or emotionally charged stories that are not relevant to their health context. Possessing this information and deciding which information to use is demanding since it requires that the information-seeking patient should raise some questions. *Is the information reliable? Who wrote it? Is there a hidden agenda? Is it outdated? What does it mean? How does the information relate to my situation? How do I apply the knowledge?* However, to raise these questions, the patient needs a set of skills called health literacy.

5.1.1   What Is Health Literacy?

In the 1990s, American researchers found a link between health and skills such as reading and numeracy, also referred to as 'literacy'. Studies showed that individuals with poor literacy also had difficulty taking their medication correctly and had less knowledge about their health situation even though information had been provided to them. In addition, they had insufficient ability to follow up procedures they had to do at home [1]. In Europe, attention to this link between literacy and health outcomes has become more prominent since the turn of the millennium. Since it was recognised that the ability to understand information varies according to the information topic, this has been referred to as health literacy. There are numerous definitions of health literacy in the literature. A shared characteristic of these definitions is their focus on skills to obtain, process, and understand health information and services considered necessary to make appropriate decisions regarding their own or their child's health [2].

> Health literacy is linked to literacy and entails people's knowledge, motivation, and competencies to access, understand, appraise, and apply health information in order to make judgments and take decisions in everyday life concerning healthcare, disease prevention, and health promotion to maintain or improve quality of life during the life course [2].

5.1.2   The Prevalence of Low Health Literacy

No doubt that health literacy is a relatively new and exciting concept, but how common is struggling with health information? Population surveys have shown that a large proportion of adults lack basic health literacy skills. For example, up to 60% of Australian adults had problems understanding health-related materials, such as instructions on a medicine label [3]. A national survey from the United States found that 43% of American adults are at risk for low health literacy [4]. In Europe, an international study including eight countries found limited health literacy in 47% of adults [2]. The health literacy levels varied between the European countries, finding 61% of adults in Bulgaria and 29% in the Netherlands with inadequate health literacy. A recent national survey from Norway found low health literacy in 33% of the adult population [5].

These surveys have identified some predictors of poor health literacy. People with low health literacy often have poorly self-reported health and experience challenges in meeting with health professionals. People with chronic diseases, low education, financial challenges, and old age are more likely to have problems understanding health-related information [6]. The World Health Organization has recently pointed out that health literacy can play a crucial role in reducing social inequalities in health. WHO even suggests that health literacy may substantially impact individuals' health in line with the more known factors such as income, education, ethnicity, and work situation [7]. Health literacy affects people's health in three crucial areas: access to health services, the interaction between patient and health professional, and self-behaviour [8].

5.1.3   Case Presentation: A Person with Low Oral Health Literacy

Alma Peterson is a 72-year-old widow. She grew up in a remote village and ended her formal education before high school. Alma worked part-time in a diner after the children left home, but she had to retire early due to muscle aches. She is diagnosed with type 2 diabetes and hypertension. Alma has been smoking since her late teens. In general, Alma finds it challenging to adapt to the modern and digital society. She is often confused about the health-related information she reads in her magazines or hears from her friends at the local café. Alma has a somewhat complex history related to oral

health. She did not have access to oral health services regularly growing up and has experienced pain and loss of several teeth due to caries over the years. As a result, Alma avoids dental treatment and only goes if the pain is unbearable. One of her grandchildren recently commented on her bad breath, and she built the courage to make an appointment at the new dental clinic in town. The dentist diagnosed her with marginal periodontitis and referred her to a periodontal practice. The periodontist gives Alma quite a lot of information regarding the disease and the treatment plan. The dental hygienist introduces her to interdental brushes and tries to motivate her to quit smoking. Alma finds it demanding to establish new routines and is frustrated that yet another health issue has arisen. She feels that she has enough to take her hypertension medicaments and keep her new diabetes-related diet. Furthermore, she is worried that her teeth eventually will fall out and be replaced with dentures, which is the case with her elder brother.

5.2   A Modern Oral Health Model

From a historical perspective, the biomedical model of health and diseases has dominated all areas of health care and medicine [9, 10], including oral health. Although credited with the discovery of bacteria, viruses, and eventually vaccines, this model viewed disease and illness exclusively due to biological malfunctioning without considering other contributing factors [11]. Consequently, good oral health has traditionally been defined as the absence of oral diseases or physical oral deficiencies. Also, there have been several different definitions across countries and regions [12], which has made it unclear whether the term 'oral health' implies the same for oral health professionals and among the more comprehensive health communities. In the last decades, Western countries have experienced a shift towards a biopsychosocial health model [13], including psychological, behavioural, and social factors related to health and disease. In keeping with this development, the FDI World Dental Federation suggested an updated definition of oral health in 2016 [14]:

> «Oral health is multifaceted and includes the ability to speak, smile, smell, taste, touch, chew, swallow, and convey a range of emotions through facial expressions with confidence and without pain, discomfort, and disease of the craniofacial complex.»

5

Box (❑ Fig. 5.1)

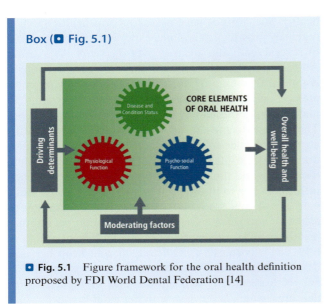

❑ **Fig. 5.1** Figure framework for the oral health definition proposed by FDI World Dental Federation [14]

'Global Oral Health aims for optimal oral health for all people and elimination of global health inequities through health promotion, disease prevention, and appropriate oral care approaches that consider common determinants and solutions and acknowledge oral health as part of overall health'.

This modern definition suggests that core elements help determine oral health status: disease and condition status, physiological function, and psychosocial function. *Disease and condition status* refers to both degrees of severity of a medical disease or condition and disease progression and conditions, including the perception of pain and discomfort. *Physiological function* refers to the capacity to perform behaviours such as talking, chewing, and swallowing. In contrast, *psychosocial functioning* refers to the relationship between oral health and psychological states that may determine whether a person interacts socially without feeling shame and uneasiness. These core elements are determined by more fundamental factors that may influence oral health, for instance, genetic and biological factors, social environment, physical environment, health behaviours, and access to healthcare services. Also, there are *moderating factors* in play that could impact a person's assessment of one's health, such as age, culture, income, experiences, expectations, and flexibility.

5.2.1 Global Oral Health

Notably, the modern definition of oral health underlines that oral health is an integral part of the general health concept, including the experience of physical and psychological wellbeing. This integration of oral health and overall health is also reflected in the recent definition of *global oral health* by the Consortium of Universities for Global Health's Global Oral Health Interest Group [15]:

Together, these definitions help us acknowledge that oral health is not an isolated concept, but a concept that coincides with other areas of health influenced by the values, norms, and attitudes found in both individuals and society. Furthermore, oral health embodies functions and aspects key to the experience of quality of life for an individual.

Perhaps most strikingly, the modern definition of oral health shifts the focus away from treating oral diseases or injuries in oral health services to acknowledging the person as a unique individual with unique experiences and needs. In this light, oral health cannot be understood as a concept that seemingly occurs in isolation within the framework of the dental office but rather as a part of all areas of the general health concept. If one considers the importance of oral health in a person's life outside of the dental office, it becomes apparent that oral health problems could influence numerous daily activities, including food intake, sleep, self-confidence, and many other specific actions and behaviours. Efforts to address these problems should arguably be multifaceted and not limited to clinical procedures or information provided within the dental office.

5.2.2 Patient Participation

Another issue worth mentioning is the emphasis on personal responsibility for one's health that is desired from health authorities. Patients' right to participate in their own health care is enshrined in the European Patient Charter [16]. Also, in line with the changes in the oral health models and society, in general, patients are expected to a more considerable degree to be an active part in the healthcare services instead of being passive recipients of health care [17]. To meet these demands, people need health literacy skills. Oral health services have a history of being paternalistic with patients trusting that oral health professionals 'know best' what to do [18], and studies indicate that patients may have strong desires to be well-informed but not necessarily want to be involved further in making decisions or problem-solving with regards to treatment choices [19].

Also, oral health professionals appear to be more critical of giving patient autonomy than dental patients are willing to take control, and dental patients seem less concerned with being involved in clinical decisions than patients from other medical areas [20]. Thus, the recent shift towards patient participation requires that both patients and health professionals acquire the mind-sets and skills necessary for this approach to be successful. For the patient, these skills include oral health literacy, and oral health professionals need to know what oral health literacy implies both within and outside the dental office.

5.3 Oral Health Literacy

Despite a large amount of research on health literacy in medicine, there has only been attention around health literacy in dentistry in the past decade. It has been recognised that the ability to understand information varies according to its content and that the person's context is crucial. While both medical and dental information is challenging for most people to understand, the context at the dental clinic differs significantly from, for example, a visit to the physician. When visiting the general practitioner for an aching shoulder, a patient can potentially walk out the door with a prescription after a few minutes without having taken off the outer jacket. In contrast, a dental patient will have to lie down in a dental chair and have instruments and cotton swabs into their mouth by oral health professionals wearing face masks and gloves.

Furthermore, as explained in ▶ Chap. 10, many patients feel uncomfortable or even anxious at the dental clinic. In sum, these aspects make the context of the dental clinical encounter unique and complex. The dental treatment situation has unique challenges compared to many other contexts where information must be disseminated, not least concerning processing new information. There are many aspects and stimuli in the clinical situation that compete for the patients' attention. For example, an anxious patient may be more concerned with observing possible threatening objects or moderating their discomfort and fear than directing attention to the information given verbally by the oral health professional. Hence, the patient does not necessarily remember what was said. Based on these challenges, oral health literacy has emerged as a separate field of research, not because there is a desire to keep the oral cavity separated from the rest of the body, but because the context is different. Oral health literacy was first defined in Healthy People 2010 by The US Department of Health and Human Services [21]:

> Oral health literacy is the degree to which individuals have the capacity to obtain, process, and understand basic oral health information and services needed to make appropriate health decisions.

It is important to note that the definition includes more than understanding – it is also about obtaining health information, interpreting it, and how this becomes the foundation for decisions that affect health. *Obtaining* oral health information can be challenging. While health personnel were the primary source of health information in the past, there are several channels for obtaining information today. TV, radio, newspapers, magazines, blogs, social media, and websites contain health information of varying quality. It can simply seem overwhelming to many people because there is so much information available.

Finding the correct information on the Internet may feel like looking for a needle in a haystack, as a simple search on the Internet can yield hundreds of thousands of sites. Health information can also be perceived as contradictory as content varies, and much of what is available in information is neither evidence-based nor written by professionals, or worse driven by commercial or non-altruistic agendas. This is not always obvious, and therefore being able to interpret health information is crucial. The definition refers to the *processing* and *understanding* of basic oral health information. Critical thinking and the ability to reflect are essential skills. Who is behind the information? Are the sources of the allegations stated? If so, are the sources valid? Is it true as long as it is health professionals or researchers who comment on something? It is not uncommon for people to base choices on something one has 'heard' from others or others 'read'. In the case presentation, we learned that Alma reads magazines and that she is sometimes confused because health information is presented differently in different magazines. She also gets upset when she hears she has periodontal disease, which caused two of her elder siblings to be edentulous. Interpretation of oral health information thus partly involves advanced metacognitive skills, and we must expect significant variation among patients. Phenomena such as scepticism towards fluoride and vaccine hesitancy can be argued to have originated in people's difficulties in revising misinformation. Although the sources of health information have increased significantly, especially since the advent of the Internet, healthcare professionals are still an essential source for many people [22]. Healthcare professionals must therefore continuously work to understand how patients are perceiving their health and interpreting the information they receive. Still, it is also of essence to help clear up misunderstandings that patients may have after, for example, searching the Internet. In the case of Alma, it would be important that the periodontist and the dental hygienist explain that a lot has happened regarding the treatment of periodontitis since her siblings were diagnosed.

As we have seen, there is a close relationship between thinking (information processing) and emotions/affect, and how this affects behaviour. Hence, cognitive capacity is a crucial prerequisite for understanding oral health. Both cognitive and affective elements and the interaction between these vary between individuals and affect the capacity to process information and make decisions. Cognitive functioning in the form of the individual's ability to acquire knowledge and intellectual thinking, so-called metacognitive skills, will be central in determining capacity. Affective elements such as values, motivation, and emotions will also be critical elements that help form the basis of oral health literacy because they affect the ability to obtain, interpret, and understand oral health information. The box below presents tasks that are typically difficult for persons with low oral health literacy.

> **Box**
> **Examples of tasks that may be difficult for a person with low oral health literacy**
> — Understanding the information on the notice card or text message
> — Figuring out how much fluoride your child requires
> — Understanding a brochure about dental erosions
> — Understanding and applying the information in a post-operative letter
> — Interpreting the sugar content in a box of cereal from the table of contents
> — Participating in choices between different substitutes for a lost tooth
> — Interpreting how to take the prescribed antibiotics

5.3.1 Factors Related to Low Health Literacy

Although one will find people with low health literacy in all groups of the population, it is essential to know which groups have the higher prevalence. So while we might categorise particular people at a population level, we must also recognise that experiences, literacy, culture and coping mechanisms, and health will also be unique to the person at an individual level. Research has identified some factors closely linked to low health literacy. Moreover, the difficulties those with decreased oral health literacy face to navigate the health system likely contribute to barriers in assessing oral health care, which could worsen existing oral conditions. Evidence suggests that oral health literacy is a mediator and not a direct factor for oral diseases [12]. Understanding what people may struggle with is essential for oral health professionals and enhances the chances of helping patients with low health literacy.

Digital skills are closely related to health literacy. In line with the changes in society in terms of how information is exchanged, banking services, social services, tax returns, job applications, etc., have become digital, and less assistance is provided face to face. This development requires more independence and specialised skills, which can be overwhelming and frustrating [7], as Alma did in the case presentation. On the other hand, digital solutions allow for the delivery of multimedia education, such as videos, voice, and print, at different reading levels, in multiple languages, using formal and informal teaching methods [23]. Furthermore, digital technologies shape how individuals and health systems interact to promote health and treat illness [24]. Therefore, the possession of general digital skills and the readiness to adopt digital health services are essential components of health literacy. However, competence in searching for digital health information is a task that may be difficult to use digital health technology and systems as a patient or caregiver. The national survey from Norway [5] found that digital skills varied according to age, level of education, and long-term illness.

There is evidence that the use of digital media for health information is more common among those who are young, educated, and wealthy [25]. It may not be surprising that digital skills are more insufficient in the older population. Moreover, age alone is a predictor of low health literacy [6]. Medical developments have led to an increase in the number of older people in the population, and today most older people have teeth. In addition to cognitive and physical impairment, it is common for older people to live with chronic diseases which require adherence to medication and medical appointments. Taking care of one's teeth may also be more challenging as the year passes. Teani et al. found that dissatisfaction with oral health in older people is a complex issue associated with oral health literacy [26]. Also, younger people with long-term illnesses have been found to have lower health literacy [6]. Knowing your medical situation and what health-promoting behaviour is required to control your disease is essential to prolong life and increase the quality of life. Therefore, it is worrying that many of these people have low health literacy.

Findings from the European population survey [6] suggest a social gradient for health literacy. Specific social groups contained higher proportions of people with limited health literacy, like those who had not finished high school and those experiencing a difficult financial situation. It is not surprising that there is a social health literacy gradient linking low health literacy with poorer health outcomes, which holds across lower-income and minority population groups [27]. A national survey describing health literacy in immigrant populations in Norway found a larger proportion of immigrants with low health literacy compared to the general population [28]. In most samples of immigrants, low health literacy was associated with low educational attainment and low economic status. The relationship is complex, but it is consistently reported in national surveys that the health literacy gradient closely follows the social gradient in health which is associated with other indicators of social and economic disadvantage. Understanding the relationships between social inequality and health literacy enables interventions that can support the ability to mediate the impact of social disadvantage [25].

There is evidence that indigenous people, at a population level, have lower health literacy than non-indigenous peoples [25, 27, 29]. Colonisation and disempowerment continue to significantly impact indigenous people on education, language, imposed cultures around health, social, and economic disadvantage, and lack of trust in mainstream health services. Shame and stigma arising from racism and inequality reduce self-efficacy and participation in health services and self-care behaviours. Poor self-efficacy – the belief in one's own competence to understand and cope – is linked to poor literacy [30]. Situations of duress compromise people's ability to absorb information as they focus on managing their 'flight or fight' responses and cope – dental care visits almost always generate duress or stress, and where trust is an issue, this will be multiplied. This can also be magnified when dealing with people who are perceived as intimidating. The cumulative effects of cultural dislocation, duress, and poor self-efficacy combine to challenge the ability to absorb and use the information and perform self-care. Oral health literacy is thus compromised [30].

It is, however, important to recognise that there is great diversity among indigenous people and immigrants. Like that of all people, their health is a product of a range of life course experiences and environmental supports and impacts that produce particular cognitions, skills sets, coping mechanisms, and cultural world views. It is essential to remind ourselves that oral health literacy is the ability of people to obtain, process, understand, and integrate health information into practice. For many, this may require reading and comprehension skills. Still, for people whose cultural background and primary language are not the same as ours, it also requires an ability to acquire and process information in culturally located ways [29]. While reading, writing, and digital skills are important, storytelling, social learning, visual, and verbal learning are more intrinsic and important for some people. In this situation, health literacy requires comprehension of the dominant language and cultural interpretation and re-location and integration into belief systems that may differ from the dominant culture and language.

5.3.2 Oral Health Literacy in a Clinical Context

In a study on patient participation in medical encounters, patients with limited health literacy skills were significantly less likely to ask questions, request additional services, or seek new information [31]. Systematic reviews regarding health literacy concluded that patients with limited health literacy have difficulty participating in shared decision-making and have poorer disease self-management [32, 33]. Without appropriate precautions or support from the oral health professional, an individuals' limited oral health literacy may compromise their ability to engage fully in healthcare interactions and participate in shared decision-making will be difficult.

Oral health literacy research has found a relationship between insufficient oral health knowledge and oral health literacy [34, 35]. Also, people with poorer self-reported oral health [36] and worse oral health-related quality of life had lower levels of health literacy [37].

Clinical studies have shown that people with limited oral health literacy had poorer periodontal health [38–40], a higher number of lactobacillus in saliva [35], and a higher number of decayed and filled teeth [36]. A significant relationship between low oral health literacy and oral health behaviour have also been found [41, 42].

Previous research indicates that patients with low oral health literacy are more likely to miss healthcare appointments than patients with higher health literacy levels [43–45]. Oral health professionals should use multiple methods to confirm appointments and ask the individual patient for their preferred method. Furthermore, Jones et al. [46] found that people with low oral health literacy visit the dentist less frequently than people with higher oral health literacy. Furthermore, Silva-Junior et al. [47] found that low literacy patients had higher use of emergency oral health services.

Parents and other caregivers are essential for children's oral health. They are in charge of meals, snacking, and other health-related behaviours like tooth brushing and visits to the dental clinic. A higher prevalence of untreated dental caries was found among preschool children whose caregivers had a low degree of oral health literacy [48, 49]. Vann et al. [46] found that children of mothers with adequate oral health literacy had better oral health and oral health habits than children of mothers with poor oral health literacy. Marquillier et al. [50] suggest that parents' knowledge and oral health literacy are the key predictors to be preferentially targeted to reduce social inequalities in health. Therefore, oral health professionals must continue to educate parents and caregivers when visiting their child's dental clinic.

> **Box**
> **Research has identified factors associated with oral health literacy**
> - Parents' or caregiver's oral health literacy affects children's oral health status and oral health behaviour
> - Adults with higher oral health literacy have better oral health behaviour
> - People with low oral health literacy have insufficient oral health knowledge
> - Low health literacy patients have more infrequent check-ups, more missed appointments, and higher use of emergency oral health services
> - Oral health status like periodontitis, dental caries, lactobacillus in saliva, decayed teeth, filled teeth are associated with low oral health literacy
> - People with low oral health literacy have poorer self-reported oral health and worse oral health-related quality of life

5.3.3 What Can Oral Health Professionals Do?

On the one hand, we now know that the patients' oral health literacy is a barrier to understanding information. On the other hand, it can be argued that poor communication skills or lack of adaptation of advanced health information by the oral health professional are an equally important barrier to patients' comprehension of health information in a clinical context. A national study in the United States found that three out of four dentists pointed out shortcomings in their competence in patient communication due to a lack of training during their education [51]. This emphasises the importance of teaching patient communication and training such skills in clinical practice in the education of oral health professionals. It is essential to underline that patients have a right to participate in decisions about current examination and treatment methods. However, comprehension of health information is a prerequisite to participating in such decisions and taking responsibility for one's health and the health of children/relatives. Therefore, healthcare professionals must adapt the information about the individual's health to the patient's prerequisites for understanding. Oral health professionals must consequently adjust the information to the patient's oral health literacy. Health literacy influences our patients' health in many ways, including access to health services, the interaction between patients and health professionals, and individual behaviour and choices [8].

5.3.4 Strategies Aimed at Low Oral Health Literacy Patients

The first step in meeting the challenges with low oral health literacy patients at the dental clinic is to improve communication [52]. For optimal communication, however, both the patient and the dental professional need communication skills. Many factors help determine how good one is at communicating, including personality, language skills, listening ability, and formulation ability. There is a limit to what we can do at the dental clinic to change the patient's communication skills, but we can adjust ourselves and adapt to the patient's prerequisites for understanding. This applies to both assumptions or conditions that may affect the dissemination of knowledge; for example, the patient is short of time and is stressed, and the patient's 'inner', and perhaps more stable, prerequisites such as level of knowledge and personality. Dental professionals must help patients improve or maintain their oral health, and the relationship between patients and the oral health professionals is crucial for this to be successful. The experience of understanding information provided while also being understood in return is a fundamental component of a relationship of trust between oral health professionals and patients. It is common to assume that understanding health information indirectly affects health status because better choices can be made regarding health, whether for prevention or treatment purposes. It is also conceivable that experiencing understanding and trust in the relationship between the oral health professional and the patient has direct health effects by reducing stress and discomfort associated with the ailments. Spending time creating a positive relationship with the patient before saying 'open your mouth, please' is a valuable investment that can positively affect the patient's attitudes and personal efforts, both short and long term. There is a need to ensure that two-way communication and learning lead the interaction – that the practitioner will learn from the patient about their cultural understanding and interpretation as a starting point. Enabling this requires openness, empathy, respect, and an ability to 'walk alongside' the person, especially when culture and language context is different from our own. Collaboration and participatory approaches – a shared interest – are needed to enable two-way learning [27]. Health literacy from the patients' world view can be fostered when we provide a clinical environment that is easy to navigate that truly enables shared and informed decision-making and autonomy – that which is culturally safe for the patient – for without cultural safety, there is no clinical safety or health literacy [29, 30].

A patient-centred approach is recognised as an essential dimension in today's healthcare services. Ask me 3™ [53] is a patient education programme designed to promote communication between healthcare providers and patients to improve health outcomes. The programme encourages patients to understand the answers to three questions: (1) What is my main problem? (2) What do I need to do? (3) Why is it important for me to do this? Oral health professionals should always encourage their patients to understand the answers to these three questions. Studies show that people who understand health instructions make fewer mistakes when taking their medicine or preparing for a medical procedure. They may also get well sooner or be able to manage a chronic health condition better.

In a study by Toibin et al. [53], patients exposed to the Ask Me *3*™ intervention, even for a very short time, felt entitled and empowered to question and seek clarity on issues that concern them during healthcare consultations – facilitating parity in the therapeutic relationship. The questions patients asked during consultation highlighted their concerns and thus elicited targeted answers, while the teach-back confirmed how much the patient understood. This method may improve treatment outcomes with fewer dental visits.

Still, a recent systematic review has revealed a lack of understanding of the importance of patient-centred care in the dental health service [54]. A patient-centred approach will help shift the focus away from pure biomedical thinking and more towards biopsychosocial thinking, which recognises the patient's autonomy and integrity. In this way, oral health professionals can be sensitive to the patient's individual preferences, needs, and values that must be considered in all decisions. In addition, research suggests that patient-centred approaches lead to increased patient satisfaction [55]. Furthermore, patient-centeredness may increase job satisfaction among healthcare professionals and contribute to a decline in the number of complaints directed at healthcare professionals [56].

Box

Researchers recommend selecting sensitive measures and methods to patients' oral health literacy [53, 57, 58].

Terminology and oral communication	Speaking a simple language free of difficult dental words, avoiding closed-ended questions (e.g. yes/no questions), facilitating the patient's participation in the conversation, and opening up to questions from the patient
Visual aids	Utilising models, posters, X-rays, and photos to supplement oral communication
Digital aids	Multimedia education, such as videos, voice, and print, at different reading levels, in multiple languages
Teach-back or 'show me'	After explaining or demonstrating, you can ask the patient to show you or teach you back to ensure the message or procedure is understood
Ask me 3	A summary with the patient by asking these questions: (1) What is the main challenge of your oral health? (2) What should be done? (3) Why is this important?

A written summary can serve as a to-do list that patients can take home to repeat the most critical elements from the consultation. This can be used actively to invest in the ending described in more detail under 'the four good habits' presented in ▶ Chap. 6.

5.3.5 A Model of Oral Health Literacy as a Risk

Several models describe how to deal with the challenges of poor health literacy in clinical practice, but few of these have been empirically validated in clinical contexts. The conceptual model of health literacy as a risk proposed by Nutbeam [8] was tested in a clinical dental context in an RCT study by Stein et al. [59]. Nutbeam's model was adapted to the oral health setting, as explained in ☐ Fig. 5.2.

According to this model, an 'oral health literacy friendly' dental clinic has employees who recognise that many people have poor oral health literacy. The employees are then aware of the challenges this can entail. Even before the patient has arrived at the clinic, the dental

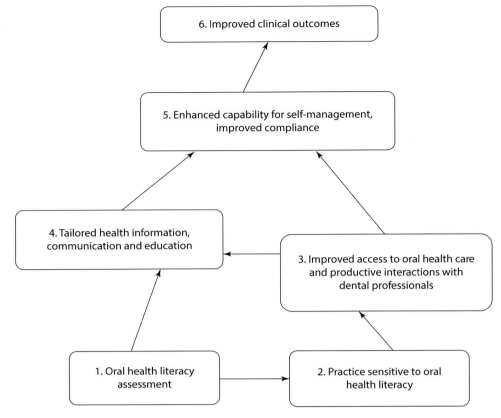

◼ **Fig. 5.2** *The conceptual model of health literacy as a risk,* proposed by Nutbeam [8]. (Adapted to oral health literacy by Stein et al. [59])

nurse has thought about this when contacting patients or paediatric patients' parents by telephone, and also when formulating the text on the notice card or the content of the text message. The dental nurse also remembers this when contacting patients in the waiting room or the reception. The model is based on assessing the patient's health literacy level. This is measured with validated methods for research purposes, but these are too extensive and time-consuming to use in clinical practice. However, an alternative is using the characteristics of people with low health literacy to pinpoint individual patients that may be at risk.

One can thus expect to find more people with low oral health literacy in certain groups of the population, such as the elderly, the chronically ill, the low educated, and the financially disadvantaged. Therefore, paying particular attention to these patients is essential, although it is essential to remember that low oral health literacy exists in all populations. Perhaps the most crucial task will be to examine oral health literacy by talking to the patient and carers and listening to what they tell you. Once the patient's oral health literacy has been assessed, communication, health information, and training in oral hygiene articles can be adapted to the patient's level. Other factors such as age, fine motor skills, and language skills must also be considered. The model further states that individualised, tailored communication

and education will lead to the patient having increased opportunities to take care of their teeth, promoting oral health, and preventing oral health diseases. The main aim of the model is that the described measures will lead to better oral health for the individual. The RCT study by Stein et al., where this model was tested, found that the intervention group had significantly improved plaque control and gingival conditions compared with the control group 6 months after baseline. This may indicate that poor oral health literacy as a risk factor for poor oral health can be reduced by using this model in clinical practice.

Summary

Oral literacy influences our patients' health in many ways, including access to oral health services, the interaction between patients and health professionals, and individual behaviour and choices. Unfortunately, many patients have poor oral health literacy, perhaps as many as every other or third. People with low oral health literacy often find examination and treatment at the dental clinic challenging, especially understanding verbal messages from the dental team. They may also find it challenging to interpret and evaluate the reliability of dental health information from various sources, such as the Internet. Individuals with poor oral health literacy are found in all groups within the population. Still, there are more among the elderly, the chronically ill, the low educated, and people in a financially difficult situation.

At the dental clinic, one must expect to communicate and listen to the patient to assess the patient's oral health literacy. Patients have the right to participate in the choice between, for example, various tooth replacements. There are several steps oral health professionals can take to increase the likelihood that people with poor oral health literacy will understand important information and instructions. It is recommended to use visual aids in communication with patients and use the teach-back method to check if the patients master the use of, for example, interdental brushes. The Ask me 3 method may be used to check if the patient has understood what you have talked about. (1) What is the main challenge of your oral health? (2) What should be done? (3) Why is this important? A summary in the form of bullet points adapted to the individual patient can be a to-do list and take-home message. To fully address low oral health literacy challenges, making health information easier must be a priority for oral health professionals, the health sector, and the authorities.

References

1. Parker R. Health literacy: a challenge for American patients and their health care providers. Health Promot Int. 2000;15:277–83.
2. Sørensen K, Van den Broucke S, Fullam J, Doyle G, Pelikan J, Slonska Z, Brand H. Helath literacy and public health: a systematic review and integration of definitions and models. BMC Public Health. 2012;12:80.
3. Australian Bureau of Statistics. Adult literacy and life skills survey, summary results, Australia. Canberra: ABS; 2008.
4. Kutner M, Greenburg E, Jin Y, Paulsen C. The health literacy of America's adults: results from the 2003 national assessment of adult literacy. NCES 2006-483. National Center for Education Statistics. 2006.
5. Le C, Finbråten HS, Pettersen KS, Joranger P, Guttersrud Ø (2021) Health Literacy in the Norwegian Population. English Summary. In Befolkningens helsekompetanse, del I. The International Health Literacy Population Survey 2019–2021 (HLS19) – et samarbeidsprosjekt med nettverket M-POHL tilknyttet WHO-EHII. The Norwegian Directorate of Health.
6. Sørensen K, Pelikan JM, Röthlin F, Ganahl K, Slonska Z, Doyle G, Fullam J, Kondilis B, Agrafiotis D, Uiters E, Falcon M. Health literacy in Europe: comparative results of the European health literacy survey (HLS-EU). Eur J Pub Health. 2015;25(6):1053–8.
7. Apfel F, Tsouros AD. Health literacy: the solid facts. https://apps.who.int/iris/bitstream/handle/10665/128703/e96854.pdf Accessed 15 May 2021.
8. Nutbeam D. The evolving concept of health literacy. Soc Sci Med. 2008;67(12):2072–8.
9. Farre A, Rapley T. The new old (and old new) medical model: four decades navigating the biomedical and psychosocial understandings of health and illness. Healthcare. 2017;5(4):88. https://doi.org/10.3390/healthcare5040088.
10. Wade DT, Halligan PW. Do biomedical models of illness make for good healthcare systems? BMJ. 2004;329(7479):1398–401. https://doi.org/10.1136/bmj.329.7479.1398.
11. Towner E. In: Schou L, Blinkhorn A, editors. The history of dental health education: a case study of Britain. Oxford: Oxford University Press; 1993.
12. Lee JY. Lower oral health literacy may lead to poorer oral health outcomes. J Evid Based Dent Pract. 2018;18(3):255–7.
13. Yevlahova D, Satur J. Models for individual oral health promotion and their effectiveness: a systematic review. Aust Dent J. 2009;54(3):190–7.
14. Glick M, Williams DM, Kleinman DV, Vujicic M, Watt RG, Weyant RJ. A new definition for oral health developed by the FDI World Dental Federation opens the door to a universal definition of oral health. JADA. 2016;147(12):915–7.
15. Seymour B, James Z, Karhade DS, Barrow J, Pruneddu A, Anderson NK, Mossey P, Task Force for the Definition of Global Health. A definition of global oral health: an expert consensus approach by the Consortium of Universities for Global Health's Global Oral Health Interest Group. Glob Health Action. 2020;13(1):1814001. https://doi.org/10.1080/16549716.2020.1814001.
16. O'Mathúna DP, Scott AP, McAuley A, Walsh-Daneshmandi A, Daly B. Health care rights and responsibilities: a review of the European charter of patient's rights. Irish Patients Association; 2005.
17. European Commission: Together for health: a strategic approach for the EU 2008–2013. Com (2007) 630 final, 2007.
18. Schiavo JH. Oral health literacy in the dental office: the unrecognised patient risk factor. Am Dent Hyg Assoc. 2011;85(4):248–55.
19. Schouten BC, Eijkman MAJ, Hoogstraten J. Information and participation preferences of dental patients. J Dent Res. 2004;83(12):961–5. https://doi.org/10.1177/154405910408301214.
20. Benecke M, Kasper J, Heesen C, et al. Patient autonomy in dentistry: demonstrating the role for shared decision making. BMC Med Inform Decis Mak. 2020;20:318. https://doi.org/10.1186/s12911-020-01317-5.
21. US Department of Health and Human Services. A national call to action to promote oral health. Rockville: US Department of Health and Human Services, Public Health Service, Centers for Disease Control and Prevention, National Institutes of Health, National Institutes of Dental and Craniofacial Research; 2003.
22. Kennedy A, Gask L, Rogers A. Training professionals to engage with and promote self-management. Health Educ Res. 2005;20:567–78.
23. Conard S. Best practices in digital health literacy. Int J Cardiol. 2019;292:277–9.
24. Azzopardi-Muscat N, Sørensen K. Towards an equitable digital public health era: promoting equity through a health literacy perspective. Eur J Pub Health. 2019;29(Suppl 3):13–7. Baskaradoss JK. Relationship between oral health literacy and oral health status. BMC Oral Health. 2018;18(1):1–6.
25. Nutbeam D, Lloyd JE. Understanding and responding to health literacy as a social determinant of health. Annu Rev Public Health. 2021;42:159–73.
26. Tenani CF, De Checchi MH, Bado FM, Ju X, Jamieson L, Mialhe FL. Influence of oral health literacy on dissatisfaction with oral health among older people. Gerodontology. 2020;37(1):46–52.

27. Nash S, Arora A. Interventions to improve health literacy among Aboriginal and Torres Strait Islander Peoples: a systematic review. BMC Public Health. 2021;21(1):1–5.

28. Le C, Finbråten HS, Pettersen KS, Joranger P, Guttersrud Ø. Health Literacy in Five Immigrant Populations in Norway: Pakistan, Poland, Somalia, Turkey, and Vietnam. English Summary. In Helsekompetansen i fem innvandrerpopulasjoner i Norge: Pakistan, Polen, Somalia, Tyrkia og Vietnam. Befolkningens helsekompetanse, del II. The Norwegian Directorate of Health. 2021.

29. Horowitz AM, Kleinman DV, Atchison KA, Weintraub JA, Rozier RG. The evolving role of health literacy in improving oral health. In: Health literacy in clinical practice and public health. IOS Press; 2020. p. 95–114.

30. Jones K, Brennan DS, Parker EJ, Mills H, Jamieson L. Does self-efficacy mediate the effect of oral health literacy on self-rated oral health in an indigenous population? J Public Health Dent. 2016;76(4):350–5.

31. Katz MG, Jacobson TA, Veledar E, Kripalani S. Patient literacy and question-asking behavior during the medical encounter: a mixed-methods analysis. J Gen Intern Med. 2007;22(6):782–6.

32. Easton P, Entwistle VA, Williams B. Health in the 'hidden population' of people with low literacy. A systematic review of the literature. BMC Public Health. 2010;10(1):1–0.

33. Berkman ND, Sheridan SL, Donahue KE, Halpern DJ, Crotty K. Low health literacy and health outcomes: an updated systematic review. Ann Intern Med. 2011;155(2):97–107.

34. Hom JM, Lee JY, Divaris K, Baker AD, Vann WF Jr. Oral health literacy and knowledge among patients who are pregnant for the first time. J Am Dent Assoc. 2012;143(9):972–80.

35. Stein L, Pettersen KS, Bergdahl M, Bergdahl J. Development and validation of an instrument to assess oral health literacy in Norwegian adult dental patients. Acta Odontol Scand. 2015;73(7):530–8.

36. Lee JY, Divaris K, Baker AD, Rozier RG, Vann WF Jr. The relationship of oral health literacy and self-efficacy with oral health status and dental neglect. Am J Public Health. 2012;102(5):923–9.

37. Lee JY, Rozier RG, Lee SY, Bender D, Ruiz RE. Development of a word recognition instrument to test health literacy in dentistry: the REALD-30–a brief communication. J Public Health Dent. 2007;67(2):94–8.

38. Wehmeyer MM, Corwin CL, Guthmiller JM, Lee JY. The impact of oral health literacy on periodontal health status. J Public Health Dent. 2014;74(1):80–7.

39. Baskaradoss JK. Relationship between oral health literacy and oral health status. BMC Oral Health. 2018;18(1):1–6.

40. Timková S, Klamárová T, Kovaľová E, Novák B, Kolarčik P, Madarasová Gecková A. Health literacy associations with periodontal disease among Slovak adults. Int J Environ Res Public Health. 2020;17(6):2152.

41. Sukhabogi JR, Doshi D, Vadlamani M, Rahul V. Association of oral health literacy with oral health behavior and oral health outcomes among adult dental patients. Indian J Dent Res. 2020;31(6):835.

42. Mohammadi TM, Malekmohammadi M, Hajizamani HR, Mahani SA. Oral health literacy and its determinants among adults in Southeast Iran. Euro J Dent. 2018;12(03):439–42.

43. Baskaradoss JK. The association between oral health literacy and missed dental appointments. J Am Dent Assoc. 2016;147(11):867–74.

44. Miller-Matero LR, Clark KB, Brescacin C, Dubaybo H, Willens DE. Depression and literacy are important factors for missed appointments. Psychol Health Med. 2016;21(6):686–95.

45. Holtzman JS, Atchison KA, Gironda MW, Radbod R, Gornbein J. The association between oral health literacy and failed appointments in adults attending a university-based general dental clinic. Community Dent Oral Epidemiol. 2014;42(3):263–70.

46. Jones M, Lee JY, Rozier RG. Oral health literacy among adult patients seeking dental care. J Am Dent Assoc. 2007;138(9):1199–208.

47. Silva-Junior MF, Rosário de Sousa MD, Batista MJ. Health literacy on oral health practice and condition in an adult and elderly population. Health Promot Int. 2021;36(4):933–42.

48. Montes GR, Bonotto DV, Ferreira FM, Menezes JV, Fraiz FC. Caregiver's oral health literacy is associated with prevalence of untreated dental caries in preschool children. Cien Saude Colet. 2019;24(7):2737–44.

49. Khodadadi E, Niknahad A, Sistani MM, Motallebnejad M. Parents' oral health literacy and its impact on their children's dental health status. Electron Physician. 2016;8(12):3421.

50. Marquillier T, Lombrail P, Azogui-Lévy S. Social inequalities in oral health and early childhood caries: how can they be effectively prevented? A scoping review of disease predictors. Revue D'epidemiologie et de Sante Publique. 2020;68(4):201–14.

51. Rozier RG, Horowitz AM, Podschun G. Dentist-patient communication techniques used in the United States: the results of a national survey. J Am Dent Assoc. 2011;142(5):518–30.

52. Green JA, Gonzaga AM, Cohen ED, Spagnoletti CL. Addressing health literacy through clear health communication: a training program for internal medicine residents. Patient Educ Couns. 2014;95(1):76–82.

53. Toibin M, Pender M, Cusack T. The effect of a healthcare communication intervention—ask me 3; on health literacy and participation in patients attending physiotherapy. Eur J Phys. 2017;19(Suppl 1):12–4.

54. Mills I, Frost J, Cooper C, Moles DR, Kay E. Patient-centred care in general dental practice-a systematic review of the literature. BMC Oral Health. 2014;14(1):1–3.

55. Epstein RM, Mauksch L, Carroll J, Jaen CR. Have you really addressed your patient's concerns? Fam Pract Manag. 2008;15(3):35.

56. Irwin RS, Richardson ND. Patient-focused care: using the right tools. Chest. 2006;130(1):73S–82S.

57. Schiavo R. Health communication: from theory to practice. San Fransisco, CA: Wiley; 2013.

58. DeWalt DA, Broucksou KA, Hawk V, Brach C, Hink A, Rudd R, Callahan L. Developing and testing the health literacy universal precautions toolkit. Nurs Outlook. 2011;59(2):85–94.

59. Stein L, Bergdahl M, Pettersen KS, Bergdahl J. Effects of the conceptual model of health literacy as a risk: a randomised controlled trial in a clinical dental context. Int J Environ Res Public Health. 2018;15(8):1630.

Communication in Dentistry: The Four Habits Model

Jorun Torper, Kjetil Strøm, Ann Catrin Høyvik and Tiril Willumsen

Contents

6

Learning Goals

- To learn the practice of structured, targeted and effective dental consultations.
- To learn and practise the Four Habits Model and its underlying techniques and skills for dental visits.
- To get insight into the overall principles and prerequisites for patient-centred clinical communication.
- To understand and practise basic verbal and non-verbal communication skills.
- To increase reflection and self-awareness of own communication in daily clinical practice.

6.1 Why Is Learning Communication Skills Important?

There are many reasons for the importance of developing good communication skills. Proper communication skills have implications for patient satisfaction, development and maintenance of dental fear and whether patients follow the advice we give them (compliance) [1, 2]. It may also prevent patient complaints. Thus, in order to inhabit the role as a dental professional, one must learn to communicate effectively, but at the same time empathetically. Learning the professional tools is not sufficient; they also need to be integrated into one's own personal style. This is necessary to be credible to patients. Proper communication skills are also important for a professional relationship with patients as well as for satisfaction in the professional life. The dentist and patient should have a professional relationship that is based on these basic factors:

- The dentist should help the patient
- The relationship has the character of an assignment
- The assignment is of limited duration
- The dentist is paid
- The dentist has a duty of confidentiality
- The dentist adheres to norms and ethical values applicable to his profession.
- The relationship and dialogue between the dentist and the patient is not of private nature [3, 4].

> **Box**
> Overarching requirements for professional communication for dentists are:
> 1. Communication should be targeted
> 2. The dentist shall be given sufficient information to provide proper treatment
> 3. The patient shall be given sufficient information to cope with the dental situation and oral diseases
> 4. Consultations should be time-effective and with the least amount of resources

6.1.1 Patient-Centred Communication

In today's Western culture, the biopsychosocial model prevails in medicine. This model combines information on biological, psychological and social elements in the understanding of disease development and treatment (see ▶ Chap. 1). To obtain such information, we use the "patient-centered clinical method" [5, 6]. This method has been developed and practised during the last decades and involves, among other things, to explore both the disease and the patient's experience of the disease, and to work out common understanding (common ground) with the patient. Medical research has repeatedly demonstrated that the patient-centred approach is associated with improved diagnostic quality, therapeutic alliance, patient satisfaction and also with reduction of emotional distress for both the patient and the health professional [5, 7].

At Kaiser, a U.S. health organisation with ten million Americans, tailored training programmes were implemented for specialised physicians. The method gave a good and lasting effect on both the doctor's own sense of coping and patient satisfaction. In addition, these doctors spent their consultation time more effectively [8].

Within medicine, several communication models have been published in the patient-centred tradition. They represent frameworks for the dividing of a medical consultation into phases, where the basic repertoire of task-focused and relationship-building skills integrates in different ways during the interview [9, 10].

Communication methods are relatively simple to learn but can often be more difficult to use in daily practice. The Four Habits Model [11] is a method that has proved to be easy to learn, recall and practise in everyday clinical life. The method aims to make the consultation more effective and has been validated in several medical research projects [8, 12–14].

The Four Habits Model is also adapted for use in dental visits [15] as described later in this chapter.

In everyday clinical life, there are many considerations that need to be simultaneously taken care of. In practice, a patient-centred clinical method requires two mindsets to run in parallel. The "task-focused" mindset keeps control of clinical/dental quality and effectiveness. The "patient-centred" mindset keeps focus on the patient's ailments, perceptions, feelings and expectations, and works on building a good relationship.

Most dental visits have limited time for communication and trust-building, since verbal communication is inhibited by oral examination or treatment. In this context it is extremely important to use the relatively limited time to communicate in a targeted and professional manner. An established relationship may easily be destroyed if the dentist lacks self-awareness or overlooks signals from the patient. Here, both what is said (verbal communication) and body language (non-verbal communication) are of great importance.

6.1.2 Basic Principles of Dentist-Patient Communication

It is essential for professional communication to respect all patients as unique individuals. Patients meet for a dental visit with different treatment needs, ailments, concerns and expectations. At the same time, they present with different personalities and life experiences into the treatment room in the form of vulnerability and psychological wounds as well as different knowledge, attitudes and resources.

An essential part of the dentist-patient relationship is the dentist's ability and willingness to be open-minded and empathetic. It is important to never forget that dentistry is performed in an area experienced as intimate and private. The mouth is often associated with feelings such as insecurity, shame and helplessness, as well as suspicion and aggression. A competent dentist is able to manage the patient's various feelings and act professionally in front of them (see ► Chap. 1).

Dental professionals also have their own personality and life experiences. Some dentists are more sensitive and have a greater capacity for compassion than others. The capacity for establishing contact and trust differs. However, no matter how naturally gifted you are to talk to or connect with people, patient communication is still something you need to constantly train and practise to obtain competence. Self-awareness and ability to self-criticism are important characteristics in the development of this competence. A dentist should be conscious of his/her own feelings and how his/her behaviour affects other people.

Box

"To view the patient from the inside and yourself from the outside".

Exercise for daily practice: Try to view yourself through the patient's eyes and ask yourself:

Does the patient, in this very moment, have the experience that
- I am interested?
- I care?
- I want to listen and understand?
- I accept and respect him/her?
- He/she can feel safe here?

6.1.3 Autonomy and Informed Consent

All health care should be voluntary and justified in the interest of the patient, and patient autonomy is a fundamental ethical value and principle. The concept of autonomy means that the patient shall have the right to resist the authority of the dentist and to be allowed to make his/her own decisions. In other words, the patient must experience control and predictability during the treatment planning, as well as during operative treatment.

Prior to all dental treatments where multiple treatment options are available, an informed consent must be obtained from the patient.

Three components must be present for a patient to give informed consent:

> *Disclosure* requires that the dentist gives the patient sufficient information to make an autonomous decision. This includes relevant information about diagnoses and treatment options including advantages, disadvantages, costs and patient responsibilities. All information given must be adapted to the patient's level of understanding to ensure that he/she understands the information provided. This kind of understanding may be referred to as oral health literacy and is described in more detail in ► Chap. 5.

> *Capacity* pertains to the ability of the patient to both understand the information provided and make decisions. Examples of patients without capacity to consent are children, mentally disabled patients and patients with mental disorders (e.g. psychosis, dementia).

> *Voluntariness* The consent shall be given without pressure. Dental professionals can deliberately or unconsciously put indirect pressure on patients if they do not have proper communication routines (for example, if the dental professional has insufficient focus on the patient's perspective).

It is the dentist's job to ensure that the patient has understood the information provided and that the consent has been given voluntarily. It is also important that the consent should be consistent, that is, the patient should have enough time to make decisions. In the case of major decisions, the patient's final decision should not be made on the same day that he/she receives information regarding the options [16].

An informed consent implies that the consent is confirmed by an active action. The consent of the patient may be oral or written, but it must be recorded that the consent has been given, what consent has been given and to whom the consent has been given.

6.1.4 A Good Situation for History-Taking

A treatment room should protect the patient's privacy. To make patients feel comfortable enough to talk about their problems, the room should be as soundproof as possible. Positioning and distance are also important. One can roughly divide this into four zones: A distance of more than 4 metres signals the absence of a personal relationship. A distance between 1.5 and 4 metres signals personal contact but does not invite confidentiality. A distance of 0.75–1.5 metres signals proximity and allows for familiarity, while a distance of less than 0.75 metres most often is within a person's intimate zone where one is selective with whom to admit. If someone enters the intimate zone without invitation, one will instinctively move backwards to a less invasive distance.

The ideal distance in a professional interview will, therefore, be about 1–1.5 metres. Dentists can become unperceptive to the intimacy of a closer distance because they have become accustomed to working so close to their patients. It is important to remember that a patient who sits in the treatment chair has no possibility to move backwards to obtain a less invasive distance.

The possibility of eye contact is good, but one should avoid being seated directly in front of the patient. If so, the eye contact may be perceived invasive.

To be positioned at the same level contributes to equality. If the patient is seated lower than the dentist during a dialogue, he/she will instinctively feel inferior. Usually patients are placed directly in the dental chair when arriving in a dental clinic. It is important to begin with the chair in an upright position. This will give the patient an experience of sitting both comfortably and at the same eye level as the dentist. It should also be noted that with some patients such as patients with dental fear, it may be advantageous to speak in more neutral environments. This can be sitting on a regular chair by the dentist's desk, or ideally in a separate, neutral room.

6.1.5 Attentive Presence

An important part of patient communication is to be well prepared. The dentist should be updated on the dental record, as well as other relevant information. Such information may be, for example, whether the crown has arrived from the dental technician, the dental nurse is available for assistance or the risk of being interrupted by other enquiries during the visit.

In order to see, understand and react to patient experiences, the dentist needs to be mentally present. To manage this, it is important to put aside private, administrative and other professional matters before receiving a patient. It is important to train the ability to be attentively present. It involves being able to turn off disruptive mental wandering, stress and other personal emotions when meeting the patient.

6.1.6 The Professional Interview

Dentist-patient communication is neither an informal conversation where the dialogue flows freely nor where both parts talk about themselves. The communication is part of a professional relationship. In a dental visit, it is the dentist who is responsible for keeping focus on the task and for organising the exchange of information in an efficient way. At the same time, the dentist is responsible for building and maintaining relationship and trust. A clear and targeted structure built on these principles strengthens the confidence of the patient.

Professional communication has been compared to playing jazz [17]. The chords (communication skills) must be present in the background in order to improvise successfully. These skills (chords) need to be rehearsed and practised until one instinctively uses them in all situations including situations with high level of stress. It is important to remember that only when these skills are integrated into the personal style of the dentist (improvisation), he/she appears credible to the patient.

6.2 Communication Skills

Basic communication skills consist of two main categories, non-verbal (body language) and verbal skills.

The first moments of the dental visit are significant to establish relation and trust, which makes awareness of body language especially important. Our body continuously expresses something, whether we speak or not. This happens subconsciously and is very revealing. Body language overrides what we say, telling patients the truth about our feelings and attitudes, such as respect, interest and care. In fact, it only takes from about 0.25–6 seconds for patients to form a perception of our credibility, warmth, strength, competence, etc. [18]. This is especially crucial when meeting a new patient. But even an acquainted patient will be aware of the dentist's initial body language, to read his mood, stress level etc. It may be difficult to repair a bad first impression, so it is important to pay attention from the very first moment.

Facial expression, especially eye contact, expresses the most about who we are and what we feel. The gaze should be attentive but not seem invasive. We adapt to this concept by adjusting the angle between the dentist and the patient to make the patient feel comfortable. Positioning is also important. One should adapt height and distance to make sure the patient sits comfortably at an equal level during all dialogue phases of a dental visit.

Physical contact may be perceived as a strong signal. A handshake can mean a lot, especially in the face of new patients, and can signal both interest and equality. Other types of physical contact may be more problematic. For sensitive patients, a gentle touch from the dentist may be perceived as intrusive or invasive. Even handshakes may be uncomfortable for some individuals. In situations where touching may seem natural and helpful, it may be better to limit physical contact to hands, forearms or slightly on the back of the shoulder. Examples of situations where touching may be useful can be as part of an empathetic response or if the patient seems to feel insecure. If you find the patient reacting negatively to touching, it is appropriate to comment and apologise for this by saying, for example, *"I'm sorry, I guess I did something you didn't like. It's important that you let me know if there are other things as well that you want me to do differently".*

Body posture and movements are also important. Stress and unconscious movements of the dentist, such as swinging back and forth on the chair or clicking with the ballpoint pen, can interfere with the contact. The posture also signals degree of interest. If the dentist turns away from the patient, for example, to look at a screen or is very reclined with crossed arms, it may easily be perceived as lack of interest. Genuine interest may be expressed by the fact that the shoulders and legs are facing the patient and one bends slightly forward with the arms in a relaxed position.

6.2.1 Verbal Communication Skills

Verbal communication skills can be divided into two main categories. The first category intends to explore and to build relationship. The second has more focus on structure and efficiency.

6.2.2 Exploratory and Relationship-Building Skills

These skills are used to elicit the patient's perspective and contribute to relationship building and perception of safety and control.

6.2.2.1 Open-Ended Questions

Open-ended questions are important tools in the collection of relevant data from patients as well as in relationship building (see ▶ Chap. 4). Such questions invite the patient to give a narrative answer and cannot be answered with single words such as "yes" or "no". Examples include, *"How can I help you?"*, *"Can you say something more about…?"*, *"What do you think about…?"* etc.

6.2.2.2 Active Listening

Active listening is an efficient communication skill which is about giving full attention and remembering what is being said by the patient.

When you have asked an open-ended question, it is first and foremost important to be completely silent and attentive and to take the time to wait for the patient's response. Being silent is putting your own impatience aside in order to give the patient the time he needs to express himself. The information that comes after the patient has had time to think can often be very important. One of the easiest mistakes, especially if one is eager or stressed, is to interrupt the silence and go on with new questions. Another frequent mistake is to interrupt the patient while they are speaking. In a study among general practitioners, it took an average of 18 seconds for doctors to interrupt their patients [19]. A third frequent mistake is to start planning what to say afterwards, rather than paying attention and concentrating on what the patient says.

One should allow a moment of silence to think carefully before speaking. This is especially important if the patient says or does something unexpected. Experience from video recordings shows that what doctors perceive as a long thinking break, in reality is perceived neither long nor uncomfortable by the patients.

The expression "active listening" refers to a situation where the dentist has their full focus upon what the patient is actually saying. Active listening will increase the patient's feeling of being in focus and cause him to provide useful additional information.

> *Five steps in active listening: 1. Ask 2. Wait 3. Listen 4. Think 5. Talk.*

Active listening includes facilitating responses that encourage the patient to continue speaking. Facilitation can be expressed, for example, through short comments such as "hm" and "mm", often called humming, which demonstrates interest and following along, or through more active comments such as *"I am listening"* or *"please continue".* Other facilitating responses may include nonverbal skills such as nods, hand gestures and encouraging facial expressions.

Another important part of active listening is to identify and respond to verbal or non-verbal cues. That is, one not only listens for factual information, but also for potential underlying themes which need to be talked about.

When the patient expresses an unclear question or cue, it is important to respond by following up with an open exploratory question such as *"I'm not sure I understand what you mean, could you please explain?"* In this way, the dentist may explore what the patient really thinks or feels, and the patient, in turn, will experience that the dentist is interested in understanding him/her.

6.2.2.3 Reflecting

Reflecting (mirroring) is another useful technique for exploring unclear messages or for focusing on specific statements from the patient. The technique may be used by repeating some of what the patient says. Hearing the "echo" of his own statement can open up the patient's mind and perhaps bring out valuable information. One example might be when the patient's statement is *"it went quite well"*, one may reflect it with *"quite?"*

This type of technique belongs to what is called "Socratic Dialogue". By being open and exploratory, one can make the patient reflect, thus discover feelings, thoughts and resources he was not aware of. These types of questions are particularly important tools in exploring and managing dental fear problems and in motivational interviewing which is described in other chapters.

The active listening skills mentioned here are important prerequisites for bringing out the patient's perspective. These skills are also useful to capture emotional messages in order to meet them with an empathetic response and are described in more detail later in this chapter.

6.2.3 Giving the Patient Perception of Control

A basic principle and a goal for all dentist-patient communication is the process of making the patient feel that he/she is in control of the situation. This includes perception of autonomy, co-determination and predictability during both dialogues and treatment. Patients have variable need for control. In reference to the knowledge that patients with high need for control and low experience of control during treatment will be at increased risk of developing dental anxiety [20], the need for control should always be a natural and fundamental issue. In a recent article, Torper et al. [15] highlight control as an important part of dental communication in line with The Four Habits Model.

6.2.3.1 Start Control

Patients will benefit little from a pre-clinical interview if their minds are occupied with the expected dental treatment. By telling the patient, *"First we will have a talk, and when we are both ready, we will start the treatment"*,

the patient will have predictability (control) and be able to concentrate on the interview. Predictability is given simply by telling the patient what is expected to happen throughout the visit. The information should be adapted to the patient's preferences in regard to how detailed information he needs. Some patients just want to know the essence of the treatment such as one should do a survey of the gums or add a filling. Patients with either high sensitivity for pain or high need for control often benefit from more detailed information. Either way, it is important to explain what the patient can expect to experience, not just the technical details. For example, at the start of a clinical treatment, one could say: *"First I am going to use the drill to remove the old filling. There is going to be quite a lot of noise and water, but I will do my best to keep the water away with this suction"*. It is important to give the patient time to prepare before starting a procedure (start control), for example, by asking *"Are you ready?"* or *"Let me know when you are ready"*. This invites consent from the patient.

Predictability for the next consultation is also important, such as *"For the next appointment I suggest doing one of the two fillings we agreed should be replaced, is that OK with you?"* or *"Do you have an opinion on which one you want to replace first?"*. Giving the patient options increases both the feeling of control, compliance and responsibility for the treatment. This applies to all phases in the course of treatment.

6.2.3.2 Stop Control

The possibility of interrupting during treatment is essential for increasing the patient's perception of control. Since the patient has limited possibility of verbal expression during clinical treatment, one should routinely arrange for a clearly defined non-verbal stop signal.

► Example

Dentist: *"Give me a sign with your hand if you would like me to stop"* or *"I find it helpful to arrange a stop signal, which makes it easy for patients to report if there is a need to interrupt, or to ask for something. Is it OK for you that we agree to raise your left hand, or do you have other suggestions?"*

Patient: *"I think this could work for me and to raise my hand seems fine"*.

Dentist: *"Ok, then we will test this out, raise your left hand like this… The dental nurse will help us to be sure that we notice your signal"*. ◄

There is an obligation to introduce stop signals, and the signal to be used should be clearly agreed on and tested. If the patient's stop signal goes unnoticed, the trust between the patient and the dentist can easily be broken. It is also important to have in mind that for some patients the assignment of saying "stop" to an authority (as a dentist is) may be too challenging. Thus, all stop signals must be discussed and tested.

To facilitate the patient's perception of control has been described as a basic principle for all dentist-patient interaction and presupposes mastering of the previously mentioned skills. In a recent publication, Torper et al. [15] have, therefore, suggested to add facilitation of perceived control to be a fifth habit in line with the original four habits in dental practice.

6.2.4 Structuring Skills

The structuring skills intend to help the dentist keep track of information exchange and time spent during the visit.

6.2.4.1 Closed Questions

Closed (structured) questions are questions answered with *"yes", "no",* or short answers. This form of questioning is used as soon as the patient's perspective is sufficiently explored. For example, to obtain more specific diagnostic information, one may ask: *"Is the pain the worse during the day or at night?"* or *"Do you have pain in the tooth when you drink something cold?"* During medical history-taking, one may say: *"I need to know if you have any allergies. I will present a list of possible allergens, and would like you to tell me, using yes or no, if you are allergic to it".* Closed questions are used to retrieve specific, detailed information. They are important for clarifying but work poorly when exploring the patient's perspective, such as what kind of symptoms the patient has.

6.2.4.2 Transitions

Some patients are very talkative. As a dental visit usually has a limited time frame, you occasionally need to lead the interview towards the direction you want. Change of topic without losing the natural flow of communication may be challenging. Thus, it may be useful to have rehearsed some transitional formulations. An example of this is: *"Thank you. I have enough information about this issue for now. It is time to move on to the next...".* Transitions may serve as a polite way of interrupting a talkative patient to get back on track.

> **Tip**
>
> The dentist should summarise at all stages of the visit. This is especially important when transitioning between dialogues and clinical phases, and at the very end of the visit. If you have misunderstood the patient, it will be discovered quickly and can be corrected. Summarising will also be helpful to review what you have heard and to check if anything still needs to be obtained or clarified.
>
> A good advice might be: If you have doubts about what to say or do next, summarise.

6.3 "The Four Habits": A Basic Toolbox of Communication Skills

"The Four Habits Model" may serve as a structural framework of dental visits and presupposes mastering of the previously mentioned underlying set of communication skills. The four habits are invest in the beginning, elicit the patient's perspective, demonstrate empathy and invest in the end [11, 21].

According to the dental version of the model, the four habits (4H) can be applied as an overall framework for dental visits. However, as dental clinicians shift between dialogue and clinical phases, the framework of 4H may also be useful within each separate dialogue phase (example in Table). In the dental model an additional habit has been suggested, Facilitate Perceived Control, due to its crucial importance in dental visits, making it "4+1 Habits for Dentistry" [15].

6.3.1 Habit I: Invest in the Beginning

To invest in the beginning comprises three components:

6.3.1.1 Create Rapport Quickly

During a dental visit, most of the time is devoted to clinical work, and the dentist should keep in mind the importance of creating rapport immediately.

6.3.1.2 Elicit the Patient's Concerns

If you do not know the patient's concerns, ask. If the agenda has been previously agreed upon, make sure it is still established and understood. Use open-ended questions, reflections and remember listening skills.

6.3.1.3 Plan the Visit with the Patient

When all concerns are disclosed and responded to, the agenda for the current visit should be determined, considering the patient's priorities.

6.3.2 Habit II: Elicit the Patient's Perspective

If you want to know the patient's perspective, ask him. As dental health professionals, it is easy to assume things such as what the patient finds painful, expensive or important in the course of treatment. Bringing out the patient's notions of their own condition and what is necessary to do is one of the most important things in a good consultation, but it is easy to forget in a busy everyday life. It is important both in terms of choice of treatment and how well the patient follows up treatment – in addition to that the patient is met with attention, respect and care. Bringing out the patient's perspective consists of three components:

6.3.2.1 Ask for the Patient's Ideas

Studies have shown that seeing the patient's ideas and responding to them has a positive impact on how well the patient later remembers information and how well he complies with the treatment plan [22, 23]. Levinson and co-workers [24] also found that doctors who explore their patient's perspective have fewer complaints.

■ **Elicit the Patient's Expectations**

This can apply to both expectations of what will happen in the current visit, to the procedures or the final result. Knowing the patient's expectations provides opportunities to gain common ground and minimise gaps between expectations and reality. Having informed the patient about diagnosis and treatment options, it is also useful to elicit how much time and resources the patient envisions spending.

■ **Explore Impact on the Patient's Daily Life and Well-Being**

Taking the time to explore the impact on the patient's daily life and well-being has implications for patient satisfaction, adherence and trust. The degree to which the problem affects the patient's daily life can revolve around topics such as pain, function or aesthetics. Knowledge of this can be important to attaining satisfactory treatment outcome, as well as creating trust by showing interest in more aspects of the patient's life.

6.3.3 Habit III: Demonstrate Empathy

An empathetic response is required when a patient expresses concerns or other emotions, and constitutes an important element of relationship building as described in ▶ Chap. 3.

Throughout the dialogues while mapping the patient's current problem and needs and in exploring the patient's perspective, it is important to pay attention to emotional statements or hints from the patient and to meet them with an empathetic response. Empathy as a therapeutic tool is especially important when dealing with distress and fear of dental treatment, or in other situations like having to break bad news related to the diagnosis.

First and foremost, empathy presupposes an attitude of openness to the patient's feelings, which implies care about the patient, genuine desire to understand how he/she feels, and the ability to get touched. However, to be helpful to a patient, this attitude must be communicated by an empathetic response.

An emotional message from a patient is usually hidden in the small hints or perhaps through body language. When the dentist or dental hygienist works by concentrating on the patient's mouth, noticing these emotional messages is particularly challenging. The clinician is, therefore, completely dependent on noticing non-verbal signals, such as facial expressions, eyes, movements and signs of muscle tension to capture how the patient feels.

An empathetic response consists of several components. A widely used model is called NURS, which is an abbreviation for Name it, Understand, Respect and Support [25].

■ **N: "Name It"**

If you are unsure whether the message you have captured, maybe only assumes, matches what the patient is actually experiencing, you should first try to help the patient identify the feeling. You may try the tactic of careful mirroring, such as *"It sounds like this is hard for you"* or *"It seems like you are a little worried now..."*. Such statements will give the patient the feeling of being seen. He can then either confirm the assumption and you can explore it further, for example: *"Do you want to tell anything more about it?"* or in the case your assumption is wrong, you can together explore what the patient is really experiencing, which in its turn may foster a helpful, empathetic response.

■ **U: "Understand"**

When the patient's feelings have come to light, one expresses understanding, such as *"I can fully understand this must be difficult for you"*.

■ **R: "Respect"**

It is important to acknowledge and legitimise the patient's feelings. For example: *"It is no wonder you are struggling with this, as it can be a demanding process"* or *"From what you have told me about your past experiences, it is not strange you find this difficult"*.

■ **S: "Support"**

Furthermore, you should express support and willingness to find solutions within the professional framework at your disposal. An example of this might be, *"I will do everything I can to make this easier for you"*. At this point, you should further explore what might be helpful to the patient: *"Do you have any thoughts about what I can do to help you?"*

A mnemonic which helps to remember the abbreviation NURS is "one NURSes the emotions". An empathetic response may range from a simple non-verbal action, such as handling a napkin in the case of tears or a soothing touch of the arm in case of distress, to a deeper verbal response.

The NURS mnemonic may also be expanded with an E (explore) to NURSE (see ► Chap. 4).

6.3.4 Habit IV: Invest in the End

A successful ending is when the patient leaves the clinic or advances to the next phase of the visit with good insight into what has been done and what to expect further.

The patient should get an overview of the diagnoses made and the treatment carried out. This is best checked by summarising the phase you have finished and checking if the patient has caught up with the most important, for example, by asking if the patient has any additional information or questions.

Finally, at the end of both the current phase and the visit, it is important to discuss what is to happen further. To ensure the patient leaves the clinic without unresolved questions or concerns, one should conclude the phase or visit by inviting remaining questions.

6.4 Structuring the Dental Visit and Implementation of the Four Habits (Illustrated by Verbal Examples)

Most often the dental visit consists of one or more clinical phases in which the dentist's hands and instruments prevent the patient from expressing himself verbally. Therefore, the visit needs to be divided into dialogue and clinical phases.

The duration of these phases may vary depending on the current purpose of the visit, e.g. an emergency visit, the first visit including history-taking or a planned follow-up session. Sometimes dialogue phases need to be extended to deal with special situations or tasks. Independent of task, all dialogue phases should follow a certain core structure, based on the framework of the Four Habits Model.

Each dialogue phase has its own purpose and should be effectively exploited to get the most clarification while the patient is sitting upright and is able to partici-

pate equally in the dialogue. This makes it easier to elicit the patient's perspective such as concerns or needs for adjustments during subsequent clinical phases. This will prevent confusion and diminish the risk of interruption or complications during clinical treatment and facilitate efficiency and quality of dental care.

6.4.1 The Pre-clinical Interview Phase

The pre-clinical phase can be brief or protracted, depending on the degree of familiarity with the patient, the complexity of his problem(s) and the amount of information exchange needed to solve it. Either way, the framework of the four habits is relevant in this phase. See ◘ Table 6.1.

With the knowledge that patients have a varying degree of distress prior to a dental visit, it is especially important to invest in the beginning to put the patient at ease as quickly as possible and facilitate access to his concerns and expectations. At this stage, it is primarily the patient who should be given the chance to speak since he is the expert of his problems and needs. Accordingly, at the beginning of this phase, there is the need for relationship-building skills, such as exploratory and active listening skills.

The first seconds of the visit are significant to creating rapport, especially through the use of non-verbal skills, such as facial expression, positioning and a handshake. Introduce yourself to everyone in the room who is not familiar with who you are. In case of a delay, you should excuse it right away; however, no explanation is needed due to confidentiality. The patient should be assisted with placement of clothes or belongings and be seated in an upright position, in a consultation or dental chair, at the same level as the dentist. The opening line might be, e.g. *"Hello and welcome, please sit down. I am sorry for the ten minutes delay. I am curious about how it has been for you since the treatment we did last month?"*

As soon as rapport is created, you should elicit the patient's current concerns by use of open-ended questions such as *"How can I help you today?"*, followed by active listening and responding to what comes up.

As soon as all concerns are disclosed and responded to, the agenda for the current visit should be determined, considering the patient's priorities. *"OK, I understand that the most urgent for you today is to get the broken tooth repaired, which we should be able to finish within the time scheduled. In case there will be any spare time, is there anything else you would like to address today?"* If the agenda has been previously agreed upon, make sure it is still established and understood.

◼ **Table 6.1** The Four Habits, including components and objectives applicable in the pre-clinical interview phase. The table is derived from the original medical model [11]

Habit	Habit components	Aim
Preparation		Confidence, increased efficiency
I Investing in the beginning	Create rapport quickly Elicit the patient's concerns Plan the visit with the patient	Establish a welcoming atmosphere and put the patient at ease Facilitate faster access to patient's concerns Increase diagnostic accuracy Promote mutual goals and frames of the visit Minimise waste of time Promote trust and predictability
II Elicit the patient's perspective	Ask for the patient's ideas Elicit the patient's expectations and requests Explore the impact on the patient's life and Well-being	Increase diagnostic accuracy and prevent conflicts Promote trust Reduce anxiety and distress Strengthen collaboration and compliance Facilitate shared decision-making and successful outcome
III Demonstrate empathy	Be open to the patient's emotions Make an empathic statement Convey empathy non-verbally	Promote trust and alliance Prevent dental anxiety and distress Ease clinical procedures and prevent interruptions
IV Invest in the end of pre-clinical interview	Review and summarise relevant information, agenda and requests Invite questions Close the interview and facilitate perceived control before proceeding into clinical position	Promote predictability Strengthen trust and alliance Reduce distress and anxiety Ease clinical procedures by preventing confusion and interruptions

"Last time we talked about starting with the crown on your lower left. Are you still tuned in to this plan or has something more urgent come up in the meantime?"

To gain common ground, the patient's perspective must be elicited (habit II). Relevant core issues are described earlier in this chapter, and examples of these may be: *"What do you think might be causing the pain?"* or *"In what way have the difficulties affected your eating habits and nutrition?"* At this point you should also explore whether the patient has certain requests, needs or expectations regarding the forthcoming agenda, e.g. *"Is there anything you want me to pay special attention to during the visit?"*

If the patient is new to the clinic, the pre-clinical interview has to be expanded, primarily to map relevant medical and oral history. Here you will need closed questions and structuring skills to get a hold of what you are aiming at in an efficient way.

Potential treatment-related problems, distress and anxiety should also be routinely explored at this point. Patients may have various problems related to treatment, ranging from neck- or breathing-problems, autonomic and psychosomatic reactions, such as gagging or fainting, to various degrees of dental anxiety or phobia. Elaboration and handling of such problems must be done in an upright equal position to prevent complications and traumatic experience during the forthcoming clinical phases. Since addressing vulnerability and dental anxiety may trigger resistance or shame, this topic should be brought up in a sensitive and trust-building way to let the patient comfortably disclose concerns on his own premises. This might be done by open-ended explorative questions, such as *"To make your treatment as comfortable as possible, I wonder if there is something you find particularly difficult when receiving dental treatment?"*

If the patient discloses distress or anxiety, either directly or perhaps by hints or non-verbal signs, it is important to explore further and collaborate with the patient to find adaptations and coping strategies to ease the treatment situation.

In case of severe anxiety or phobia, this interview section should be further expanded as described in ▶ Chaps. 11 and 12. In such cases as a rule, it is necessary to plan an alternative course together with the patient and to treat the anxiety in advance of the clinical treatment.

Throughout this pre-clinical interview, it is important to practise habit III such as to pay attention to emotional statements or hints from the patient, demonstrate empathy and take time to deal with what obstacles or problems may arise.

6.4.2 Closing the Pre-clinical Interview and Transition to Clinical Phase

Whether the pre-clinical interview has been short or expanded to explore further information or handle particular challenges, it is important to invest in the end (habit IV) before reclining the dental chair into treatment position. All relevant information, decisions and requests should be summarised, finished and dealt with, and the patient should be invited to ask questions. An example: *"OK, then we have got the medical information needed for your treatment, thank you! We agreed to start taking a look at the painful tooth, and possibly take an X-ray to find out what can be done. Is there anything else you would like to ask before we start?"*

As much as possible should be clarified while the patient still has the opportunity to express himself verbally, both in terms of diagnostic exchange, what to expect in the subsequent clinical phase, and in terms of possible needs the patient might have related to the treatment.

Providing predictability and control is important in transitioning to the clinical phase, and the degree of predictability should be tailored to the patient's individual needs. Regardless of the degree of needed control, one should routinely check if the patient is ready to be reclined into treatment position and remind him of the opportunity to stop during the clinical phase if needed. If the patient is new, one should introduce and explicitly demonstrate a non-verbal stop signal such as *"If you need to stop along the way, or to tell me something, you can give me a signal with your left hand, like this"*.

safety, communication can be further limited to practical instructions, such as *"I start by examining the tooth in the upper jaw, can you please open your mouth a little wider?"*, supplementary diagnostic questions, such as *"Does it hurt when I knock this tooth?"* or informative comments needed. Nevertheless, one should always be open to the possibility of unexpected reactions from the patient and be ready to handle them.

Some patients, especially those with a high degree of needed control, prefer continuous updates about what is going on and what to expect, whereas others only prefer headlines of the forthcoming procedures. If the patient's preference is unknown, a brief assessment may be useful: *"Now I will start examining the teeth. Would you like me to consecutively inform you of my findings, or would you rather wait for a summary at the end?"*. If the patient wants information consecutively, it is important to report what looks healthy, not only what you find or suspect to be pathological.

If clinical procedures involve discomfort or pain, it is particularly important to prepare the patient to what may be unpleasant or painful, *"I will move this probe carefully into the pocket between your gum and tooth, to measure the infection. This may cause some discomfort"*. In such situations, habit III is essential, such as to pay attention to non-verbal signs of pain or emotions, convey empathy and encourage limit-setting. For example, *"It seems this is uncomfortable for you. Please remember to give me a sign if you need me to stop, and we will figure out how to continue"*. This provides an opportunity for the patient to communicate what he needs and to facilitate adaptations.

6.4.3 The Clinical Examination Phase

Practising the four habits should be continued throughout the visit, by providing relevant information and predictability (habit I), focusing on the patient's perspective (habit II), responding to emotional hints (habit III) and summarising and inviting questions along the way (habit IV).

The first clinical phase usually consists of an oral examination, which can either be brief (such as an X-ray or rapid examination of a specific problem), or lengthy in case a more comprehensive clinical examination is needed to complete the diagnosis. Necessary investments have been made in advance, while the patient is still in an upright and equal position to ensure adequate predictability and adjustments during the clinical examination. Remember to obtain consent to begin by asking, for example, *"Now I will examine your teeth, are you ready?"* With a well prepared patient who has a sense of

6.4.4 The Shared Decision-Making Phase

As soon as the clinical examination has revealed or confirmed the diagnosis, the aim is to reach an agreement on a treatment plan and to establish an alliance on how to cooperate on the treatment's execution. The dentist and the patient are to negotiate in order to find the best solution [26]. The degree of patient participation in the choice of treatment has to vary, depending on circumstances. This dialogue may sometimes be quickly done with little discussion with the patient, for example, in case of a simple reparative treatment. At other times, in the event of extensive treatment regimens, the discussion may be more comprehensive and time-consuming.

In this dialogue, it is also important to invest in the beginning (habit I) by first and foremost placing the patient in an upright position and removing the dentist's facemask to facilitate equal dialogue. Language and pace should be adapted to the patient's level of dental

◻ Table 6.2 Steps of shared decision-making [27]

Steps	Examples
1. Diagnosis 2. Treatment options 3. Advantages, disadvantages, risks, patient's responsibilities 4. Check patient's comprehension 5. Elicit patient's goals, preferences and expectations 6. Discuss 7. Decision 8. Reinforce decision 9. Record decision	*"These X-rays show".* *"In such cases, the most durable solution is....* *.. But there are also other options...".* *"We'll take a look at what these options entail...".* *"Do you have any questions about from what I've mentioned so far?"* *"What do you think about these options?"* *" Is there anything else you need to clarify regarding these options to make a decision?"* *"Have you made your decision?"* *"I think you made a good choice".* Write agreed decision in the patient's record.

knowledge (see ▶ Chap. 5). It may also be useful to have informative resources available, such as a mirror, models or drawing equipment.

As the patient should be an active participant in the decision-making process, you will need to practise open-ended skills, silence and active listening skills. Nevertheless, structural skills must be used as well to perform the steps needed to ensure informed consent, including patient's perception of control. The steps are outlined in ◻ Table 6.2.

One starts by delivering diagnostic information relating to the patient's symptoms and concerns, such as *"The probable reason of your pain is an inflammation around the tooth"*.

At this point one should elicit the patient's perspective (habit II), which includes checking the patient's knowledge in order to more easily adapt further information to the patient's level. For example, ask, *"Do you know what periodontitis is?"* or *"Do you remember anything from the last time you got a root canal treatment?"* Provide information about causality and consequences of the patient's condition.

Next, appropriate treatment options should be presented in an understandable way, as orderly and straightforward as possible. For each treatment option, one must inform about the advantages, disadvantages and other implications, including the patient's responsibility for succeeding with the treatment outcome.

Throughout the entire dental visit, it is important to check the patient's comprehension and invite questions, such as *"Do you have any questions about what I have mentioned so far?"* It is also appropriate to break down the information to give the patient time to digest the information and opportunity to ask questions.

Before starting the discussion, one should check the patient's own expectations and treatment goals using open-ended, exploratory questions such as: *"What do you think about these options?"* or *"As you can see, these options differ in price, durability and appearance. What is most important to you?"*

During this discussion, several aspects of the patient's perspective should be explored, such as personal preferences, priorities and potential barriers. In the case of sensitive topics, one should meet them with an empathetic response (habit III). One example might be if the patient is struggling with limitations or lack of resources in planning, it may be appropriate to say: *"I understand your resistance to going through this periodontal surgery, as it is quite demanding"*.

In case of breaking bad news, it is especially important to take the time to focus on the patient's perspective. Bad news should be presented directly in the most neutral way possible, followed by silence to await the patient's reaction. The patient's reaction to the message is crucial for how to proceed. For example, *"Unfortunately, this tooth cannot be saved"* (silence). Within 30 seconds, a reaction often comes. If the patient does not react, one can continue with: *"What do you think about that?"* If the patient reacts emotionally, one proceeds with an empathetic response, e.g. *"I understand that this is a tough message; many people get distressed by losing a tooth. However, together we will work out a best possible solution for you"*.

The treatment decision should be made by the patient to ensure the requirement for informed consent as well as for the patient to perceive control and being part of the decision-making process. It is, therefore, important to invite questions from the patient in order to clarify the most before the patient's final decision.

Once the decision has been made, it is important to reinforce the decision, especially if the patient has been uncertain, such as: *"I think you made a good choice, based on what you have told me about your preferences"*.

When each diagnosis and its treatment plan has been discussed, all decisions made during the discussion should be summarised, followed by making plans for implementation and cooperation with the patient. Here you may need to review the patient's responsibility to succeed with the plan chosen. This often also involves motivation and instruction in change of oral health behaviour (▶ Chaps. 7 and 8).

Before moving on to the dental treatment itself, one should invest in the end of the dialogue (habit IV). Here, one summarises and invites questions, such as *"OK, then we agreed to do the urgent treatment of the painful grinder today and proceed with the restorative treatment in the next session. As we talked about, cleaning the root canals may be painful, so we agreed you should receive an anesthetic in advance. Is there anything else you would like to ask before we get started?"*

Before reclining the dental chair and putting the facemask on prior to treatment, all decisions should be clarified in order to give the patient predictability and perception of control. This includes clarifications of any adjustments to be made to cope with the forthcoming procedures, such as anaesthetic, need for assistance to suction, breaks and stop signal. The degree of desired predictability during treatment should also be clarified during this phase while the patient can still express himself verbally.

6.4.5 Clinical Treatment Phase

During treatment one continues practising the principles described in the previous section "The clinical examination phase". The goal is to make the patient relax and to enable the dentist's concentration on technical precision, quality and efficiency.

The clinical treatment phase includes less opportunity for verbal exchange than other phases, and dental clinicians often develop their own personal style when it comes to verbal utterances during treatment. Regardless of personal style, the primary focus should always stay on the patient, his individual need for predictability and his experience.

Even with anaesthesia, many procedures may still be unpleasant or exhausting. Therefore, it is crucial to pay attention to a patient's experience and practise habit III (demonstrate empathy). This involves awareness of non-verbal signs of pain or emotions, conveyance of an empathic response and encouragement to limit-setting if needed, such as: *"It looks as if your jaw is tired, which is quite understandable after such a long effort. Remember to give a signal with your left hand if you need a break".*

> Sometimes during a treatment phase, it may be necessary to pause to discuss something unexpected that has occurred during the procedure. This may also be in the form of a reaction from the patient, such as gagging, dizziness, hyperventilation, fear or tension. In such cases, one should elevate the patient to a comfortable position, provide space and time to deal with the problem and explore solutions on how to proceed.

6.4.6 End of Visit Phase

Regardless of the current assignment and duration of dialogues or clinical treatment.

performed, all dental visits require certain investments in the end (habit IV) to ensure that the patient leaves the clinic in a good mood and without any unre-solved questions or concerns. This includes elevating the patient into an upright, equal position and the use of relationship-building, exploratory and active listening skills as well as structuring skills.

In the case of painful or exhausting treatment experience, a "debriefing" is important. Here one can acknowledge the patient's efforts, which can open possibilities for the patient to let off steam, such as *"Thanks for your endurance, I hope it was not too hard for you?"* If emotional hints or reactions are disclosed, it should be met by an empathetic response and be given space to be dealt with. This may foster opportunities for future adjustments.

As soon as the patient has gathered, one summarises the achievements of the session, and what to expect next, to ensure that the patient leaves the clinic with a perception of control and predictability. An example may be: *"Now we are done with the first step of cleaning the root canal. It is filled with a bactericide material and covered with a temporary sealing on top of the tooth. Technically, everything went as expected, but such a procedure can cause some soreness or pain afterwards. It is a normal reaction, which usually calms down within a day or two. But feel free to get in touch with me if you need it!"* or *"Is there anything you would like to ask before we make a plan for further treatment?"*

Before the patient leaves, you should review all agreements, given advice and instructions, and if necessary, reassure the patient of the availability for further support. For example: *"I recommend that you avoid chewing the first couple of hours. We have set up a control session in three weeks, and if the inflammation is decreased by then, the tooth may be permanently restored. If anything comes up in the meantime, please call".*

Summary

Professional communication is essential in dental visits. Patient-centred communication focuses on exploring both the clinical diagnoses and how the patients perceive their situation in order to work out a common understanding. Due to limitation of time the communication should be targeted to ensure sufficient information exchange needed to provide proper treatment.

Professional dentist-patient communication entails deliberate switching between relationship-building and task-focused tools, both of them consisting of non-verbal and verbal skills. Non-verbal skills comprise body language. Verbal communication is divided into exploratory and relationship-building skills on one hand and skills focusing structure and efficiency of the visit on the other. Exploratory and relationship-building skills comprise open-ended questions, silence, active listening, reflecting and giving the patient perception of control. Closed questions, transitions and summaries are examples of skills that help the dentist structure the consultation and keep track of the information exchange.

The Four Habits Model is a basic tool that may serve as a structural framework for all dental visits, both for the visit as a whole, and within each separate dialogue phase. The first habit (I) "Invest in the beginning" comprises creating report quickly, eliciting the patient's concerns and planning the visit with the patient. The second habit (II) "Elicit the patient's perspective" entails bringing out the patient's assessments and expectations and the possible impact on the patient's life and well-being. The third habit (III) is to "Demonstrate empathy". To respond emphatically is about putting in words what the patient conveys, expressing understanding and showing respect and support. The fourth habit (IV) "Invest in the end" recommends that the dentist sums up what has been obtained so far, provides predictability and invites the patient to ask questions.

The dental visit entails switching between dialogue phases and clinical phases. The aim of the pre-clinical interview phase is to create rapport, elicit the patient's concerns, record medical history and agree on a plan for the visit. Subsequently an oral examination takes place, followed by a new dialogue phase where the treatment plan is discussed. It is important that an informed consent is obtained and documented before commencing to the clinical treatment phase. Throughout the entire visit it is of utmost importance to facilitate the patients' perception of control.

References

1. Armfield JM, Heaton LJ. Management of fear and anxiety in the dental clinic: a review. Aust Dent J. 2013;58(4):390–407.; ; quiz 531. https://doi.org/10.1111/adj.12118.
2. Woelber JP, Spann-Aloge N, Hanna G, Fabry G, Frick K, Brueck R, et al. Training of dental professionals in motivational interviewing can heighten interdental cleaning self-efficacy in periodontal patients. Front Psychol. 2016;24(7):254. https://doi.org/10.3389/fpsyg.2016.00254.
3. Vassend O. Kommunikasjon og pasientbehandling. Oslo: Spartacus Forlag AS; 1997.
4. Nerdrum P. Profesjonalitet i arbeid med klienter. In: Nerdrum P, Opsand OP, editors. Fra veldedighet mot profesjonalitet, barnevernslinja ved Norges kommunal og sosialhøgskole 25 år. Oslo: Norges kommunal og sosialhøgskole; 1998. p. 33–53.
5. Smith RC, Fortin AH, Dwamena F, Frankel RM. An evidence-based patient-centered method makes the biopsychosocial model scientific. Patient Educ Couns. 2013;91(3):265–70. https://doi.org/10.1016/j.pec.2012.12.010.
6. Steward M, Brown JB, Weston W, McWhinney IR, McWilliam CL, Freeman T. Patient centered medicine. Transforming the clinical method. 3rd ed. London: Radcliff Medical Press; 2014.
7. Rao JK, Anderson LA, Inui TS, Frankel RM. Communication interventions make a difference in conversations between physicians and patients: a systematic review of the evidence. Med Care. 2007;45(4):340–9. https://doi.org/10.1097/01mir.0000254516.04961.d5.
8. Stein T, Frankel RM, Krupat. Enhancing clinician communication skills in a large healthcare organization: a longitudinal case study. Patient Educ Couns. 2005;58(1):4–12. https://doi.org/10.1016/j.pec.2005.01.014.
9. Fortin AH, Dwamena FC, Frankel RM, Smith RC. Smith's patient-centered interviewing: an evidence-based method. 3rd ed. New York: Mc Graw-Hill Medical; 2012.
10. Silverman J, Kurtz S, Draper J. Skills for communication with patients. 3rd ed. Boca Raton: CRC Press, Taylor & Francis; 2013.
11. Frankel RM, Stein T. (2001). Getting the most out of the clinical encounter: the four habits model. J Med Pract Manage. 2001;16(4):184–91. PMID: 11317576.
12. Gulbrandsen P, Krupat E, Benth JS, Garratt A. "Four Habits" goes abroad: report from a pilot study in Norway. Patient Educ Couns. 2008;72(3):388–93. https://doi.org/10.1016/j.pec.2008.05.012.
13. Jensen BF, Gulbrandsen P, Dahl FA, Krupat E, Frankel RM, Finset A. Effectiveness of a short course in clinical communication skills for hospital doctors: results of a crossover randomized controlled trial (ISRCTN22153332). Patient Educ Couns. 2011;84(2):163–9. https://doi.org/10.1016/j.pec.2010.08.028.
14. Lundeby T, Gulbrandsen P, Finset A. The expanded four habits model. A teachable consultation model for encounters with patients in emotional distress. Patient Educ Couns. 2015;98(5):598–603. https://doi.org/10.1016/j.pec.2015.01.015.
15. Torper J, Ansteinsson V, Lundeby T. Moving the four habits model into dentistry. Development of a dental consultation model. Do dentists need an additional habit? Eur J Dent Educ. 2019;23(2):220–9. https://doi.org/10.1111/eje.12421.
16. Strand GV, Lygre GB, Hede B. Informert samtykke. Nor Tannlegeforen Tid. 2013;2013(123):106–10.
17. Haidet P. Jazz and the 'art' of medicine: improvisation in the medical encounter. Ann Fam Med. 2007;5(2):164–9. https://doi.org/10.1370/afm.624.
18. Willis J, Todorov A. First impressions: making up your mind after a 100-ms exposure to a face. Psychol Sci. 2006;17(7):592–8. https://doi.org/10.1111/j.1467-9280.2006.01750.x.
19. Beckman HB, Frankel RM. The effect of physician behavior on the collection of data. Ann Intern Med. 1984;101(5):692–6. https://doi.org/10.7326/0003-4819-101-5-692.
20. Logan HL, Baron RS, Keeley K, Law A, Stein S. Desired control and felt control as mediators of stress in a dental setting. Health Psychol. 1991;10(5):352–9. https://doi.org/10.1037//0278-6133.10.5.352.
21. Krupat E, Frankel R, Stein T, Irish J. The Four Habits Coding Scheme: validation of an instrument to assess clinicians' communication behavior. Patient Educ Couns. 2006;62(1):38–45. https://doi.org/10.1016/j.pec.2005.04.015.
22. Neumann M, Scheffer C, Tauschel D, Lutz G, Wirtz M, Edelhäuser F. Physician empathy: definition, outcome-relevance and its measurement in patient care and medical education. GMS Z Med Ausbild. 2012;29(1):Doc11.

6

23. Tan AS, Moldovan-Johnson M, Parvanta S, Gray SW, Armstrong K, Hornik RC. Patient-clinician information engagement improves adherence to colorectal cancer surveillance after curative treatment: results from a longitudinal study. Oncologist. 2012;17(9):1155–62. https://doi.org/10.1634/theoncologist.2012-0173.

24. Levinson W, Roter RS, Mullooly JP, Dull VT, Frankel RM. Physician-patient communication. The relationship with malpractice claims among primary care physicians and surgeons. JAMA. 1997;277(7):553–9. https://doi.org/10.1001/jama.277.7.553.

25. Smith RC. The patient's story. Integrated patient-doctor interviewing. Boston: Little Brown and Company; 1996.

26. Truglio-Londrigan M, Slyer JT, Singleton JK, Worral P. A qualitative systematic review of internal and external influences on shared decision-making in all health care settings. JBI Libr Syst Rev. 2012;10(58):4633–46. https://doi.org/10.11124/jbisrir-2012-432.

27. Chambers DW, Abrams RG. Dental communication. East Norwalk Connecticut: Appleton-Century-Crofts; 1986.

Behaviour Change for Oral Health

Peter Prescott, Koula Asimakopoulou and Jostein Paul Årøen Lein

Contents

7.1 Introduction

Every dental practitioner will meet patients who have issues with behaviour that contribute to reduced oral health and health in general. Examples include high sugar consumption and a lack of dental hygiene. The dental practitioner will soon learn that helping people to change their behaviour can sometimes be complicated. It is not unusual that patients have difficulty changing behaviour even though the dental practitioner advises them to do so. Even when facing serious oral health problems, some patients struggle to perform seemingly mundane tasks like brushing their teeth. We know that helping patients establish good dental habits and oral health behaviours can have a large impact and reduce the need for more intensive dental health care. This chapter will provide a framework for understanding challenges patients encounter in changing behaviour and presents the ways in which the dental practitioner can assist patients in changing behaviour.

> **Learning Goals**
> — Learn the connection between motivation, decision-making and behaviour
> — Learn how to establish health-promoting behaviours and how to maintain them
> — Learn how to structure consultations with the aim of helping patients to better oral health through behaviour change

7.2 Dental Health Care and Habits

A person's behaviour outside the dental surgery is important for maintaining or improving oral health. On the one hand, reducing behaviours like the intake of acidic and sugary foods and beverages or quitting smoking can have beneficial impacts on oral health. On the other hand, dental health can be enhanced by beginning with new behaviours (learning a skill), modifying/adjusting behaviours (improving technique), or increasing the frequency of existing behaviours (doing something more often and on a regular basis). In fact, it is arguable that very little of what dentists and their team do in the dental surgery will succeed unless the patient has the skills, opportunity and motivation to maintain it. It follows then that an individual's behaviour outside the dental surgery is paramount in maintaining the work that the dental team has performed in the person's oral cavity.

Personal dental care can be said to consist of a collection of both simple and complex intentional behaviours that require a certain amount of effort to perform.

Through repetition, and subsequently the formation of a habit, brief and simple cleaning behaviours can be performed on a regular basis without meticulous decision-making and mobilisation of effort. Habitual behaviours are easier to perform because they are at a large part performed automatically. However, even when good dental habits are established, a certain amount of effort is often necessary to initiate the behaviour. Brushing one's teeth in the proper manner is a rather uncomplicated behaviour, but a certain amount of conscious willpower and self-discipline is necessary to do it regularly on a daily basis.

When it comes to smoking, we suggest that the dental practitioner primarily addresses motivation for change by giving relevant information and electing the patient's own concerns about the effects of smoking on oral health. A short exploration of the patient's capability, opportunity and willingness to undertake "stop smoking" can also be in order.

In the COM-B model – see Fig. 7.1 – [11] it is suggested that behaviour will only be performed if the person meets all three criteria:

1. They are capable of performing the behaviour, that is, if they have skills to engage with the behaviour (capability).
2. They have the physical (e.g. time) and social environment (e.g. exposure to messages and ideas) opportunity to engage with the behaviour.
3. They are motivated consciously (e.g. they have made the decision and then planned the behaviour) or automatically (e.g. they are supported by habits or emotional processes) to perform the behaviour [1]. The patient can profit from simple professional advice about reducing the intake of certain foods and beverages, along with stopping the use of tobacco. Detailed and well-meaning practitioner attempts at life-style change can be interpreted as context discordant and experienced by the patient as unwanted, unrequested, invasive and a violation of autonomy (see ▸ Chap. 8 for more information about violation of autonomy).

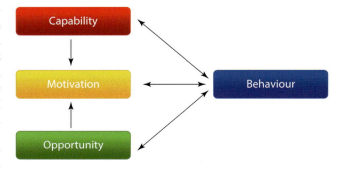

Fig. 7.1 The COM-B model. (Adapted from Michie et al. [11], p.4)

While reducing or stopping behaviours is important, the main focus of this chapter is on adapting and repeatedly performing behaviours that contribute to oral health. Three central components of intentional behaviour are discussed: motivation, decision-making and implementation/maintenance [15].

Oral health consultations are comprised of content (which issues to address) and approach (how to address these issues). An important goal is to increase the patient's active involvement in dental health care. We describe a structure for brief interventions that may facilitate communication and collaboration between the patient and the dental health expert.

7.3 Intentional Behaviour Change

Dental health habits are generally established in childhood under the guidance of caretakers, usually parents. The child is reminded countless times of the importance of taking care of their teeth. Instructions are repeated and accompanied by demonstrations along with supervised practice of brushing technique. Often, the result is longstanding behaviour patterns and durable habits maintained throughout adulthood. However, the acquisition of habits in childhood does not necessarily result in sustained performance of oral health behaviours. Effort may be required to preserve well-established behaviours if difficulties or obstacles arise. Some children, teenagers, and adults need to change their behaviour intentionally in order to establish or re-establish healthy habits.

 Intentional Behaviour Involves Three Main Tasks
- Becoming motivated
- Making a deliberate decision
- Implementing the behaviour and maintaining it over time

Although these tasks are inter-related, each has distinct characteristics. Decision-making requires motivation. Motivation and decision-making are the basis for taking action.

Decision-making and implementation of behaviour are connected to each other in two ways. On the one hand, it is difficult to envisage performing an intentional behaviour that is not preceded by a decision. On the other hand, a person may run through the behaviour in his or her head and evaluate how realistic performing it is before making a decision. After implementation, deliberate renewal of motivation and repeated decision-making are skills which can contribute to consistent, long-term performance.

7.3.1 **Becoming Motivated**

Information and knowledge about positive and negative consequences of different behaviours are the basis for motivation. Motivating information can originate from one's own experience or from outside sources (what one reads, hears about, or is told). Information can be purposely sought after, stumbled over or presented directly or indirectly by other people. Dental professionals are important and trusted sources of information about the connection between caretaking of one's teeth and the likelihood and severity of negative dental health. They are also important sources of information about positive consequences of healthy dental behaviour.

The way information is presented and discussed can either increase or decrease the likelihood of the patient attending to, thinking about, reflecting on, considering and assessing it. See the ▶ Sect. 7.3 in this chapter for suggestions about how to address aspects of dental health behaviour in a constructive manner.

> It is important to note that information is necessary but not sufficient for behaviour change to take place. For example, knowing about the benefits of and how to run a marathon is of course not sufficient unless the person also has the physical and psychological opportunity to undertake this task. Giving people information is important and necessary but only where the dental team have established that there is lack of knowledge and that the information given is relevant to the person's needs.

Being motivated can be equated with having reasons for performing a behaviour. Motivation revolves around present or future concerns about negative conditions such as: cavities, bleeding gums, gingivitis, periodontitis, enamel damage, halitosis and loss of teeth. Motivation can also be a result of worries about pain, difficulty eating or drinking, extensive dental procedures, expense of dental care or appearance of teeth. People vary when it comes to what motivates them. For some people, non-health issues predominate. Others are motivated by thoughts about positive future dental condition, for example, of having strong nice-looking teeth and healthy gums, or of feeling unencumbered in social interactions. And sometimes, what motivates one person at one time may fail to motivate them at another.

A person must believe that a specific consequence is actually important if such a consequence is going to have a motivating impact [8]. It is one thing to be aware of a consequence of, e.g. insufficient personal dental care, it is another to actually be truly concerned about this.

When Johnathan was in his teens, he knew that the condition of his teeth and gums could suffer if he didn't use toothpicks to clean between his teeth. He was not very concerned about this since it was something he felt wouldn't happen for many years. He was, however, very bothered by the thought of having bad breath and used toothpicks regularly to prevent this.

Emotion is often a signal that a consequence is important. Thoughts about negative conditions that result in unpleasant emotions such as worry indicate importance and concern. Thoughts that give rise to pleasant emotions such as pride, satisfaction or relief suggest that a person really cares about the future positive condition of his or her teeth.

Providing information and advice are perhaps the most frequent motivational strategies used in clinical practice although the effects of information and advice have been argued to be just one of the three COM-B components that support behaviour change. At the same time, the way information and advice are presented is of importance. Approaches that promote collaboration between the dental team and the patient have the largest impact on behaviour [8]. Work on delivering patient-centred care in dentistry has outlined the various levels of information and choice that may be given at any one consultation [14] noting that involving patients in a collaborative manner must lie at the heart of any consultation.

A suggested step by step format for a collaborative patient-centred consultation style is presented in the ▶ Sect. 7.3 later in this chapter.

Eliciting the patient's own concerns and worries is a useful and important motivational strategy. Increased motivation for performing healthy dental behaviours can be a direct result of the patient expressing, discussing and reflecting on concerns and worries [12]. This can be achieved by asking about and elaborating the patient's experiences and thoughts about dental health issues:

Box 7.1
— Ask about concerns about teeth, gums and dental health
  – *Have you noticed anything negative about your teeth that you would like to discuss? Do you have any concerns about your teeth or gums?*
— Explore importance of a concern
  – *Is this something that is important to you? Do you think about it from time to time? Are you worried about the future condition of your teeth?*
— Explore the connection between concerns and dental health behaviour
  – *Do you think that you can do something to take better care of your teeth and keep them in good condition or prevent something bad from happening?*

At this point it is worth exploring the concept of motivational interviewing (MI) for behaviour change. MI is a patient-centred style of communication and overall philosophy of care. MI includes explicit behavioural techniques that are designed to help people explore their inherent ambivalence about new behaviours in a non-confrontational manner. The main authority figures behind the concept, Miller and Rollnick (1996), propose that people are naturally ambivalent (e.g. I want to have straight teeth but I do not want to wear my orthodontic appliance), and this ambivalence, it is suggested, can be used to support people in engaging in health behaviour change. Whilst there is some evidence that MI in fields outside dentistry can be helpful for such behaviour change (Lundahl et al. 2013), there is currently not a great deal of good quality evidence that MI is an effective method for change in oral health settings (Cascaes et al. 2014; Gao et al. 2014; Asimakopoulou and Newton 2018).

Checklists are efficient ways of identifying dental-related concerns and can help the patient become more aware of reasons for taking care of his or her teeth. Another advantage of using checklists is that it is often easier for a person to identify than recall concerns.

1. Present and future concerns

Please check the boxes if you have these dental health concerns:		Have experienced this	Worried that this might happen
1	Negative reactions from other people		
2	Bleeding gums		
3	Not being able to eat certain foods		
4	Embarrassment or shame		
5	Avoidance of smiling		
6	Avoidance of talking		
7	Bad conscience – feeling guilty		
8	Gum disease		
9	Bad breath		
10	Worrying, anxious about condition of teeth/gums		
11	Expenses for dental care		
12	Losing teeth		
13	Drilling and fillings		
14	Root canal fillings		
15	Cavities		

7

Please check the boxes if you have these dental health concerns:		Have experienced this	Worried that this might happen
16	Pain		
17	Way my teeth look		

2. Hopes about having strong and healthy teeth in the future

Imagine yourself a few years in the future after having taken good care of your teeth. Please check the boxes below that represent what you envisage	
1	Nice smile
2	Talk freely
3	Strong teeth
4	No or few cavities
5	Low cost of dental care – money saved
6	Satisfied with myself for taking good care of my teeth
7	Don't have to worry about my teeth
8	Fresh breath
9	Teeth look nice
10	Can eat whatever I want
11	No pain
12	Better conscience
13	Good role model for others, i.e. children

Tip

Motivational effect can be strengthened if the practitioner encourages the patient to discuss his or her concerns and hopes in more detail: *"I see you have checked a few things… I wonder which are most important for you, and if you could say a little bit more about them?"*

7.3.2 Decision-Making

Just discussing concerns and worries can lead to a decision that results in improved dental health behaviour. Focusing explicitly on decision-making can also be help-

ful and increase the likelihood of initiating behaviours. Decision-making can be thought of as the gateway between thinking about the condition of one's teeth and actually performing dental health care behaviours.

> ❯ Decision-making is a complex process with three major components: (1) making one's mind up about the importance of concerns; (2) looking ahead and planning what to do; (3) an acceptance, willingness or commitment to put in the effort necessary to ensure dental health.

While motivation focuses on the patient's concerns and reasons for taking care of his or her teeth, decision-making takes the process a step further. Decision-making includes consideration of how important the patient's concerns are and can lead to the patient making up his or her mind about performing dental health behaviours.

Emotions are important for decision-making. Feelings of distress or worry, along with factual thoughts about the condition of one's teeth, are the impetus for action. Emotions are, however, by nature often transient. They can change swiftly or dissolve gradually. When the sense of emotional urgency dissipates, the patient may no longer feel the need to implement a behaviour. In order to preserve a decision, a person needs to be explicit about prioritising dental health. The behaviour in question must consciously be put high on the person's list of everyday activities and chores that are to be performed.

Important components of decision-making are looking ahead and planning. One aspect of planning is to set behavioural goals (what to do, when to start, how often, for how long). Another aspect is thinking about procuring needed materials and utensils. Looking ahead also implies evaluating one's ability to perform a behaviour. This is of special significance when the behaviour is complex, demanding or complicated. Most dental health behaviours are relatively simple, and the main difficulty is performing them consistently over time. In other words, before deciding, one must believe that it is feasible and realistic to repeat taking care of one's teeth every day for the rest of one's life [9].

The last, and perhaps the most crucial, element of decision-making is a willingness to accept the effort, cost and possible discomfort that accompanies dental health behaviours. This willingness is at the heart of decision-making and can be expressed as a commitment to endure and persevere in the face of everyday obstacles and difficulties.

Johnathan was worried about food remnants between his teeth and, therefore, motivated to increase his cleaning efforts. He thought that it would be a good idea to use toothpicks after eating and before going to bed and felt that although it would be worth the effort even though being a bit bothersome. He was willing to accept the cost of toothpicks although finding it to be a bit expensive. He bought several packs of toothpicks and placed them in visible and easily accessible places. Using toothpicks was easy and straightforward, but as an afterthought searched YouTube for information on effective ways of doing it.

7.3.2.1 Exploring Decision-Making in Dental Consultations

When addressing decision-making, the health professional balances between giving well-founded advice and exploring the patient's own perspective and thoughts. The consultation needs to be conducted in a direct manner but tempered by an understanding of a universal aspect of human behaviour and interaction: It is easy to give, but surprisingly difficult to follow advice.

With this in mind, the GPS model of supporting decision-making in oral health has been proposed and tested in periodontal disease patients: G stands for 'goal setting', P stands for 'Planning' and S stands for 'Self-monitoring'. A consultation guided by the GPS model supports the patient's decision to commit to behaviour change by first setting a SMART goal (where SMART stands for S-pecific, M-easureable, A-chievebale, R-ealistic and T-ime specific).

The second step would be for the patient to plan when, where and how they will perform the behaviour, along with a "Plan B" of how to address barriers to change if and when they occur. Patients are supported in developing a specific If … → Then … plan, where having set a SMART goal, they are asked to say when, where and how they will perform the behaviour followed by exploring possible difficulties they may experience in executing the plan. Acknowledging that making a plan is not a guarantee that life will not get in the way alerts patients to the idea that plans can be modified when 'life' happens, and that this need not mean the end of their behaviour change efforts. So, an If … → Then … plan asks them to consider what may happen to undermine achieving their SMART behaviour goal. This planning component of the GPS plan is crucial because it acts as a safety net for the patient.

> ► **Example**
>
> *Sarah decided to brush her teeth every Friday evening at 11 pm after watching the news on the TV and before settling in bed. She usually went out with friends on Fridays and needed a different plan when coming home tired after partying all night. She made and imagined following the following If→ Then plan: "If I stay out all night on a Friday and I come back home tired and sleepy I will brush my teeth while using the toilet before going to bed".* ◄

The third component of the GPS model is about self-monitoring where the person keeps track of the frequency of their performing the behaviour. In the case of brushing or interdental cleaning, this could be that they simply tick a diary kept on their bathroom mirror every time they brush and/or floss their teeth. Data from two randomised controlled trials have shown that the GPS model is effective in supporting oral health behaviours in periodontal disease patients and in fact can reduce plaque and bleeding scores at 4 and 8 weeks [3].

The steps in the GPS model should be delivered within an environment that is accepting and respecting of the patient's autonomy [13]. We have provided below some ways in which this environment may be achieved.

- Set an agenda, explain the purpose and ask for permission:
  - *"An important part of taking care of one's teeth is to make up one's mind to really do it. Would it be all right if we talked a bit about this?"*
- Ask about the importance of concerns and reasons for wanting to change:
  - *"To do what it takes to take care of your teeth, you have to feel your concerns about dental health are important. I was wondering about <u>how</u> important dental health is for you. On a scale from 0 to 10, 0 being completely unimportant and 10 extremely important? Is it important enough to put it on your daily to-do list?"*
- Explore behaviour plans for future behaviour
  - *"It's helpful to have a concrete plan … for example, what you are going to do, how often, and when will you start. You might want to think a bit about difficulties that can pop up and how to overcome obstacles and barriers that can stop you from doing what you have decided on. Do you have any thoughts along these lines?"*
- Explore willingness to exert effort and persevere
  - *"Taking care of your teeth in recommended ways requires a bit of effort. The most common challenge is that it is a lifelong project… taking care of your teeth in the right way, every day, several times a day, day in and day out... How willing and determined are you to do this? Is taking good care of your teeth something you feel half-hearted about or something you're determined to do, something you'll do no matter what?"*

7.3.3 Implementing and Maintaining Behaviour

There are two main dimensions in performing dental care behaviours: (1) knowledge and skills and (2) maintenance of behaviour.

7.3.3.1 Knowing What to Do and Having the Skills

Dental health depends on having knowledge about what behaviours to do and possessing the skills to perform them. Dental health behaviours can be done incorrectly, ineffectively or even in a damaging manner. The dental health professional's expertise is important in assisting the patient acquire proper techniques.

The simplest way to influence behaviour is to instruct the patient about what to do and how to do it. Instructions are particularly important if the patient lacks basic knowledge about healthy behaviours and how to perform them.

However, it is advisable to explore the patient's existing skills before giving instructions. Pausing to inquire about the patient's thoughts around the instructions provided is also time well spent.

> **Tip**
>
> In addition to verbal or written guidelines, demonstrating what to do is worth considering. Specific demonstrations of technique are surprisingly often necessary. Verbal instructions can be understood and carried out in a very different fashion than the practitioner intends. Demonstrations ensure that the patient really knows, for example, how to brush or to use toothpicks and dental floss in the correct manner.

Finally, it is possible to ask the patient to demonstrate how he or she performs specific behaviours. This allows the dental professional to give feedback, either confirming the patient's technique or suggesting adjustments.

7.3.3.2 Carrying Out and Maintaining Healthy Behaviours

Dental health care behaviours are in general not complicated skills. Proper technique is important, but the necessary behaviours are relatively straightforward. The main challenge is following through and actually performing the behaviours. Following a routine, using reminders, renewing motivation, repeated decision-making and identifying and overcoming barriers are strategies that can increase maintenance over time.

7.3.3.3 Put Dental Health on the Schedule of Daily Activities

It is often necessary to mobilise a certain amount of effort to carry out intentional behaviours. Even relatively simple caretaking of one's teeth requires self-discipline. Dental behaviours are not performed because they are enjoyable, but because they are fixed items on our daily schedules. Routines help us execute behaviours regardless of whether we feel motivated to do them or not. Having a routine reduces the effort and mental energy needed for initiating behaviours. If the behaviour is given any conscious thought at all, it is often just as a short message to self: "I'll do it".

> **Tip**
>
> A simple way to establish a routine is to connect brushing one's teeth to specific situations, after breakfast, before going out, before going to bed.

7.3.3.4 Visual Reminders

Another way to increase the likelihood of performing dental health care behaviours is to make sure that equipment and materials are clearly visible. Tools being out of sight, in a cabinet or drawer, create a small barrier to carrying out the behaviour. Visual reminders such as having a toothbrush, toothpaste, floss, fluoride rinse and toothpicks readily available on a shelf or by the sink serve as cues for behaviour. Other reminders can also be helpful – for example, a "brush your teeth today" note or a picture of a smile with healthy teeth taped to the bathroom mirror.

7.3.3.5 Refresh Motivation

Mentally revisiting dental health concerns, what one wishes to avoid or achieve, can refresh motivation. However, mechanical repetition of the reasons for taking care of one's teeth can quickly become an empty, meaningless ritual. When reviewing concerns, the patient should take a few seconds and focus on the importance of these issues and the feelings they activate. One interesting strategy to refresh motivation is to consciously remind oneself of the reasons for dental health behaviours while performing them; in other words, saying "I'm building strong teeth" to oneself when brushing or rinsing.

7.3.3.6 Renew One's Decision and Use Self-Instructions

Consciously giving oneself simple self-instructions like *"This is what I'm going to do"* or *"I've made up my mind and will do it no matter what"* is a way to renew commitment to continued efforts. Self-instructions in specific situations or circumstances are also helpful. These will often be formulated as an intention to implement a behaviour: *"After breakfast I use a toothpick and clean between my teeth". "Before leaving the house I will go to the bathroom and brush my teeth". "If I don't feel like using mouthwash before bedtime, I'll remember how pleased I am when I do it anyway"*.

7.3.3.7 Positive Reinforcement: Crediting the Effort

Pausing from time to time and recognising that one is doing a good job can function as positive reinforcement. Acknowledgement of effort can result in feeling satisfied or proud which, in turn, contributes to increased likelihood of future behaviour. Another form of positive reinforcement is the pleasurable sensation of passing one's tongue over freshly brushed clean teeth.

7.3.3.8 Overcoming Dips in Motivation and Self-Sabotaging Thoughts

Drops in motivation that undermine the performance of behaviour are to be expected. Loss of motivation can manifest as indifference, inertia, reduced energy, unwillingness or resistance that typically occurs and intensifies just before performing the behaviour. Accompanying these changes in motivation are automatic thoughts: *"I'm too tired, doesn't matter if I skip it today, don't feel like it, too much of a bother, I'll do it tomorrow"*.

> Fluctuations in motivation and self-sabotaging thoughts are common and everyone experiences them from time to time (Beck 2020). Even motivated, committed and competent people encounter them before executing even simple behaviours. Just being aware of the occurrence of drops in motivation and self-sabotage thoughts is helpful.

Awareness can lead to developing a plan. One useful strategy to counteract the effects of reduced motivation comes from behavioural activation, a treatment for depression [10]. The main idea in behavioural activation is that depressive symptoms can be relieved by becoming more active. However, increases in depressive symptoms such as inertia and lethargy as well as negative thoughts often occur just prior to initiating a beneficial activity.

> **Tip**
>
> One way to overcome dips in motivation and increased negativity is "acting from the outside in". Instead of allowing negative thoughts and unpleasant internal states to determine behaviour, the patient follows his or her predetermined plan and uses self-instructions like *"Don't wait until I want to do it, just get started"*. The activity is carried out regardless of negative thoughts and feelings.

7.3.3.9 Mental Rehearsing: Using Visualisation and Imagery

Running through behaviours by using visualisation and mental imagery makes it easier to actually follow through with what one has planned to do [5]. Professional actors and athletes use these techniques to improve performance. The capacity to picture oneself performing a caretaking behaviour can help mobilise resources that facilitate the implementation and maintenance of dental health. With practice, visualisation can become a helpful method of preparing for and overcoming difficulties and obstacles. The effectiveness of visualisation can be increased by including several sensory modalities in the mental image of executing the behaviour. The patient can be encouraged to create an elaborate mental picture of the situation in which the behaviour is carried out by including sights, sounds, odours, temperature, kinaesthetic and tactile elements. The more detailed the image is, the better [7].

7.4 Structuring Discussions About Oral Health

Consultations about oral health are a question of content (what to talk about) as well as style and approach (how to talk about dental health). Thus far in this chapter, we have mainly addressed the content of intentional dental health behaviour – motivation, decision-making, implementation and maintenance. We will now look more closely at how to structure dental consultations.

7.4.1 Balancing Expert Information and Eliciting the Patient's Existing Resources

Strengthening the patient's existing resources relating to motivation, commitment and concrete ideas about how to improve and maintain dental health is a vital component in consultations. This strategy can be overlooked, however, in a busy dental practice. Just telling the patient what to do can become the default method of promoting healthy behaviours.

Activating patient resources, though crucial, is often not sufficient. Most patients profit from new and relevant information about why and how to take care of their teeth. New information is essential if the patient lacks knowledge or has a faulty understanding of personal dental care behaviours. The effect of providing information can be enhanced by both preparing that a message is forthcoming and taking time to explore the patient's understanding and perception of information, recommendations or suggestions.

Both providing information and activating the patient's existing resources are laudable. The expert practitioner often does both, alternating between advising and providing information, and eliciting, elaborating and acknowledging the patient's existing knowledge and competency.

7.4.1.1 Increasing the Patient's Active Participation in Dental Care

The structure for consultations presented below increases the likelihood of the patient paying attention to, remembering and attributing importance to the topics which are addressed. It also enables confirming and reinforcing the patient's knowledge, resources and pre-existing healthy behaviours.

7.4.1.2 Cooperation and Avoiding Discord Between the Dental Health Professional and the Patient

The steps laid out below aim to facilitate cooperation and make dental health a shared endeavour. In addition, they prevent unnecessarily providing information, advice and demonstrating techniques, of which the patient already is aware.

> ❯ A word of caution is in order when it comes to addressing the connection between behaviour and health. It can be relatively easy for the patient to interpret conversations about dental health behaviour as criticism or even blame. The health professional can be perceived as judgemental and depreciating. This can lead to feelings of shame or guilt about being inadequate, or irritation or even anger and thoughts of being treated in a depreciating fashion by the dental practitioner. The patient can become defensive. This hampers receptiveness to, and acceptance of information, and undercuts the patient's willingness to be candid and cooperative in discussing healthy behaviour.

7.4.1.3 Four Steps for Structuring Dental Consultations

Dental health consultations are typically short, only allowing for brief or minimal interventions. Brief interventions focus typically on one or two aspects of intentional change - either motivation, decision-making, concrete skills, ways to maintain change or overcome obstacles. More comprehensive interventions addressing multiple issues simply repeat the steps several times.

> **Box 7.2**
> 1. Set an agenda, present a rationale and ask permission
> 2. Elicit the patient's input
> 3. Confirm and provide new information
> 4. Elicit the patient's viewpoint

This structure constitutes a framework that can be deviated from when appropriate. The practitioner must strive to be flexible and modify interventions according to the patients' needs and responses.

> ▶ **Example**
>
> 1. Set the agenda, give a rationale, and ask for permission
>   - *It can be a bit difficult to stick to good intentions to take care of your teeth. Most people experience this from time to time. I wonder if we could talk about ways to make it easier to follow through. Would that be all right with you?*
> 2. Elicit the patient's input
>   - *One thing that a lot of people experience is that motivation varies, and they don't feel like doing what they know they should. Have you ever experienced this and what happens when you do?*
> 3. Confirm and provide new information
>   - *Thinking about the reasons for taking care of your teeth is a good strategy. It also sounds like you just make up your mind to do what you should do. Some people find it helps to say something to themselves like "It doesn't matter if I don't feel like doing it, I'm just going to do it. I'll be pleased afterwards".*
> 4. Elicit the patient's viewpoint
>   5 *What do you think about this? Is it something that could be a bit helpful?* ◄

> ▶ **Example**
>
> 1. Set the agenda, give a rationale, and ask for permission
>   - *So, what I'm going to do now is to check your teeth and then we can talk about how things are. Ok?*
> 2. Elicit the patient's input
>   - *Before I begin… do you have any concerns about your teeth? Is there anything in particular you would like me to check?*
> 3. Confirm and provide new information
>   - *Your teeth are in good condition, but I can see that the enamel is a bit worn in places. I also noticed that your gums bleed a bit. It looks like you have mild gingivitis.*
> 4. Elicit the patient's viewpoint
>   - *I don't know if you were aware of this, but I'm interested in what you think about it.*
> 5. Set the agenda (give rational and ask for permission)
>   - *There are some things that you can do to reduce these problems.*
> 6. Elicit the patient
>   - *But maybe you already have some good ideas of what to do.*
> 7. Confirm and provide new information
>   - *Using a softer toothbrush can help, that's a good idea. Other things are brushing softer but for a bit longer, using toothpicks in the right way and rinsing regularly with a fluoride mouthwash. Also be careful about drinking carbonated beverages or food with low pH value.*
> 8. Elicit the patient's viewpoint
>   5 *Which of these things would you like to talk more about?* ◄

Summary

This chapter has provided a framework for understanding how you as a dental practitioner can help your patients to establish behaviours that will lead to reduced oral health problems and promote good oral health. First, by learning how habits form human behaviours, and how motivation influences decision-making. The differences between establishing new behaviours and maintaining health-promoting behaviours were described. In the last part of the chapter it is described how a dental practitioner can structure consultations with their patients to help them achieve an increased oral health.

7

References

1. Asimakopoulou K, Newton JT. The contributions of behaviour change science towards dental public health practice: a new paradigm. Community Dent Oral Epidemiol. 2015;43(1):2–8. https://doi.org/10.1111/cdoe.12131.

2. Asimakopoulou K, Newton JT, Daly B, Kutzer Y, Ide M. The effects of providing periodontal disease risk information on psychological outcomes – a randomized controlled trial. J Clin Periodontol. 2015;42(4):350–5. https://doi.org/10.1111/jcpe.12377.

3. Asimakopoulou KG, Nolan M, McCarthy CCL, Newton JT. The effect of risk communication on periodontal treatment outcomes: a randomized controlled trial. J Periodontol. 2019;90(9):948–56. https://doi.org/10.1002/JPER.18-0385.

4. Beck JS. Cognitive behavior therapy. 2nd ed. New York: Guilford Press; 2011.

5. Conroy D, Hagger MS. Imagery interventions in health behavior: a meta-analysis. Health Psychol. 2018;37(7):668–79. https://doi.org/10.1037/hea0000625.

6. Gillison FB, Rouse P, Standage M, Sebire SJ, Ryan RM. A meta-analysis of techniques to promote motivation for health behaviour change from a self-determination theory perspective. Health Psychol Rev. 2019;13(1):110–30. https://doi:10.1080/17437199.2018.1534071

7. Hagger M, Conroy D. Imagery, visualization, and mental simulation interventions. In: Hagger M, Cameron L, Hamilton K, Hankonen N, Lintunen T, editors. The handbook of behavior change. Cambridge: Cambridge University Press; 2020. p. 479–94. https://doi.org/10.1017/9781108677318.033.

8. Hagger M, Hankonen N, Chatzisarantis N, Ryan R. Changing behavior using self-determination theory. In: Hagger M, Cameron L, Hamilton K, Hankonen N, Lintunen T, editors. The handbook of behavior change. Cambridge: Cambridge University Press; 2020. p. 104–19. https://doi.org/10.1017/9781108677318.007.

9. Luszczynska A, Schwarzer R. Changing behavior using social cognitive theory. In: Hagger M, Cameron L, Hamilton K, Hankonen N, Lintunen T, editors. The handbook of behavior change, vol. 2020. Cambridge: Cambridge University Press; 2020. p. 32–45. https://doi.org/10.1017/9781108677318.003.

10. Martell CR, Dimidjian S, Herman-Duun R. Behavioral activation for depression: a clinician's guide. New York: Guilford Press; 2010.

11. Michie S, van Stralen MM, West R. The behaviour change wheel: a new method for characterising and designing behaviour change interventions. Implement Sci. 2011;6(1):42. https://doi.org/10.1186/1748-5908-6-42.

12. Miller WR, Rollnick S. Motivational interviewing: helping people change. 3rd ed. New York: Guilford Press; 2013.

13. Ryan RM, Deci EL. Self-determination theory: basic psychological needs in motivation, development, and wellness. New York: Guilford Press; 2017. https://doi.org/10.1521/978.14625/28806.

14. Scambler S, Asimakopoulou K. A model of patient-centred care—turning good care into patient-centred care. Br Dent J. 2014;217(5):225–8. https://doi.org/10.1038/sj.bdj.2014.755

15. Schwarzer R, Hamilton K. Changing behavior using the health action process approach. In: Hagger M, Cameron L, Hamilton K, Hankonen N, Lintunen T, editors. The handbook of behavior change. Cambridge: Cambridge University Press; 2020. p. 89–103. https://doi.org/10.1017/9781108677318.007.

Additional References

Asimakopoulou K, Newton T. Success with motivational interviewing techniques in the dental clinic: a case for the use of iMI-GPS. Dental Update. 2018;45(5):462–7. https://doi.org/10.12968/denu.2018.45.5.462.

Cascaes AM, Bielemann RM, Clark VL, Barros AJD. Effectiveness of motivational interviewing at improving oral health: a systematic review. Rev Saude Publica. 2014;48(1):142–53. https://doi.org/10.1590/S0034-8910.2014048004616.

Gao X, Lo ECM, Kot SCC, Chan KCW. Motivational interviewing in improving oral health: a systematic review of randomized controlled trials. J Periodontol. 2014;85(3):426–37. https://doi.org/10.1902/jop.2013.130205.

Lundahl B, Moleni T, Burke BL, Butters R, Tollefson D, Butler C, Rollnick S. Motivational interviewing in medical care settings: a systematic review and meta-analysis of randomized controlled trials. Centre for Reviews and Dissemination (UK); 2013. https://www.ncbi.nlm.nih.gov/books/NBK159484/.

Miller WR, Rollnick S. Motivational interviewing: preparing people to change addictive behavior. London: The Guildford Press; 1996.

Self-Determination Theory – Autonomy Support and Improving Oral Health

Anne Elisabeth Münster Halvari

Contents

⊚ Learning Goals
- Learn about the importance of autonomy and self-regulation in self-determination theory (SDT) in order to improve oral health
- Learn about why autonomy is one of the most important of moral pillars in biomedical ethics, professionalism and *informed consent* related to oral health choices and challenges
- Learn about the three basic psychological needs (BPN) in SDT, and how they are connected to autonomy support, learning, motivation and mastery of oral health
- Learn about how to give patients *autonomy support* related to their own oral health challenges
- Learn about the *internalisation process* and how different motivational regulations are related to different oral health behaviours

8.1 Introduction to Self-Determination Theory (SDT)

Self-determination theory (SDT), developed by Edward L. Deci and Richard M. Ryan [1], is a modern empirical macro-theory of human motivation. SDT [2] is one of the most researched and applied theories of human motivation in the field of psychology.

Motivation lies in the human nature. When we are motivated, we are active, engaged and curious. We are inspired, and we want to learn, develop and master new skills. Most people want to make great efforts, but it is also clear that some individuals are passive and alienated [3].

> **Box**
> Motivation represents both *energy* and *direction* of a behaviour [1]. Motivation plays an uttermost and central role in learning, leadership, teaching, counselling and guiding processes related to behaviour change [4, 2].

SDT is anchored in Carl Rogers [5] and his humanistic perspectives such as unconditional positive regard, authenticity, warmth, empathy and patient centeredness, thus being sensitive to patients' psychological and social needs.

The SDT theory can explain how and why motivation is important in most contexts and situations [6].

Further, SDT is concerned with how dental professionals can give autonomy support and how this generates patient's autonomous motivation, self-regulation and relevant oral health changes.

Autonomous motivation and self-regulation, in SDT research, have shown positive impacts on oral health

changes, decrease in dental anxiety, increase in well-being and oral health-related quality of life besides maintaining positive dental health behaviour over time [7–10].

A fundamental issue in SDT is how dental professionals are able to implement counsel and guide *autonomy support* in a non-controlling and non-conditional way [11].

SDT represents patient centredness and a holistic patient view by focusing on the biopsychosocial model by Engel and Williams & Deci [12, 13].

> **Box**
> Autonomy-supportive guidelines refers to SDT's three basic and fundamental psychological needs (SDT-BPN): autonomy, competence and relatedness.
>
> Supporting the three SDT - needs has shown positive effects on patients' health-promoting and preventive behaviours and oral health status [10].

> ❯ "*Autonomy support instantiates the type of provider behavior that is widely advocated by adherents to the biopsychosocial approach to medicine*" [13, p. 767].

When implementing SDT in oral health interventions, we can understand more about what lies behind motivational processes related to changes in oral health behaviour, patient's well-being and oral health quality of life. This is fundamental in order to be able to help patients in a better way in the future to manage oral health challenges [10, 14].

8.1.1 Ethical Considerations Using Autonomy

The concept of autonomy has become increasingly accepted in all health contexts and has become one of the most important of moral pillars. This is considered an ethical mandate for medicine [15].

Autonomy support is a factor that makes SDT particularly useful in health care contexts because it is consistent with biomedical ethics [16], medical professionalism [17] and informed consent [17, 18]. Clinical practitioners are, therefore, obligated to respect autonomy regardless of the theoretical frame they are using [15]. Emphasis on patient autonomy has been widely embraced in physician charters [17].

Biomedical ethics claims that autonomous motivation and self-regulation are important health outcomes in itself. SDT is, therefore, consistent with tenets of clinical practice as medical professionalism and principles of biomedical ethics.

8.1.2 Autonomy and Self-Regulation

Autonomy is derived from the Greek words "autos" (self) and "nomos" (rule). Autonomy refers to *self-regulation* and *self-endorsement* [19]. Autonomous people experience ownership of their behaviour [2].

When people are self-ruled and self-motivated, they will be able to make volitional and personal choices which generate their own energy, implicitly feeling vital and moving forward [20].

> *"SDT is concerned about how autonomy develops, and how it can be either diminished or facilitated by specific biological and social conditions. SDT has attention on the interplay between inherent tendencies toward integrated vital functioning, but also pays attention to peoples vulnerabilities to being controlled"* [19, p. 1562].

8.2 Basic Psychological Needs (BPN)

SDT focuses mainly on three basic psychological needs (BPN): competence, autonomy and relatedness. BPN are fundamental for personal growth, optimal functioning, well-being and quality of life. The satisfaction of BPN is essential for people to be fully functioning, actualise their potentials, to flourish, and being protected from stress, ill-health and maladaptive functioning [2].

Deci and Ryan [1] point out that our behaviour is governed by a desire to cover and satisfy the three inner BPN [3]. BPN can help explain why only some behaviours will enhance well-being and some will produce pathological consequences, for example, somatisation.

The three BPN are universal and fundamental to all people in all cultures [2].

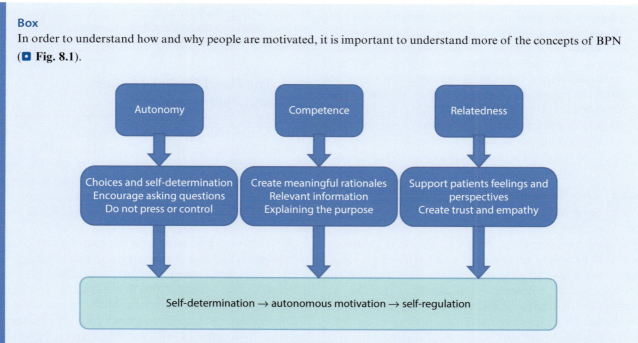

■ **Fig. 8.1**   The model shows the three basic psychological needs in SDT; autonomy, competence and relatedness, represented in SDT's guidelines for *autonomy support* [21]. Supporting psychological needs generates integration of autonomous motivation and self-regulation

8

8.2.1 The Need for Autonomy and Self-Determination

The need for autonomy is related to when you feel you can execute personal, important and volitional choices willingly. Persons feel they have a personal and valued ownership of their behaviour. The need for autonomy implies the need to experience that one is in control over one's own actions, thus self-initiating and self-regulating these actions. According to Deci and Ryan [1], individuals have an inner need to perceive themselves as the source of their own actions. Internally self-controlled and autonomous persons want to act on the basis of voluntariness related to their own interests, engagements and integrated values [1, 2, 21]. The need for autonomy means that we experience self-determination, and it contributes to make more self-conscious and more aware (mindful), strategic and meaningful choices [2]. When patients can make their own autonomous choices and develop valued and rational competence fitting into their own self, they become more and more self-regulated and appropriately competent related to their own goals and a given behaviour [21].

▶ Example

Example of support for the need for autonomy: When patients experience receiving support for the need for autonomy, they will experience that they can freely and effortlessly convey their own thoughts, reflections and feelings. Thus, they will more easily be able to ask questions and tell about their own needs and choices. Patients experience that they can more openly discuss different treatment options with dental personnel. In this way, patients feel that they have the opportunity to make more autonomous, competence- generating and relatedness-building, self-determined and self-regulated choices. The patients experience that they more easily can be themselves and that they honestly and authentically master to convey, for example, their own frustrations by not being able to lie down in the dental treatment chair or express clearly about pain experiences or other discomforts that can occur in treatment situations [22]. ◀

8.2.2 The Need for Competence and Mastery

The need for competence refers to the need to master and thus be able to experience oneself as a self governed chief who is able to solve challenges and tasks, perform an appropriate behaviour and, therefore, be able to achieve the desired goals and results. Competence refers to the need to experience making important and relevant effects in the environment. Patients who feel the oral health competence need supported, know themselves as effective and skilled when executing tasks related to oral health challenges [1].

The need for competence is also related to when you feel capable and effective in interactions with people in the environment. Persons who seek optimal challenges make efforts along with strategic thinking until they master their challenges and along with this personal growth is a result [2].

The need for competence represents individuals' desire to feel they have appropriate knowledge and at the same time perceive themselves as capable, competent and able to develop and bring about reasoned, important new skills [23]. A supported competence need involves an understanding of how to attain various external and internal outcomes, and at the same time feeling efficacious in performing the requisite behaviors.

▶ Example

Example of support for the need for competence: When the need for competence is supported in dental treatment situations, patients experience that they master taking care of their dental health. They are able to perform their own dental home care qualitatively well. They will use their effort to master their oral challenges well, and they experience mastering the challenges in a meaningful and appropriate way. ◀

Research has shown that positive feedback provides satisfaction for the need for competence, which signifies direct and concrete effect on mastering in different situations, thus enhancing more intrinsic autonomous and self-regulated motivation. Negative feedback conveys negative effects and tends to thwart the need for competence and thus undermine intrinsic autonomous self-regulated motivation [2].

8.2.3 The Need for Relatedness and Belonging

The need for relatedness is about sharing intimacy and to establish close emotional bonds and attachment with other people depending on interpersonal, friendly and warm relationships. Relatedness need is about feeling socially connected and being engaged in giving and receiving of care and attentiveness from significant people in one's life.

Relatedness, belonging and socialising are basic human needs that help develop the opportunity for close relationships built on mutual trust, respect and benevolence, accept and recognition. Being able to experience that someone cares about you establishes social ties and when someone can be present for you, it is of significant importance in order to satisfy wellness and support for the relatedness need. Experience of cohesion with the environment and society in general is of great importance for relatedness need satisfaction [2]. Relatedness and belongingness involve developing secure and satisfying connections and collaborations with significant and important persons [24].

Example of support for relatedness: When the need for relatedness is supported, the patient experiences he has a good connection and relationship with dental personnel. Patients feel safe, well, natural, authentic and relaxed in the treatment situation. Experiencing a pleasant atmosphere that helps patients feel comfortable with the dental personnel is important when building relatedness and collaboration around dental health challenges. The patients experience that the dental personnel both see them as a person and listen to what they convey during the entire treatment session. In this way, patients experience dental personnel as friendly, aware and attentive, which supports the relatedness need. ◀

When all the three BPN are met and satisfied, patients are able to develop sufficient inner autonomous and self-regulated motivation, and they are now able to learn optimally and master challenges related to their own dental health and sustain long-lasting oral health promotion and preventive behaviour [2].

Thus, for the dental personnel, it is important to be able to satisfy all the three BPN of patients. This can be done when using the SDT guidelines (see later in this chapter).

Behaviours which lead to satisfaction of the three BPN will enhance autonomous motivation and self-regulation, personal growth and well-being [2].

The need support promotes positive emotions and more autonomous motivation to continue a given behaviour even though this behaviour sometimes can be challenging, strenuous or even boring [2].

When dental personnel are able to provide highly individualised and differentiated counseling that satisfies the three BPN, this will facilitate integration of more autonomous motivation and self-regulation. In this way, patients are more likely to achieve their oral health goals. When dental personnel thwart or frustrate psychological needs in dental treatment, negative oral health consequences will arise [25].

8.2.4 Need Thwarting – Need Frustration

Dental professionals who do not take into consideration patients' individual differences or support BPNs will undermine patients personal growth. This hindering or thwarting of BPN will be associated with lower autonomous motivation, less self-regulated motivation, difficulties in mastering oral health challenges and diminished well-being [2].

Autonomous motivation will not be facilitated when need-thwarting or need-frustrating situations arise in the course of treatment. Thwarting of BPN is a consequence of dental professionals who want to control their patients. Control are for example, negative evaluations, withdrawal of attention and criticism. Controlling personnel lead patients to become more vulnerable and this may lead to dental anxiety. As a consequence of this control, patients often will avoid dental appointments [26].

Examples also include dental professionals who dominate the conversation, minimise the patient's choices, instruct the patient on what he/she "should or must do" or give few or no rationales for reflection. This will not be in line with giving autonomy support [15].

Examples When Patients Feel Their Needs Thwarted
— When the need for *autonomy is thwarted*, patients experience less choice and feel their actions are other-initiated [27]. They may feel that dental personnel will do what they want themselves and will not listen to patients when they sit in the chair.
— Thwarting of *the need for competence* means that patients experience that they are not capable of acting effectively to attain desired results [23]. For example, when the teeth are being examined, patients may feel underestimated and/or humiliated.
— Thwarting fulfillment of *the relatedness need* will involve an experience of <u>not</u> being safely attached to and understood by dental personnel [24]. An example is when a dental practitioner does not see the patients needs, but only sees the teeth.

8.3 Guidelines for Autonomy Support

Autonomy support is consistent with support of the three BPN [2]. SDT guidelines can provide a basis for appropriate guidance to promote, enhance and change dental health behaviour besides preventing and decreasing dental anxiety, increasing dental well-being and oral health quality of life [10]. Research shows that patients can learn to become more autonomously motivated and self-regulated.

8.3.1 Autonomy Support

Autonomy support is a motivating style, and it is an important issue in SDT. Autonomy support is connected to how the three BPN (autonomy, competence and relatedness) are addressed and supported in diverse contexts [2]. Autonomy support can facilitate more self-determined regulation for uninteresting activities like tooth brushing [28].

> Autonomy support is about when dental personnel are non-judgemental, aware of the patient's feelings and perspectives, provide appropriate explanations and rationales when self-determined choices are given, and at the same time focus on minimising pressure and control in all situations [2, 26].

Autonomy support concerns making the patients more aware and involve them in their own oral health situation and encourage them to become more self-determined related to choices and decisions. Dental personnel listen to the patients' own reflections, stimulate them to ask questions and they ask questions in order to stimulate additional reflections, thus opening up for a more meaningful dialogue. Autonomy supportive dental professionals will stimulate and promote more autonomous self-regulation and self-directed motivation towards patients' own dental health goals [2].

Integration of appropriate dental health behaviour will, according to Deci and Ryan [21], depend on whether significant persons like dental personnel and the environment provide sufficient autonomy support.

Providing choices implies that patients are being involved in planning and discussions related to different treatment or behavioural options together with dental personnel. When patients feel they can talk more freely and authentically with their dental professionals, it will be easier for them to decide on what is the best alternative and solution for themselves [22].

8.3.2 Autonomy – Guiding to Choice Rather Than Control

Developing autonomous motivation, self-regulation and self-management is challenging work in many health care contexts, but first and foremost, it is all about not pressing or controlling the patient's feelings, thoughts, choices, goals and behaviours [29].

> **Box**
>
> Controlling aspects can be: pressure to behave in certain ways, argue (disagree), convince, seduce, humiliate, ignore, underestimate, confront, not being responsive, withhold information, setting conditions, push to make choices, pressure to decide and expecting patients to make choices before they are ready for it, decide for the patients or give direct advices without asking. All of these controlling elements will contribute to decreased autonomous regulation, decreased feelings of competency and relatedness, besides often increased dental anxiety.

Resistance and low autonomous motivation are natural reactions along with many change processes. It is worth to remark, if dental personnel are too eager to focus on change or outcomes, it will create a feeling of control and pressure. Patients have to feel they are going through the change process in their own way and in their own rhythm. Outcome-focused dental personnel who follow their own treatment goals instead of focusing on patient's own goals for treatment, will be using a controlling style. This feeling of pressure will not be in line with autonomy support.

> **Tip**
>
> When counselling, dental professionals can be trained to develop awareness and emphasis on avoiding words as: "you could, you should or you must do" in order to be less controlling.

Autonomy support gives patients a sense of being in their own control, they are their own chief, and therefore, they feel they are in charge. This is because autonomy relates to self-control. Dental professionals can teach patients to feel in control in many ways. For example, to raise their hand in order to stop treatment, they can hold their own saliva-ejector, or hold their own X-ray holders in order to feel in control. When dental professionals stimulate patients to make choices and be more self-determined in treatment, can lead patients to be more self-conscious. Thus, over time, patients can learn to be more able to make more relevant and autonomous choices for themselves. When patients have a feeling of being in control, can result in a more authentic dialogue, because patients now feel more recognised and believed in. Because of this, patients now can express their feelings and thoughts more freely and directly. Patients will feel more in control when dental personnel ask more open-ended questions instead of close-ended questions. Asking questions about how patients are feeling, thinking and reacting in dental treatment sessions is important in order to understand and be able to communicate properly about patients needs. Dental personnel can train patients to be more aware of their own thinking and reactions. This is important in order to make appropriate plans together. These conversations can hopefully lead to more autonomous motivation in patients, being more aware of choosing of oral health promotive behaviour, which implies prevention and decrease of dental anxiety, increase in oral well-being and oral health quality of life [7–9, 26].

Dental professionals can provide patients with advices or recommendations when it is done in an autonomy supportive way. Dental professionals have to have in mind that it is easy for patients to view dental personnel as authorities, and therefore, understand and interpret their words as controlling, even if it is not meant to be [11].

> **Box**
>
> Deci and Ryan say that autonomy support does not mean: **"telling them what to do and expecting them to do it"** [11, p. 4]. This attitude will turn autonomy support into control, undermine patients' autonomous motivation and decrease optimal health behaviour. Deci and Ryan convey [11] that there is no evidence that a controlling style produces positive health effects.

Dental professionals are experts in their field, and therefore, they need to provide relevant, evidence-based and understandable information along with structure for their patients [2]; this in order to give patients informative, comprehensive, personally useful and appropriate information about their oral health challenges, health risks, and consequences regarding the patients' own health goals. Important questions are: "What are the patients concerned about?" "What is important to inform patients about?" and "What is necessary to have an appropriate conversation around?" Informed consent is important to have in mind when giving this information [30].

When patients are given the opportunity to actively participate in a dialogue and reflect upon the pros and cons related to what they feel and think are important issues that matter for themselves they often will feel more involved, and hopefully more secure, satisfied and comfortable with their choices.

Feedback is importantly related to autonomy and mastery in executing different behaviours. It is only when we provide opportunities for willingness and choice that development of intrinsic autonomous motivation and self-regulation can be realised [7].

Research shows that when patients have the opportunity to make their own choices, long-lasting changes in behaviour can occur [31].

> **Box**
>
> Dental professionals can be trained to provide more involvement and meaningful dialogues with their patients, containing different opportunities for choices, in order to develop increased autonomy and competence.

8.3.3 Competence – Providing Meaningful Rationales and Explaining Purposes

Competence is about creating a meaningful rationale. Meaningful and appropriate rationales have to be constructed in collaboration with the patients. The patients have to understand why a behaviour is important to perform. A meaningful and appropriate rationale is for example explaining: *"Why is it important to brush our teeth?"*

When dental personnel guide patients to change behaviour, it is important to provide meaningful and appropriate justifications.

Patients who feel sufficiently informed can develop relevant competence and mastery in order to make significant and appropriate choices for themselves. Dental personnel can encourage exploration when choices are to be made and thus help with appraisals and decisions. Dental personnel, who are counselling in order to give the patients the possibility to develop experience of self-regulation, self-control, personal valuable competence and efficiency of the activity, will probably succeed more often in helping patients to improve their oral health.

A constructive collaboration between patients and dental personnel is a valuable opportunity to build trusting relationships and to activate and motivate patients in order to develop their own meaningful and appropriate competence.

It is important for dental personnel to familiarise with the perspectives and assumptions that form the basis for patients being able to understand and apply knowledge and information that is provided in oral health care contexts, and thereafter build new perspectives and more effective competence together with patients [8, 32].

> **Box**
>
> *What sort of competence is necessary to be developed for different patients?*

It is important to support patients' own progress (in most cases, this takes time) related to their own autonomous goals they are pursuing and when self-determined competence is developing at the same time.

To improve perception of competence, the tasks ought to be tailored to the capacity, ability and resources of the patients, but at the same time one can give support to patients optimal challenges and believe in their ability to achieve their own goals [2]. With optimal challenges and goals, dental personnel show confidence in patients' efficiency, believing they can manage their own oral health challenges.

The experience of being able to choose and being able to make self-determined decisions relates to the experience of being competent and this leads to the patient's personal growth [14].

Dental professionals who optimise competence and support needs will significantly be contributing to patients, making a greater effort to learn more about their oral health and improve their own skills. This can contribute to better perception of their own ability, their own effects on oral health, and thus facilitate more autonomous self-regulated motivation [33].

Research supports the importance of supporting the patient's autonomous motivation, competence conceptualisation and development of new skills and how patients can use their capacities efficiently to emphasise greater control over their oral health and the factors that create promotion of oral health [7].

For dental professionals, it is important to consider what relevant competence is especially important for different patient groups to learn about?

> *"The highest quality of conceptual learning seems to occur under the same motivational conditions that promote personal growth and adjustment"* [34, p. 326].

8.3.4 Relatedness – Acknowledging the Patient's Feelings and Perspectives

Dental professionals, who take into consideration patient's feelings, perspectives and respect their frame of reference, will support relatedness and the feeling of belonging. Along with this understanding, dental personnel have to be nonjudgemental [35].

Empathy is central and important in the feeling of relatedness. Dental professionals who emphasise empathic and compassionate styles will be able to take into consideration the patient's feelings, experiences and personal considerations in an easier way.

Dental professionals who listen carefully, are present, aware/mindful, sensitive, attentive and supportive of the patient's own thoughts, experiences, feelings, actions, goals and behaviours will give support to the need of relatedness.

When dental professionals are aware, pay extra attention to, and take into consideration every step in the treatment session [36], they learn more of the patient's own feelings and reactions, besides they become more aware of their own feelings and reactions to these issues. For example, personnel have to take into consideration when patients expresses their feelings and reac-

tions related to their experience of pain and discomfort, anxiety, traumas, depression, or other vulnerabilities.

Importantly, emphasising these factors can lead to increased levels of confidence and trust between patients and dental personnel, which in turn could help patients overcome fear and anxiety. Thus, this increases the patients feeling of confidence and trust [37].

Facilitating a near, accepting and warm relationship can create better cooperation and safer treatment alliances which is an important prerequisite for all patient and health personnel relationships. Focus on developing and building relatedness, related to trust and confidence, will affect learning and self-training positively and result in patients becoming more autonomously motivated, self-determined and self-regulated. This will in turn facilitate oral health competence and oral health promotion (see Nutbeam, [38], and ▶ Chap. 5).

> The context is characterised by mutual respect when dental personnel communicate with their patients. Dental professionals who take into consideration the patient's challenges, values and plans related to taking care of their own dental health will build more consistent and valuable relations with patients. While patients learn about their own oral health and how they can relate to this in the best possible way, the need for relatedness is important to take into consideration for dental personnel [7–9, 26, 32].

Dental professionals who create predictability and structure [39] will often contribute more to patients' engagement and desire for more involvement in future activities. Positive feedback is needed for relatedness, feeling of mastery and developing competence and supporting development of more autonomy and self-regulation. Patients choosing to be more self-determined is directly connected to patients being able to take more responsibility for their own choices related to oral health. In general, dental professionals who take into account patients' individual differences when counselling, using SDT related to autonomous motivation in learning processes, more often succeed in motivating the patients taking their own relevant oral health changes. Lack of time and stress will be a threat when patients are learning about oral health promoting issues and tasks.

Research has shown that relevant health changes are likely to occur and last over time when dental personnel are autonomy supportive and patients have integrated and accepted the options, opportunities and information given in a counselling dialogue, often followed up over time [2]. Autonomy support will facilitate internalisation of more autonomous motivation and at the same time prevent and decrease dental anxiety [26].

Research shows that when people are autonomously motivated they are more deeply engaged and productive, and they are more freely and willingly developing their own appropriate competence capital. Being autonomously motivated gives patients the possibility to make better plans in order to gain their own chosen oral health goals [40]. Autonomous motivation is related to fuller and more optimal functioning, which is essential for personal growth and mental health [21, 41].

SDT gives the opportunity to understand more of how significant persons can support and contribute related to how patients can develop optimal health function, increase their own health by using their own capacities and resources, increase general health, mental and psychological well-being and general quality of life [2].

8.4 Internalisation Process

The internalisation process is unique in SDT [1]. This process gives the possibility to understand different *qualities* of motivation. This quality is reflected in how and to what extent and degree a person is regulating his or her behaviour autonomously. Ryan and Deci [2] maintain that motivation is qualitatively different if a person is extrinsically versus intrinsically regulated, controlled versus autonomously motivated, and these concepts are predictors of health behaviours, well-being, and quality of life. Many theories of motivation have treated motivation, when only focusing on the amount of motivation, but SDT is the only theory which differentiates between qualitative types of motivation [42]. Quality of motivation

is, therefore, a main theme in SDT related to the internalisation process.

Internalisation and integration is a process when a person is active and can transform an external regulation into more inner self-regulated behaviour connected with the self and their own values [43]. This process is successful if the behaviour functions optimally, when people can be able to identify with the importance of autonomous self-regulations, assimilate these regulations into their sense of self, and thus fully accept them as their own.

Autonomous self-regulation will contribute to patients being able to give more effort, have greater engagement and persistence with health behaviours [15] and oral health behaviours [32].

The internalisation process is presented as a continuum (◘ Fig. 8.2). This internalisation continuum shows how a person's behaviour, by different qualities, can become more autonomously self-regulated, or how persons can move up and down on this continuum.

Different extrinsic forms of regulations represent the internalisation process in SDT. The SDT refers to *four different types of extrinsic motivations* in the internalisation process. The four external forms start as an initiation from the outside, for example, from persons or norms from cultural contexts. In this way, the internalisation process starts from the "outside". When individuals have become autonomously and inner motivated, they have integrated a behaviour through the internalisation process. Intrinsic motivation represents behaviour sustained with engagement and without external rewards. The rewarding experiences lie within people and we can say they are the most genuine intrinsically-motivated individuals. Amotivation refers to missing or lack of motivation [2].

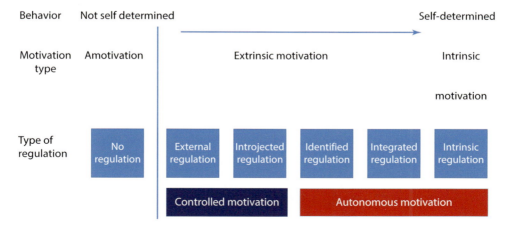

◘ **Fig. 8.2** The Internalization Continuum [2, p. 193]

8.4.1 Amotivation

Amotivation represents no regulation, no motivation and lack of intentions to act [2]. Patients will think they will *not* be doing anything, because nothing will lead to desired outcomes anyway. They feel powerless and helpless. The patients seem uninterested and indifferent. They lack the feeling of competence and mastery, either in a sense of efficacy or they have a feeling of lack of self-control [44]. A motivated patients often develop anxiety and depression [2].

> ▶ Example
>
> *Example of an amotivated patient:* He feels powerless and helpless, perhaps because having to "fix his teeth" feels like too much of a challenge. ◀

8.4.2 Four Different Types of Extrinsic Motivation

Deci and Ryan [1] describe four different types of extrinsic motivation. Below we will consider all four regulations. Extrinsic regulations are intentional and motivated.

External and introjected regulations are called controlled motivation, while identified and integrated regulation are called autonomous motivation [45].

The process of internalisation shows how a behaviour that was originally initiated by an external influence, eventually can end up with more self-determined and autonomously motivated behaviour, which corresponds to a person who acts more self-regulated [45].

8.4.2.1 External Regulation

External regulation is the first of the four extrinsic motivations and the least self-determined motivation. The behaviour is controlled by external stimuli, which means that the behaviour is initiated by other people or of a context outside the person. The individual's behaviour is mainly governed by a desire related to a reward or to avoid punishment. In this regulation, other people's assessments or judgements of what the person is thinking, feeling or doing, become important [46].

Behaviour, like brushing the teeth, starts as an external regulation. Thus, this behaviour starts as an external "requirement". Demands to perform an action can come from parents, family or friends but can also be a normative demand that lies in the environment or in the culture. Brushing our teeth is, therefore, not governed by an independent autonomous motivation from the beginning but can become an integrated, accepted and valued behaviour over time.

> ▶ Example
>
> *Example of a patient with external regulation:* Brushing is performed out of duty. Patients often want to "satisfy" dental personnel by being a "good" and clever patient. Patients perform their dental home care in order to avoid criticism or to get praise from dental personnel. ◀

8.4.2.2 Introjected Regulation

Introjected regulation is the second type of extrinsic motivation on the internalisation continuum and is still characterised as controlled motivation. Patients have partially accepted the behaviour as their own. Introjected regulation is conceptualised as "partial internalisation" [28] and refers to patients who have "taken in" the behaviour, but who have not fully accepted it as their own. The behaviour is not self-regulated. The behaviour is still not integrated.

The patient acts mainly due to bad conscience like *shame* and *guilt*. The patient experiences that he *should* or *must* act in certain ways. Or, patients do not perform the behaviour they feel they should have executed. Introjected patients often feel an inner stress and pressure themselves to act.

> ▶ Example
>
> *Example of a patient with introjected regulation:* The person experiences that he should or must brush his teeth, but he really does not like to perform this behaviour. The brushing act is often executed in a mechanical and instrumental way and often performed as a self-imposed duty. Or they *refrain from doing the behaviour*, but at the same time they feel guilt and shame by not doing this behaviour. ◀

8.4.2.3 Identified Regulation

This is the third type of extrinsic regulation. Identified regulation is the first autonomous regulation. The behaviour is now self-determined, self-regulated and the patients are therefore self-motivated. Persons feel the behaviour is important to execute for themselves, and they recognise and accept the underlying value of a behaviour. The internalisation process is now fuller than with an introjection.

> ▶ Example
>
> *Example of a patient with identified regulation:* The patient thinks that it is important to perform regular dental home care in an efficient and quality-conscious manner. The patient thinks it is important to care for his teeth and meet regularly with dental personnel. Patients naturally think it is important to achieve their own oral health goals; besides, they are concerned about their own oral well-being and their oral health quality of life. ◀

8.4.2.4 Integrated Regulation

This regulation represents the last of the four extrinsic regulations. This is the most autonomous and self-regulated of the external regulations. The behaviour is now fully integrated within the person's sense of self. The behaviour is consistent and in harmony with the person's value system and other personal goals. We say the behaviour is *integrated* into their own value system.

Patients now experience the behaviour as their own and self-chosen and they think the behaviour is important and valuable to perform. Dental behaviour is executed out of self-interest and patients are valuing the behaviour. The priorities lie in the good feelings and experiences with doing this behaviour. When the behaviour is integrated, dental personnel *do not have to inform the patients about why it is important to do this explicit behaviour,* because patients now know themselves. Integrated behaviour is usually maintained over longer periods of time.

The behaviour is accepted and connected to the underlying value of this behaviour. This behaviour is *executed without conflicts* and it is more easy for these patients to take personal responsibility for their own oral health challenges [7, 28]. The result is integrated autonomously self-determined motivation.

> ► **Example**
>
> *Example of a patient with integrated regulation:* The patient values performing dental home care regularly, efficiently, qualitatively and consciously. Patients can reflect upon why oral health promotion is valuable and important and what type of behaviours which leads to good oral health. Patients have high awareness about how to care for their own dental health. Patients' attitudes and beliefs are carried out in the best way and they will be eager to solve their own dental challenges and problems. Patients will follow up their own dental visits regularly and take responsibility as a natural habit in an appropriate manner to achieve the best possible oral health. Patients often do their own research around oral health issues and tasks to perform. They ask questions and are eager to learn about their oral health and they want to solve their own challenges. They are now autonomous and self-motivated (self-regulated). ◄

8.4.3 Intrinsic Motivation

This is the motivation Deci and Ryan [1] describe as the most genuine. This intrinsic regulation is as highly autonomous motivation and the activity starts from within a person. Therefore, it differs from the four extrinsic regulations/motivations which are initiated from outside a person. Intrinsic motivation is characterised when a person chooses, on an independent basis the behaviour that he or she finds interesting and wants to perform. As an example, we can observe the intrinsic motivation in infants who grab a rattle *without being told if it is an important behaviour.* According to Ryan and Deci [2], intrinsic motivation is our natural motivation that arises spontaneously, is exploratory and is stimulated and initiated by our own curiosity and a feeling of mastery is followed when we executing optimally challenging tasks.

Intrinsic motivation comes from within a person and it reflects an inner driving force, energy and vitality which leads to behaviours that we really want to engage in. Here, the only reward is when executing the performance (for example, mountain climbing). The feelings of flow, spontaneity and authentic enjoyment that accompany the performance are characteristics related to genuine intrinsic motivation [2].

8.5 Self-Determination Theory and Dental Health Research

Several of the studies from Halvari et al. [7–10, 14, 22, 26, 32] refer to autonomy support versus controlling dental personnel and how this is related to different patient motivation.

Autonomy support is positively associated with the patient's oral well-being, reappraisal and decrease of anxiety, oral well-being and oral health-related quality of life and increased dental health, as reduction of plaque and gingivitis, and attending dental treatment. When patients perceive dental professionals as controlling, the results are shown to be the opposite. The results from these studies show that autonomy-support from dental professionals give important and valid results over time. Building relevant oral health competence and mastery is important in order to contribute to more autonomous motivation, improved oral health, thereby helping patients to feel more wellness related to their oral health and understand how they can increase the oral health quality of life [10].

Summary
- This chapter has provided a theoretical framework using self- determination theory (SDT).
- First, the chapter gives a brief introduction of SDT.
- Further, the importance of autonomy is presented as a professional and ethical issue. Autonomy is

8

directly related to *informed consent* which is a duty for all dental professionals to provide.

- Autonomy is importantly related to *professional patient care*, thus it is important to integrate into all dental health care contexts.
- *Autonomous motivation* implies to be self-determined, self-regulated, self-ruled and self-motivated.
- The three *basic psychological needs (SDT- BPN);* competence, autonomy and relatedness are described thoroughly and related to examples in the dental field.
- Supporting SDT-BPN is shown to be fundamental in order to create a motivational climate and to facilitate internalisation of a behaviour.
- The SDT-BPN are essential to be included and taken into consideration when dental professionals give autonomy support.
- **Autonomy support and support of basic psychological needs are:**
  1. Focus on patient-centred communication.
  2. Building oral health relevant competence with choices and options related to patients own oral health challenges.
  3. Building relatedness, empathy and trust related to successful prevention of pain and understanding of patients vulnerabilities.
  4. Support of patient's feelings and perspectives. Patients are given self-control (autonomy). They are not pressured or controlled to do something they do not want to do.
- Dental professionals who emphasise empathy, friendliness, acceptance, patient's involvement and personal choices in relation to patient's competence building, learning and personal growth will support relatedness, autonomy and mastery of oral health.
- Competence-building and sufficient oral health understanding is appropriate in order to be able to promote, prevent and reduce oral health problems.
- Dental personnel can *counsel, guide, teach and train* patients to be more autonomously self-motivated by using guidelines related to *autonomy support.*

- Patients can learn to be more autonomous, self-motivated and self-regulated, conscious and intentional about their oral health behaviour.
- Self-determined and autonomously motivated behaviour is in line with promotion of oral health.
- The chapter shows with examples how dental personnel can learn to give autonomy support and be less controlling.
- A model (◻ Fig. 8.3) shows how autonomous support versus controlling dental personnel is associated with psychological and mental health outcomes in patients.
- The *internalisation process* in SDT is described with examples from the dental field, helping dental personnel to understand different motivational processes.
- The internalisation process shows qualitatively different motivations related to the *integration of a behaviour.* This quality is reflected in how and to what extent and degree a person is regulating his or her behaviour autonomously.
- Autonomously motivated patients will develop more long term goals and maintain more relevant dental behaviour over time.
- This chapter shows how dental professionals can use SDT research and the understanding of qualitatively different motivations and regulations and integrate the practical consequences into the dental health field.
- By focusing on how important autonomous motivation is and how this relates to human behaviours, we can probably be able to help more patients in the future. This is in order to help patients to better succeed in managing their own oral health challenges.
- An important issue to understand more of in the future, is how SDT and motivation influences patients' attitudes, behaviours, choices and goals.
- A theory like SDT is concerned about the what, how and why of motivation [45]. Because of this, SDT has been increasingly used in many health research designs [15].

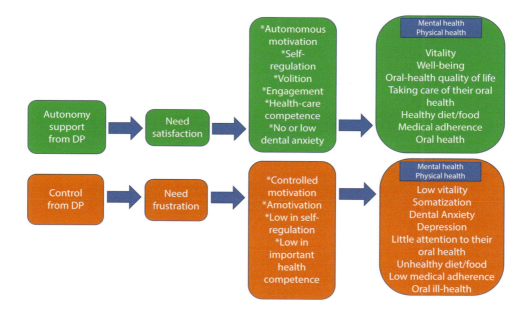

Fig. 8.3 This oral health promotion model is supported by a lot of research [2]. This model shows how autonomy support versus control given by dental professionals will influence the three SDT-Basic Psychological Needs; autonomy, competence and relatedness, and how satisfaction versus frustration of these SDT - needs will imply different motivations and regulations and different positive versus negative outcomes related to mental and physical health

References

1. Deci E, Ryan R. Intrinsic motivation and self-determination in human behaviour. Rochester, New York: Springer; 1985.
2. Ryan RM, Deci EL. Self-determination theory: basic psychological needs in motivation, development, and wellness. NY: Guilford Publications; 2017.
3. Ryan RM, Deci EL. Self-determination theory and the facilitation of intrinsic motivation, social development, and well-being. Am Psychol. 2000;55(1):68.
4. Niemiec CP, Ryan RM. Autonomy, competence, and relatedness in the classroom: applying self-determination theory to educational practice. Theory Res Educ. 2009;7(2):133–44.
5. Rogers CR. On becoming a person: a therapist's view of psychotherapy. Boston: Houghton Mifflin Company; 1961.
6. Ryan RM, Deci EL. Brick by brick: the origins, development, and future of self-determination theory. In: Elliot, A. (Ed.) Advances in motivation science. Vol. 6. Pp. 111–56. Cambridge: Elsevier, 2019.
7. Halvari AEM, Halvari H, Bjørnebekk G, Deci EL. Motivation and anxiety for dental treatment: testing a self-determination theory model of oral self-care behaviour and dental clinic attendance. Motiv Emot. 2010;34(1):15–33.
8. Halvari AEM, Halvari H, Bjørnebekk G, Deci EL. Motivation for dental home care: testing a self-determination theory model 1. J Appl Soc Psychol. 2012;42(1):1–39.
9. Halvari AEM, Halvari H, Bjørnebekk G, Deci EL. Oral health and dental well-being: testing a self-determination theory model. J Appl Soc Psychol. 2013;43(2):275–92.
10. Halvari AEM, Halvari H, Deci EL. Dental anxiety, oral health-related quality of life, and general well-being: a self-determination theory perspective. J Appl Soc Psychol. 2019;49(5):295–306.
11. Deci EL, Ryan RM. Self-determination theory in health care and its relations to motivational interviewing: a few comments. Int J Behav Nutr Phys Act. 2012;9(1):1–6.
12. Engel GL. The need for a new medical model: a challenge for biomedicine. Science. 1977;196(4286):129–36.
13. Williams GC, Deci EL. Internalization of biopsychosocial values by medical students: a test of self-determination theory. J Pers Soc Psychol. 1996;70(4):767.
14. Halvari AEM, Halvari H, Deci EL, Williams GC. Autonomy-supportive dental treatment, oral health-related eudaimonic well-being and oral health: a randomized clinical trial. Psychol Health. 2019;34(12):1421–36.
15. Patrick H, Williams GC. Self-determination theory: its application to health behavior and complementarity with motivational interviewing. Int J Behav Nutr Phys Act. 2012;9(1):1–12.
16. Beauchamp TL, Childress JF. Principles of biomedical ethics. New York: Oxford University Press; 2001.
17. Cassel CK, Hood V, Bauer W. A physician charter: the tenth anniversary. Ann Intern Med. 2012;21:290–91.
18. Woolf SH, Chan EC, Harris R, Sheridan SL, Braddock III CH, Kaplan RM, et al. Promoting informed choice: transforming health care to dispense knowledge for decision making. Ann Intern Med. 2005;143:293–300.
19. Ryan RM, Deci EL. Self-regulation and the problem of human autonomy: does psychology need choice, self-determination, and will? J Pers. 2006;74(6):1557–86.
20. Ryan RM, Deci EL, Vansteenkiste M. Autonomy and autonomy disturbances in self-development and psychopathology: research on motivation, attachment, and clinical process. Dev Psychopathol. 2016;1:385–438.
21. Deci EL, Ryan RM. Handbook of self-determination research. Rochester, NY: University of Rochester Press; 2004.
22. Halvari AEM, Halvari H, Deci EL. The roles of patients' authenticity and accepting external influence, and clinicians'

treatment styles in predicting patients' dental anxiety and avoidance of dental appointments. Eur J Psychol. 2020;16(1):45.

23. White RW. Motivation reconsidered: the concept of competence. Psychol Rev. 1959;66(5):297.

24. Baumeister RF, Leary MR. The need to belong: desire for interpersonal attachments as a fundamental human motivation. Psychol Bull. 1995;117(3):497.

25. Deci EL, Ryan RM. Facilitating optimal motivation and psychological well-being across life's domains. Can Psychol. 2008;49(1):14.

26. Münster Halvari A, Halvari H, Deci E. Attending and avoiding dental appointments: do "bright" and "dark" motivational paths have a role? Int J Dent Hyg. 2018;16(2):286–97.

27. DeCharms R. Personal causation: the internal affective determinants of behavior/R. Charms. New York: Academic Press; 1968.

28. Deci EL, Eghrari H, Patrick BC, Leone DR. Facilitating internalization: the self-determination theory perspective. J Pers. 1994;62(1):119–42.

29. Vansteenkiste M, Niemiec CP, Soenens B. The development of the five mini-theories of self-determination theory: an historical overview, emerging trends, and future directions. In: Karabenick, S, & Urdan, T. C. (Eds.), The decade ahead: theoretical perspectives on motivation and achievement (Pp. 105–65). Bingley, UK: Emerald, 2010.

30. Kadam RA. Informed consent process: a step further towards making it meaningful! Perspect Clin Res. 2017;8(3):107.

31. Ryan RM, Patrick H, Deci EL, Williams GC. Facilitating health behaviour change and its maintenance: interventions based on self-determination theory. Eur Health Psychol. 2008;10(1):2–5.

32. Münster Halvari AE, Halvari H, Bjørnebekk G, Deci EL. Self-determined motivational predictors of increases in dental behaviors, decreases in dental plaque, and improvement in oral health: a randomized clinical trial. Health Psychol. 2012;31(6):777.

33. Jang H, Reeve J, Deci EL. Engaging students in learning activities: it is not autonomy support or structure but autonomy support and structure. J Educ Psychol. 2010;102(3):588.

34. Deci EL, Vallerand RJ, Pelletier LG, Ryan RM. Motivation and education: the self-determination perspective. Educ Psychol. 1991;26(3-4):325–46.

35. Ryan RM, Lynch MF, Vansteenkiste M, Deci EL. Motivation and autonomy in counseling, psychotherapy, and behavior change: a look at theory and practice 1ψ7. Couns Psychol. 2011;39(2):193–260.

36. Kranstad V, Søftestad S, Fredriksen TV, Willumsen T. Being considerate every step of the way: a qualitative study analysing trauma-sensitive dental treatment for childhood sexual abuse survivors. Eur J Oral Sci. 2019;127(6):539–46.

37. Tessier D, Sarrazin P, Ntoumanis N. The effect of an intervention to improve newly qualified teachers' interpersonal style, students motivation and psychological need satisfaction in sport-based physical education. Contemp Educ Psychol. 2010;35(4):242–53.

38. Nutbeam D. The evolving concept of health literacy. Soc Sci Med. 2008;67(12):2072–8.

39. Taylor IM, Ntoumanis N. Teacher motivational strategies and student self-determination in physical education. J Educ Psychol. 2007;99(4):747.

40. Van den Broeck A, Vansteenkiste M, De Witte H, Lens W. Explaining the relationships between job characteristics, burnout, and engagement: the role of basic psychological need satisfaction. Work Stress. 2008;22(3):277–94.

41. Ryan RM, Deci EL, Grolnick WS, La Guardia JG. The significance of autonomy and autonomy support in psychological development and psychopathology. In: Cicchetti, D., & Cohen, D. J. (Eds.). The developmental psychopathology: Theory and method (pp. 795–849). Hoboken, NJ: Wiley, 2006.

42. Deci EL, Ryan RM. Self-determination theory: a macrotheory of human motivation, development, and health. Can Psychol. 2008;49(3):182.

43. Ryan RM, Rigby S, King K. Two types of religious internalization and their relations to religious orientations and mental health. J Pers Soc Psychol. 1993;65(3):586.

44. Pelletier LG, Dion S, Tuson K, Green-Demers I. Why do people fail to adopt environmental protective behaviors? Toward a taxonomy of environmental amotivation 1. J Appl Soc Psychol. 1999;29(12):2481–504.

45. Deci EL, Ryan RM. The" what" and" why" of goal pursuits: human needs and the self-determination of behavior. Psychol Inq. 2000;11(4):227–68.

46. Ryan RM, Connell JP. Perceived locus of causality and internalization: examining reasons for acting in two domains. J Pers Soc Psychol. 1989;57(5):749.

Children

Contents

Positive Encounters for Children to Prevent Dental Anxiety – Theory and Practice

Helen Rodd, Anne Rønneberg, Therese Varvin Fredriksen, Ingrid Berg Johnsen and Zoe Marshman

Contents

© The Author(s), under exclusive license to Springer Nature Switzerland AG 2022
T. Willumsen et al. (eds.), *Oral Health Psychology*, Textbooks in Contemporary Dentistry,
https://doi.org/10.1007/978-3-031-04248-5_9

Learning Outcomes

This chapter aims to provide the reader with the following learning outcomes:

- Understanding of how a child develops in relation to social and emotional milestones
- Ability to apply this knowledge to the dental setting, recognising the importance of security, attachment, habituation and facilitation and how these relate to developmental-supported practice
- Knowledge of how to establish positive dental encounters through simple behaviour management strategies such as "tell show do"
- Insight into the experiences and behaviours of dentally-anxious children
- Awareness of the principles of guided self-help cognitive behavioural therapy and its application for children with dental anxiety

9.1   Understanding Child Development

9.1.1   Overview

Over the years, a greater understanding of child development, in all its complexity, has radically changed how we view and understand children. Much of this knowledge has come from the field of developmental psychology; the study of how individuals evolve and change throughout life and the processes and elements that underlie these changes. We now recognise that children are active contributors to their own development and the perceptions they have of the world. Because child development is so complex, no single theory can explain it all. Furthermore, there is the fundamental question of how nature and nurture interact to shape the development process. Genetic inheritance, referred to as nature, relates to characteristics received from our parents such as physical appearance, personality and intellect. Nurture refers to the environment, both physical and social, and how this may influence our development. Other broad concepts that interplay to shape a child's development as a whole include: cognitive development (capabilities such as perception, attention, language, problem solving, reasoning, memory and conceptual understanding); social development (growth of emotions, personality, self-understanding, relationships with family members and later with peers) and motor development.

An understanding of these aspects is fundamental to how we exercise parenting, what pedagogic approaches are used in school and what legal rights are afforded to children [1]. It is also important that healthcare workers have an appreciation of the key aspects of child development and behaviour to better inform their interactions with children and parents. The following sections will,

therefore, aim to provide the reader with a deeper understanding of how to manage children at different stages of their development.

9.1.2   Social Development

9.1.2.1   Attachment Theory

One aspect of child development, that has particular relevance to the dental setting, is the attachment style that each child demonstrates. Attachment relates to the formation and development of social and close interpersonal ties between a child and its caregivers which, in turn, greatly influences how a child will build relationships as an adult. The theory was developed by psychiatrist and psychoanalyst John Bowlby (1907–1990) through his study of children who were separated from their parents during the Second World War. According to Bowlby, all children have a biological need to seek attachment for survival and development. Fundamentally, children who form attachments have a better chance of survival than those who do not. Based on this assumption, he developed the attachment theory that frames the understanding of emotional development from birth into adulthood [2, 3]. Attachment theory focusses on what is going on *between* the child and the caregivers and how the quality of that relationship influences the development of the child. Attachment, therefore, has two interfaces; the first is the child's attachment to the caregivers, and the second is the caregivers' *bond* to the child. Children are born with a repertoire of specific behaviours (e.g. crying, eye contact, mimicry, smiling) with the purpose of promoting closeness to the caregiver. For example, when the child smiles, most parents will respond by smiling back at the child. This is known as attachment behaviour; behaviour initiated by the child that promotes closeness and contact with the child's significant others [2].

Children need protection and care to survive, and therefore attach themselves to their caregivers, regardless of how well or poorly they are treated. However, the quality of the attachment and bonding depends on the emotional interaction between the child and the caregivers (see the descriptors A–D below) [2]. For example, a child who has warm and attentive parents will form a secure and confident attachment with them, knowing that they will always be there when he/she needs them. In contrast, a child whose parents are abusive or neglectful and erratic in their behaviour will understandably struggle to know how to react to and bond with their parents [2]. Children learn throughout their childhood about themselves, their emotions, how to interact with others and what kind of help and support they can expect from their surroundings. Researchers have proposed that children (along with their caregivers) broadly fit into one of the four main attachment styles, which may resonate with the experiences of dental health professionals in their everyday practice [3].

A. Avoidant Attachment

The child has little experience of the attachment figure being there if needed, so has learnt to deal with the world mostly by themselves. The child may seem independent and confident in many situations, but this is more a reflection of being forced to manage frightening situations alone, rather than because they actually feel safe. The attachment figure is described as withdrawn, dismissive, often angry and can appear "uncomfortable" with any physical contact.

B. Secure Attachment

The child knows that the attachment figure is accessible, responsive and helpful in difficult/frightening situations. The child explores the world freely, knowing that their safe haven is accessible if needed. The attachment figure is often described as warm, accepting and attentive.

C. Ambivalent Attachment

The child has mixed experiences of getting help and support from their attachment figure, so does not know if they are safe or not. These children seek help and support when they don't really need it, but rather because the attachment person may need it. The children seek contact and closeness in a way that inhibits their independence. The attachment person is often described as anxious or unpredictable, sometimes warm and loving, sometimes cold and dismissive.

D. Disorganised Attachment

The child appears chaotic, afraid and difficult to understand because they display contradictory behaviours. The child has no clear strategy for interacting with the attachment person, because the child does not know if the attachment person will harm them or not. They have often experienced that the attachment person can be intimidating and dangerous. The attachment person, who is supposed to protect and comfort the child, is also the one that can hurt and be threatening to the child.

These four categories describe the quality of the bond between the child and the attachment person/s. Attachment style is considered one of the most important risk/protective factors in child development and acknowledges the key role of caregivers in shaping the child's development [2]. Attachment behaviour becomes especially visible when the child is placed in an unfamiliar situation (such as in the dental setting) that is perceived as unsafe, unpleasant or painful for the child and/or the attachment person. However, it is not possible to assess a child's attachment style from just a few observations in the dental clinic; a child might have a secure attachment style, but if the accompanying parent is highly dentally anxious, they may not be able to appropriately respond to the child's needs. The child might be hungry, just had a bad day at school, or the caregiver might have had problems with parking, have a headache or had a conflict at work. Many things can affect the child's and the caregiver's behaviour and responsiveness. Even so, it is useful to be aware of the different attachment styles to better understand pre-cooperative behaviours and to take into consideration child-parent interactions during the dental visit.

9.1.3 Emotional Development

Balancing against their need for safety is a child's inherent curiosity and urge to explore the world. Children who feel "safe" tend to have greater motivation and energy to explore and learn than children who feel insecure and unsafe. A term used in child psychology is a "safe-haven" which may be offered by parents/caregivers and is essential to supporting children to develop in an emotionally healthy way. Children tend to regulate their emotions by shifting between exploring and asking for support/safety. These cycles are important in terms of helping children to manage their emotions by themselves in the future.

Adequate regulation relies on adults responding appropriately to a child's signal for need and this is very evident in the dental setting. Parents who, for example, prepare their child for their first clinic visit by role playing the dentist-patient encounter and introduce the unfamiliar situation in a safe environment make the visit less unpredictable and scary. Parents can also facilitate children's acceptance of dental equipment (e.g. light or mirror) by using a curious and encouraging tone of voice to engage the child's urge to explore. These are good examples of interactions that help the child to regulate their negative and positive feelings in the dental treatment situation.

9.1.3.1 Circle of Security

Another psychological concept relevant to the dental encounter is the "The Circle of Security" (COS) [4]. This visual map, developed by Hoffman and colleagues (2006), depicts how secure parent-child relationships can be supported and strengthened (◘ Fig. 9.1). It provides a framework for children's attachment and explorative behaviour in various situations, and it is a useful aid for parents and other adults working with children. The COS demonstrates how children, through repeated experiences within the circle, become more confident in themselves in different situations and in their relationships with other people.

9

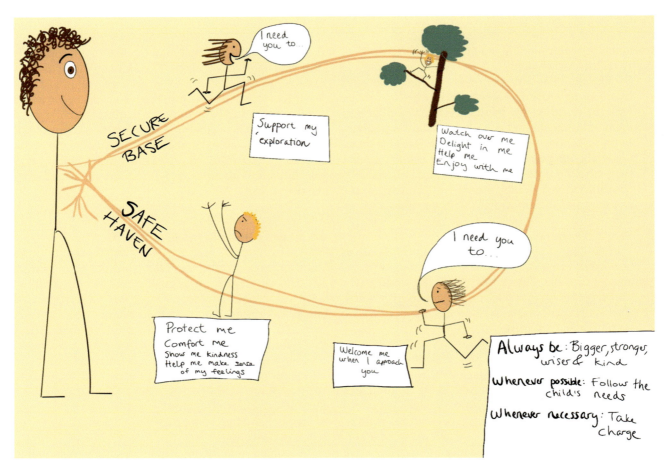

◼ **Fig. 9.1**   The Circle of Security (Hoffman et al., 2006) using illustrations provided by Berg Johnsen (2021)

The hands in the illustration symbolise the child's attachment person/s which is, in effect, the child's safe haven or secure base. The child takes help from his or her safe haven/secure base for regulation, exploration and protection.

When the child is "positioned" at the top of the circle, they are exposed to a world they want to discover, explore, learn and master. It is crucial that the child is free to explore in this way to develop autonomy, and their safe base shares the excitement of their discoveries. It is also important that caregivers support this developmental step, even when the child is hesitant.

However, when the child is at the bottom of the circle, he/she needs physical and mental support. They may have been frightened or sad and it is important their safe haven is available to them to provide comfort and emotional regulation. With this support from their caregiver/s, the child learns that it is ok to share their emotions and to seek support from others.

A common feature during early childhood is the alternate switching between exploration and safety within the COS. When exploring, young children often cast a glance at their attachment figures to ensure their safe haven is still there. If they discover something interesting such as the control buttons on the dental chair, they can physically approach them to take a closer look (i.e. explore the world). But, if the nurse turns on the suction unit unexpectedly, the loud noise (i.e. a scary sound, a danger) may trigger the child's attachment behaviour, maybe they start to cry or cling to their attachment figure. In these situations, it is important that the attachment person is responsive and recognises the child's need for comfort and safety. When the child receives support in the form of physical closeness, acceptance and explanation of his/her experience, it does not take long before he/she is again ready to explore the world, with an open and curious mind.

9.1.3.2 Attachment in Action at the Dental Clinic

Let's look at a case study to illustrate how a dental visit can trigger the attachment system in a young patient.

Paul is a 4-year-old boy who normally sits in the dental chair by himself and just accepted a dental examination with a mirror. You need to take some dental radiographs and follow the "tell, show, do" approach. While you are getting the equipment ready, Paul starts to look worried, which his mum notices, and says "Paul it's okay". But Paul slides down from the dental chair and rushes over to his mother. She recognises her young son's signals for reassurance, and puts her arms around him, and speaks in a calm voice: "You are being such a good boy, can we help the dentist take some pictures of your teeth?" Paul looks down, crosses his arms, frowns and hides in his mother's arms. His mother holds him for a little while and then says: "I'll be really close by, watching you have your pictures taken, and it will be really quick.

Do you remember when your brother had a special picture of his arm? That was ok wasn't it?" Paul reluctantly lets his mother place him back in the chair. You position the X-ray tube closer to Paul while telling him that his pictures will appear on the computer screen, so he can see them afterwards: "and you might be able to see where your big teeth are growing". His mother agrees and says it will be exciting to see the new big teeth. With more reassurances from you and his mother, you are able to take the radiographs. When Paul is finished, he looks pleased and expectantly at his mother. She smiles at him proudly and says: "What a superstar, you were such a brave boy!" When you show Paul his teeth on your computer screen, he peers at them with interest and announces: "look, those are my big teeth!"

The first visit to the dental clinic is a new experience for a young child and, understandably, will often trigger the attachment system, as the child does not know if this is a safe or unsafe place to be. An awareness of where the child is on the COS will hopefully give some insight as to their underlying needs in the dental setting. It is worth noting in ◘ Fig. 9.2 that the use of the terms "bigger and stronger" in relation to the dental professional is suggesting they are

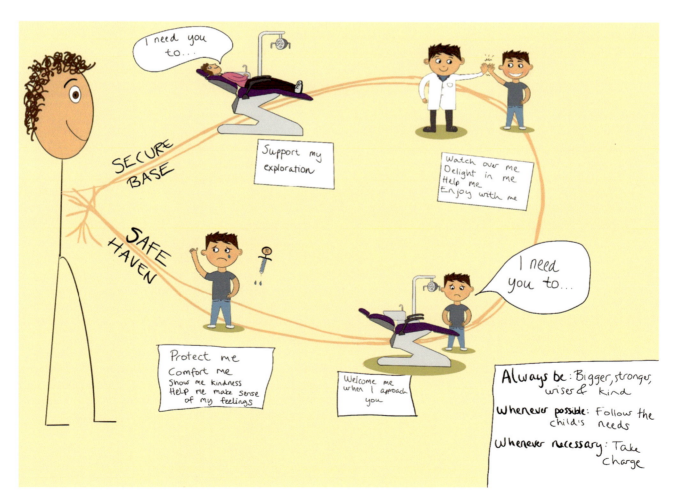

◘ **Fig. 9.2** The Circle of Security (Hoffman et al., 2006) applied to the dental setting using illustrations provided by Berg Johnsen (2021)

taking on a protector role, rather than one of authority or power. For example, if the child is on the top of the circle, they may demonstrate their explorative and inquisitive behaviours by picking up dental instruments or climbing/bouncing on the chair. In this instance, the dental professional needs to take charge and be bigger and stronger in order to protect the child from potentially hurting themselves, whilst acting in a kind and wise manner. Another illustration of the COS may be where a child refuses to open their mouth and expresses anger and protest; in this case, the behaviour can be explained by "pushing" the child to the top of the circle when they are naturally aligned to the bottom of the circle and need help to become emotionally capable of co-operating. Instead of labelling the child as naughty or uncooperative, we should instead look for the underlying causes of the child's behaviour.

We need to ask ourselves:

— *What is the child trying to achieve by this "unhelpful" behaviour?*
— *What can we say and do to turn this dental encounter into a positive developmental step for this particular child?*
— *What can we do to help the child to move from a "position" underneath the circle (safety-seeking zone) to the upper part (exploratory zone)?*

Some young patients can be challenging and, on occasions, it might be difficult for the clinician to feel genuine empathy for these children. But, by using the COS, we can overcome our own irritation and frustration and, instead, see the fear and insecurity that often lies behind the protest.

A safe haven is a prerequisite for a good treatment experience, but there will be considerable variance in what constitutes a safe haven for individual children. An important consideration is the child's temperament. Typically, cautious children need more time and support in a new situation than children who are intrinsically more open and curious. We will now look at how children's temperaments impact on their behaviours including those displayed at the dental clinic.

9.1.3.3 Temperament

A child's temperament can be described as the typical way in which they respond to the world. Interestingly, children's individual temperaments are apparent from the moment of birth and tend to remain constant throughout their lives. Temperament is considered to have, in part, a genetic basis although no clear inheritance patterns have been identified for specific temperament traits.

The following scenario illustrates how children's temperaments can prompt vastly different reactions in relation to a new bicycle.

Case Studies

Mehdi is a careful boy. He looks at his new bike with some trepidation. He gradually approaches it and pushes it along the path. It takes several days for him to actually get on it and a few more days before he dares take his feet off the ground.

Anna is a curious, active and adventurous girl. She's keen to try out her new bike and sets off on it straight away, even though she is very wobbly. Eventually, she gets the hang of it and speeds down the hill shouting with excitement.

Peter is active and impatient. He hastily grabs his new bike and tries to get going. His father wants to show him how to use the pedals, but Peter doesn't have time to pay attention and gets frustrated and irritated when the pedals do not seem to work. He leaves the bike in anger and tears. After a few days, and a great deal of frustration, Peter gets the hang of things and heads down the road with quick and purposeful pedaling.

Broadly speaking, children's temperaments can be categorised into three main types: easy (as Anna in the example above), reserved (as Mehdi) and difficult (as Peter) [5]. Children with easy temperaments are mostly cheerful, have steady sleeping and eating patterns, readily adapt to new situations, are open to strangers, show moderate emotional reactions in stressful situations and are easy to calm down when they become angry, scared or sad. This group makes up about 40% of all children [5]. Children who are described as having a difficult temperament comprise those with inconsistent sleeping and eating patterns, those who tend to pull away in new situations, can seem negative and suspicious, show strong emotional reactions and are difficult to calm down when they become angry, scared or sad. This group makes up about 10% of all children. The third group (15%) includes children referred to as reserved. These are children who need time to feel safe in new situations, they can cry and become troubled, but do not react as forcefully as children described as having a difficult temperament.

A child's temperament is of utmost importance in shaping not only how they face the world, but also how the world and the environment respond to the child. For the infant, it is the closest caregivers (parent/s) who are the "world" and they are usually well attuned to their child's temperament. Through positive interactions, most parents learn to work *with* their child's temperament. In contrast, some may appear to work *against* their child's temperament by trying to change them. Working *with* the child is not the same as always letting them have their own way. Caregivers should still set boundaries, make decisions, and take a leadership role, but at the same time considering the child's specific needs.

9.1.3.4 Developmental-Supported Treatment

Having presented a brief overview of some key aspects of children's emotional and psychosocial development, we will now consider what age-adjusted interventions can be adopted by dental health professionals to support their young patients. Ideally, children should start attending the dentist from a young age (1–2 years) along with their family so that it becomes a familiar and non-threatening environment for them.

9.2 Preparing for a "Successful" Dental Visit

It is common for dental health services to send out information (paper/electronic format) to prepare the child and family for their pending visit, especially if they are new patients. This information might tell the child/caregivers what to expect. If possible, it is nice for the patient to be told in advance about the clinician they will be meeting and photo board of the dental team in the waiting room will help the child to feel more prepared. It may also be helpful if the dental team has some pre-visit "social" information about new patients, in much the same way that a medical history is sought. One suggestion might be to ask the child and/or caregivers to complete a brief "*about me*" questionnaire which would allow the dental team to meet the child in a way that is most sensitive to their individual needs and to readily establish a good rapport. A more detailed discussion and communication aid to seek specific information about a child's worries and requests is provided later in the chapter.

9.2.1 Pre-school Children (2–5 Years)

Case Study

Simon is a 4-year-old boy and visits the dental clinic for the first time with his father. He is playing in the waiting room, whilst holding onto his favourite soft toy, a little rabbit. When you ask Simon and dad to follow you into the clinic, Simon holds his arms up and his father carries him into the surgery. Simon turns away when you say "hi" to him. The father strokes Simon on his back and tells him that there are lots of nice things to see here and a special magic chair. The father takes a seat with Simon on his knee. Simon hides his face but slowly starts to investigate the room more and more. You ask him what his rabbit's name is, but he remains silent. So, you start to talk to his father and show them both the dental mirror and explain how it is used for counting his teeth. Simon gradually becomes more interested and holds the mirror in his hand. You encourage him to look at this rabbit's teeth with the mirror. You then ask if Simon would like a ride in your chair, and you demonstrate the buttons that move the chair up and down. He looks at you briefly and turns away. "Maybe your bunny would like a ride", you suggest. Simon looks at his father who agrees that is a fun idea. Simon leaves his father's lap and holds his rabbit on the chair while you take it for a ride, and he shouts "again" when you bring the chair back down.

As illustrated in the above scenario, it is usually the parents who help very young children to evaluate and confirm what is safe and unsafe in unfamiliar situations such as the dental clinic. At this age, it is completely normal for children to be apprehensive about different objects in the dental setting such as bright lights, dental instruments in the mouth, strange smells and tastes.

During pre-school years, children have a very short attention span, so it is important to give brief and simple messages and explanations. It is also worth remembering that children learn through play and fantasy, and this can be effectively incorporated in your approach.

Even when children are doing something they enjoy, little ones can easily become distracted and head off in a different direction. When conversing with a pre-school child, themes change rapidly and the child may alternate between periods of engaging and not engaging, so it might be necessary to repeat yourself several times before the child understands your message. Although pre-school children are developing their language skills and learning to communicate more effectively, their conversations are still limited to concrete events and episodes and they are not able to fully express themselves.

A term frequently applied to children during this early pre-school period is the "terrible twos or threes". This description relates to the common occurrence of a young child protesting (physically and/or verbally) at being asked to do something perfectly reasonable but something they do not want to do at that point in time. For example, they might scream and refuse to put a hat on when it is freezing outside. This behaviour might also emerge during a visit to the dental clinic. However, the term is not ideal as it indicates, unfairly, that the child's behaviour is calculated to manipulate and sabotage. Rather, it should be considered a normal stage of child development where the child's protest is part of their emerging autonomy: they begin to understand the concepts of "being a separate me" and "I can influence my surroundings".

9.3 Top Tips for Managing Pre-school Children

We are not saying that it is easy to carry out a dental examination and treatment for very young children, but by following some simple steps, it can be a positive experience for the child, their parent/s and the dental team.
1. Building a Relationship

Start by building a relationship in the waiting room. Bend/sit down to establish eye contact on the same level as the child (◘ Fig. 9.3). This makes you seem less intimidating and helps the child feel safer in the situation (remember the Circle of Security). It is the child who "plays the leading role", so engage them before greeting the parent. Even when speaking to the parent, continue to make the child the centre of the conversation and actively involve them. Most children respond positively when friendly adults show an interest in them.
2. Make the Parents Part of the Team

Parents know their child best and are the child's most important supporter. They can, therefore, be invaluable in helping the dental team make the child's visit a positive one. Ask their advice about how best to manage their child. Most parents appreciate being involved in supporting their child and are happy that their insights are sought.
3. Use Play

Try to make the visit fun. You could give the dental instruments' names and/or attributes and engage the child in this imagery: e.g. the slow hand-piece might be "Mr Tickle-Bump"; the cotton rolls might be "squishy sausages". A dental glove can be blown up to make a

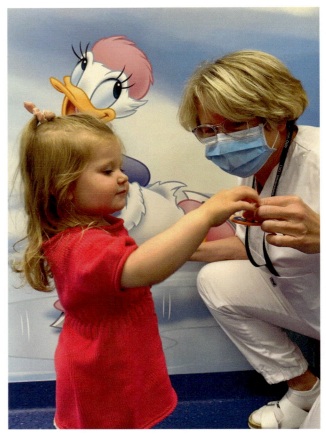

◘ **Fig. 9.3** Dr. Rønneberg establishes rapport with her young patient by adopting a non-threatening pose

balloon animal (◘ Fig. 9.4) and given to the child to hold. By naming instruments like this, you make them more familiar, engaging and fun.
4. Encourage the Child to Sit in the Dental Chair on His/Her Own

Most children can sit in the chair by themselves and this provides a great opportunity to experience self-efficacy. The parent may sit in a chair next to the child, holding their hand if necessary, so the child feels safe to explore the chair (i.e. positioned on top of the Circle of Security). If the child insists on sitting on the parent's lap, go with it. The lap is the support that makes the task safer to explore, and that is the most important thing at this stage.
5. Use the "Knee-to-Knee" Dental Examination

Young children frequently sit on their parent's lap as it provides a comfortable and safe haven. The knee-to-knee method for examining a toddler's teeth is simply a progression from this secure position, whilst affording the dentist good visual access. First, explain the concept to the parent/child, clarifying that you and the parent

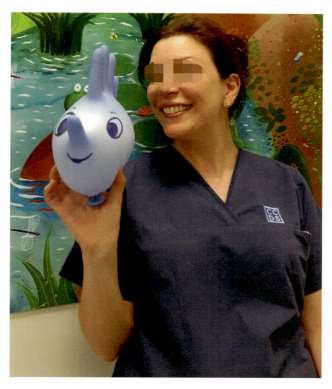

Fig. 9.4 An unused dental glove can be blown up and tied with floss to create a balloon animal as a reward for a young child

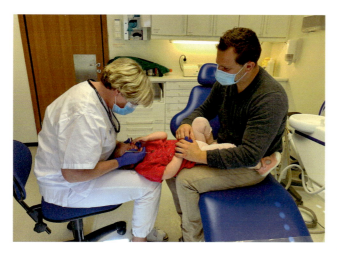

Fig. 9.5 Use of the knee-to-knee approach to facilitate a "safe" dental examination of young children

will be safely "holding" the child and that the child may initially cry, but the examination is necessary and will be very quick. The parent and dental professional sit facing each other, with their knees close together. The child first sits on their parent's lap, facing them, with their legs on either side of their parent's waist. The child is then placed backwards with their upper body and head resting on the clinician's lap (Fig. 9.5). This knee-to-knee

position allows the child to look up into their parent's face (which is reassuring) while the parent holds their child's hands to keep them still in a safe manner [6].
6. Don't Forget "Tell-Show-Do"

Every paediatric dental patient should be managed with appropriate behavioural management techniques (BMTs), irrespective of their vulnerabilities or treatment needs, right from the outset. The use of BMTs has an undisputed place in preventing the development of dental fear and anxiety and is a cornerstone of paediatric dentistry. A simple and frequently used BMT involves a "Tell-Show-Do" approach, which can be used in conjunction with stepwise systematic learning in conjunction with positive reinforcement [7]. "Tell-Show-Do" can be adopted for any patient, but obviously needs to be age and/or intellectually appropriate. First, the clinician explains in a calm voice, using simple and age-appropriate language, what procedure they would like to do (and why). They then show the child what is involved, check if the child is happy to proceed, and then they can undertake the procedure.

The method can be viewed as a staircase; the first step may simply be sitting in the dental chair. The next step could be asking the child to open their mouth widely, before progressing to having a dental mirror inside their mouth. Further up the "stairs" the child should experience the sensation of a probe (or another dental instrument) on their fingernail and then a tooth. The next step is blowing air on the child's hand and then in their mouth. If there is still positive acceptance, the next step could be a clinical examination. If the child continues to give positive feedback, a further stepwise introduction to prophylaxis and fluoride varnish could be undertaken. Using this method, the clinician may further introduce different procedures such as the use of rubber dam or local anaesthetic. The fundamental principle of the "Tell-Show-Do" method is that you should not move to the next step until you have positive acceptance. It is important to reinforce the child's positive acceptance and coping by providing feedback at every step. The "Tell-Show-Do" approach may be successfully adapted for all ages, but when managing pre-school children, it is important to avoid long verbal explanations of things, but to rely more on visual and tactile demonstrations. The use of age-appropriate language and metaphors is also crucial to meet an individual child's level of understanding and experience. When you show a young child how the instruments work, you trigger their curiosity (remember the Circle of Security) and the child can create an understanding of what to expect. Make a goal (the next "step") that is achievable for the child as positive experiences will build self-efficacy for the future.

9

Case Example of "Tell-Show-Do"

Mohammed is a timid 3-year-old boy who is attending the dental clinic for the first time. Initially, you chat to Mohammed while he sits on his father's knee. You then ask him if he would like a ride in your special "magic" chair so you can look at his teeth. You **tell** him that the chair will move up and down while he sits on it, and it can go flat like a bed. You then **show** him the foot pedal and show him how you press it to make the chair go up and down. He can then hear the noise it makes and see how it moves. You might even ask him if he would like to press the button? The next step is to encourage him to sit in the chair, so you can take him for a ride (**do**). You might even invite him to say "stop" when he wants the chair to stop, so he can feel in control.

---

7. Give the Child Time

Time is a precious resource for the dental team, but some children do need additional time to "warm up" and feel safe in unfamiliar situations. Others may be starting to develop their autonomy and need more "space" to make decisions for themselves. It is especially important for pre-school children that they are given short breaks, when needed, as their attention span and reserves are quite short at this age. Always try to plan your time effectively and according to the child's needs.

8. Be Bigger, Stronger, Wiser and Kind

Some children and situations will severely test your patience. But remember that children rarely want to be difficult towards strangers for no good reason. Their pre-cooperative behaviour and negative emotions may stem from many things such as being tired, hungry or feeling unsafe. Imagine the COS and place the child either at the top or bottom and try to think of the child's needs rather than focussing on the perceived negative behaviours. Picture the child's expression as a smoke detector that tells you something is burning; you just need to find out what made the alarm go off.

9.3.1 Primary School-Aged Children (6–12 Years)

Case Scenario

Nadia (9-years-old) arrives at the clinic. She needs a filling for the first time. When you meet her in the waiting room, she sits close to her mum and looks away when you say "hello". Nadia appears hesitant and uneasy when entering the clinic. When she sits down, you observe tears in her eyes, she breathes fast, and is clenching her fists. "Thank you for coming to see us Nadia, but have you been worrying about this visit?", you ask. She nods her head and looks down at the floor. "Have you talked to your mum about what we were planning to do today?" you enquire. "Yes", she replies. "I have to have a needle….". "Have you ever had one before?" "Yes", she replies. She looks at you and says: "I had to have a needle from the school nurse and when I had a blood test at the doctor's" "Okay, then you know something about how it feels to have a little injection?" "Yes…", Nadia replies hesitantly "but I have never had one in my mouth before". "Well that's fine and might be why you were worried about coming here", you say. "Will it hurt a lot?" "Well actually it's easier than the one you had at the doctor's; I always use a magic cream first on your gum so that you will only feel a tiny scratch, or even nothing at all. But it does taste a bit nasty, so we will have a drink of water ready for you" you explain. "So would it be ok with you if I just show you the things we will be using and we can check you are happy with everything first". "Ok", Nadia replies. She sighs and leans forward towards you.

Throughout their school-aged years, children need activities and play to convey the nuances of their experiences and to process new information properly. The child still "sees" the world in a different and more immediate manner than adults, and their understanding of events is closely related to their own personal experiences of these events. It is during this period that children start to develop rules and ethical codes and appreciate the consequences of their actions/behaviour. Behaviours are viewed as either right or wrong, depending on the rules that they have learnt. For example, children know that it is wrong to tell a lie and would, therefore, characterise a liar as a bad person. Additionally, at this age, children perceive rules and principles as absolutes and would not agree to them changing through a process of social agreement. So, if a dentist informs a child patient that he/she is only going to "wobble" a tooth (and gains trust for this) but, in actual fact, goes ahead and extracts it, this may be a very negative experience for the child. They will deduce from this event that "the dentist lied to me, people who lie are bad, dentists are bad".

9.4   Top Tips for Managing Primary School-Aged Children

1. Modify your communication approach

Take the time to talk to the child about non-dental topics and ideally without wearing your protective mask and glasses. This allows them to gain a first impression of you. Show, explain and ask the child questions in a way that they are invited to engage. If the child is shy and does not answer, give them time to warm up. It is important to adjust your communication style and topic of conversation to the personality and maturity level of the child.

2. Prepare the child for what is planned, be honest and predictable

Explain what is planned for the current assessment/treatment visit in short and simple language. It is important that the child and parent get a picture of what is going to be done and approximately how long it will take. This information frames the appointment and makes it more predictable, which in turn, makes the pending experience feel safer. Ensure your terminology/language is age-appropriate and use drawings or models to aid the child's comprehension. Always check if the child understands before you start a procedure. Remember that children also have the right to be heard and express their views and we need to support those with specific learning needs so that they can also be "heard" [1].

3. Agree on a stop signal with the child

Give the child a stop signal to use if needed such as lifting an arm. This action serves as both a stop signal and a distractor from the dental procedure. By giving the child a stop signal, you give them a sense of control which may help them to feel safer when exposed to unfamiliar sensations. If the child uses their stop signal, it is obviously very important to stop when it is safe to do so, give the child a break, and to explore why the child needed you to stop.

4. Use play actively

Play is still an important element to children of this age, so use play as a mediator to make a connection with the child, increase positive feelings and make the unfamiliar more familiar. The child will then be more likely to associate their visit with something safe, enjoyable and fun.

5. Let the child choose if the parent accompanies him/her in the clinic or waits outside

The positive and negative influences of parental presence on a child's behaviour/anxiety in the dental surgery have stimulated a lively debate over the years [8, 9]. Although there are cultural and societal differences in terms of the importance placed on parental accompaniment, most dental health professionals would encourage the input of parents to support their child. However, the child has a right to choose whether, or not, they wish to be accompanied by their parent while they have treatment [1]. It is also important to focus your communication on the child. If the parent dominates, shift your attention back to the child, asking them direct questions and choosing a topic of conversation relevant to them.

6. Make agreements with the child and keep them

Make agreements with the patient and parent about what is to be done and how it will be done and then stick to that agreement. This builds trust between you and the child and you and the parent. The trust gives you a solid foundation for more challenging interventions in the future. Do not stretch the agreement even if the parent suggests it (e.g. "can you just do Ruby's last filling today as well, so I don't have to take any more time off work").

7. Invest in the end of the appointment

Make sure the appointment ends in such a way that the child leaves with positive feelings. Even if the appointment did not go as you hoped, it is important to summarise the things that you thought the child had done well, as well as asking them/their parent for their opinions as to what had gone well. This builds self-efficacy and motivation for future appointments at the clinic: "I am sorry your tooth hurt you a bit at the end of treatment today and you became sad. But you did a very good job by telling me how you felt by using the stop signal. And you were so still when you had the numbing liquid, that was brilliant. Next time we will give you a little more of the numbing liquid, so your tooth doesn't hurt. Will that be ok, do you want to ask me anything before you go?"

8. Be bigger, stronger, wiser and kind

As with little children, primary school-aged children can also challenge your patience and provoke feelings of frustration when they decline treatment. Although it may be tempting to tell them to behave like a "big" boy/girl, we still recommend that you view their behaviour within the Circle of Security framework. This will help you to find out what is really going on behind the protest and pre-cooperative behaviour. Often you will find the need to feel safe (as the child is frightened of something) and/or has low self-efficacy.

9.4.1 Adolescents (13–18 Year-Olds)

Case Study

Paulo (15-years-old) arrives at the clinic with his mum. He is hunched over this phone with his hood up when you enter the waiting room. You say "hello" but he barely answers. He and his mum follow you into the surgery and you sense he is very uncomfortable when sitting in the dental chair and looks pale and jittery. He answers your questions with monosyllables, with little eye contact. You explain that you are just going to put the chair back to check his teeth. He suddenly says "no, I don't want my teeth checked" and sits forwards. His mum snaps at him "Paulo, I'm not having this again, just open your mouth and don't be stupid". Paulo mutters something rude under his breath but does not sit back in the chair. You say "It's not a problem Paulo, let's just put the chair up and we can have a chat". You suggest that Paulo might be feeling worried, and it is completely normal, and it is completely normal to feel some fear at the dentist, especially when meeting someone new. You explain that our bodies can react in strange ways when we are worried, making us feel faint or sick or even angry. "Is this something you recognize?" Paulo confirms with a "'yes". "Thanks for telling me, why don't we make a plan together so you don't feel like this next time?" Paulo makes eye contact with you when he answers "Yes". You then turn to his mum and ask her how she feels about coming to the dentist, she says she is "scared-stiff". You suggest that it might be easier if she sits in the waiting room next time, if that works better for Paulo and her, and you will come and talk to her after the check-up. Both, Paulo and his mum, think this is a good plan.

Adolescence is a time of rapid development, especially in the early stages. This is a time when the young person sees increasing facets of the world which may challenge their already established views of themselves and society around them. A lot of what Piaget (1896–1980) would have referred to as accommodation is going on in this period of development. The young person experiences constant conflicts between their existing worldview and contradictory new experiences [10].

It is worth remembering that some teenagers may react immaturely (relative to their chronological age) when facing authority figures and challenging situations. Indeed, there is considerable variation in children's maturity and understanding during this adolescent period. It is, therefore, always helpful to talk to your adolescent patients prior to dental treatment to gain some insight into their maturity levels, and thus better adjust your communication approach. Sometimes, we overestimate their level of maturity as adolescents might have advanced language skills and comprehension, but there may also be areas where they lack experience and have misperceptions. In contrast, this age group do not like being patronised by being "talked down to" or being excluded from decisions that affect them.

9.5 Top Tips for Managing Teenagers

1. Establish a rapport

Invest a few minutes chatting to your young patient before you start any actual treatment. You could ask about their school, family or outside interests. Adjust your language and approach according to their maturity level, not too childish and not too complicated. Remember the four good habits described in ▶ Chap. 3.

2. Be honest and predictable

Explain what you are going to do, offer to demonstrate aspects of it and then do exactly what was agreed. Even if your intentions are good, holding back information may compromise establishing trust and a good relationship. So, be honest about what you are doing and confirm the young person is happy for you to proceed.

3. Ask them how they really are

As a health care professional, you have a duty of care to be vigilant in identifying and addressing any safeguarding, social or wider health problems that your young patient might be experiencing. If you have concerns about mental health conditions such as eating disorders, neglect, domestic violence, substance abuse or other issues, find the time to talk to the young person in confidence. You will then need to seek advice on the next course of action, but the key thing is that you took the time and interest to look beyond just the child's dental needs.

4. Use "Tell-Show-Do" when needed

Not all young people have experienced every type of dental treatment or know what that procedure entails. The basic principles of the "Tell-Show-Do" method should, therefore, be adopted for every new dental procedure, regardless of the patient's age. Gradual habituation when introducing new procedures is essential to prevent the development of dental fear and anxiety.

5. Agree on a Stop Signal

Give the young person the opportunity to stop the treatment if needed. This communicates that you respect and acknowledge that he/she knows best about their tolerance limits. If the stop signal is used, it is important that you stop, find out why the young person needed you to stop and amend your approach accordingly.

6. Respect young people's autonomy when giving health advice

It is important to educate young people about their health (i.e. increase their health literacy) in a way they can make their own informed and un-coerced decisions. Oral health education (tooth brushing, diet advice, smoking cessation, etc.) must be delivered in a positive, engaging and non-condescending manner, whilst accounting for wide variance in levels of comprehension. Rather than reprimanding those with sub-optimal health habits, try to find out why, for example, they don't brush their teeth twice a day, and whether they actually want to improve their practices. When motivation is established internally, there is more chance that the person will succeed in their behaviour change.

7. Be bigger, stronger, wiser and kind

This approach is just as important when dealing with adolescents as it is for younger children. Some of the adolescents you meet may, initially, seem unlikeable. They can appear rude, aggressive, dismissive or indifferent towards their own oral health and the advice you offer. However, these behaviours may simply be hiding the underlying feelings of embarrassment, insecurity or fear. The young person may have unconsciously decided that it is better to reject you and make you feel bad before you can criticise them.

9.6 Dental Anxiety: Understanding the Anxious Child

9.6.1 Background to Child Dental Anxiety

Dental anxiety (DA) is extremely common in children, with a 2020 systematic review reporting a global pooled prevalence of around 24% [11]. Dental anxiety is a term used to describe a state of apprehension and/ or catastrophising, together with a feeling of lack of control, in relation to a dental encounter. It is distinct to dental fear (a relatively normal response, which is experienced by lots of children) and dental phobia (a severe and incapacitating response) although the three terms are sometimes, incorrectly, used interchangeably [11, 12]. Numerous studies have attempted to identify the key risk factors for the development and maintenance of childhood DA, but questions remain about this complex construct [12]. In general, DA appears to be more common in younger (pre-school) children and

those with caries, but further research is needed to elucidate the effect of gender and socio-economic status, past dental experience and parental factors [11, 13]. It is also important to recognise that some children are simply dentally anxious, but others may have concomitant mental health conditions (depression, eating disorders, experienced child maltreatment (▶ Chap. 11)) and/or other specific anxieties (e.g. social phobia).

Regrettably, DA is associated with several negative oral and general health outcomes [11]. Children with DA tend to be irregular dental attenders, often presenting only when they are experiencing acute symptoms. Consequently, these children may have poorer oral health and oral-health related quality of life than their non-anxious peers [11, 14]. They may also have greater reliance on pharmacological interventions, such as sedation or general anaesthetic (GA), in order to accept dental treatment, a reliance which may persist into adulthood [15, 16]. From a service provider point of view, the management of children with DA has obvious economic and capacity implications. Furthermore, some dental health professionals report an increase in their own stress and anxiety levels when trying to provide treatment for very anxious patients [17, 18].

A challenge when trying to measure (quantify) children's DA is the heterogeneity of instruments that are available with some focussing on trait anxiety and others on state anxiety [19]. Although several self-report measures have been validated for use with children, they tend to have a limited focus of enquiry and lack a theoretical basis [19]. There is also the argument that quantitative assessments of DA only give limited insights into children's experiences and perspectives of DA. For that reason, it is helpful to present some findings from qualitative studies as described below.

9.6.2 Children's Experiences of Dental Anxiety

It is clear from participatory research with children that they share some similar anxieties about the dentist. An interview-based study with dentally-anxious British children found that they recounted vivid descriptions of previous traumatic dental episodes and described a variety of emotions in addition to anxiety (including anger, shame and embarrassment) [20]. They reported physical symptoms of shaking, sweating and feeling faint and frequently described the tactics they used to try to avoid dental care (pretending to be ill or downplaying any symptoms). Interestingly, they often imagined that really bad things might happen to them such as the dentist making a mistake and taking the wrong tooth out or choking on something or even getting germs from dental equipment.

» "What if they do something wrong? They slip, and then I swallow something and it chokes and I die?" (Michael, 13 years)

In order to successfully treat children with this degree of DA, clinicians may need to use approaches additional to the excellent behaviour management strategies described earlier. There is now growing interest in the application of cognitive behavioural therapy (CBT) in the dental setting with some promising findings for the management of dentally anxious children.

9.7   Cognitive Behavioural Therapy

9.7.1   What Is It and How Does It Work?

CBT is described as a problem-based "talking therapy" which aims to provide key knowledge (psychoeducation) and teaches coping skills with the intention of altering unhelpful thoughts or behaviours. There is a good evidence-base to support its effectiveness in treating children, who have a range of anxiety disorders, from the age of around seven years upwards [21]. The delivery of CBT can vary widely from purely self-help formats (such as online) right through to multiple sessions with a clinical psychologist depending on the level of need. There are also options of engaging in CBT alone, as a family unit or in group sessions.

9.7.2   CBT for Children in the Dental Setting

It is only relatively recently, however, that the application of CBT for dentally anxious children is being recognised; with a systematic review finding that CBT was more effective in reducing DA and improving cooperation compared to behavioural management techniques [22]. Studies conducted in Sweden have provided compelling evidence for the effectiveness of both face-to-face and psychologist-guided Internet-based CBT (ICBT) in reducing children's DA [23, 24]. Following these interventions, children described how their views of dentistry had changed and how they had new feelings of being in control and safe, which improved their ability to undergo treatment (including acceptance of intra-oral injections) despite their fears [25].

However, the costs and availability of expert psychologists prohibit the widespread use of CBT for child dental anxiety in many countries. Furthermore, it is not feasible for primary care dentists alone to deliver complex psychological interventions within most health systems [26]. To improve general access to CBT in non-specialist services or general dental practices, a "stepped care" approach can be used, where children are offered the least intensive form of CBT initially and then these are "stepped up" for children whose anxiety does not respond to these low intensity treatments [27]. With this in mind, a simple self-help CBT intervention "Your teeth, you are in control" has been developed for delivery by dental professionals [28]. This intervention aims to use a range of evidence-based psychological techniques for the reduction of DA in children with guidance provided by dental professionals. The intervention includes a self-help guide for children aged 9–16 years with accompanying resources for parents and the dental team (to be used as hard copies or accessed online). It was developed using a "person-based" approach involving dentally anxious children, parents and dental health professionals to ensure the perspectives and needs of children were taken into account. A study was conducted in which 48 children with self-reported DA were given the intervention by paediatric dentists in hospital and primary care settings. After three treatment visits, children reported a significant reduction in anxiety (measured using the Modified Child Dental Anxiety Scale) and better health-related quality of life. Additional findings were improved attendance rates and maintenance of anxiety reduction one year later [29]. Use of this guided self-help CBT approach was also found to be feasible and effective in a general dental practice setting; the effect size of this reduction in anxiety was large [30].

9.7.3   Using the "Your teeth, you are in control" Intervention

The intervention is designed for use with children, aged 9–16 years, with mild to moderate dental anxiety, no urgent treatment needs but requiring a course of treatment. The dental professionals delivering the intervention typically undergo a two-hour training session and it is crucial that the child remains with the same clinician throughout the course of treatment, as establishing trust is integral to a successful outcome. The intervention is based on the five areas model of CBT (◘ Fig. 9.6), with the overall aim of breaking the perpetual cycle of negative thoughts, feelings and behaviours [31]. For example, imagine a 14-year-old who needs to see a new dentist for an emergency appointment because she has toothache (situational factors). She keeps thinking that the dentist is going to hold her down and pull her tooth out without her permission (unhelpful thoughts). Because of these thoughts, she starts to feel helpless and trapped (altered feelings). In turn, these negative feelings cause her to be rude to the dentist and she denies having had any pain (unhelpful behaviours). When she eventually sits in the dental chair, she can feel her heart thumping and she feels sick (altered physical symptoms). She starts to catastrophise that she is going to faint and the dentist will laugh at her; and these unhelpful thoughts, feelings and behaviours will continue unless she is supported to find a way of coping with them and breaking the cycle.

The resource works by incorporating the following key "ingredients":

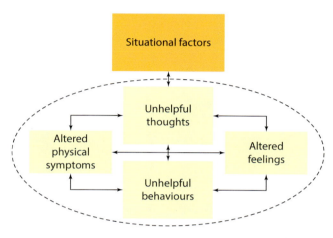

Fig. 9.6   The five areas model of CBT (Williams and Garland, 2002)

– Helps children, parents/carers and dental team members understand the factors that may be maintaining the child's dental anxiety
– Includes factual information on the dental team and basic procedures
– Describes a variety of cognitive and behavioural tools/strategies that children can use to help them feel less anxious (e.g. challenging unhelpful thinking, goal setting/graded treatment planning, relaxation exercises)
– Suggests activities to increase children's feelings of control and self-efficacy in their ability to undertake dental treatment (including a "message to dentist" (◼ Fig. 9.7) and signed stop signal agreement)
– Prompts them to reflect on what went well about each visit to build a memory bank of positive experiences
– Provides structure and guidance on how to incorporate the use of individualised positive reinforcement techniques into dental treatment/visits
– Promotes effective communication and shared decision-making between children, parents and dental team members

The following case study of a very anxious 10-year-old girl illustrates the steps involved in using this simple, but effective intervention.

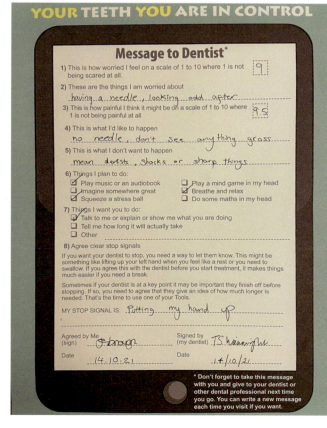

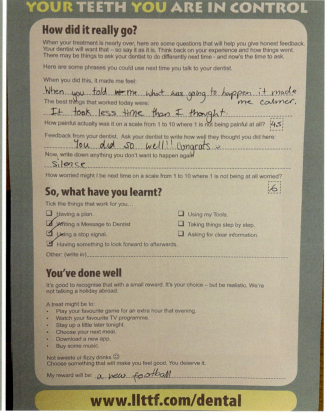

Fig. 9.7   Example of a completed "Message to Dentist" sheet

Case Study

Ella was referred a hospital dental service as her dentist thought she may have caries. However, she had always been too scared to allow a thorough examination, despite attending from a young age.

Step 1: Identify the anxiety, normalise it, introduce the intervention and agree the plan for next visit

At her first visit to the dental hospital, she would not speak directly to the dentist. She kept her gloves on and her hood up. Her parents didn't understand why she was so anxious. However, further questioning revealed that she had severe social anxiety. The dentist explained that she did not need to look at Ella's teeth until Ella agreed to this. However, she stressed she wanted to help Ella not feel anxious about visiting the dentist, keeping the focus away from potential treatment. Ella and her parents were given the "Your teeth, you are in control" guide and the accompanying parent guide and were asked to complete the "message to dentist" sheet for the next visit when it was agreed she would brush her teeth, without the dentist looking at her

Step 2: Review "Message to the dentist", discuss worry/pain score and specific situational factors, agree coping tools, stop signal and sign agreement, consider rewards for progress, agree plan for next visit

At her next visit, Ella had read the "Your teeth, you are in control" guide with her mum and had completed the "message to dentist" sheet. Her main concern was "things falling down her throat and choking". The dentist reassured her, talked about her coping plan and agreed a stop signal. Ella brushed her teeth as agreed and said she would have a check up with a mirror and an X-ray at her next visit. Her mum said she could do some baking as a reward for making good progress.

Step 3: Review plan for that visit and confirm coping strategies. Reflect what went well at the end of the visit and plan for the next one. Congratulate achievements.

At her third visit, Ella took her gloves off and hood down and made direct eye contact with the dentist for the first time. She wanted to see all the dental instruments before they were put in her mouth. She said she wanted to do maths puzzles in her head to give her something else to think about. She had a check up with a mirror and a radiograph. The dentist noticed that she had a large overjet and needed an orthodontic referral and impressions. Ella was given the trays for the moulds to practice with at home, so she would not worry about things going down her throat. The dentist promised to introduce her to the orthodontist next time.

Step 4: Review plan for that visit and confirm coping strategies. Encourage self-reflection to build a positive memory bank and re-complete anxiety and anticipated pain scores

When Ella attended the orthodontist four months later, she was noticeably more confident. Her family had supported her by talking about the visit the night before. She had brought the "Your teeth, you are in control" guide and "message to dentist" sheet with her. She accepted the impressions and photos happily. Her mother (and the dentist) was amazed by this progress. Ella's self-report scores of her own dental anxiety had significantly reduced. Ella reported that she was still fearful of dental treatment, but now felt she had greater trust in the dentist and could cope if she was prepared for what was going to happen and was given control in decision-making.

Clearly there is great potential for innovative approaches that embrace technology, psychology and the skills of the dental team to reduce children's dental anxiety and improve their lifetime experience of treatment. Hopefully, increased awareness and uptake of self-help or online CBT resources, training for dental professionals in low intensity psychological techniques and integrated working across multidisciplinary teams will provide acceptable, accessible, clinically effective and cost-effective improvements to the care of children with dental anxiety.

Summary

As dental health professionals, we meet many different children and adolescents, each with their individual history, attachment style, temperament and past experiences of general health and dental care services. This chapter has introduced concepts around normal psychological development with a focus on attachment and interaction. It has hopefully demonstrated how this knowledge may be applied in the dental clinic to promote positive encounters for children and their families from the outset. It is our responsibility to give children and adolescents the assurance of safety, predictability (control) and mastery, so they feel able to accept the planned dental treatment and will establish a lifelong pattern of optimum oral health and dental attendance.

References

1. UN General Assembly. Convention on the rights of the child. United Nations; 1989. Accessed 1 July 2021

2. Ainsworth MS. Infant–mother attachment. Am Psychol. 1979;34:932–7. https://doi.org/10.1037/0003-066X.34.10.932.

3. Bowlby J. Attachment and loss. London: The Hogarth Press and Institute of Psycho-Analysis; 1969. p. 428.

4. Hoffman KT, Marvin RS, Cooper G, et al. Changing toddlers' and preschoolers' attachment classifications: the circle of security intervention. J Consult Clin Psychol. 2006;74:1017–26. https://doi.org/10.1037/0022-006X.74.6.1017.

5. Thomas A, Chess S. Temperament and development. Oxford: Brunner/Mazel; 1977.

6. Fux-Noy A, Shmueli A, Herzog K, et al. Attitudes of EAPD members toward using the "knee-to-knee" position. Eur Arch Paediatr Dent. 2020;21:687–91. https://doi.org/10.1007/s40368-020-00514-0.

7. Holst A, Crossner CG. Management of dental behaviour problems. A 5-year follow-up. Swed Dent J. 1984;8:243–9.

8. Crossley ML, Joshi G. An investigation of paediatric dentists' attitudes towards parental accompaniment and behavioural management techniques in the UK. Br Dent J. 2002;192:517–21. https://doi.org/10.1038/sj.bdj.4801416.

9. Shroff S, Hughes C, Mobley C. Attitudes and preferences of parents about being present in the dental operatory. Pediatr Dent. 2015;37:51–5.

10. Gebhardt S, Grant P, von Georgi R, et al. Aspects of Piaget's cognitive developmental psychology and neurobiology of psychotic disorders – an integrative model. Med Hypotheses. 2008;71:426–33. https://doi.org/10.1016/j.mehy.2008.03.042.

11. Grisolia BM, Dos Santos APP, Dhyppolito IM, et al. Prevalence of dental anxiety in children and adolescents globally: A systematic review with meta-analyses. Int J Paediatr Dent. 2021;31:168–83. https://doi.org/10.1111/ipd.12712.

12. Seligman LD, Hovey JD, Chacon K, et al. Dental anxiety: an understudied problem in youth. Clin Psychol Rev. 2017;55:25–40. https://doi.org/10.1016/j.cpr.2017.04.004.

13. Klingberg G, Broberg AG. Dental fear/anxiety and dental behaviour management problems in children and adolescents: a review of prevalence and concomitant psychological factors. Int J Paediatr Dent. 2007;17:391–406. https://doi.org/10.1111/j.1365-263X.2007.00872.x.

14. Coxon JD, Hosey MT, Newton JT. The impact of dental anxiety on the oral health of children aged 5 and 8 years: a regression analysis of the Child Dental Health Survey 2013. Br Dent J. 2019;227:818–22. https://doi.org/10.1038/s41415-019-0853-y.

15. Taskinen H, Kankaala T, Rajavaara P, et al. Self-reported causes for referral to dental treatment under general anaesthesia (DGA): a cross-sectional survey. Eur Arch Paediatr Dent. 2014;15:105–12. https://doi.org/10.1007/s40368-013-0071-2.

16. Haworth S, Dudding T, Waylen A, et al. Ten years on: is dental general anaesthesia in childhood a risk factor for caries and anxiety? Br Dent J. 2017;222:299–304. https://doi.org/10.1038/sj.bdj.2017.175.

17. Moore R, Brødsgaard I. Dentists' perceived stress and its relation to perceptions about anxious patients. Community Dent Oral Epidemiol. 2001;29:73–80.

18. Rønneberg A, Strøm K, Skaare AB, et al. Dentists' self-perceived stress and difficulties when performing restorative treatment in children. Eur Arch Paediatr Dent. 2015;16:341–7. https://doi.org/10.1007/s40368-014-0168-2.

19. Porritt J, Marshman Z, Rodd HD. Understanding children's dental anxiety and psychological approaches to its reduction. Int J Paediatr Dent. 2012;22:397–405. https://doi.org/10.1111/j.1365-263X.2011.01208.x.

20. Morgan AG, Rodd HD, Porritt JM, et al. Children's experiences of dental anxiety. Int J Paediatr Dent. 2017;27:87–97. https://doi.org/10.1111/ipd.12238.

21. James AC, James G, Cowdrey FA, et al. Cognitive behavioural therapy for anxiety disorders in children and adolescents. Cochrane Database Syst Rev. 2015;2015:Cd004690. https://doi.org/10.1002/14651858.CD004690.pub4.

22. Gomes HS, Viana KA, Batista AC, et al. Cognitive behaviour therapy for anxious paediatric dental patients: a systematic review. Int J Paediatr Dent. 2018;28:422–31. https://doi.org/10.1111/ipd.12405.

23. Shahnavaz S, Hedman E, Grindefjord M, et al. Cognitive behavioral therapy for children with dental anxiety: a randomized controlled trial. JDR Clin Trans Res. 2016;1:234–43. https://doi.org/10.1177/2380084416661473.

24. Shahnavaz S, Hedman-Lagerlof E, Hasselblad T, et al. Internet-based cognitive behavioral therapy for children and adolescents with dental anxiety: open trial. J Med Internet Res. 2018;20:e12. https://doi.org/10.2196/jmir.7803.

25. Shahnavaz S, Rutley S, Larsson K, et al. Children and parents' experiences of cognitive behavioral therapy for dental anxiety–a qualitative study. Int J Paediatr Dent. 2015;25:317–26. https://doi.org/10.1111/ipd.12181.

26. Newton T, Asimakopoulou K, Daly B, et al. The management of dental anxiety: time for a sense of proportion? Br Dent J. 2012;213:271–4. https://doi.org/10.1038/sj.bdj.2012.830.

27. Williams C, Martinez R. Increasing access to CBT: stepped care and CBT self-help models in practice. Behav Cognit Psychotherapy. 2008;36:675–83. https://doi.org/10.1017/S1352465808004864.

28. Porritt J, Rodd H, Morgan A, et al. Development and testing of a cognitive behavioral therapy resource for children's dental anxiety. JDR Clin Trans Res. 2017;2:23–37. https://doi.org/10.1177/2380084416673798.

29. Rodd H, Kirby J, Duffy E, et al. Children's experiences following a CBT intervention to reduce dental anxiety: one year on. Br Dent J. 2018;225:247–51. https://doi.org/10.1038/sj.bdj.2018.540.

30. Bux S, Porritt J, Marshman Z. Evaluation of self-help cognitive behavioural therapy for children's dental anxiety in general dental practice. Dent J (Basel). 2019;7(2):36. https://doi.org/10.3390/dj7020036.

31. Williams C, Garland A. A cognitive–behavioural therapy assessment model for use in everyday clinical practice. Adv Psychiatric Treat. 2002;8:172–9. https://doi.org/10.1192/apt.8.3.172.

Family Violence and Child Maltreatment

Anne Rønneberg, Jenny Harris, Therese Varvin Fredriksen, and Tiril Willumsen

Contents

Family violence may be an act of violence between a parent and a child, violence between family members, violence between current or former intimate partners as well as between siblings. Maltreatment includes harm, neglect or threat to a child.

In this context, this chapter focusses on the importance of childhood as a crucial time period in an individual's development. The World Health Organization (WHO) has highlighted the health sector's important role in addressing child maltreatment (child abuse and neglect) in order to promote children and young people's wellbeing and to assist all to reach their potential. Adverse childhood experiences (ACEs) have negative impacts on child development and, furthermore, may cause irreversible and, sometimes, lifelong damage. The impact of ACEs is well documented through studies from both the USA and Europe [1–3].

This chapter will discuss how we may become concerned about a child or a young person regarding family violence, witnessing violence or maltreatment and how to respond when suspicion occurs.

Regarding adults, dental personnel have an obligation to act on suspicion of all kinds of domestic violence as well. The chapter elaborates several aspects of domestic violence and how to address this difficult issue in a dental setting.

Learning Goals
- Be able to recognize signs of child maltreatment
- Be aware of the current legislation regarding child maltreatment according to the United Nations Convention on the Rights of the Child (UNCRC)
- Know how to fulfil our obligations as healthcare providers according to the UNCRC
- Understand domestic violence including the phases in a cycle of abuse
- Know how to fulfil our obligations as healthcare providers according to the Universal Declaration of Human Rights (UDHR)

10.1 Child Maltreatment

10.1.1 Rights of the Child

The United Nations (UN) Convention on the Rights of the Child (UNCRC) [4, 5] is an international convention. Nearly all countries in the world have ratified the UNCRC and several have incorporated the UNCRC in their national law by statutory provision, which gives the UNCRC the same status as other statutory regulations and with supremacy over concurring statutory provisions. Health professionals in some countries are man-

dated by their national legislation to report suspicion of child maltreatment to the child welfare services (CWS, also variously known as social services, children's services, children's social care) and, sometimes, also to the police. In other countries, there is no mandatory reporting but a clear ethical obligation to do so.

The UNCRC defines the child as a person under 18 years of age. In order to help all children to reach their full potential, early intervention and fulfilment of the United Nations Convention on the Rights of the Child (UNCRC) is an obligation of all health professionals. The UNCRC includes four General Principles:
1. Non-discrimination (Article 2)
2. Best interests of the child (Article 3)
3. Right to life survival and development (Article 6)
4. Right to be heard (Article 12)

Regarding health professionals' actions and professional behaviour, which are crucial for safeguarding vulnerable children, Article 19 should be highlighted:

> *1. Parties shall take all appropriate legislative, administrative, social and educational measures to protect the child from all forms of physical or mental violence, injury or abuse, neglect or negligent treatment, maltreatment or exploitation, including sexual abuse, while in the care of parent(s), legal guardian(s) or any other person who has the care of the child.*

> *2. Such protective measures should, as appropriate, include effective procedures for the establishment of social programmes to provide necessary support for the child and for those who have the care of the child, as well as for other forms of prevention and for identification, reporting, referral, investigation, treatment and follow-up of instances of child maltreatment described heretofore, and, as appropriate, for judicial involvement.*

10.1.2 Types of Child Maltreatment

Child maltreatment is defined by the Center for Disease Control and Prevention report 2008 and Gilbert et al. as "Any act of commission or omission by a parent or other caregiver that results in harm, potential for harm, or threat of harm to a child. Harm does not need to be intended" [6, 7].

Violence is defined as any act directed at another person which through this act injures, inflicts pain, intimidates or violates and causes that person to do something against his/her will or to stop doing something he/she wants.

Domestic violence is a term used for many different abusive actions such as when a person is subjected to or witnessing physical or psychological violence or threats between family members or former family members, like between a parent and child and/or siblings and between caregivers. Regardless of the child's age, it is important to define the different types of maltreatment or combinations thereof.

Physical abuse is intentional use of physical force, with or without an implement, against a child that results in, or has the potential to result in, physical injury with harm to the child's health, survival, development and/or dignity. It may include actions such as hitting, kicking, punching, beating, stabbing, biting, pushing, throwing, pulling, dragging, shaking, strangling, smothering, burning, scalding and poisoning.

Sexual abuse is any completed or attempted sexual act, sexual contact, or non-contact sexual interaction with a child by a caregiver (includes substitute caregivers in a temporary custodial role e.g. teachers, coaches, clergy, and relatives), which a child may or may not fully comprehend, is unable to give informed consent to, or for which they are not developmentally prepared.

Psychological (emotional) abuse is intentional behaviour that conveys to a child that he/she is worthless, flawed, unloved, unwanted, endangered, or valued only in meeting another's needs. It can include blaming, belittling, degrading, intimidating, terrorising, isolating or otherwise behaving in a manner that is harmful, potentially harmful or insensitive to the child's developmental needs, or it can potentially damage the child psychologically or emotionally. Witnessing **domestic violence** and **intimate partner violence** has been additionally classified as exposure to emotional or psychological abuse.

Extensive research on domestic violence has revealed how damaging it is for children to witness violence between their caregivers, even if they are not being directly abused themselves [8–10].

Today, we know that the harmful effects may include developing attachment difficulties, mental disorders, social adjustment difficulties and even suicidal acts. Parental care capacity, the atmosphere before and after the violence, worries about what might happen to the parents (divorce, kill each other) and if the child experiences carrying the secret of violence alone are all factors in addition to the violence that has an impact on the child's functioning. Vu et al. found that the child adjustment difficulties persisted and increased in follow-up measures ten years later [9].

Neglect is the failure to meet a child's basic physical, emotional, medical/dental, or educational needs; failure to provide adequate nutrition, hygiene, or shelter or failure to ensure a child's safety. It includes failure to pro-vide adequate food, clothing, or accommodation; not seeking medical or dental attention when needed; allowing a child to miss large amounts of schooling; and failure to protect a child from violence in the home or neighbourhood or from avoidable hazards. Childhood neglect can be as damaging, or perhaps even more damaging to a child, than physical or sexual abuse [6]. Sometimes, the mouth becomes focus of abuse and neglect. Receiving dental care and getting help to maintain good oral health is one of the basic needs of a child [11, 12].

Dental neglect is defined by The British Society of Paediatric Dentistry [13] as "the persistent failure to meet a child's basic oral health needs, likely to result in the serious impairment of a child's oral or general health or development", explaining further that "this definition focusses on identifying unmet need rather than on apportioning blame" so that the dental team can plan for the family to receive the support they need. "Children have a right to good oral health, which forms an integral part of their general health" [14]. Other definitions, taking a global perspective, recognise that to meet a child's oral health needs requires that "reasonable resources are available to the family or caregiver" [15]. Evidenced by a systematic review of the international literature, features of dental neglect include: failure or delay in seeking dental treatment, failure to comply with or complete treatment, failure to provide basic oral care and co-existent adverse impact on the child, for example, dental pain or swelling [15].

One should be aware that different kinds of child maltreatment may overlap; children may be victimised repeatedly and in many various ways.

10.1.3 Safeguarding and Protecting Children

"Safeguarding" is a term used to describe a broad range of measures taken to minimise the risks of harm to children, to protect them from maltreatment and to enable all children to have the best outcomes. Different countries vary in their approach. As Kojan and Lonne [16] have described, some place emphasis on "child protection" – managing risk and protection from harm – while others focus on "child welfare" – prevention, early intervention and supportive measures for children and families. In turn, "These differences influence practitioner's intervention strategies and how the needs of children and parents are met" [16]. In this chapter, we have chosen to use the term "child welfare services" (CWS) instead of "child protection services" but readers should be aware of varying emphasis in their own national contexts and workplace settings.

10.1.4 Dental Professionals and Child Maltreatment

Dental professionals are well placed to identify children at risk of maltreatment. Injuries resulting from physical abuse are frequently located in the face, head and neck region. Literature reports physical abuse to the head and neck in the range from 59% to 76% of maltreated children. Given this high prevalence of injuries to the head and neck, caused by physical violence, all dental professionals should pay extra attention to such injuries [17–19].

Furthermore, severe untreated dental caries may be a predictor of maltreatment, particularly neglect. Children living with household dysfunctional problems, intimate partner violence, domestic violence and in general exposure to adverse childhood experiences are more likely to have poor dental health and more decayed teeth and toothache [20, 21]. Kvist et al. reported that children investigated because of suspected child maltreatment had significantly higher prevalence of caries, had experienced more dental treatment and had higher irregular attendance at dental appointments compared with a control group [22]. Dentists should be concerned and assess for neglect if high caries incidence is not related to obvious causes such as severe illness or other known causalities.

Organisation and funding of paediatric dental services vary between countries. In some Scandinavian countries and the UK for example, the state provides free dental care for children. In other countries, the family is responsible for paying for dental care or for contributing to dental insurance schemes. In the Nordic region of Europe, almost all children are enrolled in the Public Dental Health Service (PDHS), which means that they are regularly summoned to appointments in the PDHS. Thus, the dental team has a unique opportunity to detect different kinds of child maltreatment and to collaborate with the child welfare services (CWS) to safeguard the child.

■ How to Explore Signs of Suspected Maltreatment in Children

Detecting different types of child maltreatment is challenging. One needs to bear in mind that unfortunately not all parents act in the best interests of their children. People are capable of committing cruel and horrifying acts against individuals at all ages. As dental professionals, it is important to have a holistic approach.

■ Taking a History and Examining the Child

Both careful history taking and a thorough examination of the head and neck area are essential. Do not forget to look at the extremities and the body in general. For documentation, it is important to be accurate when writing in the patient's record and to differentiate clearly between facts and opinion.

The possible physical and behavioural signs of child maltreatment are shown in ◘ Table 10.1. These may also have a completely different explanation so you will need to ask yourself questions to clarify if there is reason to be concerned. In relation to observations of physical injuries, typical sites of accidental and non-accidental (abusive) injuries are shown in ◘ Fig. 10.1a and b. To become familiar with the typical appearance of accidental and abusive injuries, further reading is advised. A selection of images is available on the Child Protection and the Dental Team website hosted by the British Dental Association at ► www.bda.org/childprotection and further examples in comprehensive clinical textbooks are available from medical libraries.

All injuries must be assessed and interpreted in the context of the explanation given. Dental professionals need to consider several aspects and ask themselves questions like:

» *Do the child and the parents give matching explanations?*
> *Is it possible that the injury has been inflicted?*
> *Can you say anything about how long it has been since the injury happened?*
> *Has there been a delay seeking treatment?*
> *If violence was the cause, can you say something about the type of violence?*

Further, the child's interaction with their accompanying parent or carer should receive attention, together with observations of the parent or carer's attitude such as any apparent signs of anxiety, distress or disinterest or a history of missed dental appointments.

Behavioural signs of child maltreatment might be different for different children. There are no signs that are present exclusively when exposed to violence. Some children react with hyperactivity, restlessness, aggressiveness and impulsive behaviour. Other children are hypoactivated where passivity, indifference and emotional distance dominate. Others switch between the two behaviour patterns described. It is an advantage to observe and speak to the child on several occasions, although you should not delay taking action if concerned they are at immediate risk.

For further reading, see the CPDT (Child protection and the dental team) website ► https://bda.org/childprotection

◪ **Table 10.1** Possible Signs of Child Maltreatment

Possible signs	Analyse the worries

Physical:
    Bruises (pattern, colour, site)
    Burn and cut injuries
    Bite-marks
    Eye injuries
    Intra-oral injuries
    Injuries with a particular pattern, unlikely explanations or stories that change
    Delays in presentation
    Untreated injuries
    Severe caries that cannot be explained by illness or other known causalities
    Sleep and eating difficulties
    Frequent complaints of somatic pain (e.g. stomach and headaches)
Psychological:
    Restlessness and irritability
    Clingy behaviour or rejecting contact and closeness
    Dental fear and anxiety with unknown causality
    Dissociation
    Sadness and withdrawal
    Overly eager to please or compliant behaviour
    Unexpected reactions when touched
    Loses abilities previously established (e.g. bladder control)
    Use of drugs
    Self-harm
Worrying factors in parent's behaviour
    Delays seeking health care when child is injured or ill
    Demonstrates aggressive, argumentative or threatening behaviour
    Fails to put the child's needs above his/her own needs
    Admits inflicted harm, but often only partial ("I hit him, but not hard")
    Seems indifferent to the child, lacks compassion towards the child and gives inadequate responses of the child
    Has unrealistic expectations to the child
    Makes fun of and is condescending of the child
    Seems depressed and not emotionally involved
    Threatens the child
    Appears intoxicated with alcohol or drugs
	What is your gut feeling?
	What signs have you observed and registered?
	What has the child expressed?
	What have the parents explained?
	Write down the worries and what they are based on
	Have the worries been consistent over time and each time the child has been at the clinic?
	Discuss the worries with an experienced colleague and/or your leader or supervisor
	Summarize the observed signs, the child's condition, the interaction between the child and parents at the clinic and your knowledge about the family
	Have the concerns/worries increased or decreased after the conversation with the child?
	Choose the next step
	    Your concerns have decreased, and no action is acquired at this time
	    Worries are the same or have increased, and action is acquired

■ **Differential Diagnoses**

Different disease conditions may be confused with physical abuse. Inflicted cigarette burns may be mistaken for impetigo or herpes labialis (cold sores). Birthmarks like Congenital Dermal Melanocytosis (blue spot) and haemangiomas may be confused with bruises. Bruising may be a sign of systemic diseases such as a bleeding disorder. Therefore, referral and collaboration with paediatricians or the child's family doctor should be considered, not least to exclude differential diagnoses.

Another important differential diagnosis is enamel mineral disturbances, which could be mistaken for severe caries. Worsening of a child's caries situation may also be a consequence of long-term illness. Obtaining a thorough and updated medical history is essential.

10.1.5 Communicating with the Child

It is good practice to talk with the child alone away from the parent or carer, as appropriate to age. You should ask open questions. Avoid leading questions which could inadvertently prompt or encourage the child to answer in a certain way. If they disclose abuse, you should always take it seriously. However, you should never promise to keep a secret. Nevertheless, you can promise that you will move forward together, keeping them informed of your intentions.

Sometimes professionals become concerned about the welfare of a child because of a single observation or something the child expresses, but more often this happens after several worrying observations over time. On

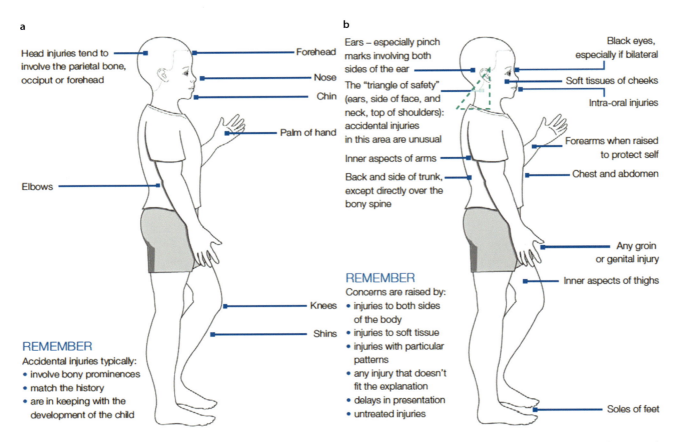

a

Head injuries tend to involve the parietal bone, occiput or forehead — Forehead

Nose

Chin

Palm of hand

Elbows

Knees

Shins

REMEMBER
Accidental injuries typically:
• involve bony prominences
• match the history
• are in keeping with the development of the child

b

Ears – especially pinch marks involving both sides of the ear

The "triangle of safety" (ears, side of face, and neck, top of shoulders): accidental injuries in this area are unusual

Inner aspects of arms

Back and side of trunk, except directly over the bony spine

Black eyes, especially if bilateral

Soft tissues of cheeks

Intra-oral injuries

Forearms when raised to protect self

Chest and abdomen

Any groin or genital injury

Inner aspects of thighs

Soles of feet

REMEMBER
Concerns are raised by:
• injuries to both sides of the body
• injuries to soft tissue
• injuries with particular patterns
• any injury that doesn't fit the explanation
• delays in presentation
• untreated injuries

Fig. 10.1 Typical sites of **a** accidental injury and **b** non-accidental (abusive) injury. (Figure reproduced with permission from Harris et al. [14])

occasions, there may be time to plan in advance for a conversation with the child before deciding on further action:

1. What is the purpose of the planned conversation? What information is necessary to explore further with the child? Be specific what information you need to evaluate your concern.
2. Formulate how the conversation should start and how you will introduce the reason for the appointment. You may find it helpful to note your questions on paper. A comprehensible introduction for the child would be to repeat what the child has told you earlier, what you have observed, seen and heard. Refer only to what the child has expressed.
3. Think through what kind of child this is. A quiet, reserved child or a restless child? Prepare in order to make the meeting as safe and comfortable as possible. Maybe having paper and coloured pencils available would be useful to help the child to settle.
4. Evaluate if your concern is of a character that there is a risk of threats or reprisals for the child in talking to you. They may be afraid of what will happen to them or to their parents if they tell. They may be

ashamed or think they have done something wrong. If necessary, contact child welfare to seek advice.

General principles in this sort of communication:
- Show interest, receptivity and neutrality
- Invite conversation based on how the child responds
- Ask the child what has happened in a caring manner
- Use the child's own words, be curious and exploratory with your questions
- Use open questions (not leading)
- It is not your role to ask a lot of details (Child Welfare or the Police are the ones who investigate). It is sufficient to uncover concerns about maltreatment – you do not have to be certain it has occurred.
- Reflect back what the child says and allow them time to speak. Use "hmm...", "yes", "do you want to tell me more" to support the child in answering the questions
- Be attentive and ensure you have enough time to avoid rushing the child to answer
- Facilitate confidentiality and trust
- Never promise the child that what he/she tells you can be a secret between the two of you

- You might consider creating an informal security agreement or contract with the child: an agreed follow-up plan for further action and safeguarding. Remember, the child chose you to confide in because they consider you are a trusted person.
- Always remember that it is the child/young person who reveals, not the professional

---

Tips

Questions inviting to report violence:
- "I have noticed that you have some bruises on your left arm and neck. What happened? How did you get the bruises?"
- When someone has such injuries that you have, it is a possibility they have experienced something they find difficult to speak of, but also difficult to carry as a secret. Do you recognize yourself in some of this?
  - What is the most dangerous thing that can happen if you talk about it?
  - What is the most dangerous thing that can happen if you do not talk about it?

■ **Reaching a Decision**

Having taken a history, examined the child, observed the interaction between the child and their parent or carer and, when appropriate, talked to the child themselves, it is time to decide what to do next. If you conclude that you still have concerns about the child's welfare, you will need to take further action and share information with other professionals. You will also need to remember your responsibility to ensure that the child receives the dental treatment they need, especially in cases of dental neglect.

10.1.6 How To Proceed When Worried that a Child Is Exposed to Maltreatment

■ **Working with Child Welfare Services (CWS)**

Given the high prevalence of untreated dental caries and injuries to the head and neck in maltreated children, dental professionals should always be vigilant [17–19]. Once concerns have been identified, communication and collaboration with child welfare services (CWS) are essential for safeguarding children. When the CWS investigates suspicion of child maltreatment, they have to collect as many pieces of the "jigsaw puzzle" as possible from the different professionals involved with the child in order to build a more complete picture of what is going on in the child's life (■ Fig.10.2). The perspec-

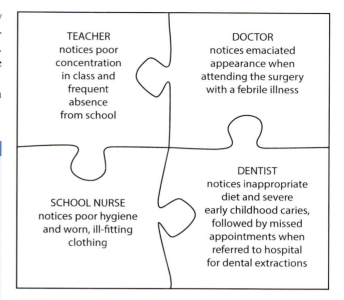

■ **Fig. 10.2** When information from different sources is shared, a more complete picture of concern emerges. (Figure reproduced from Harris J & Welbury R in Welbury, Duggal & Hosey (Eds), *Paediatric dentistry, 2018* with permission of Oxford University Press through PLSclear)

tive of healthcare personnel who meet children both in preventive healthcare situations and when receiving treatment for disease or accident makes an important contribution to the CWS investigation.

The precise arrangements for communicating concerns to CWS will vary between countries. You should have local protocols and contact details readily available, prepared in advance and kept up-to-date. You must follow legislation on information sharing, which usually allows you to discuss your concerns with CWS in the best interest of the child. You should make clear what is fact and what is opinion. You can also document any strengths you have observed while working with the family. It is good practice to follow up a telephone discussion with communication in writing within 48 hours. Normally, it is advised to inform parents or carers of your concerns and your intention to share information, but in some circumstances that is inadvisable, for example, when that might put the child at greater risk or when parents or carers are being violent or abusive. Generally, being open and honest from the start results in better outcomes for children.

Many countries in Europe have mandatory reporting legislation for suspected child maltreatment to the CWS. In cases where there is suspicion of a criminal act, one should additionally make a report to the police. Several countries require the CWS to provide feedback to health personnel after receiving a referral regarding suspicion of child maltreatment. Unfortunately, professional uncertainty and lack of national guidelines have

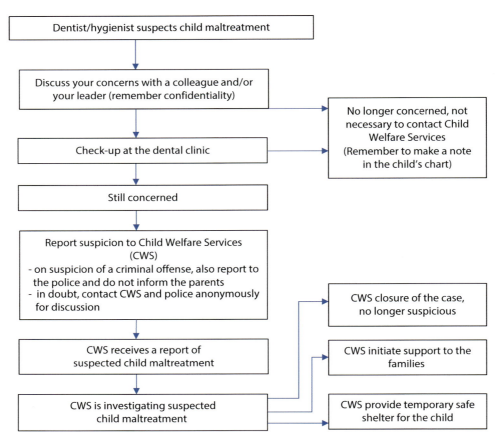

Fig. 10.3 Flow chart illustrating the process from suspicion of child maltreatment to possible action

been identified as a barrier to safeguarding children in an adequate manner [23]. Regular training and clear policies and procedures help reduce uncertainty among health professionals and strengthen clinicians in their daily practice. ◘ Figure 10.3 illustrates the process from suspicion to possible action. In all steps, be aware of the importance of writing thorough notes in the child's chart. A case may be closed due to lack of evidence. If there is still suspicion or suspicion arises years later, the child's chart will be of great importance.

> **Box**
>
> **The Barnahus Model (Which Literally Means "Children's House" or "Child Advocacy Center")**
>
> Barnahus originates in the Child Advocacy Model adopted in the US in the 1980s. It was firstly implemented in 1998 by Iceland followed by other Nordic countries (Sweden in 2005, Norway in 2007, Greenland in 2011, Denmark in 2013) under the name "Barnahus" or "Children's House" (► https://www.barnahus.eu/en/about-barnahus/). In the US, centres are run privately, but in Iceland and in Scandinavia, they are implemented as part of the public legal,
> health and social systems. In 2020, Scotland announced its intention to open a similar Child's House for Healing.
>
> The main purpose is to provide a child-friendly justice approach. At the Barnahus, children are medically examined and forensic interviews are conducted in child-friendly surroundings, rather than in a police station or courtroom. Designed to look like a family home, the atmosphere is welcoming and supportive.
>
> At "Barnahus", children from 3 to 18 years or mentally impaired adults can be referred after having witnessed or been the victim of violence, sexual abuse, suspicion of violence associated with genital mutilation, forced marriage or honour-related violence. The idea is that the individual meets all the various interdisciplinary professionals in one place at the Children's House. Interviews are undertaken by qualified police personnel, specially trained in interviewing children and judges sitting in separate rooms observe interviews in real time via a video link. Defense attorneys, legal-aid attorneys, appointed guardians as well as police attorneys and investigators may also be present. Experienced paediatric doctors

and nurses along with specially-trained dentists conduct medical examinations at the Children's Houses. Clinical forensic oral examination at Children's Houses is a new professional procedure for dentist's examination of teeth, oral cavity, head and neck. A Norwegian study concluded that cross-professional interaction in the Children's Houses is an important factor in successfully safeguarding the child or young person. As the various professions work together, sharing knowledge, it provides better insight and understanding of the child's circumstances, enabling effective planning to keep them safe and support their recovery [24].

10.2 Traumatized Children Grow Up to Be Adults

Individuals who have experienced maltreatment in childhood have a higher risk in adult life of being victims of violence, being sex offenders themselves, having high-risk sexual behaviour and having problems with drug abuse as adults [25]. In a dental context, sexual abuse may be associated with poor oral health and dental fear and anxiety [26].

In a life span perspective, maltreatment during childhood causes increased economic costs related to medical expenses, legal costs and lost productivity. This substantial economic burden is amounted by the WHO and Fang et al. to approximately 124 billion annually, approximately 1% of the national GDP in the USA [27]. This lifetime costs are greater than both stroke and type 2 diabetes [27].

10.3 Domestic Violence – Adults

Domestic violence includes the term intimate partner violence and is defined by the UN as:

> A pattern of behaviour in any relationship that is used to gain or maintain power and control over an intimate partner.

This kind of violence can occur among heterosexual or same-sex couples and does not require sexual intimacy [28]. Domestic violence may also occur in all other domestic relationships like between siblings, between adult children and their elderly parents, or between caregivers and persons with mental illness or physical or cognitive disabilities. In this chapter, we focus mainly upon partner violence, but it is important to bear in mind that all kinds of violence may occur in other domestic relationships as well.

A growing body of empirical research has demonstrated that domestic violence and intimate partner violence involves different categories of violence that can be differentiated with respect to partner dynamics, context and consequences.

The phenomenon is a serious health problem in all parts of the world and occurs in all cultures and within all socioeconomic levels.

WHO reports that "Worldwide, almost one third (27%) of women aged 15-49 years who have been in a relationship report that they have been subjected to some form of physical and/or sexual violence by their intimate partner".

In the National Intimate Partner and Sexual Violence Survey in USA, 16,507 adults (9.086 women and 7.421 men) were interviewed in 2010. More than 1 in 3 women (35.6%) and 1 in 4 men (28.5%) reported to have experienced rape, physical violence, and/or stalking by an intimate partner in their lifetime [29].

In 2020, the number of murdered people in Norway was 31, and 42% of them the victim and the perpetrator had a close relationship [30].

Knowledge about normal reactions and the dynamics of a violent relation is important for health professionals to understand the patient and to provide sufficient help.

10.3.1 Categories of Intimate Partner Violence

When the general public thinks about domestic violence, it is likely they think in terms of physical assault that results in visible injuries to the victim. This is only one type of abuse among several categories of abusive behaviours. Lethality involved with physical abuse may place the victim at higher risk, but the long-term damages of the person that accompanies the other forms of abuse is significant and important to be aware of. Often one person is victim of several types of violence.

The literature reveals somewhat different categories and overlapping definitions across countries and institutions. The categories used here are mainly based on those described by the UN [28].

10.3.2 The Dynamics of Domestic Violence

In some relationships, the violence is episodic, for instance, when there is a conflict between the couple (Situational Couple Violence). Even if violent episodes rarely occur, the abuse may still influence the relation-

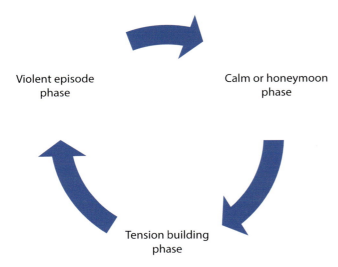

■ **Fig. 10.4**   Cycle of Violence

ship to a large extent. If the power is unbalanced, the victim of abuse remembers the episodes and possibly adjusts his/her behaviour to prevent another episode of violence (latent violence). In other relationships, the violence creates an imbalance of power and control and permeates the everyday life. The abusive partner uses intimidating, strong social control, hurtful words and behaviours to control his or her partner.

Once a serious episode of violence has occurred and entered the relationship or family, this has a great traumatic potential and creates systems. The risk of new violence can control everything the victim does. Having experienced violence means that you know it can happen again. Violence is then present all the time by virtue of its possibility. In such cases, the family has entered a system of violence. The onset of violence in the family changes the family system and creates a system in which interaction and communication are organized in relation to the violence and the possibility of new violence. Latent violence can affect both adults and children in a family.

Walker was, in 1979, the first to describe the dynamics in violent relationships in three distinct phases called the cycle of violence, see ■ Fig. 10.4 [31].

1. Tension building phase (latent violence)
   The tension between the couple is building up. The risk of another violent action controls the victim. The abusive partner may feel tense, irritable, frustrated, disgusted, self-righteous, jealous and act verbally abusive, fits of anger or be complete silent, acting controlling, arrogant, possessive and/or demanding. The victim may feel angry, unfairly treated, hopeless, tense, afraid, humiliated, disgusted, and/or depressed while being nurturing, submissive, "walking on eggshells" and afraid to express their own feelings and at the same time watchful of the

atmosphere, focused on avoiding behaviour or situations that may provoke another violent incident.
2. Violent episode phase
   The tension escalates and reaches a level that leads to an incident of violence. The violent partner may feel angry, enraged, "right", jealous, frustrated and be dangerously violent with a deliberate desire to hurt or kill his/her partner. The victim may feel frightened, trapped, helpless or numb and may try to protect him-/herself, hit back, submit helplessly, escape and seek help.
3. Calm or honeymoon phase
   The violence ends and tension drops. The abusive partner may feel remorseful, apologetic, promise to change, yet forgetful of the degree of violence, or rather self-righteous and unable to understand why the partner is still angry or afraid. The victim may feel angry but relieved, guilty, offer excuses for the batterer, be hopeful the violent episode was the last one and in denial of the seriousness of the incident.

Victims of domestic violence often remain in the abusive relationship for a variety of underlying reasons such as the victim's learned co-dependency, the escalated risk of violence if the victim leaves the batterer, feelings of guilt, insecurity and concern for the children's well-being. Therefore, it often takes many attempts to end the relationship for good. Without an intervention, the frequency and severity of the abuse tends to increase over time.

► **Case Example**

Susan and Frank have five children together ranging from early primary to high school age. They met in a social setting and began dating. Susan noticed that Frank could get angry and frustrated easily. When Susan was pregnant with their first child, the abuse started as name-calling. Frank would call her "fat and ugly" and a "loser" if he felt he was not getting his own way. Initially, Susan would fire back her disapproval, but over time, she became so diminished by the abuse that she said and did nothing, which would enrage Frank even more.

They had a joint bank account that Susan's salary was paid into. If she did not pay the bills immediately, Frank would clear out the account.

As time went by, Frank's abuse became physical. He frequently spat on Susan, pulled her hair, dragged her through the house, smashed her head into the wall and threw drinks over her. There were many such occasions in front of the children. During another pregnancy, Frank strangled Susan because she had discovered he had been cheating on her. She managed to kick him away from her but miscarried afterwards.

Susan put up with the abuse in the interests of preserving the family as Frank had threatened to get a court order to take the children if they separated. Frank had convinced Susan that she was the cause of his behaviour and the court would see it that way too. Frank's behaviour went through cycles of being friendly and engaged followed by angry and violent. He claimed he had depression. Frank tried to isolate Susan from her family and friends. Despite her family and friends' extreme concerns of her wellbeing, Susan would not listen to their criticism of Frank.

When Susan felt Frank's violence and abuse had become extreme, on her sister's advice, she sought a protection order. The domestic violence support service at the court helped her prepare the application. Susan obtained a temporary protection order, but after pressure from Frank, she failed to appear at the final hearing, and the application was dismissed.

Frank told Susan he loved her, wanted a happy family life and wanted them to try again to make the relationship work. She found Frank charming when he was in this mood and agreed to get back together. However, the physical and emotional violence started again immediately, as well as socially isolating Susan from her family and friends and controlling the family finances. One day, Susan's sister rang her and could hear Frank's verbal abuse in the background. She was so horrified that she called the police and asked them to check on the house. When the police arrived, Frank ranted at them blaming Susan before he left the house. The police explained that his behaviour was domestic violence and suggested to Susan that she get a protection order. Susan was so emotionally exhausted that she had to take time off work to get some help while she continued caring for the children. Susan believes the protection order probably saved her life. But, Frank breached the protection order by turning up at the children's school and sending abusive emails. Susan was able to access counselling and began learning about the cycle of violence she had endured for nearly 15 years. She realized that Frank had manipulated her thoughts and her sense of self, and she had to retrain how to think and rebuild herself as a person. Susan is beginning to feel stronger and more equipped to face the future now that she is receiving counselling support. ◄

It might take hours, days, or sometimes many months to complete the circle of violence depending on the specific couple's history. Where in the circle (◘ Fig. 10.4), a patient like Susan is on the very day of her dental consultation, may be decisive for whether she can make use of advice and help offered by the dentist.

For example, it is conceivable that Susan seeks dental help after an episode of violence (for instance, due to a dental injury). It will be important that the dentist suspects violence, asks open-ended questions related to the dental trauma and offers further consultations over a period of time. Then the dentist will be in a position to build a safe and trustful alliance. By explaining the circle of violence, the patient might recognize the pattern in her relationship and hopefully be, at a given time, capable to receive help in breaking the circle.

Another type of violence which needs attention, related to the "case about Susan", is financial or economic violence (◘ Table 10.2).

10.3.3 How to Explore Signs of Domestic Violence?

The most typical feature of violence is that it is a secret and made invisible by the perpetrator and the victim(s). The first and perhaps the biggest challenge is, therefore, making the violence visible to be able to stop it and take care of the victims when the violence comes to the surface. This is something that requires courage, a willingness to act, a high level of competence and good knowledge of the aid available for families in crisis.

While health professionals can act on the child's behalf in their best interests, adults are responsible and free to make their own decisions. Even so, it is important to talk about the issue if you suspect that a patient is being abused. To have a conversation about challenging topics like domestic violence, trust from the patient is crucial. Questions to ask might be:

- "How is it at home" or "Is everything fine at home?"
- "Sometimes when I see a broken tooth, a wound or a hematoma like this one, it might mean that someone has injured that person. Is it possible that someone has injured you?"
- "These marks make me think someone has injured you. What is it like for you at home these days? Is there anything you would like to talk about?"

How to proceed when someone answers "yes"?

It is important to state that violence is wrong by expressing sympathetic confirmatory statements that places the responsibility on the abuser and lifts the victim's dignity. These kinds of statements may be one of several interventions valuable to the victim's process.

Examples of confirmatory statements:

- "Everyone has the right to feel safe at home, I am worried about your health and safety".
- "As your dentist, I have to ask when I see signs that is associated with abuse. Unfortunately, many people are victims of abuse, but no one deserved living under such conditions".

The dental staff should have an overview of local services of help to inform and guide the patient to relevant

□ Table 10.2 Definition and Descriptions of Different Categories of Violence

Category of violence	Definitions	Examples of actions from the abuser:
Physical	Psychological violence is hurting or trying to hurt a family member through pain, injury, intimidation and abuse or to force another human being to stop doing something he/she wants or to do something against his/her will.	Pushes, slaps, bites, kicks or chokes Abandons someone in a dangerous or unfamiliar place Scares by driving recklessly Uses a weapon to threaten or hurt Forces to leave home Traps in home or keeps from leaving Prevents from calling police or seeking medical attention Uses physical force in sexual situations Damages property when angry (throws objects, punches walls, kicks doors, etc.)
Psychological	Psychological (emotional) violence is always harming, intimidating or insulting that are not directly physical in nature or ways of controlling or dominating others using an underlying power or threat	Threatens to hurt persons or pets Coercive control Insults or continually criticizes Calls names Does not trust and acts in a jealous or possessive manner Tries to isolate from family or friends Monitors where to go, whom to call and with whom to spend time Punishes by withholding affection
Financial or economical	Financial or economic violence is to prevent a person from having control of their own finances	Controls finance or refuses to share money Making or attempting to make a person financially dependent Forbids attendance at school or employment
Sexual	Sexual abuse includes all actions aimed at another person's sexuality, which, through pain, injury, intimidation or abuse, causes that person to do something against their will or stop doing something they want	Force or manipulate into having sex or performing sexual acts Sexual activities without consent (for instance when drunk or sleeping)Accuses of cheating Demands someone to dress in a sexual way Demands sex when you are sick, tired or after beating someone Ignores someone's feelings regarding sex
Stalking	Stalking may be defined as violence when it involves pattern of behaviour that serves no legitimate purpose and is intended to harass, annoy or terrorise the victim.	Repeated telephone calls Unwelcome letters or gifts Surveillance at work or other places

services (▶ https://dinutvei.no/) [32]. Such information must be easily accessible for the patients.

■ **Documentation**

Documentation of injuries, treatment and information of the patient's legal rights is important. It may be difficult to accept the patient's choice to stay in the relationship and not follow your advice. Here are some questions relevant to ask:

- I would like to help you, but of course you know what is best for you. Either way I would advise you to think through your options.

- What is the worst that might happen if you seek help?
- What is the worst that might happen if you do not seek help?
- You may contact me again if you change your mind and like me to help you.

If the patient would like help, refer the patient to the police, Support Centre or the local Crises Shelter and offer a follow-up appointment.

When violence/abuse happens repeatedly, it is likely it will happen again. Health workers are obliged to avert new incidences of violence even if the patient refuses offered help.

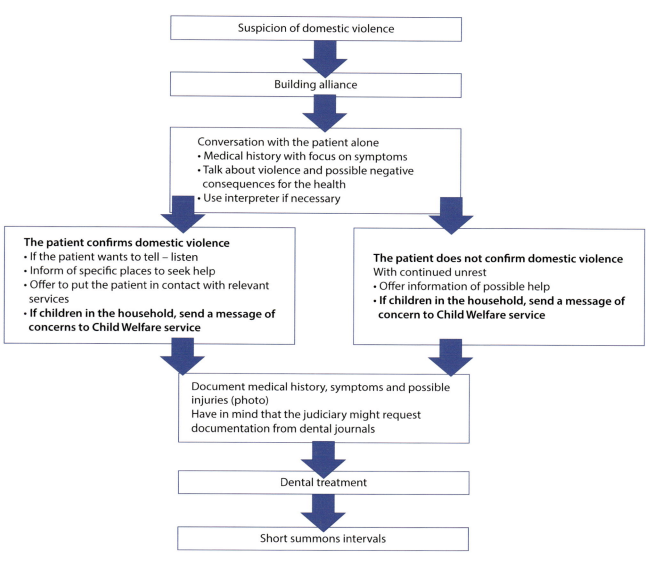

Box
Advises for Concerned Staff from the UN [28]
How you can help victims of domestic abuse?

— Listen and believe the abused person to let them know they are not alone.
— Encourage her/him to seek support through a confidential hotline to connect with a professional in the field.
— Express concern for him/her, show support, and offer referrals to available resources.
— If you have not been directly approached but have reason to believe that a colleague may be in an abusive relationship, consult with your Organization's Counselling or Ombudsman's Office >

Note: Keep in mind that a survivor often makes several attempts to leave the abusive relationship before succeeding.

10.3.4 When a Dawning Concern Becomes a Severe Worry – What to Do?

As illustrated in the flow chart in ■ Fig. 10.5, professional communication and building a good alliance with all patients is important, in particular, people exposed to domestic violence. It is important to be able to help beyond their oral health. If you have a patient in dental practice and suspect that the person is exposed to violence, it is important to document your findings. For example, medical history and possible injuries or statements that may indicate that the patient is exposed to violence. It is not always the patient will tell or confirm a possible act of violence.

Tips

Establish a dialogue and describe examples in third person form about violence and of the consequences that follows.

"I see you have an injury that reminds me of a patient of mine with a similar injury. She had been abused. I would like to help you if you have been exposed to something that is difficult for you to talk about. It is routine here to inform every patient with that kind of injuries of help services available".

> If you suspect domestic violence in a family with children, it is an obligation to contact and report your suspicion to the child welfare system, even if you have not examined the children.

It is important to adopt a listening position and not moralise. In addition, in those cases where the patient confirms being abused and declines receiving any help, it is important to exercise empathy and understanding, but at the same time encourage to proceed with the case.

When there are signs of possible abuse, more frequent follow-up consultations are justified with the purpose of building trust and for the patient to change his/her mind concerning reporting to the police and contact support services. Objective descriptions and clinical photos of possible injuries are important to be documented in the patient's journal. Such evidence is crucial in case of a lawsuit and for future dental visits. If there are new injuries in the future, the record possibly documents repetitive incidences of domestic violence.

Summary

Dental professionals have an important role in addressing child maltreatment (child abuse and neglect). Childhood is a crucial time in an individual's development. Adverse childhood experiences (ACEs) have negative impacts on child development and, furthermore, may cause irreversible and, sometimes, lifelong damage.

This chapter highlights the importance of responding when suspicion of child maltreatment occurs with focus on how to recognise, current legislation and how to fulfil our obligations as healthcare providers to the United Nations Convention of the Rights of the Child.

Further, traumatized children grow up to be adults with burdens from childhood. Individuals who have experienced different types of maltreatment in childhood have a higher risk of being victims of violence, being sex offenders themselves, having high-risk sexual behaviour and having problems with drug abuse as adults.

To explore signs of domestic violence requires courage and willingness to act and a high level of competence. The categories used in this chapter are mainly based on those described by the United Nations. The most typical feature of violence is that it is a secret and made invisible by the perpetrator and the victim(s). The first and perhaps the biggest challenge is, therefore, making the violence visible to be able to stop and take care of the victims when the violence comes to the surface.

If you suspect domestic violence in a family with children, it is an obligation to contact and report your suspicion to the child welfare system, even if you have not examined the children. Remember that without an intervention, the frequency and severity of the abuse tends to increase over time.

References

1. Felitti VJ, Anda RF, Nordenberg D, Williamson DF, Spitz AM, Edwards V, et al. Relationship of childhood abuse and household dysfunction to many of the leading causes of death in adults. The Adverse Childhood Experiences (ACE) Study. Am J Prev Med. 1998;14(4):245–58.
2. Bellis MA, Hughes K, Leckenby N, Jones L, Baban A, Kachaeva M, et al. Adverse childhood experiences and associations with health-harming behaviours in young adults: surveys in eight eastern European countries. Bull World Health Organ. 2014;92(9):641–55.
3. Anda RF, Felitti VJ, Bremner JD, Walker JD, Whitfield C, Perry BD, et al. The enduring effects of abuse and related adverse experiences in childhood. A convergence of evidence from neurobiology and epidemiology. Eur Arch Psychiatry Clin Neurosci. 2006;256(3):174–86.
4. UN convention on the rights of the child [Internet]. United nations human rights office of the high commissioner. 2016 [cited 04.03.2019]. Available from: http://www.ohchr.org/en/professionalinterest/pages/crc.aspx
5. Unicef. How we protect children's rights with the UN convention on the rights of the child unicef.: Unicef; 2019 [cited 2019 21.07.2019]. Available from: https://www.unicef.org.uk/what-we-do/un-convention-child-rights/
6. Gilbert R, Widom CS, Browne K, Fergusson D, Webb E, Janson S. Burden and consequences of child maltreatment in high-income countries. Lancet. 2009;373(9657):68–81.
7. Leeb RT, Melanson C, Simon T, Arias I. Child maltreatment surveillance: uniform definitions for public health and recommended data elements, version 1.0. . In: Atlanta (GA): Centers for Disease Control and Prevention NCfIPaC, editor. https://www.cdc.gov/violenceprevention/pdf/CM_Surveillance-a.pdf:

National Center for Injury Prevention and Control (NCIPC), part of Centers for Disease Control and Prevention (CDC); 2008. p. 148.

8. Chan YC, Yeung JWK. Children living with violence within the family and its sequel: a meta-analysis from 1995 to 2006. Aggress Violent Behav. 2009;14(5):313–22.

9. Vu NL, Jouriles EN, McDonald R, Rosenfield D. Children's exposure to intimate partner violence: A meta-analysis of longitudinal associations with child adjustment problems. Clin Psychol Rev. 2016;46:25–33.

10. Wolfe DA CC, Lee V, McIntyre-Smith A, Jaffe PG. The effects of children's exposure to domestic violence: a meta-analysis and critique. Clin Child Fam Psychol Rev. 2003;6:171–87.

11. Harris JC. The mouth and maltreatment: safeguarding issues in child dental health. Arch Dis Child. 2018;103(8):722–9.

12. Harris J, Whittington A. Dental neglect in children. Paediatrics Child Health. 2016;26(11):478–84.

13. Harris JC, Balmer RC, Sidebotham PD. British Society of Paediatric Dentistry: a policy document on dental neglect in children. Int J Paediatr Dent. 2009; https://doi.org/10.1111/j.1365-263X.2009.00996.x.

14. Harris J, Sidebotham P, Welbury R, Townsend R, Green M, Goodwin J, Franklin C. Child protection and the dental team: an introduction to safeguarding children in dental practice. Sheffield: COPDEND; 2006. [updated online 2013:[Available from: https://bda.org/childprotection. Accessed Feb 2021.

15. Bhatia SK, Maguire SA, Chadwick BL, Hunter ML, Harris JC, Tempest V, et al. Characteristics of child dental neglect: a systematic review. J Dent. 2014;42(3):229–39.

16. Kojan BH, Lonne B. A comparison of systems and outcomes for safeguarding children in Australia and Norway. Child Family Social Work. 2012;17(1):96–107.

17. da Fonseca MA, Feigal RJ, ten Bensel RW. Dental aspects of 1248 cases of child maltreatment on file at a major county hospital. Pediatr Dent. 1992;14(3):152–7.

18. Cairns AM, Mok JY, Welbury RR. Injuries to the head, face, mouth and neck in physically abused children in a community setting. Int J Paediatr Dent. 2005;15(5):310–8.

19. Valente LA, Dalledone M, Pizzatto E, Zaiter W, de Souza JF, Losso EM. Domestic violence against children and adolescents: prevalence of physical injuries in a southern Brazilian metropolis. Braz Dent J. 2015;26(1):55–60.

20. Bright MA, Alford SM, Hinojosa MS, Knapp C, Fernandez-Baca DE. Adverse childhood experiences and dental health in children and adolescents. Community Dent Oral Epidemiol. 2015;43(3):193–9.

21. Kvist TWT, Rønneberg A. Våld i nära relationer- tandvårdens roll. Aktuel Nordisk Odontologi 2017: Universitetsforlagetno. 2018:114–25.

22. Kvist T, Annerback EM, Dahllof G. Oral health in children investigated by Social services on suspicion of child abuse and neglect. Child Abuse Negl. 2018;76:515–23.

23. Rønneberg A, Nordgarden H, Skaare AB, Willumsen T. Barriers and factors influencing communication between dental professionals and Child Welfare Services in their everyday work. Int J Paediatr Dent. 2019;29(6):684–91.

24. Rønneberg A, Bie TMG, Willumsen T, Köpp UMS. Clinical forensic oral examination at «Statens Barnahus» – ways of cross-professional interaction in the best interest of the child. Nor Tannlegeforen Tid. 2019;129:884–92.

25. Søftestad S, Kranstad V, Fredriksen TV, Willumsen T. Invading Deeply into Self and Everyday Life: How Oral Health-Related Problems Affect the Lives of Child Sexual Abuse Survivors. J Child Sex Abus. 2020;29(1):62–78.

26. Willumsen T. The impact of childhood sexual abuse on dental fear. Community Dent Oral Epidemiol. 2004;32(1):73–9.

27. Fang X, Brown DS, Florence CS, Mercy JA. The economic burden of child maltreatment in the United States and implications for prevention. Child Abuse Negl. 2012;36(2):156–65.

28. United Nations. COVID-19 response what is domestic abuse? United Nations; 2021. [cited June 2021]. Available from: https://www.un.org/en/coronavirus/what-is-domestic-abuse

29. Breiding MJ. Black Intimate partner violence in the United States – 2010. Atlanta: National Center for Injury Prevention and Control of the Centers for Disease Control and Prevention DoVP; 2014.

30. NCIS. NASJONAL DRAPSOVERSIKT 2020 Drap i Norge 2011–2020/national homicide overview 2020. Norway: National Criminal Investigation Service (NCIS); 2020.

31. Walker LE. The battered woman. University of Michigan: Harper & Row; 1979.

32. NKVTS. National guidelinde – violence/nasjonal veiviser mot vold og overgrep 2016. Available from: https://dinutvei.no/

Part II

Voice of Children

The Change Factory (Forandringsfabrikken) is a nonprofit Norwegian foundation [1]. It is financed through government funding, scholarships, and donations from foundations and nonprofit organizations.

Their philosophy is built on a simple idea: Listening to what (young) people in welfare systems think about what is good help, and what should change for the help to feel good and actually help.

The Change Factory aims to get young people to identify system-changing ideas, build consensus around them, and open direct communication between service users and implementing agencies to create real change.

Youth, members of the Change Factory, have discussed oral health related issues to provide advice to all workers in dental heath services.

> **Box**
> The Change Factory youth' advice to dental professionals:
> — Tell me your name, use your first name, and tell me a bit about yourself before you put on a face mask.
> — Have friendly rooms for waiting and treatment.
> — Give me enough time for me to feel safe and not troublesome.
> — Talk to me alone.
> — Give *me* information I can understand.
> — Teach me how to take care of my teeth.
> — Ask me how I feel – and cope with my answer.
> — Be honest, but say it in a nice way.
> — Care about me — not just my teeth.
> — If you need to refer to child welfare, please first to try to do it in cooperation with me.
> — Make sure I feel safe enough to get back to you.

Reference

1. Forandringsfabrikken. About us (English) (Cited 2021 May 20). Available from
► https://www.forandringsfabrikken.no/article/about-us-english

Dental Anxiety

Contents

Understanding Development and Persistence of Dental Anxiety

Tiril Willumsen, Maren L. Agdal, and Margrethe Elin Vika

Contents

Learning Goals

- To understand dental anxiety from an evolutionary biopsychosocial perspective
- To have knowledge of the continuum from mild to severe dental anxiety
- To have knowledge about the etiology and prevalence of dental anxiety
- To understand how dental anxiety may develop and persist
- To implement knowledge of safety-seeking strategies

11.1 Introduction

The terms "dental fear" and "dental anxiety" are used interchangeably in the literature; however, in this book, "dental anxiety" (DA) is used. DA is relatively common in both children and adults. It is useful to categorize DA into none, mild, moderate, and severe. However, the term "DA," in this chapter, refers to moderate and severe anxiety.

The prevalence of DA varies in different studies, which may be due to differences in measurement modalities, samples, and research methods. In a sample of 10,900 UK adult citizens, 51% were classified with low DA, 36% with medium DA, and 12% with severe DA [1]. In a Swedish study carried out in 2013 with 3500 adult citizens, 90% had mild/no DA, 5% had moderate DA, and 5% had severe DA. Interestingly, it was also found that DA was significantly reduced from the first measurement in 1963 to 2013 [2]. In a Finnish study, it was found that severe anxiety decreased during a 10-year period for persons >34 years of age [3]. The prevalence of dental anxiety in children and adolescents varies substantially in different countries and among different age groups. Klingberg and Broberg found in a review study from 2007 that the prevalence of DA varied from 5.7% to 6.7% in children with a proxy reported level of DA, whereas the prevalence was higher (19.5% with one study included) when the child was the informant [4].

In general, anxiety disorders are more frequently reported in women compared to men, and this is also found in DA. Furthermore, the highest prevalence is between 30 and 50 years of age [5], which shows that it is important to address and treat mild-to-moderate DA in children, adolescents, and young adults.

The core nature of anxiety is a strong urge to avoid (cognitive and/or behavioral) trigger(s). For patients with DA, there are a variety of triggers in the dental office. Patients with severe DA seeking treatment in a dental anxiety clinic reported an average of 11.2 years of avoidance [6]. On the contrary, 73% (72.9%) with severe DA in a Swedish study reported regular dental visits. Avoidance behavior related to DA is a great concern for patients and for dental professionals. A vast amount of research documents that avoidance behavior related to DA has considerable negative side effects on both oral health and psychosocial well-being. Studies report that persons with severe DA have more dental caries, fewer sound teeth, and poorer oral health-related quality of life [5, 7].

Awareness should be created regarding the risk of developing avoidance behavior. Consequently, DA should have high priority as a public health concern [8].

11.2 Dental Anxiety from an Evolutionary Biological Perspective

Why are people afraid of sitting in a dentist's chair when they are not afraid of driving a car, which poses a much greater risk to our safety and survival?

This question may be explained by the fact that the dental situation, unlike driving a car, may trigger feelings of helplessness and pain, which are feelings that have been important to avoid to ensure survival. Furthermore, negative emotions connected with danger are easily learned [9, 10] and have been transferred from generation to generation. It can be seen from our evolutionary history that we have evolved into a species (humans) with excellent traits for both detecting danger and interpreting dangers with immediate relevant survival reactions. However, having the trait of "better safe than sorry" encoded in our genes may have contributed to an increased predisposition toward fear and phobia – even in situations that no longer present a danger to us. Thus, to understand dental fear and anxiety, it is important to accept that dental treatment that includes lying back, having another person in your intimate zone, and being at risk for painful experiences may instinctively and subconsciously be interpreted as dangerous. Fear reactions are natural reactions that help defend ourselves from harm and death. Providing patients with information about the body's natural reaction to danger is an effective tool in the treatment of DA and is named psychoeducation (read more in ► Chap. 12).

11.2.1 The Body's Natural Reaction to Danger

Avoidance of danger is the best way to survive. Consequently, we avoid dangerous situations, whether it is jumping into deep water when we know that we cannot swim, climbing ladders when we are afraid of heights, or seeking out situations where we have previously experienced pain.

However, in case one faces danger, there are two natural reactions that increase the potential action in the situation:

» "Fight" or "flight" is the most common response that occurs when you are close to or in a dangerous situation. You seek immediate safety by running away or hiding from the threat or you are instantly ready for a fight. This implies an activation of the autonomic nervous system. Activation of the sympathetic nervous system causes a rapid increase in cardiovascular activity where heart rate, blood pressure, and respiration increase to supply oxygen to the large muscle groups that can carry us to safety or address the danger (fight-or-flight reaction). At the same time, the parasympathetic nervous system is deactivated causing blood supply to the fingers and toes, skin, and the digestive system, and parts of the central nervous system have decreased activation, all for the purpose of directing focus and effort to escape from the danger or to fight for life if necessary.

However, not all experience an urge to run or fight. Other reactions may instinctively be used to reduce the risk of harm in the situation.

— *Freeze* may be described as a fight-or-flight reaction on hold. You prepare to protect yourself. Despite rapid physiological activation, you stay completely still to get ready for the next move. Some individuals will experience only seconds when they are scared stiff "when a sudden danger occurs," whereas some will be so for a longer time. Biologically, this may be a rational reaction, to hide, stand completely still, and hope for the dangerous animal (or human) not to detect you, but, at the same time, the autonomic nervous system is activated so that you can immediately and quickly run if detected.

— *Fawn* (used synonymously with please, flop, or submission) occurs when a person is activated, but the situation is unavoidable. The body's activation decreases and, in a way, hibernates. The term "fawn" has evolved from when deer hide their newborn fawns in tall grass so as not to be detected by predators (unfortunately, farmers do not detect the hidden fawns either when they drive their shackles on the fields). Fawns can also confuse the predator, making it believe that the animal is dead, and, for some, the hunting instinct will cease. Moreover, fawn may be the biological equivalent of mercy to those who are eaten alive by a predator; the body shut downs to avoid pain when caught and eaten.

In addition to intense and unpleasant bodily arousal, anxiety involves negative thoughts concerning the object or situation. These negative thoughts may be about the danger involved. A person who is highly anxious of spiders may often have thoughts like "The spider will run up to me and hide in my ear and I would not get it out." For an anxious person, negative thoughts usually do not just stop with the spider hiding in the ear. The thoughts will often focus on the negative feelings and unpleasant arousal the spider in the ear would evoke. "Can my body tolerate the stress of having a spider in my ear?" or "I would literally die of heart attack if the spider ran up to me and hid in my ear!" In the dental situation, many patients have negative thoughts involving feelings of intense pain, feelings of not being able to escape from the situation, etc. Moreover, in the dental situation, concrete negative thoughts about the situation are followed by negative thoughts about the possible consequences of what will happen in the dental situation. The negative thoughts involve consequences for the person's well-being like involving shame or extreme bodily reactions.

Anxiety, when the body is activated in response to danger in the near or more distant future, is also a rational reaction from an evolutionary biological perspective. Mild degrees of anxiety may be appropriate to avoid future potentially dangerous situations (for example, avoiding places where people are most likely to be exposed to danger). Anxiety can also be a source of motivation to plan how to face dangers that may occur (for example, to bring a gun on excursions to Svalbard in case of being attacked by a polar bear). The problem with anxiety is that the perceived danger may not be an actual threat, and the threat felt by the anxious person is often not obvious to others. In addition, anxiety is often followed by exhausting rumination concerning potential danger or exaggerated threat in upcoming situations.

The degree of anxiety varies on a continuum from a mild degree that does not create significant obstacles for the person to a severe degree of anxiety or phobia that will affect the person's way of living. Mild degrees of anxiety are normal and is a natural part of everyday life. It is normal to experience bodily discomfort before a job interview and a mild degree of anxiety before a dental appointment.

11.3 When the Fear Reaction Becomes Dysfunctional

Increased levels of anxiety result in an increment of extremely unpleasant bodily reactions, negative thoughts, and avoidance behaviors. When anxiety for a specific object or situation is so extensive that it significantly affects daily living, it is called a phobia. A phobia is a learned and highly exaggerated anxiety reaction. The triggers are not always obvious and do not cause strong anxiety in others than in the person with the phobia. To simplify, if you are walking in the woods and you suddenly see a benign snake in front of you, you react instinctively and jump away from the snake. Afterward, you feel a bit shaky, but you continue walking in the woods. Your reaction was a natural fear response. If you had a snake phobia, you would have high anxiety while walking in the woods. You would look out for snakes and be uncertain about your safety being in the woods. When confronted with the snake, the phobic person's preparedness for avoiding snakes would rapidly cause an alarm reaction and most possibly turn into a flight reaction. Thus, the sight of the snake would make you extremely uncomfortable, and you would have problems calming down as long as you were in the woods. As a consequence, you focus on the track looking out for snakes and walk as fast as you can out of the woods. Afterward, you would no longer dare to go for a walk in those woods (most likely, in other woods too) or you could attempt it again, despite being strongly affected by severe anxiety, by adopting some safety precautions (e.g., wearing large wellies, staring continuously at the path while walking, etc.).

> **Box**
> A specific phobia is a psychiatric diagnosis described in medical diagnostic systems. In the Diagnostic and Statistical Manual of Mental Disorders (DSM)-5, it is described as [12]:
> - Marked fear or anxiety about a specific object or situation.
> - The phobic object or situation almost always invokes immediate fear or anxiety.
> - The fear or anxiety is out of proportion to the actual danger posed by the specific object or situation and to the sociocultural context.
> - The phobic object or situation is actively avoided or endured with intense fear or anxiety.
> - The fear, anxiety, or avoidance causes clinically significant distress or impairment in the social, occupational, or other important areas of functioning.
> - The fear, anxiety, or avoidance is persistent, typically lasting for 6 months or more.
> - The disturbance is not better explained by the symptoms of another mental disorder, including fear, anxiety, and avoidance of situations associated with panic-like symptoms or other incapacitating symptoms (as in agoraphobia); objects or situations related to obsessions (as in obsessive-compulsive disorder); reminders of traumatic events (as in post-traumatic stress disorder); separation from home or attachment figures (as in separation anxiety disorder); or social situations (as in social anxiety disorder).

When diagnosed according to the DSM-5 or the International Statistical Classification of Diseases and Related Health Problems (ICD)-10 [11] criteria, the specific phobia for dental situations is named dental phobia or odontophobia. If dental phobia is established, the person will try to avoid stimuli that will trigger the anxiety. This phobia usually causes complete avoidance of dental treatment or the person may undergo dental treatment with intense anxiety and/or panic. For some, the avoidance behavior will include every instrument and procedure associated with oral health, dental examination, and/or dental treatment. Even tooth brushing or looking at or thinking about their own teeth may be avoided. Daily living may be affected since all situations that may involve cues of teeth or dentistry potentially trigger anxiety or panic attacks. Watching movies with scenes from the dental office, hearing others talk about going to the dentist, or even reading about DA may be situations that are strictly avoided.

11.4 Biopsychosocial Understanding of Dental Anxiety

The development of DA in a biopsychosocial framework is a method to understand the complexity of the contributing factors. The biopsychosocial model is grounded on the idea that biological inheritance together with personal experience in a social context are compound elements in disease development. The contributing factors within the biological, psychological, and social labels are complex and may have an overlapping contribution to the development of DA.

In a trauma-sensitive approach, it may be claimed that every person has an individual vulnerability (biological), where his/her adverse life experiences (social or environmental) and coping abilities and strategies (psychological strain) are crucial for the development of DA (◘ Fig. 11.1).

11.4.1 Biological Perspective

There is growing awareness of genetic vulnerability to DA. In a 2016 study, it was found that both DA and anxiety about pain were linked to heredity [13].

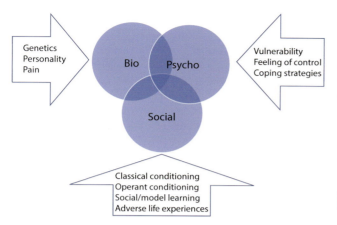

Fig. 11.1 Dental anxiety from a biopsychosocial perspective. The risk of developing anxiety increases by the number and severity of the causative factors. In the interface, the risk is the greatest

Several personality traits have been linked to the development of DA. Temperament in both children and adults, such as being shy, introverted, and impulsive, shows an increased risk [14–17]. Subjects who have a high desire for control and experience loss of control in the dental situation seem to be at a higher risk of developing DA. Neuroticism, a personality trait with a tendency to ruminate over small things and to be easily worried, vulnerability to criticism from others, and being unsure of oneself have also been linked to DA [18].

The teeth are highly innervated. At the time of tooth eruption, all teeth have large pulp chambers and are extra sensitive to pain. Thus, children and young adults are extra exposed to pain during dental treatment. Patients with congenital disorders with compromised mineralization of the teeth like amelogenesis imperfecta (AI) and molar incisor hypomineralisation (MIH) have highly pain-sensitive teeth, which may be difficult to properly anesthetize. Pain-sensitive teeth may elevate the risk of developing DA. The combination of pain-sensitive teeth and DA complicates both dental treatment and daily tooth cleaning [19]. As people grow older, their teeth often become less sensitive. This may be a biological explanation to the fact that the prevalence of DA is lower among individuals over 50 years of age.

Biological factors may be influenced by the environment in which the person lives. There is a large field of research on heritage and environmental factors. Epigenetics highlights that the expression of genes varies according to the influence of the person's environment.

11.4.2   Psychosocial Perspective

All dental patients arrive at the dental clinic with a history of different life experiences. Whereas many are robust and are able to establish a good relationship with the dentist, others are psychologically vulnerable after adverse life experiences and have attachment problem due to psychological traumas. The psychosocial perspective related to the dental situation and the development and treatment of DA is the core of this book and is elaborated in many of the chapters.

In the following, we will cite two examples to expand the perspective of the biopsychosocial understanding of DA:

> **► Example**
> Therese is a 32-year-old woman. She is shy by nature and has difficulties expressing her opinions when meeting authorities. As a child, she had "bad teeth" and she remembers the dentist was "rough" and that he always said "anesthesia is not necessary/or you have had enough anesthesia." Now, she is afraid of pain during drilling and also during injecting anesthetics. Her DA has been present as long as she can remember. She remembers that her mother talked about herself having DA and also talked negatively about dentistry in general. From the moment that Therese could decide for herself, she has only visited the dentist when in pain or for emergency treatments. Now, she has intense dental pain and is in urgent need of dental treatment. ◄

> **► Example**
> Fredrick is a 40-year-old man. He grew up in a home with domestic violence. His parents never taught him to brush his teeth properly, and, as a child, he had a lot of caries and experienced many painful dental treatments. He has always been afraid of going to the dentist. Being highly anxious, he has negative thoughts about the consequences of the anxiety and thinks that the treatment will be extremely painful. In addition, he anticipates that the dental health care provider will make negative comments about his terrible oral health. ◄

With a biopsychosocial understanding, it is obvious that people have different vulnerabilities for developing DA. However, in the end, if the patient experiences negative feelings, and feelings of fear during dental treatment, they may consequently interpret the dental treatment as dangerous, uncontrollable, and unpredictable [20]. This potentiates the risk of developing DA. Thus, dental health care providers must be aware that both direct mechanisms, such as pain, feeling of being less in control, being belittled by negative remarks, etc., and indirect mechanisms, such as personal vulnerability factors, social learning, information and instructions, etc., contribute to the development of DA.

11.5 Development of Dental Anxiety

11.5.1 Classical Conditioning

Classical conditioning, described by Ivan Pavlov in the 1890s [21], means that a biologically potent stimulus (e.g., pain from a needlestick) is paired with a previously neutral stimulus (e.g., a dental office). The pain triggers anxiety reactions. Eventually, the dental office triggers anxiety reactions even without a syringe.

Almost all patients with DA report negative experiences at the dentist [22]. There is strong evidence that pain during dental treatment is the main cause of the development of DA [23–25]. Repeated pain experiences during dentistry is an especially potent factor for the development of DA [26]. Not surprisingly, if the patient experiences a sense of lack of control and pain at the same time, the risk of developing DA increases further [27].

Studies show an association between low socioeconomic status and DA [28]. The reason for this may be that people with a lower socioeconomic status have a higher prevalence of caries [29], which, in turn, involves more dentistry with potential for negative experience classical conditioning.

> ► **Example**
>
> Robin, is a resilient 12-year-old boy. He is a clever pupil at school and has caring parents. He has now got a deep cavity in a molar and is highly motivated for treatment. During treatment, he suddenly feels intense pain and experiences immediate bodily discomfort with violent palpitations and trembling. However, he manages to go through with the dental treatment and afterward feels strong relief. He also wonders about what it would be like if it was even more painful. Could the body endure it? The next time he visits the dentist, the dentist starts polishing the filling. When he feels the vibration on the tooth, the bodily discomfort that he felt during the last treatment is reactivated. Unless the dentist takes Robin's bodily discomfort seriously and adjusts the treatment to help Robin to master the procedure, there is a risk that Robin will develop DA through classical conditioning. ◄

11.5.2 Operant Conditioning

Operant conditioning refers to the consequence that follows a certain behavior. The phenomenon was originally described by B.F. Skinner in the 1950s. Skinner's animal experiments showed how reward and punishment affected learning. Animals learned the association between their behavior and reward/punishment. Rats learned (associated) that when the green light appeared, they received a pellet if they pressed the lever. They also learned that red light predicted a mild electric shock if they pressed the button.

In operant conditioning, we basically have two ways to decrease or increase behaviors. To increase behavior, we can either positively or negatively reinforce the patients' behavior. An example of positive reinforcement is giving the patient a reward like positive vocal feedback, e.g., a high five. Negative reinforcement is when the patient exhibits a behavior that reduces or elicits a negative feeling. The two most common negative reinforcements in dentistry are active avoidance or escape from the situation. When the patient actively avoids the dental situation, the expected negative feelings in the dental situation are avoided. An example of avoidance is when the patient is afraid of the needle and the dentist suggests to postpone it to the next appointment. In contrary reinforcement where the goal is to increase behaviors, punishment is used to reduce unwanted behavior. Punishment is categorized into positive punishment where the dentist adds a behavior to unwanted patient behavior or negative punishment where behaviors/consequences are withdrawn. An example of positive punishment is when the dentist is harsh toward the patient with avoidant behavior, like when the patient turns the back to the dentist while lying in the dental chair. Punishment may also be negative with withdrawal of something the patient likes. In the treatment situation, negative punishment may be silence with lack of positive verbal feedback or denying rewards after treatment like playing computer games, going to the cinema, etc. From an evolutionary perspective, it is better for our survival to avoid something bad rather than to get an easy reward, e.g., avoiding the dental appointment instead of hoping for praise from the dentist for showing up. Avoidant behavior will feel rewarding, and the possibility of not showing up for the next appointment is increased.

11.5.3 Social/Model Learning

Rachman launched in 1977 the theory that fear can be acquired by indirect learning [30]. Social learning means that behavioral and physiological responses may be learned by observing another person's behavior in a particular situation or hearing stories about a particular situation. From an evolutionary perspective, social learning is important as it is appropriate, based on survival instinct, that a child learns to fear what his/her parents fear. This will protect the child from potentially dangerous situations. Studies on monkeys [31] show how young monkeys develop a fear of snakes when they observe other monkeys react with fear when exposed to snakes.

Up to early adolescence, parents or others in a close relationship with the child are the main models for the child's learning of fear. Children quickly perceive body language, and anxiety involuntarily expressed through a parent's body language when he/she accompanies the child to the dentist is easily transferred to DA in the child. There is a large amount of evidence that children with parents with DA more often have DA [32, 33]. Older children and adolescents are more affected by friends or information/instructions via social networks. Social learning happens when the child observes, reads, or listens to stories about other people's reactions at the dentist, e.g., "It was extremely painful," "Dentists are cruel," or "I can't stand to go there." Young patients may report on exaggerated experiences of pulling teeth or stories of fainting or pain in their teeth after starting orthodontic treatment.

Albert Bandura, a well-known behavioral researcher, claims that it is the cognitive process that distinguishes social learning from classical conditioning [34]. Positive role models with good behavior, like a secure and calm dental patient, may be used in social learning to prevent or reduce DA and to increase the desired behavior.

11.6 When Dental Treatment Feels Threatening

The physiological activations we find in fear reactions are generally the same as in other types of activations such as anger and in a normal fight–flight response.

The autonomic nervous system with sympathetic activation and parasympathetic deactivation that follows, e.g., an injection, may cause patients with dental fear to experience unpleasant fear reactions like cold sweat, numbness of the fingers and toes, nausea, indigestion, trembling, and a feeling of unreality. The patients may be frightened and misinterpret their bodily arousal as: "I feel dizzy, this must be linked to the dental treatment," or "My heart is going bananas, something must be wrong with this situation," or "My heart may not tolerate the high frequency, and it will possibly explode."

If the patient has moderate anxiety and the reactions are within his/her window of tolerance (WOT) (see ▶ Chap. 2), and the dentist is calm and the situation feels safe, then the patient will reassess the situation. Thoughts that promote learning in the dental situation are "This is not dangerous, I just hyperventilate" or "Oh, now I feel the palpitations in my fingers, it's natural." With an understanding of the situation and the anxiety response, the fear reaction will cease spontaneously.

However, when the anxiety level is extremely high, the patient is close to or above the upper limit of his WOT, and, so, the person will not be able to cognitively reassess the danger. Catastrophic thoughts such as "This is dangerous to me," "I can't get out of the situation," or "It's going to get worse" will enhance the anxiety reaction. In this manner, interpretations of the anxiety reaction will amplify the anxiety, and many patients describe that they feel trapped in a vicious circle with no control of the anxiety reaction and that it is the anxiety that controls them. In the context of the WOT, the anxiety keeps them stuck outside (above/under) their WOT and they will not be able to use possible coping strategies to reduce the anxiety reaction. When the patients are above the WOT, higher brain functions are rather limited. The dental staff have to calm down the patient to have further progress.

The higher the level of anxiety that the patient feels, the more catastrophic will the interpretations of the situation be. This is in accordance with our "better-safe-than-sorry instinct" – if danger is imminent, one should prepare for the worst. You not only interpret all signals from your body but also body language and face expressions from your surroundings (dental personnel) on the assumption that you need to prepare for a worst-case scenario. When you are terrified and are afraid that you will die of anxiety, it is difficult, if not impossible, to differentiate between a friendly, neutral, or angry face (◘ Fig. 11.2).

To feel that your anxiety determines your behavior and you are unable to control it is a scary feeling, and you get anxious of being anxious. In addition, it easily promotes feelings of shame.

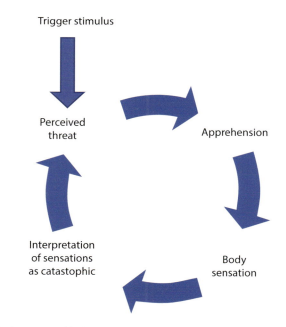

◘ **Fig. 11.2** This internal vicious circle is modified from Clark's cognitive model of panic. Dental treatment is perceived as a threat, and it shows how physiological reactions, interpretations of these, and catastrophic thoughts affect each other [35]

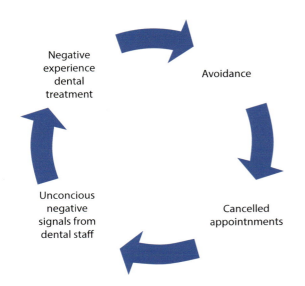

Fig. 11.3 The interpersonal circle describes how anxiety is amplified by emotions and behaviors in both patients and dental professionals

▶ **Example**

Ken, a man of 25 years, was sitting in the dental chair when he suddenly ran out of the dental clinic. When at some distance from the clinic he managed to assess the fear that triggered his reaction, he felt ashamed. In the aftermath of such an anxiety response, he experienced many emotions related to the situation including a strong sense of shame for a lack of control of his own reactions (that he suddenly ran out). He now thinks that the dentist finds him extremely troublesome, but he really likes this dentist and dreads that he will no longer be welcome at the clinic. He also dreads of future episodes of such lack of control of his own reactions (that he ran off). ◀

11.7 The Persistence Maintenance of Dental Anxiety

Maintenance of DA can be described with the help of two "vicious circles."

A relational circle describes how anxiety is amplified by emotions and behaviors in both patients and dental professionals (■ Fig. 11.3). This circle theoretically explains how behaviors, such as a highly stressful patient, a patient exhibiting behavior not easy for the dentist to understand, no show and cancellation of appointments, etc., may affect both the patient and dental staff and lead to increased stress in the treatment situation.

The following is an example:

▶ **Example**

A patient with dental anxiety has severe pain and calls a dental office at 2 pm on a Friday. Both the dentist and the dental assistant have planned to go home at 3 pm but feel obligated to offer an emergency consultation to release the patient's pain. The patient is kindly asked to be there at 3 pm, and the dental assistant underlines that it is important to be on time. The patient arrives 10 minutes late saying: "I just had to smoke a cigarette before entering, I am so nervous." The patient perceives the dental professional's subconscious negative reactions (often body language). He does not know that the negative reactions are related to him being late, and he feels that they are negative toward him, thus giving him a sense of not being welcome. In addition, he is tired due to pain, tense, and also believes that the upcoming treatment may be extremely painful. Due to his anxiety because of the pain that he is in and the dentist being in a rush to go home, the treatment is perceived as a negative experience, and this increases the risk of future avoidance of dental visits. This circle illustrates how easily negative emotions are communicated, especially nonverbally. ◀

For the dental staff, to help both the patients and themselves, it is important to accept and relate the negative emotions that anxious patients may invoke in them. First, by acknowledging and accepting these kinds of emotions in oneself, one can relate professionally to them. By suppressing them, you might express the emotions subconsciously in your body language, and the DA patients will observe and interpret you as hostile or negative based on their fear of being rejected.

Berggren and Meynert described the vicious circle of dental anxiety in 1984 (▶ Fig. 4.4). It has been tested and further developed and can today theoretically be seen as a spiral where the time aspect of avoidance of dentistry also constitutes an important component (■ Fig. 11.4).

Avoidance of dental treatment (and avoidance of daily tooth brushing as well) contributes to a deterioration of oral health. Patients are not only ashamed of their bad teeth but also because they cannot "pull themselves together and get it done." Shame and embarrassment over their teeth are problematic when meeting with dental professionals and also in familial and social relationships. Poor oral health is often a well-kept secret. A secret that they are afraid to reveal. Therefore, they may never smile, even at their children, and some hide their mouths with their hands.

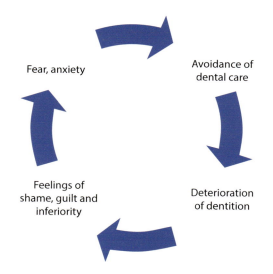

Fig. 11.4 The maintenance circle describes the development and maintenance of dental anxiety over time [23]

> The mental strain of having bad teeth and the great joy and deliverance of having her teeth rehabilitated and being able to smile was described as follows by a woman of 35 years:
> For the first time this summer I felt like a perfectly ordinary person. I could enjoy the summer, bought myself pretty clothes and could eat with others and smile. It was absolutely amazing not to think about hiding my teeth all the time.

11.8 Safety-Seeking Strategies

Safety-seeking strategies are central to the understanding of the development and maintenance of DA. The patient assures him/herself that a specific type of behavior or way of thinking is imperative to enable him/her to be able to face a phobic stimulus. For example, a patient feels that she must drink water just before and during dental treatment to prevent suffocating from anxiety during treatment. Using this safety-seeking strategy, the patient concludes afterward that it was the drinking of water that made everything go well. If the patient had skipped drinking water, she would most certainly have felt suffocated.

The phenomenon was first described by Salkovskis and employees in several articles, in 1996 [36, 37], as a model related to the maintenance of panic anxiety. The model is transferable to anxiety attacks that patients experience in the dental situation.

Salkovskis [35] categorized safety-seeking strategies into three main forms:

1. *Avoidance of situations that could conceivably trigger anxiety.* There may be thoughts like "I wasn't bitten by the big dog because I ran so fast - I have to run fast the next time I meet a dog too." or "I'm having a terribly bad day and can't go to the dentist today, but next week I'm ready." The patient avoids the dental situation because the patient does not feel well.

2. *Escape from situations after the anxiety attack has occurred.* One example might be "I didn't fall off that cliff because I was holding onto the railings. If the railing hadn't been there, I'd definitely have fallen." An example from dentistry: "I'm glad I refused to have my tooth done today. Since I refused treatment, my heart tolerated the dental visit." Here, the patient escapes from the situation by refusing treatment.

3. *Safety-seeking behavior.* This is subtle avoidance behavior to reduce anxiety attacks and prevent possible disasters. These may be the strategies that the patient becomes dependent on in order to carry out a function. "If I'm with someone when I'm driving an elevator, I'm fine. Alone I could never have made it." In the field of dentistry, this could be "Because I have a floss tied between my finger and the rubber dam clamp on the tooth, I know I can pull it out if I get it in my throat." or "Because my dentist is so amazing, I manage to do dental treatment with him/her. I would never be able to go to another dentist (the majority of other dentists are terrible)."

It is important to be conscious about the difference between making adjustments to help patients cope with dentistry and the strategies that help persist anxiety because their catastrophic beliefs are not put to test.

Summary

Anxiety in dental treatment situations is triggered and expressed in the same manner as anxiety experienced in other contexts. Anxiety reactions are instinctive and are controlled by the autonomic nervous system to increase our chances of survival. DA is a continuum of levels of anxiety, which increase in line with bodily arousal, negative thoughts, and avoidance behavior. It is important to prevent and treat high levels of fear and anxiety before these develops into a phobia, which has consequences for the person's daily living.

The biopsychosocial model is a way of understanding the etiology of DA and phobia. In classical conditioning, self-perceived negative experiences lead to a future fear response. In social/model learning, fear develops indirectly without the individual being in personal contact with the stimulus that triggers the fear reaction. From a biological point of view, one should stay away from danger; psychologically, one should choose what feels good for oneself, and, from a social learning perspective, it is wise to copy the group's experiences.

Development and persistence of dental anxiety is explained using a model with three vicious circles. One circle describes the bodily reactions during anxiety activation. A relational circle describes how anxiety is amplified by emotions and behaviors in both patients and dental professionals. A persistence circle describes how dental anxiety develops over time. Security-seeking strategies also contribute to maintaining the anxiety.

DA poses a high risk of poor oral health. With an incidence of about 10%, preventing and treating early signs of dental anxiety is highly important and should be implemented in preventive dental health care.

References

1. Humphris G, Crawford JR, Hill K, Gilbert A, Freeman R. UK population norms for the modified dental anxiety scale with percentile calculator: adult dental health survey 2009 results. BMC Oral Health. 2013;13:29. Published 2013 Jun 24. https://doi.org/10.1186/1472-6831-13-29.

2. Svensson L, Hakeberg M, Boman UW. Dental anxiety, concomitant factors and change in prevalence over 50 years. Community Dent Health. 2016;33(2):121–6.

3. Liinavuori A, Tolvanen M, Pohjola V, Lahti S. Changes in dental fear among Finnish adults: a national survey. Community Dent Oral Epidemiol. 2016;44(2):128–34. https://doi.org/10.1111/cdoe.12196.

4. Klingberg G, Broberg AG. Dental fear/anxiety and dental behaviour management problems in children and adolescents: a review of prevalence and concomitant psychological factors. Int J Paediatr Dent. 2007;17(6):391–406.

5. Schuller AA, Willumsen T, Holst D. Are there differences in oral health and oral health behavior between individuals with high and low dental fear? Community Dent Oral Epidemiol. 2003;31(2):116–21.

6. Agdal ML, Raadal M, Skaret E, Kvale G. Oral health and oral treatment needs in patients fulfilling the DSM-IV criteria for dental phobia. Possible influence on the outcome of cognitive behavioral therapy. Acta Odontol Scand. 2008;66(1):1–6. https://doi.org/10.1080/00016350701793714.

7. Armfield JM, Slade GD, Spencer AJ. Dental fear and adult oral health in Australia. Community Dent Oral Epidemiol. 2009;37(3):220–30. https://doi.org/10.1111/j.1600-0528.2009.00468.x.

8. Carlsson V, Hakeberg M, Wide Boman U. Associations between dental anxiety, sense of coherence, oral health-related quality of life and health behavior--a national Swedish cross-sectional survey. BMC Oral Health. 2015;15:100. Published 2015 Sep 2. https://doi.org/10.1186/s12903-015-0088-5.

9. McNally RJ. Preparedness and phobias. A review. Psychol Bull. 1987;101(2):283–303.

10. Seligman MEP. Phobias and preparedness. Behav Ther. 1971;2(3):307–20.

11. World Health organization (WHO) International statistical classification of diseases and related health problems (ICD). Cited 21. May 21. Available from: https://www.who.int/standards/classifications/classification-of-diseases

12. American psychiatric association. Diagnostic and statistical manual of mental disorders (DSM–5). Cited 21. May 21. Available from: https://www.psychiatry.org/psychiatrists/practice/dsm

13. Randall CL, Shaffer JR, McNeil DW, Crout RJ, Weyant RJ, Marazita ML. Toward a genetic understanding of dental fear: evidence of heritability. Community Dent Oral Epidemiol. 2017;45(1):66–73. https://doi.org/10.1111/cdoe.12261.

14. Arnrup K, Broberg AG, Berggren U, Bodin L. Temperamental reactivity and negative emotionality in uncooperative children referred to specialized paediatric dentistry compared to children in ordinary dental care. Int J Paediatr Dent. 2007;17(6):419–29. https://doi.org/10.1111/j.1365-263X.2007.00868.x.

15. Bergdahl M, Bergdahl J. Temperament and character personality dimensions in patients with dental anxiety. Eur J Oral Sci. 2003;111(2):93–8.

16. Lundgren J, Elfström ML, Berggren U. The relationship between temperament and fearfulness in adult dental phobic patients. Int J Paediatr Dent. 2007;17(6):460–8. https://doi.org/10.1111/j.1365-263X.2007.00880.x.

17. Stenebrand A, Wide Boman U, Hakeberg M. Dental anxiety and temperament in 15-year olds. Acta Odontol Scand. 2013;71(1):15–21. https://doi.org/10.3109/00016357.2011.645068.

18. Vassend O, Røysamb E, Nielsen CS. Dental anxiety in relation to neuroticism and pain sensitivity. A twin study. J Anxiety Disord. 2011;25(2):302–8. https://doi.org/10.1016/j.janxdis.2010.09.015.

19. Pousette Lundgren G, Karsten A, Dahllöf G. Oral health-related quality of life before and after crown therapy in young patients with amelogenesis imperfecta. Health Qual Life Outcomes. 2015;13:197. Published 2015 Dec 10. https://doi.org/10.1186/s12955-015-0393-3.

20. Armfield JM, Slade GD, Spencer AJ. Cognitive vulnerability and dental fear. BMC Oral Health. 2008;8:2. Published 2008 Jan 24. https://doi.org/10.1186/1472-6831-8-2.

21. Pavlov IP. Conditioned reflexes. London: Oxford University Press; 1927.

22. Berggren U, Carlsson SG, Hagglin C, Hakeberg M, Samsonowitz V. Assessment of patients with direct conditioned and indirect cognitive reported origin of dental fear. Eur J Oral Sci. 1997;105(3):213–20.

23. Berggren U, Meynert G. Dental fear and avoidance. Causes, symptoms, and consequences. J Am Dent Assoc. 1984;109(2):247–51.

24. Locker D, Shapiro D, Liddell A. Negative dental experiences and their relationship to dental anxiety. Community Dent Health. 1996;13(2):86–92.

25. Milgrom P, Mancl L, King B, Weinstein P. Origins of childhood dental fear. Behav Res Ther. 1995;33(3):313–9.

26. Skaret E, Raadal M, Berg E, Kvale G. Dental anxiety among 18-yr-olds in Norway. Prevalence and related factors. Eur J Oral Sci. 1998;106(4):835–43.

27. Milgrom P, Vignehsa H, Weinstein P. Adolescent dental fear and control. Prevalence and theoretical implications. Behav Res Ther. 1992;30(4):367–73.

28. Armfield JM, Spencer AJ, Stewart JF. Dental fear in Australia: who's afraid of the dentist? Aust Dent J. 2006;51(1):78–85. https://doi.org/10.1111/j.1834-7819.2006.tb00405.x.

29. Oscarson N, Espelid I, Jönsson B. Is caries equally distributed in adults? A population-based cross-sectional study in Norway - the TOHNN-study. Acta Odontol Scand. 2017;75(8):557–63. https://doi.org/10.1080/00016357.2017.1357080.

30. Rachman S. The conditioning theory of fear-acquisition. A critical examination. Behav Res Ther. 1977;15:375–87. https://doi.org/10.1016/0005-7967(77)90041-9.

31. Mineka S, Davidson M, Cook M, Keir R. Observational conditioning of snake fear in Rhesus-Monkeys. J Abnorm Psychol. 1984;93(4):355–72. https://doi.org/10.1037/0021-843x.93.4.355.

11

32. Blomqvist M, Ek U, Fernell E, Holmberg K, Westerlund J, Dahllöf G. Cognitive ability and dental fear and anxiety. Eur J Oral Sci. 2013;121(2):117–20. https://doi.org/10.1111/eos.12028.

33. Themessl-Huber M, Freeman R, Humphris G, MacGillivray S, Terzi N. Empirical evidence of the relationship between parental and child dental fear. A structured review and meta-analysis. Int J Paediatr Dent. 2010;20(2):83–101. https://doi.org/10.1111/j.1365-263X.2009.00998.x.

34. Bandura A. Self-efficacy. Toward a unifying theory of behavioral change. Psychol Rev. 1977;84(2):191–215.

35. Clark DM. A cognitive approach to panic. Behav Res Ther. 1986;24(4):461–70.

36. Salkovskis PM. The cognitive approach to anxiety. Threat beliefs, safety-seeking behavior, and the special case of health anxiety and obsession. In: Salkovskis PM, editor. Frontiers of cognitive therapy. New York: Guilford Press; 1996. p. 48–74.

37. Salkovskis PM, Clark DM, Hackmann A, Wells A, Gelder MG. An experimental investigation of the role of safety-seeking behaviours in the maintenance of panic disorder with agoraphobia. Behav Res Ther. 1999;37(6):559–74.

Psychological Prevention and Management of Dental Anxiety

Tiril Willumsen, Maren L. Agdal, Mariann Saanum Hauge, and Bent Storå

Contents

12.1 Introduction

Dentists can, paradoxically, be frightened when they are confronted by patients' anxiety. Research shows that many dentists feel uncomfortable and react with difficult emotions when treating anxious patients. It has also been shown that the more behavioral management methods a dentist masters, the more joy and satisfaction he or she finds in their work [1]. In other words, learning techniques for treating patients' dental anxiety in a general practice have the potential to not only help patients but also increase job satisfaction for the dentist.

In this chapter, the dentist is addressed as the one in charge of the treatment, but it is important to emphasize that cooperation between the dentist and the dental nurse is essential for a good treatment outcome. Patients' experience in a dental office is always a result of the efforts made by the full dental team, and, therefore, the knowledge described in this chapter, and in this book, is useful to all dental staff, including nurses and hygienists.

Psychological management of dental anxiety can be time-consuming. However, for providing the best possible oral health care from a lifetime perspective, it is just as essential as oral hygiene education or proper treatment of periodontitis. In addition, clinical experience shows that the time spent on dental anxiety treatment is time saved in the long run. Patients cope better with dental treatment, and canceled and postponed treatment sessions are reduced.

We will introduce Rita as an example of a patient with dental anxiety. She postpones dental treatment and finds it extremely unpleasant, but she still manages to go through with most treatments. Last year, she had a need for an endodontic procedure in a molar but chose to extract the tooth to avoid the frightening procedure.

🕿 Learning Goals
- To have knowledge of the basic elements in behavioral management of dental anxiety
- To be able to assess the level of dental anxiety
- To be able to carry out dental treatments based on a coping plan
- To have knowledge about behavioral management in combination with sedation and nitrous oxide
- To have knowledge about how to reduce patient anxiety through psychoeducation

12.2 Part 1: Basic Elements in the Prevention and Management of Dental Anxiety

This chapter relies on the knowledge of all the topics described in the previous chapters of this book. The patient has to feel respected and understood by the dental health personnel and rest assured that the treatment of dental anxiety is considered an important part of providing oral health care by the dentist. As shame is an important part of dental anxiety for many of the patients [2], a nonmoralizing attitude is important.

12.2.1 Providing the Patient with the Experience of Predictability and Control

A patient with dental anxiety will have an even greater need for predictability and control (including pain control) than patients without anxiety. In a Swedish study among patients with dental anxiety, having a "safe relationship with the dentist" and "a sense of control" were considered the most important factors by the patients in order to cope with dental treatments [3]. The experience of control is subjective and must be explored in each individual [4].

Dental treatment is at its best when the patient is confident and feels "in the driver's seat." Proper alliance, communication strategies, and structure of the consultation are essential factors for achieving this. In addition, the patient should constantly receive relevant information about the upcoming treatment. Knowing what is about to happen next has great potential for inducing feelings of safety, predictability, and control.

The patient should be met with respect and the anxiety validated during the first phone conversation prior to the patient's arrival at the clinic: "Thank you for telling me that you have dental anxiety. It is an important part of treatment in our office to deal with patients' anxiety. In the first session the dentist will have a conversation about how to give you the best possible care and if you wish, we will do an oral examination."

In a treatment process, it is useful to conclude each treatment session by discussing and planning the content of the next session, i.e., constructing a treatment plan. To further increase control and codetermination, an anxious patient may benefit from an opportunity to choose between two treatment options. "I suggest we start with the filling in the front tooth or in the upper molar, do you have any preferences?"

Box 12.1

Today's treatment:_

_____

_____

Next appointment: _____

Treatment plan next appointment:

_____

It is particularly important that the dentist makes an effort to help the patient to experience control at the start of the treatment. The professional can say "Tell me when you're ready." Predictive control will be increased by letting the patient give his consent to start the dental procedure. Such start-up control also allows the patient to prepare for the task, for example, "Focus on your breath, let me know when you're ready for me to start."

The patient and the dentist should agree upon stop signals before the treatment starts. Stop signals give patients the power to stop treatment, which gives them a sense of control. Several signals may work. For some, sounds from the throat can be a stop signal. One hand up – to signal "I need a break" or "I have to spit, breathe, itch, rinse, etc." – is commonly used. Two hands up may be used to signal "full stop." Patients who prefer stop signals may be asked "What stop signal can be OK for you to use?"

Many anxious patients are reluctant to stop the dentist during treatment. They may fear that the dentist will be annoyed or overlook their signal. Thus, it is important to test out and practice specific stop signals. Some patients have difficulty in daring to raise their hand. For these, a more passive method like holding one hand up and lowering it to signal stop could be an alternative.

Signals like these work well but are dependent upon the dentist's ability to see the patient's hands. It is a problem when the dentist is working, for example, in the upper jaw or with binocular loupe glasses and the field of vision is extremely small. Worse than not agreeing upon a stop signal is to have the opportunity to give a signal to stop but get overlooked by the dentist. Thus, cooperation with the dental nurse is essential. One person in the room must be responsible for observing signals, verbalizing them during treatment, and making sure that the stop signal is followed.

Some patients think that a dentist should be able to see when their patients need a break. This is not realistic and gives the dentist a responsibility he cannot fulfil. Studies show that treating patients with dental anxiety increases dentists' stress [5]. If the dentist is met with expectations from the patient he cannot fulfil, it may increase stress activation. The patient must be made aware that the dentist cannot be expected to know when he or she needs a break. By discussing and practicing suitable signals, both the patient and dentist will feel more secure and probably less stressed.

12.2.2 Checking Out the Alliance

There are several studies that indicate that an alliance between a professional and a patient is fundamental to achieving a successful treatment. Here, success means both the dental aspects and the treatment of the anxiety [6]. It is important to talk openly with the patient about mutual respect and emphasize the fact that teamwork is necessary if the treatment is to be successful. The patient needs to understand that the dentist takes their alliance seriously. Moreover, focusing on the alliance allows the dentist to explore it and to take corrective action if the patient–dentist relationship has got off to a bad start. Questions about the alliance should be asked throughout the treatment of patients with dental anxiety to help establish an alliance and create a safe relationship. One example is "It is important to make you feel safe and that we are working as a team, do you have any thoughts about whether I succeed in this?" (See ▶ Chap. 4 for more on the importance of the relationship during treatment.)

12.2.3 Psychoeducation

Explaining the symptoms and functions of anxiety as part of treatment is called psychoeducation. It is greatly advantageous to understand dental anxiety in order to cope with it [7]. A patient is taught that anxiety reactions are functional and natural if one is in real danger (see the previous chapter).

> ▶ **Example**

Rita and the dentist shake hands and say hello.
DENTIST: – Please take a seat.

RITA – sits down in the dental chair and the dentist observes.

DENTIST: – I can see that this is difficult for you, I also felt tremors in your hand as we shook hands, and your hand felt cold and sweaty. I would like to start out by discussing these kinds of reactions with you, is that OK?

RITA: – OK

DENTIST: – This is a natural reaction because your body perceive danger and is getting ready to escape from/handle/react to the situation. Your blood is passed to the large muscle groups in the legs and arms, there will be little blood supply to the hands and feet making them cold and sweaty. That is the only sensible reaction when you're going to escape from a dangerous animal but not just as understandable when you're stuck in a dental chair. ◄

12.2.3.1 Bodily Reactions

Often, it is a great relief for the patient to get explanations for their own bodily reactions in the context of anxiety (◘ Table 12.1).

> ▶ **Example**

A psychoeducative dialogue about tension and palpitations is as follows:
DENTIST: – What do you usually feel in your body when you're sitting in a dentist's chair?

RITA: – I feel very tense.

Table 12.1 Overview of some of the most important bodily reactions that dentists must know of in order to explain the biological function of a fear reaction to their patients

Symptom	Physiological explanation
Palpitations and increased heart rate	A lot of activity in the body because the body prepares for fight/flight
Sweat	The body gets rid of excess heat due to its high activation
Trembling	High activity in the muscles such as static training
Chest pressure/pain	Muscle tension
Dry mouth	Digestive activity is reduced, and there is an increased need for a free respiratory tract
Heat/cold sensation in the body	The blood flows to the large muscle groups in the legs and arms, and there will be little blood supply to the hands and feet, thus making them cold
Unreality sensation	Due to extreme activity in the sympathetic nervous system
Nausea or upset stomach	Digestive activity is reduced not to use too much energy
Tingling sensation in the body	Because the blood flows to the large muscle groups
Pressure on the bladder	To get rid of excess weight, the body will get rid of urine/intestinal contents in order to be able to escape faster
Feeling of breathlessness/difficulty in breathing	Hyperventilating to increase oxygen content in the blood
Dizziness and choking sensation	Due to hyperventilation, there is an imbalance between O_2 and too little CO_2 in the blood (hypocapnia)
Fainting	Vasovagal syncope – To prevent death from anxiety. To gain control over respiration and blood pressure

12

DENTIST: – You mean in your muscles?

RITA: – Yes, I'm almost above the chair.

DENTIST: – And your heart?

RITA: – Yes, it's beating fast.

DENTIST: – This happens to protect you and is part of our survival mechanism. Because of what you have experienced in the past your body experiences the situation as dangerous. The body puts the muscles in alarm position and the heart pumps full speed to make you ready to escape from or fight the danger. And it happens automatically without you thinking about it. In this way, humans have survived dangers throughout history. So, your body reacts correctly based on what you've experienced before. What we want is to give you some new experiences and eventually this situation – to be at the dentist – will not initiate the fear response as it does now. ◄

Explaining what happens when muscle tonus is increased due to anxiety is quite simple, but explaining hyperventilation is not as easy.

► **Example**

A simple explanation of the complex mechanism is as follows:

The breathing mechanism has a "breathing thermostat" that tells us when we need more oxygen. We breathe oxygen in, and it is converted into carbon dioxide (CO_2). It is the CO_2 in the blood and exhalation that determines the thermostat (how much we need to breathe). This works well during physical activity. When we use a lot of oxygen, such as when we run, the breathing rate increases. When we are anxious or stressed, the breathing rate increases in the same manner as it does when we are running, even if the body remains immobile. As a result, we breathe more CO_2 than the body needs, we exhale more CO_2 than usual, and, thus, we get too much oxygen and too little CO_2 (hypocapnia) in the blood. Nevertheless, it feels like we are getting too little air and the need to take rapid breaths increases. In addition, we tighten the muscles of the chest as a kind of a protective muscle shell (like a turtle), which also includes the chest muscles and allows us to breathe only through the upper parts of the lungs. We can get dizzy and eventually become extremely unwell and feel like we are going to lose consciousness. If this proceeds, our body's autonomous nervous system will ensure a drop in blood pressure and we will faint in order to let the body resume normal breathing (one cannot die from anxiety). ◄

12.2.3.2 Catastrophic Interpretations and Thoughts

Catastrophic thoughts are terrifying automatic thoughts that appear without reflection and are often without a hold in reality. In psychoeducation, patients should learn that these thoughts are the result of the interpreta-

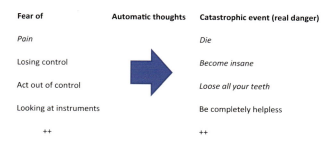

Fear of	Automatic thoughts	Catastrophic event (real danger)
Pain		*Die*
Losing control		*Become insane*
Act out of control		*Loose all your teeth*
Looking at instruments		Be completely helpless
++		++

Fig. 12.1 Usual catastrophic thoughts in the dental office

tions that one makes of a situation (see the previous chapter for details). Catastrophic interpretations are often subconscious; you just feel that you are afraid without being aware of what you are afraid of. Our tendency for catastrophic thinking has a biological explanation; for survival, it is useful to interpret a situation as more dangerous than it actually is. Your chances of surviving are increased with "better safe, than sorry" or "better to run too fast, too often, than too slowly, once" (Fig. 12.1).

To uncover catastrophic thoughts, one can start by simply asking, "What are you afraid of?"

The more severe dental anxiety the patient has, the more important it can be to follow the catastrophic thoughts until real danger occurs. Let us look at some examples of catastrophic thoughts and how to explore them.

> ► **Example**

RITA: – I'm afraid I'm going to feel pain.

DENTIST: – If so, what's the worst thing that can happen?

RITA: – I may lose consciousness due to the pain.

DENTIST: – If so, what's the worst thing that can happen?

RITA: – That I don't wake up again (real danger).

DENTIST: – How likely do you think it is that this will happen?

RITA: – Approximately 30%.

DENTIST: – Yes, then it's no wonder you're afraid to feel pain. We know that what you describe is something that in reality never happens, but if you think like you do, it's natural that you get scared. Is there another possible solution or outcome if you feel pain?

RITA: – Yes, I can as you have said give signal for you to stop.

DENTIST: – Yes…. (active listening, give her time to think)

RITA: – and then you can give me more anesthetic. ◄

The goal of exploring catastrophic thoughts is to redefine the automatic negative line of thought into a constructive line of thought. When the patient learns to think "I can tell the dentist to stop if I feel pain," then catastrophic thoughts are averted. Edna Foa writes in the manual of Prolonged Exposure that exposure is the most effective treatment for catastrophic thoughts because it allows the patient to understand through experience that these catastrophic thoughts are not correct [8]. Dental treatment will almost without exception include exposure to frightening stimuli for the fearful patient, and, therefore, if addressed adequately, it has the potential to correct catastrophic thoughts.

> ► **Example**
>
> Catastrophic thoughts:
>
> Nina fears that the dental team will not stop even if she feels terrible, either by continuing "a little more" or holding her down. Then, she will feel completely helpless.
>
> Birgit is afraid that she will sit in the dental chair, with her mouth opened higher than her rheumatism allows. She is afraid that she will have to open her mouth too wide to make room for dental instruments. She is afraid that the dentist will not listen when she needs to take a break and that she will remain in helplessness and get extreme pain in her joints afterward.
>
> Colin feels completely unprepared for what is going to happen. He thinks that he is going to be paralyzed and not be able to escape.
>
> Tracy is afraid that water or saliva will enter the back of her pharynx and suffocate her. ◄

12.2.3.3 The Anxiety Hierarchy

The purpose of establishing a patient's individual anxiety hierarchy is both to raise the patient's awareness of his/her own anxiety: "Am I more afraid of the syringe than the drill?" and to provide necessary information on systematic exposure when applicable (see the next chapter). Often, patients with dental anxiety have an unspecific description of situations and procedures that trigger their anxiety. They dread the whole dental situation. During construction of an anxiety hierarchy, patients will be able to relate to their anxiety reactions at a more specific and detailed level, including specific dental procedures, and, consequently, will be able to better think and react to each specific procedure independently. The anxiety hierarchies are highly individualized and will show the patient "how my personal dental anxiety is constructed" or "this is my dental anxiety." Patients should be encouraged to take a picture of their anxiety hierarchy and get to know it.

This hierarchy will also provide useful information to the dentist on how to best plan further treatment for this particular patient. Even when systematic exposure is not intended, it will often be useful to start with treatments at the lower end of the ladder/hierarchy. This will allow the patient to gain more confidence and the alli-

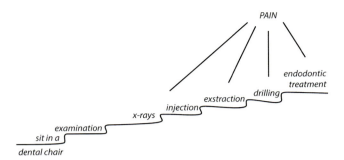

Fig. 12.2 Example of an anxiety hierarchy (Rita's). As pain is the common denominator for Rita's pain, focus on receiving injections would probably be a good start for the dental treatment

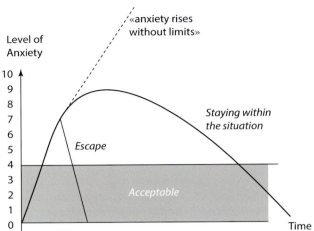

Fig. 12.3 Habituation model of anxiety. Time is represented horizontally and level of anxiety vertically. It can be seen how anxiety rises when individuals are exposed to a scary situation. The gray straight line shows a change in anxiety in an avoidance reaction, and the gray dotted line shows the activation of catastrophic thoughts established when choosing to avoid. The last line shows how anxiety develops if one stays in the situation under safe, controlled conditions

ance between the patient and the dentist to strengthen before starting the more challenging tasks at the top of the hierarchy. The patient's anxiety hierarchy is designed by putting the patient's anxiety of procedures in the dental treatment into a gradient. The dentist starts by drawing (on a paper or a board) the empty "staircase" and in continuation fills in the steps with anxiety-provoking situations of increasing severity. A good start may be to explore the "worst" procedure first, put it at the top, continue with what the best procedure is at the bottom, and eventually put it in place in the middle. The fears should be written with a pencil so that they can be changed as the patient reflects on his or her anxiety (**Fig. 12.2**).

12.2.3.4 The Habituation Model of Anxiety

The habituation model of anxiety (see **Figs. 12.3 and 12.4**) is a model used to explain the step-by-step exposure to patients. It illustrates how situations that the patient perceives as frightening gradually become less frightening if one repeats them. It should be used in systematic CBT for anxiety treatment (see the next chapter) but can also be useful for psychoeducation in patients who are to receive, for example, sedation to overcome their dental anxiety. The habituation model of anxiety should be drawn while explaining to the patient the important parts of the anxiety process:

Escape: What happens to anxiety in avoidance/escape reactions is drawn into the curve; the anxiety rises first, but the anxiety level falls abruptly if one cancels or does not show up at an appointment (gray line).

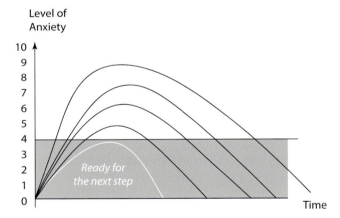

Fig. 12.4 Change in the curve model with repeated exposures. The line at 4 on the level of anxiety illustrates an imaginary patient's maximum limit of anxiety for feeling okay during dentistry

▶ **Example**

DENTIST: – You have told me about how you delay booking of dental appointments even if you know you need to go. I would like to explain how avoidance behavior in general affect anxiety, is that OK?

RITA: – OK

DENTIST: – When you get into a frightening situation, the anxiety rises abruptly, the discomfort of this often leads to

the decision to avoid the danger. As you cancel, the anxiety will fall abruptly. Instantly this feels good. You have avoided the terrifying situation and the brain interpret the escape/anxiety reduction as having succeeded in getting away from the danger -implied that the danger exists. The next time you are heading into a similar situation, your brain would like to seek the same solution, as this strategy was interpreted as successful last time. In other words, avoidance has led to increased anxiety and avoidance behavior. Is this something you can think relevant to you?

RITA: – Yes ◀

Avoidance is often a result of a feeling that anxiety can rise unlimited and that it will only continue to escalate if you do nothing to avoid the danger. So, to avoid/flight, making you think the avoidance helped you escape the danger. In this manner, catastrophic thoughts create avoidance, but avoidance also creates/sustains catastrophic thoughts.

Given the condition that you are in control, you can stay in the situation with some anxiety activation (but no more than that you can control), and the anxiety level will eventually decrease if the danger is not real. When repeated, the anxiety reaction will over time be reduced.

Metaphors are useful in the process of explaining this principle to patients. Let us go back to Rita:

► Example

DENTIST: – During treatment with us, we will try to get a feeling of control all of the time, and we're going to proceed slowly, how slowly will depend upon how you react. If your anxiety is controllable, we will be able to do regular dental treatment at once, if it is more difficult, we must consider other treatment options (see the next chapter). Anyway, we will together work out strategies to keep you in your window of tolerance (see chapter...)

To explain the principle of habituation to the dental situation, I will use a completely different example. For example, if you were afraid of heights and did not dare stand in a high ladder to paint the house. In this case we could put standing on top of the ladder as maximum fear of you (mark 10 in the drawing of the anxiety curve).

I will hold the ladder so it's safe. We would start with you trying to stand on a step that you think is a little scary for a short time, for instance 3 s and then step down. Your anxiety would be for example, 7 on the anxiety scale.

Do you understand this example?

RITA: – Yes

DENTIST: – When you have rested and become calm again, we would do the same thing again, and probably you will not be as scared as the first time. The more you practice, the less anxiety you will feel. This is habituation. When you feel safe, we can go on with the next step. In my experience this principle may be transferred to the dental situation, what do you think?

RITA: – I think so, if you go slowly, let me take breaks and I think it is worth a try. But you must make it as painless as possible.

DENTIST: – I agree, it is very important that you have minimum pain. Painful experiences may be very bad for your dental anxiety, even if you think it will work OK and you "just want to get it over with." Both of us need to be patient and work it out slowly and in full control, OK? ◄

12.3 Part 2: Coping Strategies

How patients cope with dental situations is crucial to how dental anxiety may be increased or reduced. Dental personnel who actively use strategies to improve their patients' coping will contribute to reduction of dental anxiety. In a Swedish study, Bernson et al. found that dental anxiety patients with regular recall treatment had more positive coping strategies than did dental anxiety patients who avoided dental treatment [9].

12.3.1 Giving Positive Reinforcements

When dealing with children, it is important to give praise [10]. The same goes for adults with dental anxiety, but one should be aware not to sound childish. Exclamations like "You were so clever today!" work poorly on an adult. It is better to focus on the positive effect of the interaction between the patient and dentist and make statements during the clinical treatment phase like: "When you are as relaxed as you were now, it is much easier for me to make the injection with the least amount of discomfort," preferably in combination with useful feedback like "This worked well from my view, you kept your tongue still and we got a saliva free situation when making the filling, how did you experience it?"

12.3.2 Distraction

Music played through headphones can work well as a distraction for adult patients with mild and moderate anxiety. Scientifically, the effect is questionable [11, 12]. In patients with high anxiety, no effect has been found [13]. Studies with film, both two-dimensional (2D) and three-dimensional (3D), have also been conducted but without any significant effect. Testing music in headphones or movies/computer games from patients' phones may be a good idea for patients who are motivated by these interventions. However, some patients may exhibit an opposite effect; they may feel less in control and left to themselves when they cannot hear the dentist. The dentist may ask the patient: "Did you find it calming when we tested music with your headphones?"

Another use of music is music in the treatment room for all to hear. In other contexts, soothing music has been found to affect breathing and heart rate in everyone present in the room [14].

Another distraction technique is to "move" the focus of pain by stimulating/pressing a point on the body different from the area of dental treatment. This may distract and remove attention from what is happening in the mouth. Melzack and Wall [15] found the nervous system to have a limited capacity for pain impulses. Stimulation takes up capacity in the autonomic nervous system, and pain sensation is reduced (in addition, the massage initiates increased blood flow to speed up the immune system). This may partly explain why we automatically massage ourselves in places that are painful. There are two ways of applying this, regularly used by dentists: (i) the patient uses the right fifth finger (thumb) to put pressure on the skin between the left fourth and fifth finger and (ii) the dentist cautiously squeezes the cheek with fingers holding the cheek aside while applying anesthesia.

12.3.3 Assessing Catastrophic Thoughts

Assessing and reconstructing catastrophic thoughts can be done in all phases of the treatment. At the start of the treatment, it is used to explore anxiety as described previously (see ▶ Sect. 12.2.3). Another example may be to discuss reactions in the debriefing after the treatment. We go back to Rita:

> ▶ **Example**
>
> DENTIST: – OK- now we have made the filling we planned, from my point of view this worked well. How about you?
>
> RITA: – It was far better than I expected it to be.
>
> DENTIST: – Yes, in advance you had some negative thoughts?
>
> RITA: – Yes, I thought that it would be very painful, but I experienced that you waited for the local anesthetics to work, and you also gave me an extra injection, so it was not.
>
> DENTIST: – That is good to hear, if you were to do the same procedure again tomorrow, what would you think?
>
> RITA: – I think I would fear pain, but I would think that it worked well today, and I have the opportunity to ask for more of the local anesthetics and wait until it works.
>
> DENTIST: – This is great, if you are able to think "if I get pain, I will ask for more local anesthetics" you have reconstructed your catastrophic thought of pain. It is important that you try to remember this and remind yourself of it before next treatment. ◀

12.3.4 Using the Window of Tolerance

While dealing with all levels of dental anxiety, it is important to work within the patients' window of tolerance (see ▶ Chap. 2).

12.3.4.1 Decreasing Activation When the Patient Is at the Higher End of the Window of Tolerance

The main rule is to stop and introduce coping strategies when the anxiety activation increases beyond control. The objective of these coping strategies is to bring the activation down to a level that is possible for the patient to handle and, hence, get a sense of achievement. In principle, anything that seems calming might work.

Muscular relaxation can help regain control of anxiety [16]. Several studies have shown systematic relaxation training in combination with exposure as an effective treatment for dental anxiety [17, 18].

Applied relaxation is a method developed to control bodily activation. The method is based on two basic principles: (1) the patient learns to recognize early signs of muscular tension and (2) the patient learns relaxation [19]. This method has been found to be effective in dental anxiety treatment [20]. Bodily activation during dental treatment is individualized, and it is important to figure out the bodily reactions when anxiety rises (for instance, tingling sensations in the hands, stomach ache, and tension in the shoulder muscles). Patients should learn the unique patterns of responses that arise under the influence of anxiety to help recognize personal needs during treatment (for instance, if a break is needed). Knowledge of a patient's unique reactions when a rise in the anxiety level occurs is also important information to the oral health-care personnel, since it gives valuable information about which part of the patient's body should be more closely observed during treatment to help uncover changes in anxiety levels (see ▶ Sect. 12.4.2.3). In applied relaxation, the patient, dentist, or nurse recognizes the symptoms of a rise in anxiety and initiates a break for relaxation to bring down the activation level.

Control of breathing is relevant in relaxation training since dental anxiety patients often automatically stop breathing or start hyperventilating [21]. The patient must be asked to observe his/her breathing: "Do you notice your breathing?"

It is useful to check whether the patient has experience with relaxation training or breathing exercises, and, if so, encourage them to use the same during dental treatment.

> **Tip**
>
> Three simple breathing instructions are presented here. The instructions should be given in a calm voice. Clinical experience has shown it to be beneficial if the dentist or dental hygienist gives out instructions before starting the dental procedures. During treatment, the dental nurse follows up and gives the instructions. The pace should be slow and steady.
> 1. Exhale one– two–three
> 2. Breathe and hold one–two–three and release
> 3. Breathe in wait ... exhale wait ...
>
> Body scanning is somewhat more extensive but is effective as a muscle relaxation method and still quite time-efficient.

An example of instructions during body scanning is as follows:

  Ask the patient to sit comfortably in the dental chair and give instructions in a calm and muted voice: "Focus on your toes. Feel that your toes are relaxing and that they are securely attached to the bottom of your instep. Feel your heel relaxes. Focus on your legs, feel that blood flows from the legs and that the legs relax and lie side by side in the chair. Feel your knees, the knees are completely relaxed. Focus on your thighs, feel that they lie heavy in the chair. Focus on your thighs, feel that they lie heavy and comfortably in the chair, feel that your buttocks have good support in the chair and relax. Make contact with the lower back, the middle part of the back, which ends up in the top part of the back. Your body have support in the chair and you relax. Focus on your shoulders, feel that your shoulders are as far down as possible and slightly back. Back of your head, feel that the back of your head is relaxing. Think of your forehead, focus on your forehead, forehead relaxes. Feel your cheeks, see that you can relax your cheeks. Relax in your lower jaw, let it fall and create a freeway space between the teeth in your upper and lower jaw. Let the tongue relax, you can feel that when it is relaxed it will be big and fill out the space between the teeth." ◄

We will continue with Rita and illustrate how the treatment progression may be explained by using the anxiety curve, relaxation training, and the window of tolerance. In Rita's case, her activation obviously increases, but, if in doubt, the dentist may ask "Do you feel that your activation increases or decreases when you approach a dental procedure?"

DENTIST: – I will try to explain to you how we can proceed with this. I will do that by using the window of tolerance model. We all have a level of activation where we at "at our best". It is in this activation level our brains function best, and we are best prepared for technically challenging tasks. At this activation level we are in the center of our window of tolerance. Both above and below this we have a zone where we function adequately, but the nearer we get to the limits of our window of tolerance the poorer we function. For example, it gets more difficult to give stop signals or to understand what I am saying as the unconscious part of your body and brain is in a survival situation and then getting away from danger is the most important. If you are above or below the limits of the tolerance window the activation is very unpleasant and if you don't have proper coping strategies you will feel that the anxiety is in charge, not you.

Together we will make sure that you don't get that experience. By giving you good information in

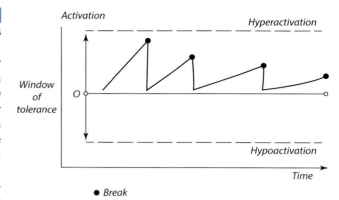

● **Fig. 12.5** A typical activation scheme when using systematic relaxation training. Time is represented horizontally and level of anxiety vertically. Zero represents an activation level optimal for feeling calm, secure, and able to cope with the situation. You start out with systematic relaxation procedures, e.g., breathing techniques or other methods of relaxation training given by the dentist or the dental nurse. When the patient feels ready, treatment starts. When the patient's activation increases, then he/she gives a signal and the dentist stops working. Instructions for systematic relaxation procedures are given. When the patient feels calm and ready, the treatment continues. It is important to teach the patient to be familiar with his/her bodily activation and to be sure that the patient feels safe and able to stop the treatment. It is also important to stop before the activation gets too high. Ideally, the patient shall stop early, as soon as he/she feels the activation starting to increase. With repeated cycles of treatment/relaxation breaks, the bodily activation and the feeling of fear eventually decreases. This method has been tested in applied relaxation training [19, 20].

advance and practicing relaxation in combination with start- and stop signals we will control your anxiety like this (draw). Your anxiety will rise. It is important for you to concentrate on observing where and how you feel the anxiety in the body, and ask me to stop when it rises, as we discussed in the coping plan (see page...). We will take breaks to work with relaxation, and when you feel comfortable and ready, we start up again. As you get used to the situation your activation will decrease and usually the need for breaks will be reduced. In this way slowly and calmly, we will get your dental treatment done. How does this sound to you, do you feel like trying?

RITA: – I think this sounds a bit scary, but at the same time I think it is worth a try (● Fig. 12.5). ◄

12.3.4.2 Increasing Activation When the Patient Is at the Lower End of the Window of Tolerance

A main rule is to stop when anxiety activation decreases beyond control and introduce coping strategies.

  The objective of the coping strategies is to increase activation, "wake up" the patient, and make the patient be more at present.

  The most common problem with decreased activation in dental care is parasympathetic activation.

Parasympathetic activation may result in a sudden decrease in blood pressure and result in fainting or almost fainting [22]. Ordinary symptoms are dizziness, cold sweating, and a fear of "disappearing." It is when receiving injections that these reactions are most often seen.

Applied tension is like applied relaxation developed by Öst and Sterner [23]. In contrast to applied relaxation, applied tension aims to counteract the fall in blood pressure by increasing the blood pressure by tightening the big muscle groups in the legs, thighs, buttocks, stomach, chest, and back. It is based on two basic components: (1) the patient learns to tighten the large muscles and (2) the patient learns to recognize the early signs of a fall in blood pressure (for instance, feeling dizzy, cold, sweaty) [23].

The dentist shows the patient how to tense the large muscle groups in the body by increasing the tension in the legs, buttocks, hands, and arms over 15 s.

> **Tip**
>
> Applied tension:
>   DENTIST: Draw both hands into your fists. Pull your fists into your chest and hold for 15 s, squeezing as tight as you can, I will count to 15, then you shall relax for 30 s. We will follow this procedure 5 times.

It may be useful to hold a mirror in front of the patient to observe how the increased blood pressure will make the face redder.

During the injection, the patient pulls his/her fists toward his/her chest squeezing as tightly as possible. To further increase blood pressure, the patient may lift up his/her legs and move the feet in the air and, in this manner, activate muscles in the legs and the stomach. This method is effective in physically increasing activation and might have additional benefits as a distraction.

More seldom, but all the same maybe more easily overlooked, is decreased activation. It primary affects traumatized patients. Decreased activation occurs when the patient approaches a fawn condition. From a trauma perspective, this may be called submission or dissociation (see ▶ Chap. 2). This is a complex reaction and will be described in more detail in other chapters.

Grounding techniques are strategies that can be used to help patients focus on what they observe in their present environment to wake up and be present and detached from the past. All senses may, in principle, be used. It is important to know that these strategies are individualized and what works for one patient may not work for another. Thus, these strategies should be discussed in advance. Often, patients have used strategies in other situations that can be used in the dental office as well. Some easily accessible strategies are mentioned here:

> **Tip**
>
> "Keep your feet on the floor, can you feel that you have contact with the floor"
>   "Feel how you sit in the chair, how you are in contact with the material of the chair"
>   "Rub your hands against your thighs. Feel the pressure on your skin."
>   "Can you tell me the time and date of today."
>   "Focus upon the body – curl and stretch your toes". Body scanning maybe useful here.
>   "Look around the room, spot three blue things, focus on the details."
>   "Touch this object, focus upon whether it is smooth or rough, hard or soft." A stress ball (see picture) may be helpful in this context.
>   "Can you identify some pleasant smell that arouses good associations or something unpleasant that you don't like?"
>   "Can you describe sounds that you can hear?"

12.3.4.3 Observing Patients' Presence in the Present

If patients are at a risk of staying above or below their window of tolerance, it is important to remember that their presence in the present is the antithesis of flashbacks and reliving bad experiences.

If the patient is hyperventilating or due to other reasons "disappearing" above – or below – the window of tolerance, it is recommended to establish eye contact and control breathing: "Look at me and breath in the same manner as me, in through the nose and out through the mouth."

Another effective task is to "talk the patient to the present"; this is especially important in flashbacks:

> ❯❯ It's 26 June 2020 (date today). You're in the dentist's office, you're here in Oslo (name the location). You are safe, and we are taking care of your teeth.

12.4 Part 3: Daily Practice

This section will focus on how to organize dental treatment when patients have dental anxiety.

12.4.1 Emergency Treatment

Many patients with dental anxiety seek dental treatment only in case of urgent needs. Patients in an emergency should always receive help with their pain. Sedative premedication and adequate local anesthesia as well as

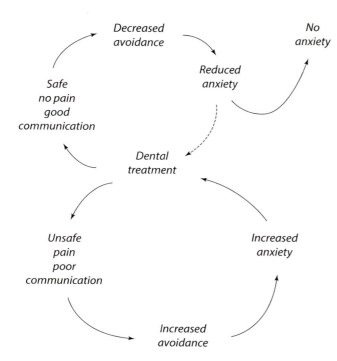

Fig. 12.6 The window of opportunity. Every dental treatment session has an oppertunity to modify dental anxiety, the figure is a modified version of Nermo et al. [24]

pre- and postoperative pain control are essential here. An emergency situation is an opportunity to motivate the patient to address the dental anxiety problem. Even in emergency situations, an appropriate treatment plan including both operative dentistry and psychological management of dental anxiety should be worked out. Treatment should never be decided without taking the patient's anxiety into consideration; the main goal should always be that the patient returns for further treatment. Often, dental anxiety patients have negative experiences in emergency situations with stressed dental professionals and little time for adequate pain control (see interpersonal circle; ▶ Chap. 12). On the other hand, if the emergency generates positive experiences, there is a potential for reducing dental anxiety. In a study among adolescences from Norway, Nermo et al. found that large treatment needs in combination with low pain experiences decreased dental anxiety [24]. One positive dental experience may turn a vicious negative cycle of dental anxiety into a positive circle, which leads to overcoming the anxiety (▶ Fig. 12.6).

12.4.2 Elective Treatment

A friendly welcome and a minimum amount of waiting time is a good start. Talking to the patient in a neutral area makes the patient more relaxed and may be a better atmosphere for preclinical discussion.

12.4.2.1 The Preclinical Phase

An appropriate treatment plan including both operative dentistry and psychological management of dental anxiety based on shared decision-making should be outlined. The dentist is responsible for fulfilling all components of an informed consent in a manner that the patient experiences ownership of the plan (see ▶ Chap. 6).

Patients may want more comprehensive treatments once they understand that they are able to cope with the dental treatment situation than they were able to prior to the treatment. To increase patients' motivation, it is important to initiate a treatment plan according to their preferences. Patients' preferences are probably a good starting point for the treatment, and the dentist should take into consideration the patients' requests, for instance, to improve aesthetics or eliminate pain.

Patients with dental anxiety often look at dental treatment as "black" or "white" or "success" or "failure." Thus, it is important to make clear that there are several ways to solve dental challenges. For example, one might say: "We have several options concerning how to get your dental treatment done. I suggest we start by doing this slowly with focus upon proper information and that you are in full control all the way. If you still feel uncomfortable, we have other options; for example the use of a sedative tablet, we may choose to spend more time on a more systematized treatment aimed at treating your anxiety or I can refer you to a specialist dental fear clinic."

12.4.2.2 Assessment of Dental Anxiety

Assessment of dental anxiety should be part of the general anamnesis. A question like "What's it like for you to get dental treatment?" is a good starting point.

> ▶ Example
>
> RITA: – I don't like dental treatment; in fact I have dental anxiety
>
> DENTIST: – Thank you for telling me, it is important to know, and I would like to know your thoughts about what made you develop dental anxiety.
>
> RITA: – My dentist as a child held me down during treatment, it was awful.
>
> DENTIST: – I see, we know that such behavior from dental staff is very powerful for establishing anxiety. Do you remember anything else from the treatment?
>
> RITA: – Yes, it was extremely painful.
>
> DENTIST: – That is a vicious combination, feeling helpless due to being held down in combination with pain, how was your social support?
>
> RITA: – What do you mean?
>
> DENTIST: – How did the dentist and the nurse react and were you alone?

RITA: – They became angry at me. My mother was there, and she was angry too.

DENTIST: – This was a very bad start, how was your dental anxiety after this?

RITA: – I have never liked dentists after that, as an adolescent I had a dentist that was OK, but as an adult I have only been to emergency treatments when in pain and it has always been painful. ◄

In addition to asking, it is beneficial to use a validated questionnaire, which may well be completed in advance. The dentist is obliged to go through the results together with the patient; otherwise, the patient will feel neglected.

The Modified Dental Anxiety Scale (MDAS) is extremely easy to use and has been shown to correspond well with patients' anxiety levels [25]. The MDAS is available in many languages, see: https://www.st-andrews.ac.uk/dentalanxiety/.

Another useful questionnaire may be the Index of Dental Anxiety and Fear-4c (IDAF-4c) [26]. This is a more comprehensive questionnaire that provides more specific information.

12.4.2.3 Devising a Coping Plan with the Patient

Coping techniques are beneficial for anxious patients [9]. A coping plan is a tool that can be used to ensure that the dental professionals and the patient agree on the framework of treatment. The aim is to make an individual "recipe" to ensure the best possible dental treatment situation (◘ Fig. 12.7).

◘ Fig. 12.7 Coping plan exemplified by Rita

Coping plan for *Rita*

The aim of the coping plan is to facilitate a best possible treatment situation during dental treatment.

WHAT the dentist/dental hygienist/dental nurse needs to know about me (background, cause of fear, special needs, triggers):

- *I was held down during painful dental treatment as a child and have had dental anxiety as long as I can remember. Even getting an injection is painful.*

My catastrophe thoughts/ what I'm most afraid of:

- *Pain. When in pain, the dentist won`t stop, telling me I should manage this. This will leave me feeling helpless/ridiculous.*

What increases my   anxiety?

- *Expectations and feelings of pain and to feel out of control during treatment.*

What do I do if I feel the anxiety rises (my coping strategies)?

- *Focus om breathing, give a stop signal and ask the dentist to take a break, if pain give me more local anesthesia*

My bodily reactions when anxiety rises (to be observed by the dentist/dental hygienist/dental nurse):

- *Muscular tension maybe best to observe by watching my arms and hands. In addition: sweating, short breathing. I tend to become quiet and obedient to what the dentist tells me*

Relevant adaptions (breaks, quality of dialogue, explanation, counting during treatment, etc.):

- *Explain everything to me, use enough local anesthetics, listen when I have worries, give me opportunity to take a break.*

Stop signals:

- *I raise my left hand when my anxiety rises,or I want a beak*

Routine in case of cancellations/no show:

- *Send me an SMS the day before, and if I don't show up give me a call*

Utilizing a coping plan can create a win-win situation: the patient becomes more confident that the dentist understands his/her needs and the dentist will have relevant information and feel more secure when trying to respond to the specific needs of this unique patient. It is important to stress that this is a flexible plan that can be used during treatment.

The process will probably be best and most efficient if the dentist asks open-ended questions and discusses coping techniques based on the patient's former experiences with coping strategies during dentistry or in other contexts. Working together with the coping plan provides the basis for a more efficient treatment and, consequently, may act as a time-effective task.

12.4.2.4 The Clinical Examination Phase

The clinical examination phase has a great potential for testing both reactions to having the dentist's instruments and fingers in the oral cavity and for practicing start/stop signals.

Many patients feel anxious about the probe since they have experiences of unpredictable pain when dentists have examined their teeth with a probe. As a ground rule, the probe should be used only when necessary and when the patient is prepared for it. Focus should be on giving an adequate explanation of why and when a probe is needed. Many patients benefit from the knowledge that scratching is an unpleasant sound but means that the tooth is healthy.

It is also important to provide patients with a realistic picture of their own dental status to increase their feeling of being in control.

> ► Example
>
> "I will start in the right side of the upper jaw and I will all the way tell you what I find. I start with the back tooth, it has a big hole, but it can be repaired, the next is the sixth year molar, is very broken so it's probably lost, but the two next ones it seem healthy, the canine is also absolutely fine and it's very good as the canine is a very important tooth in the dental arch" etc. ◄

To increase control further, a hand mirror may be useful. As the mouth is so highly innervated, small changes (a swelling or a lost part of a filling) are enlarged and feel huge. The mirror may help check in with reality, challenging the fantasy and catastrophic thoughts. Ideally, all dental anxiety patients should test using a hand mirror during the dental examination, and many patients have found this to be beneficial, even if they did not think so initially. Many patients are reluctant to use a mirror, and the dentist should undermine the importance of using a mirror during examination and treatment. It is important that the patient her/himself holds the mirror so that she/he can decide how much she/he

wants to see. Mirrors fixed on the unit may be counterproductive. The patient may feel compelled to look.

12.4.2.5 The Clinical Phase of Dental Treatment

Tell–show–do is an effective method when introducing children to dentistry [27]. The concept of explain–ask–show–do is based on tell–show–do and applied in relaxation and is well-suited for anxious adult patients. The dentist explains the procedure and what the patient is expected to experience and answers any questions that the patient may have. Then, the dentist asks for permission to move on to "show" and "do." If the patient's dental anxiety is moderate, then this may be the first method to check out. If the anxiety is more severe or the patient does not benefit adequately, then more elaborate psychoeducation and coping strategies described earlier in this chapter should be introduced.

Many patients with anxiety have reported dentists as being supportive at the beginning of treatment, but, eventually, the dentist "forgets my anxiety and just keeps going." To counteract this development, it may be useful to plan the dental treatment as a work with many subtasks. Between each subtask, the patient should be "reset" physically and mentally and get ready to take on the next part of the treatment.

The more anxious the patient is, the more subtasks are needed (■ Fig. 12.8).

> Tip
>
> Explain–ask–show–do should be used in this combination:
> – Explain–ask–show–do
> – + Proper communication (see ► Chap. 6)
> – + Systematic relaxation training (see ■ Fig. 12.5)

12.4.3 Psychological Management in Combination with Pharmacological Sedation

The use of benzodiazepines or nitrous oxide gas has been shown to be useful tools for patients with dental anxiety [16, 28–30]. General anesthesia may also be a treatment option in patients with severe dental anxiety problems.

However, sedation and general anesthesia should always be a supplement to psychological management. In patients with dental anxiety without complex comorbidities (cognitive impairment, chronic psychiatric diseases, etc.), a successful treatment outcome is to cope without sedation. Sedation may still help us reach this goal, since treatment sessions while sedated, when

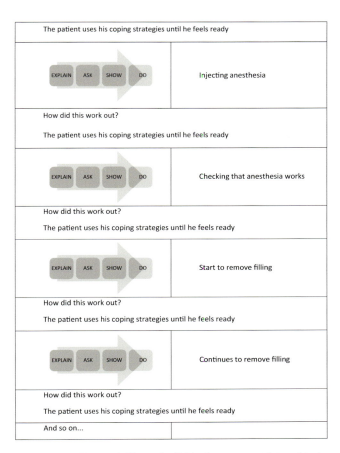

The patient uses his coping strategies until he feels ready

| EXPLAIN ASK SHOW DO | Injecting anesthesia |

How did this work out?

The patient uses his coping strategies until he feels ready

| EXPLAIN ASK SHOW DO | Checking that anesthesia works |

How did this work out?

The patient uses his coping strategies until he feels ready

| EXPLAIN ASK SHOW DO | Start to remove filling |

How did this work out?

The patient uses his coping strategies until he feels ready

| EXPLAIN ASK SHOW DO | Continues to remove filling |

How did this work out?

The patient uses his coping strategies until he feels ready

And so on...

◘ **Fig. 12.8** How to deliberately divide the treatment into subtasks and use "explain–ask–show–do"

combined with adequate psychological management, can provide good experiences. Moreover, clinical evidence shows that these good experiences may increase confidence and patients may after some sessions be able to expose themselves to treatment also without being sedated. The downside is that being sedated may also inhibit learning, implying that exposure while sedated is less efficient than it would have been without sedation.

Some indications are as follows:

Need for dental treatment in combination with high dental anxiety and/or low motivation.

Comprehensive dental treatment (for example, surgical interventions or large-scale prosthetic preparations).

Strong gagging reflexes.

A relatively short half-life is desirable for dental treatment. Some of the medications recommended, such as midazolam, have an extremely short half-life and the effect may decrease toward the end of the treatment. However, the drug may be highly beneficial as the anxiety most often is the highest at the start of a treatment; this is particularly true for patients with a fear of injections.

Benzodiazepines can also be used as a premedication to improve sleep the night before treatment. A patient

who arrives at the clinic exhausted from lack of sleep due to worries and fears has less resources for working with anxiety reactions and coping strategies.

It should be noted that patients may experience hallucinations during sedation. Therefore, to ensure the patient's safety and prevent false complaints, the dentist should always be assisted by at least one dental nurse.

> **Tip**
>
> Pharmacological sedation should always be used combination with psychological management:
> - Pharmacological sedation
> - + Explain–ask–show–do
> - + Proper communication (see ▶ Chap. 6)
> - + Systematic relaxation training (see ◘ Fig. 12.5)

12.4.4 Cooperation with the Patient's Doctor/Psychologist

Rita has relatively understandable dental anxiety. In cases where the patient has a more complex background and/or dysfunctional personality traits, it is beneficial to cooperate with the patient's physician, psychologist, or therapist. The dentist may consult with the physician, psychologist, or therapist (provided the patient gives consent) or a common consultation may be arranged. Clinical experiences show beneficial outcomes by making the dentist and physician, psychologist, or therapist gain better understanding of each other's treatment arrangements. If the patient is in the middle of a psychological treatment, it may be wise to adapt to anxiety/dental treatment in the process of the psychological treatment. When the patient's dental anxiety is part of general mental problems, it may be beneficial to plan appointments with the therapist before or after the dental appointment.

> **Box 12.2**
>
> **A clinical psychologist treating adult patients with severe dental anxiety**
>
> by Ulla Wide, licensed psychologist, Clinic of oral medicine, Public Dental Service, Region Västra Götaland, Sweden
>
> I work at the Clinic of Oral Medicine, Public Dental Service. My assignment includes anamnestic interviews, treatment planning, and delivering individual CBT for adult patients with severe dental anxiety/phobia. I work in a multiprofessional team with dentists, dental nurses, and dental hygienists, with regular team meetings and collaboration for both the assessment and the treatment of patients.

12

When I meet a new patient, the patient has already met a dentist for an anamnestic interview (no clinical examination) and has answered screening questionnaires, now available to me. Two hours are scheduled for my interview, including time for administration. Usually, patients react with strong emotions, both anxiety and sadness, but also with hope on realizing that help exists. After the interview, I meet the dentist to plan for both CBT and dental treatment, including managing acute oral treatment needs. Since most patients have a deteriorated oral status, the CBT and dental treatment must be sensibly integrated. Our primary goal is to cure patients' severe dental anxiety/phobia.

The exposure-based CBT is adapted for each patient following a behavioral functional analysis and includes progressive relaxation and cognitive restructuring. Many patients also need trauma-related interventions, self-assertiveness, and applied tension techniques. I meet the patient for eight 50 min sessions, for 2–3 months, at the dental clinic in a fully equipped dental room. Graded exposure, the most important CBT intervention, is achieved using the dental room with all instruments available. However, most important is the use of film scenes of a non-dentally anxious individual undergoing dental treatment. My patient views the scenes sitting in the dental treatment chair, and I sit beside, sharing the view. The last session includes a prevention program and planning of the continued treatment with the dental team and, thereafter, referral to general dentistry. I deliver the eight-session CBT in one sequence, and, thereafter, the patient (without the psychologist) attends dental treatment with the dentist who performed the assessment. The dental treatment is a form of behavioral experiment, in CBT terminology.

12.4.5 Common Reactions in Scared Patients

Patients can be perceived as difficult or demanding if you do not understand why they react as they do. To react adequately, it is important to understand some of the most common patient reactions.

Patients who cancel: Patients who delay or cancel treatment sessions as avoidance strategy enhance development and maintenance of dental anxiety.

Patients who are angry and/or naughty: When the anxiety levels are high, it is difficult to distinguish between anger and fear. Milgrom characterized a group of dental anxiety patients as "goers but haters" [31]. These are patients who from the very beginning express aggressiveness such as starting the conversation with "I hate dentists." Some patients do not acknowledge their anxiety. They say "I'm not afraid," while their body language expresses anxiety.

Patients who are suspicious: Patients who have a complex case of dental anxiety often are distrustful of dentists. Dental health staff can be accused of evil intent, which can be perceived as highly unreasonable. It is useful to remind yourself that the underlying feeling may be anxiety and that the patient very rarely has a desire to be "difficult." Other patients are suspicious of almost everyone they meet as part of their personality or personality disorder.

Patients who cry: Crying is an emotional expression that may feel shameful to adults. However, it may be helpful to cry when in need of it, and dental professionals should be emphatic and always say, "It is totally OK to cry" or feel free to ask an open question about how patients want their crying to be taken into account. This is highly individualized. Some patients think that it is okay to keep going with the treatment even if they cry, whereas others need time to reconsolidate. The main thing is to make crying harmless.

Summary

Adequate psychological management of dental anxiety is important to treat and prevent anxiety and, consequently, to prevent poor oral health. Whatever the method, the patient rarely gets completely rid of his/her anxiety but can learn to endure, understand, verbalize, regulate, deal with, and live with it and not let it control the patient's choices. Treatment may be successful, but the risk of relapse is relatively high.

- The more knowledge about anxiety treatment, the better the treatment that can be offered and the safer the patient and the dentist feel.
- The dentist–patient relationship has a decisive impact on the results of dental anxiety treatment and must have high priority.
- The patient should be in "the driver's seat" and given control over his/her treatment situation.
- An individual coping plan is a useful and time-efficient tool.
- Explain–tell–show–do provides predictability and control throughout the treatment.
- Sedation should never be used alone but as a supplement to psychological management of dental anxiety.

References

1. Strom K, Ronneberg A, Skaare AB, Espelid I, Willumsen T. Dentists' use of behavioural management techniques and their attitudes towards treating paediatric patients with dental anxiety. Eur Arch Paediatr Dent. 2015;16(4):349–55.

2. Moore R, Brodsgaard I, Rosenberg N. The contribution of embarrassment to phobic dental anxiety: a qualitative research study. BMC Psychiatry. 2004;4:10.

3. Bernson JM, Elfstrom ML, Hakeberg M. Dental coping strategies, general anxiety, and depression among adult patients with dental anxiety but with different dental-attendance patterns. Eur J Oral Sci. 2013;121(3 Pt 2):270–6.

4. Logan HL, Baron RS, Keeley K, Law A, Stein S. Desired control and felt control as mediators of stress in a dental setting. Health Psychol. 1991;10(5):352–9.

5. Ronneberg A, Strom K, Skaare AB, Willumsen T, Espelid I. Dentists' self-perceived stress and difficulties when performing restorative treatment in children. Eur Arch Paediatr Dent. 2015;16(4):341–7.

6. Lutz W, Leon SC, Martinovich Z, Lyons JS, Stiles WB. Therapist effects in outpatien psychotherapy. J Couns Psychol. 2007;54(1):32–9.

7. Armfield JM, Heaton LJ. Management of fear and anxiety in the dental clinic: a review. Aust Dent J. 2013;58(4):390–407; quiz 531.

8. Foa EB. Prolonged exposure therapy: past, present, and future. Depress Anxiety. 2011;28(12):1043–7.

9. Bernson JM, Hallberg LR, Elfstrom ML, Hakeberg M. 'Making dental care possible: a mutual affair': a grounded theory relating to adult patients with dental fear and regular dental treatment. Eur J Oral Sci. 2011;119(5):373–80.

10. Davies EB, Buchanan H. An exploratory study investigating children's perceptions of dental behavioural management techniques. Int J Paediatr Dent. 2013;23(4):297–309.

11. Moola S, Pearson A, Mejia G. A comprehensive systematic review of evidence on the feasibility, appropriateness, meaningfulness and effectiveness of management of dental anxiety and dental fear in paediatric and adult patients. JBI Libr Syst Rev. 2012;10(56 Suppl):1–26.

12. Bradt J, Dileo C, Magill L, Teague A. Music interventions for improving psychological and physical outcomes in cancer patients. Cochrane Database Syst Rev. 2016;8:CD006911.

13. Lahmann C, Schoen R, Henningsen P, Ronel J, Muehlbacher M, Loew T, et al. Brief relaxation versus music distraction in the treatment of dental anxiety: a randomized controlled clinical trial. J Am Dent Assoc. 2008;139(3):317–24.

14. Triller N, Erzen D, Duh S, Petrinec Primozic M, Kosnik M. Music during bronchoscopic examination: the physiological effects. A randomized trial. Respiration. 2006;73(1):95–9.

15. Melzack R, Wall PD. Pain mechanisms: a new theory. Science. 1965;150(3699):971–9.

16. Gordon D, Heimberg RG, Tellez M, Ismail AI. A critical review of approaches to the treatment of dental anxiety in adults. J Anxiety Disord. 2013;27(4):365–78.

17. Berggren U, Hakeberg M, Carlsson SG. Relaxation vs. cognitively oriented therapies for dental fear. J Dent Res. 2000;79(9):1645–51.

18. Lundgren J, Carlsson SG, Berggren U. Relaxation versus cognitive therapies for dental fear – a psychophysiological approach. Health Psychol. 2006;25(3):267–73.

19. Ost LG, Sterner U, Fellenius J. Applied tension, applied relaxation, and the combination in the treatment of blood phobia. Behav Res Ther. 1989;27(2):109–21.

20. Willumsen T, Vassend O. Effects of cognitive therapy, applied relaxation and nitrous oxide sedation. A five-year follow-up study of patients treated for dental fear. Acta Odontol Scand. 2003;61(2):93–9.

21. Appukuttan DP, Tadepalli A, Victor DJ, Dharuman S. Oral health related quality of life among tamil speaking adults attending a dental institution in Chennai, Southern India. J Clin Diagn Res. 2016;10(10):ZC114–ZC20.

22. Ayala ES, Meuret AE, Ritz T. Treatments for blood-injury-injection phobia: a critical review of current evidence. J Psychiatr Res. 2009;43(15):1235–42.

23. Ost LG, Sterner U. Applied tension. A specific behavioral method for treatment of blood phobia. Behav Res Ther. 1987;25(1):25–9.

24. Nermo H, Willumsen T, Johnsen JK. Prevalence of dental anxiety and associations with oral health, psychological distress, avoidance and anticipated pain in adolescence: a cross-sectional study based on the Tromso study, Fit Futures. Acta Odontol Scand. 2019;77(2):126–34.

25. Humphris GM, Morrison T, Lindsay SJ. The modified dental anxiety scale: validation and United Kingdom norms. Community Dent Health. 1995;12(3):143–50.

26. Armfield JM. Development and psychometric evaluation of the Index of Dental Anxiety and Fear (IDAF-4C+). Psychol Assess. 2010;22(2):279–87.

27. Brahm CO, Lundgren J, Carlsson SG, Nilsson P, Hultqvist J, Hagglin C. Dentists' skills with fearful patients: education and treatment. Eur J Oral Sci. 2013;121(3 Pt 2):283–91.

28. Ogle OE, Hertz MB. Anxiety control in the dental patient. Dent Clin N Am. 2012;56(1):1–16, vii.

29. Willumsen T, Vassend O, Hoffart A. A comparison of cognitive therapy, applied relaxation, and nitrous oxide sedation in the treatment of dental fear. Acta Odontol Scand. 2001;59(5):290–6.

30. Hauge MS, Stora B, Vassend O, Hoffart A, Willumsen T. Dentist-administered cognitive behavioural therapy versus four habits/midazolam: An RCT study of dental anxiety treatment in primary dental care. Eur J Oral Sci. 2021;129(4):e12794.

31. Milgrom P, Weinstein P, Heaton LJ. Treating fearful dental patients a patient management handbook. Third ed. Seattle, Washington: Dental Behavioral Resources; 1996. 2009.

12

Dentist-Administered CBT for Dental Anxiety

Mariann Saanum Hauge, Tiril Willumsen, and Bent Storå

Contents

Learning Goals
- To be able to recognize patients who may benefit from D-CBT
- To understand the rationale behind D-CBT
- To gain knowledge about how to use the D-CBT manual

13.1   An Evidence-Based Treatment Method for Dental Anxiety

13.1.1   Cognitive Behavioral Therapy (CBT)

Cognition refers to thinking or more explicitly "all forms of knowing and awareness, such as perceiving, conceiving, remembering, reasoning, judging, imagining, and problem solving," and cognitive psychology is the "scientific study of mental processes such as attention, language use, memory, perception, problem solving, creativity, and thinking" [1] (▶ Chap. 1). Cognitive therapy was developed by Aron T. Beck and Albert E. Ellis in the 1960s [2], and, today, the term includes several slightly different treatment methods.

> CBT presupposes the following:
> - Cognitive activity affects behavior
> - Cognitive activity can be supervised and changed
> - Behavioral change can be achieved through changing cognitions [3]

13.1.2   CBT in the Treatment of Dental Anxiety

Cognitive behavioral therapy (CBT) is the best documented psychological treatment for a number of psychological disorders, including anxiety [4, 5]. CBT has both a cognitive and a behavioral component. The cognitive component of CBT focuses on changing negative cognitions. A patient that suffers from social anxiety may experience thoughts like: "everybody will look at me and dislike me," which can prevent him from going to the supermarket. If thoughts about how people think about him are altered, then this may enable him to go shopping again. The behavioral component is, on the other hand, directed primarily toward the behavior, e.g., if the patient practices by going to the supermarket, he will understand through experience that the negative thought was untrue (everybody did not stare), and, in this manner, a behavioral change might in fact lead to a change in the way of thinking [4].

CBT has been well-established as an effective treatment for both dental anxiety and intraoral injection phobia [6–10]. In most studies on CBT for the treatment of dental anxiety, interdisciplinary teams of psychologists and dentists are responsible for the treatment [7]. However, Agdal et al. obtained good results from dentist-administered CBT of oral injection phobia after assessment by a psychologist. Haukebo et al. described a similar treatment model for dental phobia with promising results [9], and Willumsen showed that CBT with focus on cognitions and relaxation administered by a dentist without assessment of a psychologist had comparable and positive effects, even from a 5-year perspective [11, 12]. The authors of this chapter have obtained favorable long-term results with the use of D-CBT as depicted below [10, 13].

13.1.3   What Is New in D-CBT?

The D-CBT manual has been adapted from manuals of CBT used in treatment of anxiety and interdisciplinary treatment of dental anxiety [14]. A novel feature is that the method is adjusted to fit within the framework of a general dental practice and to be administered by a dentist without the imminent support of a psychologist. What is also new is a detailed practical treatment manual.

13.2   Treatment Requirements

13.2.1   Manualized Treatment

Even when therapists utilize a manualized method, research shows deviations from the manual during treatment and also that the effect of treatment is reduced when the manual is not adhered to [5]. The manualized treatment described later in this chapter must therefore be administered in its original form to ensure a predictable result of treatment. D-CBT has been tested against a combination of the Four Habits Model and midazolam in a randomized controlled trial (RCT) in a general dental practice. The manual can be downloaded from the web resources of the University of Oslo The University of Oslo, Faculty of Dentistry. Practical manual D-CBT. https://www.odont.uio.no/iko/om/organisasjon/fagavd/pedodontiatferdsfag/rutiner-og-metoder/kommunikasjon-og-tannbehandlingsangst/ and is available in the Supplementary section of the corresponding article [10, 15].

13.2.2   Dentist Requirements

Dentists who educate themselves and train for use of D-CBT must have detailed knowledge about oral health psychology. Reading this entire book (not just some chapters) may serve as basic knowledge.

Therapist characteristics impact the treatment results to a considerable degree, even when the treatment is manualized [16]. This means that it is not sufficient to adequately learn a manualized method to achieve a good outcome of treatment. Dentists learning D-CBT must also receive training in establishing a good rapport with patients and strive to induce hope.

A dentist should not start treating patients with D-CBT if incompetent or not interested in achieving competence in the requirements that are described below. However, when unable to deliver the proper treatment, it is a professional's ethical duty to refer patients with the need for anxiety treatment to personnel with the adequate competence [17].

> **Box**
>
> The code of ethics for dentists in the European Union (2.10) is as follows:
>
> The dentist must undertake only those treatments that he/she is competent to perform, and must refer a patient if a recommended treatment is beyond their competence. [17]

13.2.3 Practical Training

Practice is necessary for optimal performance of D-CBT and should be rehearsed through role play and video recordings accompanied by competent guidance. It is preferable that the first patients present with uncomplicated dental anxiety.

13.2.4 A Clear Definition of the Role of the Dentist

The dentist is not supposed to act as a psychologist but more like a counselor that can aid in moving the patient forward through a systematized method and positive reinforcements. The dentist should not involve himself or herself in psychological issues other than dental anxiety, except for health conditions relevant to the dental anxiety treatment.

13.3 When Is D-CBT Applicable?

- D-CBT is appropriate for youth and adults that find it hard to go through with dental treatment or in other ways struggle to take care of their oral health due to anxiety.
- D-CBT is not suitable for patients not motivated for treatment or for patients that have problems communicating with the dentist (due to, for example, language difficulties or weakened cognitive skills).
- D-CBT is not always advisable if the patient has numerous other complaints. This could be, for example, a life crisis, physical or psychological disease, or substance abuse. If this is the case, it might be useful to collaborate with other health personnel in taking care of the patient or sometimes wait until a better suited moment in time. Oral health must be taken care of using, for example, sedation or general anesthetics while waiting for a better opportunity to treat the patient's anxiety.

Exposure treatment with D-CBT requires that the patient confronts his/her anxiety. This may be extremely challenging. However, for many patients, positive side effects are seen in other aspects of their life. Studies have shown increased quality of life and enhanced psychological health after CBT for dental anxiety and injection phobia [13, 18]. An individualized assessment of the ability to follow through with treatment, of the individual cost of the treatment, and of the potential for personal gain should be carried out in close collaboration with the patient. This evaluation is necessary when deciding, with the patient, whether D-CBT would be the right choice of treatment.

Although D-CBT has been reported to be a robust treatment method suitable for a heterogeneous sample of dental anxiety patients, including patients with traumatic life experiences [10], it is important to keep in mind that complications may occur. Thus, it is recommended to have an emergency plan ready. Studies show that patients often do not tell dental personnel about their traumatic experiences [19]. This is reason to believe that traumatic experiences increase the risk that negative reactions may be triggered by the treatment situation. Reactions that may arise are long-lasting dissociation, anxiety, and nightmares. The patient's physician or psychologist can be important collaborators in the development of an emergency plan. Another option can be to establish an agreement with psychologists in the vicinity of the clinic to assure access to proper help if needed.

During exposure in D-CBT, in principle the patient should always be inside of his/her window of tolerance. Being outside of the window of tolerance can be beneficial to treatment effect when the patient copes well, but, if the patient cannot be helped back into the window of tolerance relatively fast, then D-CBT should be reassessed and other treatment alternatives considered.

13.4 Practical Arrangements

The manual is designed to be administered by a dentist and is completed in five consultations with a total duration of a maximum of 300 minutes. The appointments should be scheduled within a tight time frame to prevent relapse of anxiety between consultations. Weekly sessions are often suitable, and it might be useful with fixed weekdays and hours. The treatment can be conducted in a dental office. It may, however, be advantageous to complete the first appointment in a neutral room since this might ease the attendance for the patient. The intervention should not be interrupted by distractions (e.g., the secretary coming and going, telephones ringing, the use of a personal computer (PC)). It is important to stay within the time schedule and thereby allow for adequate closure of each consultation. It can be useful to talk about the schedule before and during the appointment. An example on how to talk about the time schedule: "This is good, now we have 20 minutes left to work further."

13.5 Step-by-Step Use of the D-CBT Manual

The manual will be illustrated through the treatment of Kristin.

13.5.1 Before the First Treatment Session

> ► Example
>
> Kristin's husband contacted the clinic on behalf of his wife. She is a 36-year-old woman who last saw a dentist 7 years ago. A dental nurse, Linda, listened to Kristin's husband, gave him positive feedback for helping his wife out in this matter, explained how D-CBT works, and offered a first appointment for explaining how the treatment is carried out. ◄

13.5.2 The First Treatment Session (60 Minutes)

> ► Example
>
> When entering the waiting room, Kristin is greeted by Linda and given a health form and the Modified Dental Anxiety Scale (MDAS) questionnaire. The dentist invites her into the dental treatment room.
>
> Kristin is seated in a regular chair alongside the PC desk instead of the dental chair. She immediately says that it felt easier to enter the dental office when she knew the plan for the first appointment was to talk with the dentist rather than undergo regular dental treatment. ◄

13.5.2.1 Establishing a Good Relationship

Establishing a good relationship is a continuous task. However, the first few minutes or even seconds give a first impression that, if the patient feels seen and understood, can make a robust platform. For many patients, it can be advantageous to start out with a bit of small talk, keeping in mind the principles on how to build an alliance (► Chap. 4) and the Four Habits Model for adequate communication (► Chap. 6). It is beneficial to ask open-ended questions.

> ► Example
>
> DENTIST: – It is really good that your husband has encouraged you to come here today, how did you find our office?
>
> KRISTIN: – He has been trying for some time now to make me seek treatment for my dental fears, and finally he succeeded. We have heard about you from our friend Brittany. She recommended you.
>
> DENTIST: – Thank you, that was kind of Brittany, and I will do my best to fulfill your expectations. It is very important that we are honest with each other. I want you to keep in mind that if anything doesn't work out well for you, I would appreciate it if you told me immediately. Otherwise, I might not understand that something is wrong, and consequently I may not be able to adjust the treatment to your needs.
>
> We work with a specific treatment method that I would like to tell you about, but first I would like to hear more about your background and your motivation. I can see that according to this MDAS questionnaire, your scores om dental anxiety are 19, which indicate a quite serious dental anxiety. I would very much like to know how this anxiety developed. ◄

13.5.2.2 Background, the Patient's Problem, and Motivation

It is important to let patients tell their story and show empathy for the experiences they choose to share with the dental personnel. However, the dentist has the responsibility to try and keep the focus on issues directly related to the dental anxiety. The patient should be made aware that only the headlines of their life experiences are important to offer adequate dental anxiety treatment.

Earlier treatment attempts and the degree to which they were useful to the patient may also be important background information. Coping strategies learned in other psychological therapies might be successfully employed in further D-CBT.

KRISTIN: – I had a lot of cavities growing up, and dental visits were always painful. I also had bad experiences with the orthodontist; he was rough, and the treatment was painful. And once I was held down by the dental nurse and my mother, while the dentist removed a tooth that was not fully anesthetized. From the time that I was old enough to decide for myself whether to attend or not I have only visited dentists when I have been in pain, and I think that it has always been awful.

DENTIST: – I can see why dental treatment is difficult for you. These episodes must have challenged your sense of personal safety. Traumatic incidents like these may severely influence your level of anxiety when you are in a dental chair. Your history with the dentist could make anyone anxious of dental treatment.

DENTIST: – Do you have other traumatic experiences that could have affected your dental anxiety? This could be for example accidents, abuse, being bullied etcetera?

KRISTIN: – I was bullied in primary school. At the age of 10 I was diagnosed with ADHD, and I have always had difficulties "fitting in" with classmates.

DENTIST: – This is important information in our context. Has it ever occurred to you that there could be a connection between the harassment and the dental anxiety?

KRISTIN: – No, I have never thought about that.

DENTIST: – I think this is an important part of your history and it may be relevant to your dental anxiety. I think it is very important that we focus on your sense of control in the dental situation. We will never do anything to you that you have not previously consented to. Have you ever been treated for dental anxiety, or for other anxieties before?

KRISTIN: – No

DENTIST: – OK, do you have other anxieties or phobias?

KRISTIN: – I fear snakes and spiders, but not to an extent that it prevents me from doing any activities that I like to do.

DENTIST: – OK that is good to know. We can offer you several options for dental treatment, including our treatment program D-CBT, depending upon your treatment goals. Do you have any thoughts about the best way that we can help you?

KRISTIN: – I want to get rid of my anxiety, so that I can be able to attend regular dental visits.

DENTIST: – It seems like you could benefit from the treatment program D-CBT. ◄

13.5.2.3 Psychoeducation

The patient's individual symptoms of anxiety are mapped. In this manner, the patient becomes more conscious about individual reaction patterns and learns to identify signals like stomach pain and sweaty hands as signs of anxiety. This insight can in itself be anxiety-reducing. An explanation of the symptoms based on human's natural fear response is provided. This normalizes the patient's reactions, as described in ► Chaps. 11 and 12.

DENTIST: – We will now explore your reactions during dental treatment. How does your body feel when you are in a dental chair?

KRISTIN: – I feel very tense!

DENTIST: – Do you mean that you feel tense in your muscles?

KRISTIN: – My body tightens up completely. I am completely exhausted after appointments.

DENTIST: – And your heartbeat?

KRISTIN: – My heart beats fast.

DENTIST: – This happens to protect you, and an increased heart rhythm is a part of a human beings' repertoire of survival mechanisms. Your body perceives the situation as dangerous, and consequently puts the muscles into high alert, and your heart beats fast to make you ready to flee from or fight the danger. It is completely normal that your body reacts this way to a perceived threat. This process happens without conscious thought, through the part of our neural system that is automatically regulated. This way man has survived dangers throughout all ages. So, in other words, your body reacts adequately considering your past experiences. What we want is to provide you with new experiences in the dental office, to let your body experience that the dental treatment situation is not dangerous, even though your body says that it is. And eventually, with practice, being in a dental office will not initiate the fear response as it does now. Does this make sense to you? ◄

13.5.2.4 Cognitive Restructuring

The patient's involuntary thoughts about frightening events that might take place in conjunction with dental treatment are called catastrophic thoughts. In D-CBT, these thoughts are explored to increase the patient's awareness about those scenarios that frighten the patient the most. In this manner, the patient will gain better access to these frightening and anxiety-driven scenarios. The increased awareness allows for discussion and rationalization around the catastrophic thoughts.

► **Example**

DENTIST: – What are you afraid of during dental treatment?

KRISTIN: – I am afraid that the treatment will be terribly painful.

DENTIST: – How painful do you think drilling would be on a scale from 0-10?

KRISTIN: – I think it could be about 8.

DENTIST: – How probable is it that you would experience a pain of 8 when drilling, do you think?

KRISTIN: – I don' know, maybe about 30% chance.

DENTIST: – Is there any way to prevent painful treatment?

KRISTIN: – I could ask for more anesthetics. I think it would be painful even so, but maybe it would be a little better. ◄

The patient's personal experiences are also explained using known causal connections related to dental anxiety. This will give the patient a better explanation to, and a better understanding of, the reasons why dental treatment has become a trigger to the fear response. This may further normalize the patient's fearful response.

► **Example**

DENTIST: – Your dental story is loss of control, helplessness and at the same time you experienced pain. This must have felt like a dangerous situation. We know that the combination of pain and loss of control is very potent for creating anxiety, particularly for children. Anxiety has a biological purpose – to keep you from danger. Anxiety gives bodily reactions like withdrawal to protect you from experiencing this danger again. That is what the fear response was made for; to keep you out of harm, and as you see, it functions exactly the way it is supposed to. ◄

13.5.2.5   Method and Coping Techniques

In this section, the patient's individual anxiety is further explored. The patient learns about the processes that trigger his/her anxiety the most. This increased understanding facilitates the process of finding the right steps in exposure training. First, the anxiety hierarchy is established as explained in ► Chap. 12. It is essential that the patient is in the driver's seat in this process and that the dentist acts as a facilitator. Kristin's anxiety hierarchy looks like this:

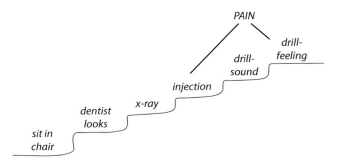

► **Example**

DENTIST: – It was great that we through this process managed to construct how YOUR anxiety looks like. As you can see the most frightening procedure to you is the sound and feeling of the drill. And that the drill may cause pain. We know for sure that pain accelerates anxiety. I think we shall focus upon two elements in our treatment. The first element is to be able to do dental treatment without pain, meaning we must work on giving you adequate local anesthesia. The other element is your fear reactions to the sound/feeling of the drill. As the sound of the drill is so connected to pain, I suggest starting out our dental anxiety treatment with exposure to the sound and feeling of the drill with a minimal risk of pain. In my experience the use of a rubber cup for polishing teeth can accomplish this. My suggestion is that we start out using a drill with rubber cup. What do you think?

KRISTIN: – Well, it sounds good, but I am a bit worried.

DENTIST: – Yes, that is why the challenges ahead will be separated into smaller task, and it is important to find a suitable first task. When you gain confidence in relation to the first task, we may go on to the next task. You will be an active part all the way and you will be in control of decision making on how and when to proceed. If there is no anxiety present there will no anxiety to reduce, but if the situation is too anxiety provoking it will be difficult for you to think rationally and you will have less capacity for learning. Therefore, we should start with a procedure that provokes your anxiety moderately. ◄

The dentist explains the anxiety curve to help the patient understand the rationale behind the stepwise exposure (see ► Chap. 12). After explaining the curve, it is important to transfer the curve to the patient's situation.

▶ **Example**

DENTIST: – In D-CBT, you will see that the frightening situation gradually becomes less frightening upon repetition. The acceptable anxiety level is different in every person, and we will try to find yours. First, we must decide what task or step you would like to practice first, then for how long the exercise should last. Afterwards we do the planned exercise, and I will ask you how elevated your anxiety level was on a scale from 1-10. We repeat the task until you feel comfortable with this step of the procedure before going on to the next step. How does this sound to you? ◀

In this phase, it is important to introduce coping strategies (see ▶ Sect. 12.3). In Kristin's case, this included the use of start and stop signals and strategies to decrease activation when at the high end of the window of tolerance (see ▶ Sect. 12.3.4).

▶ **Example**

DENTIST: – First, we must work out a way that you can say STOP to me, for instance that you raise the left hand- or we can find another signal.

KRISTIN: – I think it is a good idea to use the left hand to signal when I need to stop.

DENTIST: – Fine, and how can we ease your bodily stress?

KRISTIN: – From what we talked about; I think it can be helpful with breathing techniques

DENTIST: – I agree, lets rehearse

Linda, the nurse, gives instructions for breathing by using the "Exhale- one- two –three" method (see ▶ Chap. 12). Kristin quickly manages to control her breathing when given instructions, and she says that she wants Linda to help her "remember to breathe" during appointments. She tells the team that her acceptable level of fear during treatment is 3-4 on a scale from 0-10. ◀

13.5.3 End of the First Session: Evaluation, Alliance Check, Home Lessons, and Further Plans

At the end of each appointment, 5–10 minutes should be reserved for evaluating that day's progress and to plan the next appointment. An alliance check is also included in all D-CBT sessions. Discussing the relationship with the patient openly shows the patient that the dentist values this element. The dentist is also given an opportunity to discover and correct misunderstandings.

▶ **Example**

DENTIST: – Do I treat you with respect? Do you feel that I take your concerns seriously? Do you feel that we are a team (against the problem)? ◀

Home tasks should be part of the treatment whenever the patient accepts them. It is beneficial to be creative and find personally adjusted assignments.

Box

Some suggestions for home tasks include the following:
- Rehearse breathing techniques
- Watch educational videos about anxiety (necessary to give specific recommendations on quality material)
- Practice laying back on a chair with the mouth open.
- Record the sound of a drill on the patient's cell phone to allow him/her to listen to it at defined intervals at home
- Let the patient bring home dental equipment to be used at home (mirror, probe, impression spoon)
- Practice applied tension (when fainting is a threat – see ▶ Chap. 12)

▶ **Example**

Kristin is apparently happy with her first appointment. She says that the atmosphere and style of communication made her feel quite safe. She felt that she was met with respect, taken seriously, and the dentist had managed to make her feel a part of the team working together to combat anxiety. The first home tasks were breathing exercises, in addition to watching an educative video about anxiety.

DENTIST: – OK, let us work on the plan for the next appointment. My suggestion is to start with observing the drill with the rubber cup in place and then start working with the sound. The first task with sound could be with the drill positioned around here, about a meter away from you, and I could start the sound for 3 or 5 seconds. How does that seem to you?

KRISTIN: – A bit scary, but I will try, and I think 3 seconds is enough.

DENTIST: – Good. If it turns out that you cannot manage to do what is planned, you should still come to the next appointment. In that case, we will find a new, and more suitable, task for you. We will never do anything that we have not agreed upon.

You will be the one in the driver's seat and in control of the exercise.

KRISTIN: – OK, I think am ready for a new treatment session

DENTIST: – Good, now we have agreed that we will do exposure to the sound of the drill in the next appointment. I will hold the drill around here, about a meter away from you, in about 3 seconds and then we will see what happens to your anxiety. Gradually we will try to do the drilling closer to the mouth, but not until you feel ready to do it. Does this seem OK?" ◀

The dentist writes the plan for the next appointment and assigns home tasks along with key words about that day's treatment in the written treatment manual. The patient is encouraged to take a photograph of this page by a cell phone or, if this is not possible, the dentist provides a photocopy.

13.5.4 The Second, Third, and Fourth Appointments

The three middle sessions are quite similar in content, as described below.

13.5.4.1 Start of the Sessions: Psychoeducation and Cognitive Restructuring, Continued

In the sessions' first minutes, the treatment plan agreed upon in the former session is repeated. The present catastrophic thoughts and bodily signs of anxiety are also explored and recorded. Restructuring of the thoughts and psychoeducation is repeated. If there is a need for adjustments of the original plan, because of high anxiety or other reasons, a new plan is made.

▶ Example

Kristin's second appointment was scheduled exactly 1 week after the first one. She started by telling us that her pulse had been 107 in her pulse watch when entering the office. However, she had slept well the previous night. She felt ready to do what we had planned at our last appointment. ◀

13.5.4.2 Exposure Training

When starting the first exposure, it is always appropriate to show the equipment and explain its functions. Many patients are at this point curious and often discover that the equipment is not quite as scary as they thought it was.

Giving explanations is an integral part of the exposure. Describing the sound of the drill, why we have different speeds and different burs, and how this affects

sound and vibration is an integral part during exposure to the drill. The patients might not want to know or see, and it may be necessary to explain how knowledge most often decreases anxiety. What is known is generally less frightening than the unknown.

Sight is an important sense that should be part of all exposure training. A handheld mirror may therefore be vital during exposure in the mouth. Reluctance to use a mirror is not uncommon, and, it is, in these cases, important to highlight the advantages. Many patients, despite their initial skepticism, will be positively surprised by a feeling of enhanced control when using a mirror. By holding the mirror themselves, the patients will have control and be able to choose whether to watch or not.

All activities are initiated with a detailed explanation by the dentist about the next task and after obtaining an explicit consent from the patient that it is okay to move forward as suggested. The length of each exposure is decided by the patient (the sound of the drill in 3 seconds or 5 seconds?). The anxiety level is supervised by asking the patient and by being attentive to bodily signs of anxiety. Exposure is repeated until the anxiety level decreases to the value decided upon in the first appointment (or an adjusted value). Thereafter, the length of exposure is increased or one moves one step up in the anxiety hierarchy.

The anxiety will decrease with repeated exposures. The pace will differ massively between the patients. If anxiety levels no longer decrease, then it is necessary to take one step back and find a new task that is a little less demanding to the patient. The dentist should be supportive and always encouraging. The progress is demonstrated to the patient to increase the feeling of success and motivation for further treatment. To expose oneself to anxiety-provoking stimuli is hard work, and it is essential that the patient see value for that work.

▶ Example

DENTIST: – OK, you have seen the drill and touched the rubber cup, I will now hold the drill here (points about one meter in front of the patient), start the drill and count to 3.

Take a couple of deep breaths as we have practiced and say OK when you are ready.

KRISTIN: – (Breathes) OK

DENTIST: – 1-2-3, (places the drill back to the unit). How was this? On a scale from 110, what was your anxiety level?

KRISTIN: – Oh, I would say 8.

DENTIST: – OK, I think we should try the same exercise one more time. Try to find a comfortable position in the chair, try to relax in your shoulders and breath while I count to 3. Please let me know when you are ready to proceed.

KRISTIN: – OK, I'm ready.

DENTIST: – 1-2-3. How was this? On a scale from 1-10, what was your anxiety level?

KRISTIN: – Hmmmmm, maybe 6.

DENTIST: – That is great, why do you think it went down from 8 to 6?

KRISTIN: – Well, I knew what to expect and I think I managed to control my breathing better too.

DENTIST: – Good, let us try again!

The exercise is repeated until Kristin's score is 3.

DENTIST: – Very good, now I think you may be ready for a next step, I will suggest counting to 5 while doing the same exercise.

KRISTIN: – OK

They repeat the step until Kristin's score is 3.

DENTIST: – Very good, now I think you may be ready for another step. I will suggest that I hold the drill inside your mouth without touching any teeth while counting to 3 or 5.

(At this point, a handheld mirror should be offered to the patient.)

KRISTIN: – OK, I would like to start with counting to 3.

They repeat until Kristin's score is 3.
And so on…
The next steps could be:

1. Placing the rubber cap on the buccal surface of the tooth
2. Moving the rubber cap on the buccal surfaces of several teeth
3. Moving the rubber cap on the lingual surfaces of several teeth

Demonstrating the achievement to Kristin,

DENTIST: – When we started today your anxiety was 8 when hearing and seeing the drill on 1 meter's distance. Now you are able to let me polish your tooth with the drill inside your mouth with anxiety levels no higher than 4. Did you believe this when you came today?

KRISTIN: – No, not really.

DENTIST: – This is very good; can you see that this works?

KRISTIN: – Yes.

DENTIST: – Yes, and this is how we will continue to work with new tasks. You have challenged yourself in a very good way today!

KRISTIN: – I feel very proud of myself! What should we do next?

DENTIST: – It is important for you to remember that when the teeth have adequate local anesthesia the feeling and sound of the drill will be very similar to the feeling and sound you have experienced today. There are drills with water with higher speed that have a different sound and feeling, but we will expose you to them as well. The water may feel painful because of the temperature. Thus, before we practice with these drills, we should use local anesthetics and, therefore, I will suggest making injections as our next task. ◄

During exposure, elements from psychoeducation or information on coping strategies are repeated when suitable.

13.5.4.3 End of the Sessions

The dentist documents in the written manual what the patient was exposed to, for how long, and the patient's anxiety the first time it was done and the last time.

► Example		
Exposure, activities	**Anxiety level**	
	Start	**End**
Drill with rubber cup on 1 meter's distance, 5 sec	8	3
Drill with rubber cup on buccal surface of teeth, 5 sec	7	3
Drill with rubber cup on lingual surface of teeth, 5 sec	6	4

◄

At the end of each appointment, 5–10 minutes should be reserved for an evaluation of that day's progress, assign home tasks, and plan the next appointment. An alliance check is included in all the sessions.

► Example
Homework
Watch recorded movie clip of the drill 3 times per day

Examples include breathing, watching movie clips or photographs of a syringe or drill, talking to someone about the anxiety, and finding out more about individual catastrophic thoughts.

Plan for the Next Appointment

> Explain procedures and place anaesthetics (by drop technique)
>
> Continue exposure to the drill, 3-5 se intervals while polishing a filling in an upper left molar

A copy of the page is given to the patient either by taking a photograph of it with a cell phone or by photocopying the page. ◄

► Example

In the third appointment, Kristin says she has slept well again but that she felt tension when driving to the office. She is afraid that her anxiety will be extremely high, but she is ready to try to expose herself further to a local injection of anesthetics. She is tense at first, but her anxiety level still never exceeds 8. She uses the handheld mirror, and, in the end, she allows the dentist to polish a composite filling in the anesthetized area of her mouth. This is carried out in a stepwise manner, while she watches in the mirror. The plan for the next appointment is to drill a cavity in a premolar in the upper right side of her mouth.

In the fourth appointment, Kristin tells us that she has come directly from a meeting at work and that she has not had the time to think about the fact that she was about to receive dental treatment. She worries about how the drilling will be, but she remembers that polishing went well the last time, and this calms her down. She watches in the handheld mirror as the anesthetic is applied, and as we start stepwise exposure to the drilling. With increasing time intervals, we first drill into the air inside her mouth, thereafter, touch the tooth, and finally drill without needing intervals at all. Her anxiety is monitored at all times, and Kristin is in charge of the progression, deciding when she is ready for new intervals. She is not afraid of the filling procedure, and this is conducted only with explanations. At the end of the appointment, she is extremely relieved about how well everything went. She says that she is convinced that dental treatment is no longer something to be afraid of. She thinks that it went well because we were calm, we explained well, she could see what happened in the mirror, and also there was very little pain involved. ◄

Box

The dentist should help and encourage the patient to face frightening tasks and not push the patient toward challenges that are perceived as overwhelming. If the patient feels overwhelmed, it is important to recognize it and adjust further process. It is crucial not to stop exposure when anxiety levels are elevated since this might add to the patient's anxiety. Appointments should be planned to make sure that the conclusion of the exposure training is with a task that renders success. Accordingly, one should never start new and challenging tasks if only a few minutes are left of that day's appointment.

13.5.5   The Fifth and Last Session

The last treatment session starts in the same manner as do sessions 2, 3, and 4, but 20 minutes is saved at the end of the appointment to conclude the treatment.

Standard D-CBT requires five sessions. However, this must be individualized. If the patient shows steady progress, extra sessions may be beneficial. If the progress is weak or D-CBT is not sufficient to render the patient capable of receiving ordinary dental treatment, then other treatment alternatives must be considered. Referral to an interdisciplinary team of psychologists and dentists for further anxiety treatment should be the preferred option. Dental treatment under general anesthesia or under conscious sedation should also be considered to gain control over oral treatment needs.

13.5.5.1   Coping Plan

Making a summary of the treatment conducted and a plan for further treatment is part of the D-CBT and lets the patient reflect on what he/she has achieved (see ► Chap. 12). Both the dentist and patient must construct a coping plan in close collaboration. The plan provides the patient with a tool that is useful for her/himself as well as for any future dentist that he/she will meet.

The final plan is documented in the patient's dental record, but, maybe even more importantly, it should be made available to the patient in paper or electronically.

► Example

Coping plan for Kristin

The aim of the coping plan is to facilitate the best possible treatment situation during the dental treatment.
WHAT the dentist/dental hygienist/dental nurse needs to know about me (background, cause of fear, special needs, triggers):

- *I was held down as a young girl and I have been afraid of dentist after that happened. My dental anxiety is much better now and if the dentist lets me have control, I think it will work out fine.*

My catastrophic thoughts/what I'm most afraid of:
- *What I fear the most is the sound of the drill and pain. It is important to be fully anesthetized.*

What increases my anxiety?
- *Losing control, hearing the drill and pain*

What do I do if I feel the anxiety rises (my coping strategies)?
- *If I want the dentist to stop, I will raise my left hand. Take a brake and focus upon breathing*

My bodily reactions when anxiety rises (to be observed by the dentist/dental hygienist/dental nurse):
- *Signs of stress would be easy to detect, my facial expression would change, and I would hold on hard to the chairs side rests.*

Relevant adaptions (breaks, quality of dialogue, explanation, counting during treatment, etc.):
- *Dental personnel can help me by giving enough anesthetics, and to do it drop by drop. They can also explain and prepare for what will happen. A handheld mirror is helpful and music in the background is nice. I can help by letting the dentist know if anything hurts or something does not feel ok.*

Routine in case of cancellations/no show:
- *I want to come back for appointments every 6 months, and if I must move a scheduled appointment, I will never cancel it, just move it to a new date.* ◄

Summary

In this chapter, we have introduced a treatment method for dental anxiety, designed for the use by dentists. D-CBT is an evidence-based treatment method that requires the use of a practical manual. The objective is to reduce patients' dental anxiety. The important treatment components are psychoeducation, cognitive restructuring, and exposure training.

Adequate relational skills and good theoretical knowledge within oral health psychology is a prerequisite for all dentists working with patients with dental anxiety. For dentists wanting to build competence within D-CBT, practical training is also needed. This should include role play and the use of video recordings.

References

1. APA Dictionary of Psychology. Washington, DC: American Psychological Association; 2007.
2. Beck AT. Cognitive therapy. A 30-year retrospective. Am Psychol. 1991;46(4):368–75.
3. Dobson KSD, D.J.A. Historical and filosophical bases of the cognitive -behavioral therapies. In: Handbook of cognitive-behavioral therapies. Third ed. New York: Guilford press; 2009.
4. Epp AM, Dobson KS. The evidence base for cognitive-behavioral therapy. In: Handbook of cognitive-behavioral therapies. Third ed. New York: Guilford press; 2009.
5. Shafran RC, Clark DM, Fairburn CG, Arntz A, Barlow DH, Ehlers A, Freeston M, Garety PA, Hollon SD, Ost LG, Salkovskis PM, Williams JMG, Wilson GT. Mind the gap: improving the dissemination of CBT. Behav Res Ther. 2009;47(11):902–9.
6. Armfield JM, Heaton LJ. Management of fear and anxiety in the dental clinic: a review. Aust Dent J. 2013;58(4):390–407; quiz 531.
7. Wide Boman U, Carlsson V, Westin M, Hakeberg M. Psychological treatment of dental anxiety among adults: a systematic review. Eur J Oral Sci. 2013;121(3 Pt 2):225–34.
8. Vika M, Skaret E, Raadal M, Ost LG, Kvale G. One- vs. five-session treatment of intra-oral injection phobia: a randomized clinical study. Eur J Oral Sci. 2009;117(3):279–85.
9. Haukebo K, Skaret E, Ost LG, Raadal M, Berg E, Sundberg H, et al. One- vs. five-session treatment of dental phobia: a randomized controlled study. J Behav Ther Exp Psychiatry. 2008;39(3):381–90.
10. Hauge MS, Stora B, Vassend O, Hoffart A, Willumsen T. Dentist-administered cognitive behavioural therapy versus four habits/midazolam: an RCT study of dental anxiety treatment in primary dental care. Eur J Oral Sci. 2021:e12794.
11. Hauge MS, Stora B, Willumsen T. Dental anxiety treatment by a dentist in primary care; a 1-year follow-up study. Eur J Oral Sci. 2022;e12872. https://doi.org/10.1111/eos.1287.
12. Willumsen T, Vassend O. Effects of cognitive therapy, applied relaxation and nitrous oxide sedation. A five-year follow-up study of patients treated for dental fear. Acta Odontol Scand. 2003;61(2):93–9.

13. Willumsen T, Vassend O, Hoffart A. A comparison of cognitive therapy, applied relaxation, and nitrous oxide sedation in the treatment of dental fear. Acta Odontol Scand. 2001;59(5):290–6.

14. Foa E, RothBaum EA, Barbara Olasov Rauch S. Prolonged exposure therapy for PTSD. Oxford University Press Inc; 2019.

15. University of Oslo, Dental faculty. Practical manual for dentist administered cognitive behavioural therapy for treatment of adult patients [updated 2022 cited 2022 July 7]. Available from: https://www.odont.uio.no/iko/om/organisasjon/fagavd/pedo-donti-atferdsfag/rutiner-og-metoder/d-cbt-manual-engelsk.pdf.

16. Lutz W, Leon SC, Martinovich Z, Lyons JS, Stiles WB. Therapist effects in outpatient psychotherapy. J Couns Psychol. 2007;54(1):32–9.

17. Code of ethics for dentists in the European Union: Council of European Dentists; 2017. Available from: https://cedentists.eu/ced-code-of-ethics.html.

18. Agdal ML, Raadal M, Ost LG, Skaret E. Quality-of-life before and after cognitive behavioral therapy (CBT) in patients with intra-oral injection phobia. Acta Odontol Scand. 2012;70(6):463–70.

19. Willumsen T. Dental fear in sexually abused women. Eur J Oral Sci. 2001;109(5):291–6.

13

Blood–Injury–Injection Phobia

Maren Lillehaug Agdal, Karin Goplerud Berge and Margrethe Elin Vika

Contents

14.1 Introduction

Painless dentistry – is it too much to promise? What if it is too frightening for the patient to receive a dental injection? Some patients perceive dental injections to be extremely painful, often accompanied by significant physical discomfort due to both pain and anxiety. The pain together with bodily discomfort and negative thoughts make it nearly impossible for persons with intraoral injection phobia to receive an anesthetic injection. Knowing that pain during dental treatment is one of the greatest risk factors for the development of dental phobia, the dentist potentially faces a dilemma. How should the dentist meet and treat patients who refuse to receive anesthesia due to their anxiety? How can the dentist help the patient overcome the intraoral injection anxiety? It is a prerequisite that a good relationship must be established. To enable patients to share their negative thoughts and feelings about receiving an injection, the patients must feel that the dentist is respectful and that they can trust the dentist. When the therapist knows what the patient is afraid of, a systematic, controlled, and gradual exposure to the syringe, needle tip, and anesthesia can help the patient change their irrational thoughts about the perceived danger of getting a dental injection. Being able to receive anesthesia is a necessity to experience painless dental treatment.

This chapter describes what characterizes blood–injury–injection (BII) phobia, the possible reasons why this phobia develops, maintenance factors, and how it differs from odontophobia. Treatment of BII phobia is illustrated with a case study.

🎓 Learning Goals
- To understand the reasons behind the development of BII phobia
- To describe the maintenance factors of BII phobia
- To illustrate an example for the treatment of BII phobia

14.2 Possible Causes of Blood–Injury–Injection Phobia

From an evolutionary perspective, BII phobia may have evolved to prevent exposure to life-threatening injuries such as stings, which could potentially lead to life-threatening infections, and larger injuries that could lead to major blood loss. Preventing infections and injuries to the body is basically lifesaving and thus is a functional behavior. However, if the individual, at all costs, avoids situations that can lead to injury such as wounds and stings, then BII phobia may develop.

In the modern society, situations where blood and injuries are involved are rare. However, contrary to earlier times, injections have become an important part of today's society, for example, through childhood vaccination programs and through medical treatments for many diseases. Recently, we have seen the importance of vaccines when the world is facing a pandemic threat. It is important that the majority of the population takes the vaccine. Avoidance of injections due to anxiety may constitute a worldwide problem. However, why does the phobia develop? A genetic predisposition for development of BII phobia has been suggested [1]. Refusal to receive injections is normal in young children. Negative experiences with severe physical discomfort due to pain and fear when receiving a vaccine may be the cause for later development of BII phobia. Children who have experienced an anesthetic injection at the dentist's will, to a greater extent than children who have not received an anesthetic injection, avoid dental treatment if they know that the dental treatment involves injections [2]. This illustrates the importance of interacting with the children in such a manner that they feel cared for and safe in situations involving injections and anesthesia at the dentist's. Understanding and regulating the bodily discomfort associated with vaccines or injections is important because of the negative thoughts that usually accompany fear. Therefore, health professionals should address fear and bodily arousal with knowledge and understanding to prevent the child from developing injection anxiety/phobia.

BII phobia has a complex clinical expression, and it differs significantly from most other phobias, in that it is often associated with:
- Experience of pain [3]
- Fainting [4–6]
- Disgust – an emotional response described as nausea, malaise, etc. [7]

In BII phobia, perceived pain during previous exposure is an obvious explanatory model for the development of the phobia. The pain element distinguishes BII phobia from other phobias. Pain is a significant trigger for avoidance. Mineka and co-workers [8, 9] have described that suddenly perceived and unexpected danger is perceived as more stressful than expected danger. Similarly, one can expect that a sudden feeling of pain that coincides with an unexpected fear response accompanied by a feeling of lack of control, to a greater extent than pain alone, leads to phobia. People with BII phobia tend to overestimate the pain associated with a needle's penetration and have less tolerance for physical pain and discomfort [3, 10]. Another important factor is that pain, anxiety, and loss of control have a potentiating effect on each other.

Although pain is often a component of BII phobia, it is not always the trigger for this phobia. The autonomous nervous system is divided into the sympathetic and parasympathetic branches. Box 14.1 illustrate the diphasic activation of the automatic nerve system in patients with BII-phobia. The sympathetic nervous system is normally activated in stressful situations. The patient has increased heart rate and increased and deepened breathing and the body is ready to flee or fight. For some people, the sight (for some, even the thought of) of blood, an injury, or the sight or feeling of the needle will cause a reduced heart rate with a subsequent rapid drop in blood pressure due to parasympathetic activation. This atypical physiological anxiety response may lead to dizziness, nausea, malaise, and cold sweats and may also result in fainting (vasovagal syncope).

Box 14.1: The diphasic activation of the autonomic nerves system when a fearful patient experiences fainting
- Phase 1: Sympathetic activation, high blood pressure, and palpitations
- Phase 2: Parasympathetic activation (vasovagal response), rapid decrease in heart rate and blood pressure, and dizziness and fainting

---

14.3 Two-Phase Change in Blood Pressure in BII Phobia

This atypical reaction seen in BII phobia is described as a two-phase (or diphasic) change in blood pressure [6, 11]. The initial phase involves a rapid increase in heart rate and blood pressure, which is the classic sympathetic activation that occurs during an anxiety response. However, this phase is quickly followed by a rapid drop in heart rate and blood pressure. This sudden drop can lead to reduced cerebral blood flow and thus lead to dizziness and fainting [12, 13]. This unpleasant vasovagal response occurs more frequently in those with blood phobia than in persons with injection phobia and more often during extraoral injections (e.g., vaccines, blood tests) compared to intraoral injections [6, 14]. These differences may be explained as differences arising due to the patient's position during injections – the sitting position at the medical office compared with the reclined position at the dental office. It is also reported that the vasovagal response may occur in persons without anxiety associated with BII stimuli. Usually, the initial phase with increased heart rate and high blood pressure is not observed in these individuals. They only experience the sudden and rapid decrease in heart rate and blood pressure, compatible with the second parasympathetic phase for BII-phobic patients. For these persons, it is speculated that they may have a genetic vulnerability to this atypical drop in blood pressure.

The exact relationship between the fainting response and BII phobia is not fully understood. It has been suggested that fainting, as previously mentioned, may be an appropriate response to danger. Looking at animals, there is a remarkable resemblance to an immobile prey, which the predators lose interest in as it may be dead [15]. Furthermore, it has been claimed that a drop in blood pressure and fainting is beneficial for surviving as it minimizes blood loss and thus the risk of circulatory failure [16]. BII phobia is also often related to possible or actual tissue damage, but not always. A generalized BII phobia may elicit fainting just by the thought of blood, syringe, etc. The unpleasant feelings of dizziness and nausea may also trigger an anxiety response due to previous experiences. Having BII phobia may generalize to many parts of the person's life. Adolescents seek treatment because they cannot go to the cinemas as they are anxious that the movie will contain scenes of accidents or crimes with blood stimuli. ◼ Table 14.1 explains the functions of the autonomic nervous system. BII phobia is described as one of the least understood subgroups of phobias, for which more research is required [17]. It is pointed out that the important reasons for sparse research on BII phobia may be challenges related to fainting, disgust, and exposure treatment, where qualified medical personnel (e.g., dentist, dental nurse, doctor, nurse) are needed [18–20].

Studies also indicate that conditions such as a perceived lack of control and changes in respiration may affect the fainting response associated with BII phobia [21, 22]. Unfortunately, the experience of vasovagal syncope is for some persons the reason for their BII phobia. The social inconveniences and reactions that the person may experience by others after having fainted may be anxiety-provoking. Therefore, health-care professionals must be calm and supportive. If health-care professionals, on the other hand, appear restless and insecure as the patient is about to faint, or after the fainting, the patient may become unsure of their own safety and negative assumptions about the situation that they are in might develop. Later, the patient will have increased anxiety associated with the stimulus that triggered the fainting or may develop a more generalized anxiety associated with the situation. It is important that patients immediately after experiencing pain, anxiety, or fainting are guided in the retrospective cognitive understanding of the situation. This means that the patient is given the opportunity to understand what happened in the situation, and, if necessary, a strategy can be drawn for how to handle a similar situation in the future. For people who tend to faint, it is not uncommon to experience both psychological and emotional discomfort and thus develop negative thoughts related to fainting, in addition to the feeling of social embarrassment

Table 14.1 An overview of how different organs are affected by the sympathetic and parasympathetic nervous systems (selected organs)

Sympathetic nervous system	Organs	Parasympathetic nervous system
Increased muscle tone	Smooth muscles	Reduced muscle tone
Reduction of the pupil Increased tear secretion	Eyes	Enlargement of the pupil
Low secretion	Salivary glands	High secretion
Increased heart rate, stronger heartbeat	Heart	Slower heart rate – activation of the N. Vagus leads to reduced heart rate with consequent drop in blood pressure
Expansion of the trachea	Lungs	Tracheal narrowing, secretion
Decreased peristalsis and secretion, closes the outlet	Stomach	Increased peristalsis and secretion, opens the outlet
Increased secretion of adrenaline	Adrenal margin	No effect on the adrenal margin
Inhibits insulin secretion	Pancreas	Increased insulin secretion
Decreased peristalsis and secretion	Intestines	Increased peristalsis and secretion
Inhibits the wall muscles, closes the outlet in the digestive system	Urinary bladder	Activates the wall muscles, opens the outlet
Increased blood pressure due to increased muscle tone – dilation of the arterioles in self-directed muscles and blood vessels in the heart	Arteries/arterioles	No significant effect

and increased anxiety for the new episode of fainting. Consequently, anxiety very often leads to avoidance of situations where there is a risk of fainting. For some, this may develop into a phobia.

14.4 Model/Social/Vicarious Learning

Vicarious learning or model learning is when one learns or adapts behavior by observing the behavior of others in a similar or almost similar situation or by hearing negative or positive information about the situation

(see ▶ Chap. 10 on etiology). Both model learning and learning by hearing negative information/instructions may lead to the development of BII phobia. A negative modeling situation may be when you see others faint or have high fear or an anxiety response to situations where a syringe or blood is present. Among pupils, it is common to develop injection anxiety based on negative information from friends and fellow students. For instance, we have all probably heard of the "terrible and painful BCG vaccine" years before we found ourselves anxious with anticipation at the health nurse's office. As we stood there with our half-naked upper bodies, we could almost hear the negative words that had been said about the intense pain accompanying the sting, the characteristic inflammation that ached for weeks, and the big scar we would get afterward. We felt increasing anxiety pervading our bodies while the nurse held our arm firmly and we saw the famous long needle move toward our upper arm.

Negative information about syringes and dental treatment, such as burring, extractions, endodontics, surgical exposure of canines, and so on, is enough for some individuals to develop anxiety for similar situations, without having undergone the negative experiences. With low anxiety, the person manages to challenge him/herself in the situation. If the anxiety is high, and exceeds the patient's motivation and negative thoughts, then there is a big chance that you will do your best to avoid the situation even though you have not experienced the situation before.

14.5 Congenital Vulnerability

Personal vulnerabilities, factors achieved both congenitally and environmentally, play an important part in the personal experiences of different situations. Two patients may objectively undergo the same treatment, with the same dentist, and in the same dental environment. How they subjectively experience the situation may, however, be extremely different between the two persons. Personal experience means that two people rarely experience the same exposure equally. There are several prerequisites for a person to perceive a situation as safe and tolerable. Specific feelings and their intensity, thoughts concerning the situation, detailed knowledge about the situation, and surrounding factors such as social support are contributing factors to the personal experience of the situation.

The patient's feelings are essential for how the situation is perceived. Good feelings such as happiness, confidence, and bravery are feelings associated with positive and explorative interactions. Negative feelings often give a sense of wanting to get out of the situation or not wanting to deal with the challenges that one is exposed to. Think of yourself going into a new situation that you have never been in before. Based on what others have told you about their experiences, you feel uncertain about what is expected from you. You are confused about how trustworthy the people you are supposed to interact with are, and you are anxious about the outcome of the situation. The feelings give you negative vibrations and thoughts about the situation, while, in fact, you do not know the content of the situation. The attention you give the feelings and how you interpret them is crucial for the experience that you have in any situation.

In the context of injections, the feeling of disgust related to blood and injury on seeing or feeling syringes or injuries is a predisposing factor for the development of BII phobia [23]. Not only being sensitive to the feeling of disgust but also the person's attention to and interpretation of the disgust are important factors for how the situation is perceived [24]. The feeling of disgust may be associated with thoughts of being exposed to contaminated and contagious instruments, and, for some, these thoughts contribute to the feelings of fear [25]. Negative thoughts are linked to the possible threat of the syringe. Fearful people who have a tendency to interpret the situation as uncontrollable, unpredictable, or dangerous will more easily develop anxiety connected with the situation or to specific objects in the situation [26]. Even without having experienced negative situations or hearing others discuss a specific situation negatively, people with congenital vulnerability can perceive the situation as insecure. Especially, if the stimulus leads to a negative change in feelings and arousal. People who develop anxiety will have increased negative attention to potentially threatening stimuli unlike people who do not develop anxiety [27]. The negative attention often confirms negative assumptions about the situation. Concerning syringes, such negative cognitive considerations can be: "The dentist is going to inject the anaesthesia in a place where it can be harmful for the tissue. It was terribly painful, probably because the dentist did something wrong." Another common negative assumption is when the patient shivers due to the adrenaline in the anesthetic solution and the patient worries "Oh, why are my feet and hands shivering and my heart beating so suddenly after the injection? I'm having an allergic response. For sure!" Selective attention toward threatening factors in the situation is not intentional and is subconscious in patients with anxiety [28]. BII phobia may, for some, be more associated with disgust than fear when exposed to the phobic stimuli [29]. It is also claimed that persons with BII phobia have a lower threshold for fainting when feeling disgust, especially for the subgroup of blood phobics [30].

Pain, the intensity, and interpretation of the probable meaning of experienced pain differ from person to person. The bodily reaction, how the pain is felt, during an injection may, for some, feel like a lightning through the body, whereas others feel a local and short-lasting pinch. Pain, as more profoundly described in ▶ Chap. 3, is a sensation, which requires retraction from the trigger that elicits pain. Therefore, patients' experience of pain and how they previously dealt with it is crucial for being able to handle painful situations in the future. Moreover, having trust in being safe in spite of the pain and social support when feeling pain are important and vary from individual to individual due to congenital vulnerabilities.

A poorly developed ability to regulate negative interpretations of bodily discomfort and lack of control over intrusive negative thoughts are also vulnerability factors for the development of anxiety [31]. Cognitive vulnerability factors that contribute to the development of anxiety may be related to the persons' thoughts on how to handle the situation. Furthermore, people with low confidence in self efficacy and previous experiences of not coping new situations, will find new situations more difficult to handle than people with high coping confidence. Coping strategies and self-esteem can affect whether one develops anxiety for a stimulus or a situation [32]. Positive and active coping strategies such as actively contributing during exposure are more beneficial than withdrawal and negative thoughts such as "I just have to persevere" or "I do not know if I can handle any more" [33].

BII phobia is among the phobias with the highest degree of familial accumulation, and it is claimed that some are biologically predisposed to develop this subgroup of phobias [34]. Öst reported that 61% of adults with blood and injury phobia and 29% of those with injection phobia stated that they had a parent or sibling with a similar fear [6]. Such familial accumulations of BII phobia can also be explained by various causes. It is believed to be a genetic component of fainting that, for some, is triggered by anxiety about BII stimuli [34]. The increased frequency of fainting also applies in other situations where you may experience a sudden drop in blood pressure, such as when you get up quickly after sitting (orthostatic hypotension). The family may also have a common genetic vulnerability to the development of anxiety disorders such as increased anxiety, a pattern of more negative thoughts, or a stronger physical reaction to fear (◘ Fig. 14.1).

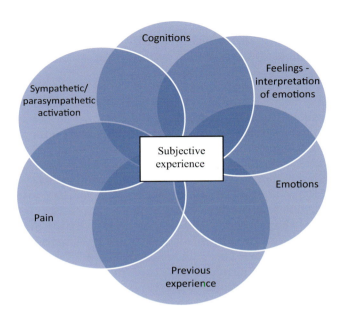

Cognitions

Feelings - interpretation of emotions

Sympathetic/ parasympathetic activation

Subjective experience

Emotions

Pain

Previous experience

Fig. 14.1 Illustration showing how a person's cognitions, emotions, pain, feelings, the autonomic nervous system, and previous experiences are important for the subjective perception of a situation. Positive or negative personal traits concerning all these elements play an important role in the subjective perception

14.6 Overlap Between BII Phobia and Odontophobia

In the Diagnostic and Statistical Manual of Mental Disorders (DSM)-5, odontophobia is categorized as a specific phobia [35]. Since dental treatment includes medical procedures (e.g., injections, tooth extractions, surgery), it has been suggested that odontophobia should be characterized as blood–injury–injection phobia [36]. This classification is debated, as research in the field is contradictory to this view and points in the direction that odontophobia can be considered a specific phobia, independent of blood–injury–injection phobia [37].

Although BII phobia and odontophobia are diagnosed as separate conditions, a significant but varying degree of overlap has been documented [38]. A larger proportion of those with a fear of dentistry have a fear of injections than a fear of blood [6, 39]. In a sample of primary school pupils in Norway, there was a relatively high overlap between high dental fear and high fear of dental injections. Approximately 58% of the pupils with a high degree of fear of intraoral injections also had a high degree of fear of dental treatment. Seen from the opposite perspective, 63% of pupils with a high degree of fear of dental treatment also reported a high fear of intraoral injections [2]. A study from The Netherlands

found that intraoral injections are one of the most anxiety-triggering stimuli during dental treatment [40]. Patients who avoid anesthesia at the dentist's due to fear of intraoral injections may be at a higher risk of experiencing pain during dental treatment. Pain and painful dental treatment have been shown to play important roles in the development of odontophobia [41]. It has been suggested that BII phobia and the experience of taking intraoral injections with high anxiety might contribute to the development of dental anxiety by the means of direct conditioning to the dental situation [42].

14.6.1 What Do BII Phobics Fear?

During the initial conversations with patients with BII-phobia, they usually exhibit an uncontrollable bodily restlessnes. The physiological part of the anxiety response prevents the patient from active participation in a conversation. They cry, they shiver, and some cannot sit still and walk across the room. You can imagine how it feels to speak calmly while an angry pit bull terrier is charging at you. Therefore, it is appropriate to start the conversation with neutral topics so that the patient's anxiety level may decrease to a level where a clinical relationship may be established. A highly anxious patient will have problems in maintaining focus and would not be able to benefit from a therapeutic conversation. It is extremely important that the patients feel that they are safe and are taken care of. Both "being safe" and "taken care of" may be controversial words because the opposite may imply that dentistry is harmful or dangerous and that the dental staff do not care or have empathy for the patient. In this context, the meaning of safe is that the patient is aware and confident that there will not be any dental treatment without the patient's consent. The meaning of "taken care of" is that the patient is seen and acknowledged for their need for comfort and support and that the dental staff have proper knowledge of how to deal with anxiety. These are key elements for the patients during the conversation in order to make them feel accepted for sharing their thoughts and feelings associated with the anxiety disorder.

During the first part of the conversation, it may be helpful to get the patients' understanding of why they have developed anxiety associated with blood, injury, and/or injections. Many patients carry negative experiences that they want to share, whereas other patients are more uncertain about the origin and etiology of their anxiety. In any case, one should support the patient and express understanding for the difficult situation they are in, which makes it difficult for them to undergo dental treatment.

A high anxiety level has three components, which are (1) a strong physiological anxiety response, (2) the patient's cognitive assessment of the situation, and (3) the avoidance of the triggering stimuli. The three components have a reinforcing effect on each other. High activation leads to both more avoidance and a stronger belief in negative thoughts, whereas negative thoughts may lead to increased avoidance and a stronger physiological response as opposed to the anxiety-provoking triggers. The negative thoughts related to the consequences of entering an anxiety-triggering situation are often of such a serious nature that they are referred to as catastrophic thoughts.

Common catastrophic thoughts have dramatic outcomes for the patient if they were true and the negative assumptions occurred. Usually, the actual catastrophe in the mind is the result of a cascade of consequences. What triggers the cascade is usually an external physical strain that is inflicted by dental professionals or the cascade is triggered by the anxiety response. Patients with catastrophic thoughts linked to anxiety responses are most often anxious about the anxiety response itself, which we may refer to as "anxiety about the anxiety."

Children's and adolescents' catastrophic thoughts regarding the consequences of taking anesthesia at the dentist's have previously been explored through psychological interviews conducted at clinics that specifically work on the treatment of dental anxiety. The thoughts vary, but, on review, they can be described in five different categories; see fact box.

14.6.2 Negative and Catastrophic Thoughts About Getting Anesthesia

14.6.2.1 Thoughts About Bodily Consequences

- I will get a heart attack because my heart is beating faster than my body can handle.
- I cannot breathe during the anxiety attack, and I may suffocate.
- The anesthesia can lead to bleeding that will not stop.
- The syringe can end up in a place that will cause permanent damage.
- Exposure to the syringe can lead to fainting and physical consequences of fainting (death, losing memory).
- Anesthesia can lead to permanent paralysis.
- Cascade of thoughts: My anxiety increases so fast that I will move reflexively, and the dentist may hit me with the syringe. Then, the needle will be inserted somewhere where it should not be inserted. The dentist will be so annoyed with me. This will have serious conse-

quences for me because then I do not think I could manage to come back due to shame. Then, I would never be able to get dental treatment, my teeth would rot, and I could not show myself to other people.

14.6.2.2 Thoughts About Psychological Consequences

- Everything is out of control, and my brain is damaged. I am going crazy!
- I will never be the same again.
- At the sight of the syringe and needle or at the feeling of the anesthetic, a panic attack can occur, which has lasting psychological consequences.
- Losing control of the body and mind will have serious consequences, as it will lead to increased anxiety.
- If I faint, I will lose my memory.

14.6.2.3 Thoughts About the Consequences of Not Being Able to Trust the Dentist

- What will they do with me and think about me when I have fainted? Then, they will probably sting me when I do not have control and cannot speak for myself, and, then, something can happen; but, I cannot describe what.
- The dentist can make a mistake, which can result in a serious injury.
- There may be a wrong substance in the anesthetic.
- It is difficult to stop the dentist, and, so, you must persevere. When you try to persevere, you can panic or have other catastrophic thoughts about anxiety.
- The dentist does things without saying what he/she is doing. Then, for example, errors or injuries may occur because the patient may move or because the dentist does not know if the patient can tolerate what is being done.
- Negative thoughts about the dentist.
- Negative thoughts related to being criticized by the dentist.
- Negative thoughts about prejudice from the dentist.

14.6.2.4 Thoughts About Pain

- The sting is so painful and lasts so long that it will never go over.
- It is so painful that I cannot stay calm, and I will never manage it again.
- My body cannot tolerate the pain.

14.6.2.5 Thoughts About the Effect of the Syringe and the Anesthetic

- I am afraid of the effect of the anesthetic itself. Will the paralysis ever go away?
- The needle may break and go through the blood stream to the heart or the brain.

- The anesthetic will lead to a serious and life-threatening allergic reaction.
- The anesthetic does not work for me, and, then, the dental treatment will hurt so much that I cannot get the treatment. This will mean that I will never be able to have my teeth fixed, I will have ugly teeth all my life, and I will not be able to have social relationships. My life would be ruined.

14.7 Cognitive Restructuring

Cognitive restructuring together with education about anxiety symptoms (psychoeducation) can help patients gain an understanding of what they are feeling and why they feel and think the way they do when they are confronted with anxiety-provoking triggers. Spending time on cognitive comprehension is also extremely important when treating children and adolescents to prevent them from developing anxiety associated with dentistry and syringes. This can be illustrated by statements from a 24-year-old patient. Before and after a diagnostic interview with a psychologist, he happened to meet the same dentist in the waiting room. Before the interview session, he made the following remark:

> ► **Example**
> "Every time I go to the dentist and have anaesthesia something happens to me. I do not know what's going on. The whole body shakes, and the heart runs wild. Am I going crazy?" ◄

The patient was diagnosed with BII phobia. He had avoided syringes for many years and had not been to the dentist or doctor due to his fear of syringes. The avoidance behavior had prevented him from going on a holiday to Africa with his family, as he was unable to take the necessary vaccines. Immediately after the interview with the psychologist, he stated:

> ► **Example**
> "Anxiety response, as if a lion is coming towards me?! Yes, that's how I feel. Maybe I'm not out of my mind after all?" ◄

Very gently and without making the patient feel bad, the reality in the catastrophic thoughts should be explored together with the patient. Here is an example of how you may address catastrophic thoughts regarding the safety of your heart. "When you sit still in the chair and your heart beats it feels bad for you and you recognise that the heart beats out of proportion to the actual activity you are in. Have you ever been questioned why it beats when you are active, like when you are hiking in the

woods? Remember that your heart doesn't know why it beats. The brain tells it to beat in case you need to flee or fight against the threat. Therefore, you can be sure that it is safe for your heart to beat – even if it doesn't feel good for you!"

After reconstructing the situation, you should try to make the patients reflect and summarize how their assumptions and perceptions of the situation, based on their anxiety, have been wrong and exaggerated.

14.8 Applied Tension (AT): To Prevent Fainting

As described, the parasympathetic activation that leads to the sudden drop in blood pressure can result in fainting or almost fainting [43]. Applied tension (AT) is a method developed to counteract the drop in blood pressure. The method is based on two main components: (1) the patient learns to tense the large muscle groups in the body (legs, thighs, buttocks, abdomen, arms, chest, and back) and (2) the patient learns to recognize the first signs of a drop in blood pressure (e.g., dizziness, paleness, cold sweats, wheezing in the ears) [44].

During instructions about AT, the therapist shows the patient how to tense the large muscle groups in the body. The patient is then instructed to hold the tension for 10–15 s and then release the tension and relax lightly for 20–25 s. This is repeated five times (◘ Fig. 14.2).

The therapist can hold a mirror in front of the patient so that the patient can see the red-color blush on the face. If a blood pressure monitor is available, the initial pressure can also be measured before the start and just after the exercise, as a cognitive feedback to ensure that the blood pressure has increased. In the beginning, the therapist may ask the patient to initiate AT during exposure when signs of a vasovagal reaction are seen or felt. The goal is, eventually, to ensure that the patient recognizes such early signs him/herself, and then starts AT. Very few patients perform AT correctly in the beginning. The therapist needs to coach the patient to help keep the muscle contraction in all the big muscle groups for as long as it takes to increase the blood pressure. Some patients are reluctant or shy in the beginning, but, when they feel the effect, they are more active and eager to do the exercise correctly. It can be useful for the patient to practice the muscle tension exercises at home a few times a day, for example, for the first week of therapy. During treatment, some patients only need a couple of contractions to avoid fainting. Other patients need longer and more series of contractions. In our clinic, we have had patients doing AT for up to 20 min and still having signs of low blood pressure, and, during the subsequent consultation, the duration needed for a good result dropped

Fig. 14.2 Illustration of how to perform applied tension

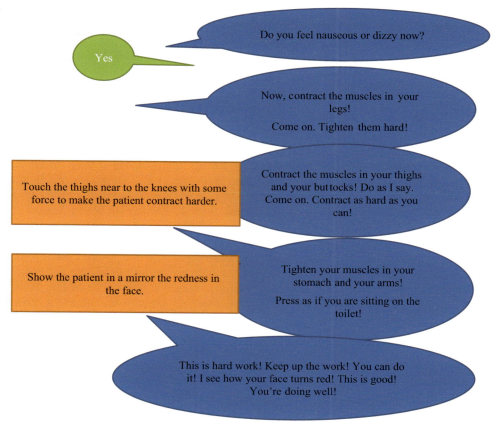

to only a couple of minutes. As a therapist, it is important that you have trust in the intervention so that you help the patient do it correctly.

The method aims to increase blood pressure to avoid fainting. In addition, there is probably a cognitive component, namely, distraction, which plays a role in decreasing the length of the drop in blood pressure. An important factor in AT is that the patient must understand the physiology behind the drop in blood pressure and the rationale for the method. It is also important that the therapist makes it clear to the patient, in advance, that fainting is not dangerous and clarifies all catastrophic thoughts that are related to fainting. AT is a quick and easy method that is suitable for both children and adults.

14.9 How to Treat BII Phobia? Case Study: Peter 33 Years Old

Peter is 33 years old and has for several years refused all dental treatments due to anxiety associated with syringes. Since he was old enough to go to the dentist alone, without being accompanied by his parents, he has avoided all dental appointments, except for emergency treatments when he has had tremendous dental pain. The fear also

applies to other situations involving syringes, and he has not been able to receive necessary vaccinations and blood samples. He avoids conversations about dentists/syringes, and he feels sweaty, clammy, and dizzy if this becomes a topic. Due to an accident during a football match, Peter needed an emergency appointment at the dentist's. During the appointment, he saw a syringe, which immediately triggered a terribly unpleasant feeling in his body. He became extremely dizzy, whereupon he fainted. This frightening experience has caused Peter to stop playing football matches even though he has always been an active football player and he likes to play football. Now, he has pain in several areas of his mouth. Peter is diagnosed with BII phobia according to the DSM-5.

The following negative/catastrophic thoughts emerge during an examination with a psychologist:

– Peter is anxious of fainting if he sees a syringe. He feels that the changes he experiences within his body prior fainting are scary. In addition, he is afraid of getting hurt if he should fall. Furthermore, he experiences shame associated with fainting and is unsure whether he would be able to return to the dentist after fainting. He also has thoughts related to the consequences of fainting because he is afraid that the brain might be damaged due to lack of oxygen.

- He assumes that the pain during the penetration of the needle will be unbearable and will last a long time, causing major consequences for his everyday life. He is not afraid of the anesthetic liquid itself, but he fears the pain during the injection. He thinks that the pain of the injection will be too heavy a burden for his heart and that he will have a heart attack.

The first session of anxiety treatment takes place at the dentist's office. There is an emphasis on building a trustful relationship, which is a prerequisite for good treatment. The dentist asks Peter how it felt to sit in the waiting room and how he feels now when entering the dental office. Peter sits in the dental chair, and the dentist asks him to reproduce, in his own words, his worst thoughts of what he might experience in the dental situation. During the conversation, the dentist does not challenge or disprove his catastrophic thoughts, but she lets Peter complete his train of thoughts. Peter is then asked to state how likely (0–100%) he believes that the content of his thoughts will happen if he gets anesthesia in his mouth.

Now, the dentist goes through the physiology of anxiety and gives Peter psychoeducation with an emphasis on interpreting and recognizing the body's signals and accompanying thoughts. She gradually connects the review of anxiety symptoms with Peter's catastrophic thoughts. Furthermore, the dentist draws and explains the anxiety curve (see page XX), which describes the association between anxiety and avoidance. The curve shows how there is a rapid and steep increased anxiety when the patient is exposed to an anxiety-inducing stimulus and how avoidance leads to transient relief from the anxiety and discomfort. If Peter, on the other hand, manages to stay in the discomfort associated with the anxiety without fleeing from or avoiding the trigger, the anxiety will, with repeated exposures, decrease. To ensure decreased anxiety during treatment, there must be a trustful relationship between Peter and the dentist in order to make Peter feel in control of the treatment situation, namely, exposures should take place gradually and they should be endured for a sufficient period of time. The difference between control of the situation and control in the situation is important. To feel control in the situation may be misinterpreted as to also have control over the anxiety. The dentist must not be vague about how the patient should let anxiety come without avoidance behavior and how he must stay in the situation along with his cognitions but with a secure and positive knowledge that he at any time can stop the ongoing exposure by showing a sign to the dentist. The significance of the team effort is also important for the dentist to emphasize. Both Peter and the dentist must contribute to reach the goal of the treatment. Where the dentist knows how to gradually and systematically pro-

vide exposures, Peter has feelings and thoughts that he may express to rewrite the understanding of the danger in the exposures.

As fainting played a part in most of the central catastrophic thoughts, it is reviewed how the vasovagal response can lead to dizziness and fainting as a result of a sudden drop in blood pressure. Peter learns how to recognize such an incipient drop in blood pressure. He says that he can feel cold sweat, dizziness, wheezing in the ears, blurred vision, and tingling in front of the eyes. He is then instructed in how the applied tension (AT) method, a method with contraction of the large muscle groups in the body, can be used to counteract a drop in blood pressure. The rationale for the method is to directly prevent fainting by increasing the blood pressure, venous back flow, and cerebral blood flow. The dentist focuses on the fact that it is not dangerous to faint, and as he is sitting safely in the dentist's chair, it is impossible to fall. Peter says that he is willing to try this technique and thinks that he will be able to recognize signs in the body if an incipient blood pressure drop occurs. It is important that Peter practices the AT so that he becomes confident in his performance and can start the exercise in all situations where he feels that there is a drop in blood pressure.

All the abovementioned elements needed for understanding the treatment must be addressed before they agree on a common treatment goal, namely that Peter should be able to receive anaesthesia when there is a need because of necessary dental treatment.

Exposure to the syringe begins with the dentist retrieving the various parts and putting them on the table in front of Peter. They look at the needle, the ampulla with the anesthesia, and the syringe. Peter receives information about pain during mucous penetration (e.g., how pain and pressure cells work with different stimuli). He is challenged to distinguish between pain and discomfort. Furthermore, the dentist focuses on getting Peter to distinguish between transient pain associated with injections and chronic pain that can cause long-term suffering. The dentist asks Peter to compare how he thinks the pain associated with the injection is to the worst pain he has ever experienced. In this context, she encourages him to grade the pain he believes the needle penetration will cause. She explains the interaction between pain experience and anxiety and how pain tolerance has a psychogenic component. This means that an increased perception of control and a lower anxiety response can lead to increased pain tolerance (more about pain in ▶ Chap. 3). Furthermore, the dentist uses a model (a skull) to explain in detail where the nerves enters the tooth and thus where it is necessary to insert the needle and how far into the gum the syringe should go to achieve the desired effect. It is important for Peter to know that there is nothing in the tissue that can be injured by the needle or by the injection. She explains how anesthesia is injected under the mucous membrane during an infiltration into the teeth in the maxilla and how the anesthetic is injected extremely slowly to prevent pain and where it is injected to ensure a good effect. Peter feels that his anxiety increases when he receives such in-depth information, something he has previously deliberately avoided. He prefers that the dentist does not say so much and tells her to "do what you have to." The dentist repeats the common goal. Is the goal to avoid discomfort or to master anxiety and overcome the fear of injections? Peter strongly wants to master his fear of injections, and the dentist makes him aware that his catastrophic beliefs are based on missing knowledge and that knowledge will help him understand what he feels during the prick of the needle and during injection. He sees that his previous choice of action has not worked out, and he wants to try a new strategy. They mount the syringe together. The dentist then shows him the surface anesthesia, and, with a sign of acceptance, she lubricates the mucous membrane. When the mucous is somewhat numbed with the topical anesthesia, the dentist uses a probe, both against the numb area and against another area in the mouth. Peter now feels the difference, and he experiences that the surface anesthesia works. This gives him positive feelings of hope that the needlestick will not be as painful as he had anticipated. Furthermore, both in this and in the next sessions, the dentist and Peter work with gradual exposure, moving the syringe closer to the mouth and mucous membrane. For each step, the degree of anxiety is stated from 0 to 100. In retrospect, this is compared with the patient's expectations and a review of current catastrophic thoughts and anxiety symptoms in the situation. AT is used when Peter feels signs of a drop in blood pressure. Once Peter seems confident in a step, the dentist suggests a new step with the syringe closer to the mucous membrane. It is not the reduction in anxiety that is important but that Peter feels that the anxiety is not dangerous. Current steps for Peter include a gradual approach to the mucous membrane with the syringe, then pushing on the mucous membrane with a needle in the area with surface anesthesia, and, further, a "mini-prick" without injecting any anesthetic. Peter constantly pays attention to the current steps in a handheld mirror. He is motivated to not think ahead but to stay cognitively in the current step. The next step can be a sting with a few drops of the anesthetic, while, for example, counting to three. Thereafter, they can agree to increase the amount of anesthesia that is given, while counting a little longer. The dentist may suggest putting a few more drops of anesthesia and then even more. Eventually, the dentist may ask Peter if it is OK to put anesthesia in different parts of his mouth. Counting is always used actively by the dentist, and Peter always agrees in advance the number she will count to at each

step. Peter experiences that the count is a time limit that gives him a feeling of being in control in the situation. In addition, he can also stop the exposure by lifting his hand as a stop signal before he has the feeling "I need to get out of this." At each stage of the exposure, anxiety and current catastrophic thoughts related to vasovagal response and pain experience must be evaluated. Is this what Peter expected would happen? The dentist focuses on the coping experience, which means that the experience in some way feels good because the anxiety has decreased or that the situation feels manageable. Moreover, the dentist tries to make Peter aware of changed thought patterns. After three sessions at the dentist's, Peter masters the anesthetic syringe, and he has managed the drill and filled a cavity. He can still, on occasion, feel signs of a sudden drop in blood pressure but feels that he has a technique to counteract this. He is no longer afraid of fainting and now sees that his catastrophic thoughts were exaggerated and anxiety-driven.

Summary

BII phobia is an obstacle to painless dentistry and may therefore cause development of dental anxiety. The phobia is characterized by strong anxiety associated with blood, injury, and/or injections. The reasons for developing BII phobia may be personal, negative, and painful experiences and also different types of vicarious learning. There is assumed to be a familial accumulation of BII phobia (compared with other phobias), which may be caused by a genetic vulnerability to this phobia. Usually, BII phobia is characterized by catastrophic thoughts related to one or more of the following areas: severe physiological and psychological consequences, loss of control, anxiety about pain, and thoughts of negative consequences of the anesthetic itself. BII phobia can be successfully treated with cognitive behavioral therapy as most other phobias. However, BII phobia is unique, in that it is associated with fainting. Fainting is perceived as an extremely unpleasant physiological and emotional response that may result in increased avoidance behavior. Fainting can be counteracted by applied tension, which is illustrated in the example with Peter in this chapter.

References

1. Wani AL, Ara A, Bhat SA. Blood injury and injection phobia: the neglected one. Behav Neurol. 2014;2014:471340.
2. Berge KG, Agdal ML, Vika M, Skeie MS. High fear of intra-oral injections: prevalence and relationship to dental fear and dental avoidance among 10- to 16-yr-old children. Eur J Oral Sci. 2016;124(6):572–9.

3. Smith NB, Meuret AE. The role of painful events and pain perception in blood-injection-injury fears. J Behav Ther Exp Psychiatry. 2012;43(4):1045–8.

4. Bienvenu OJ, Eaton WW. The epidemiology of blood-injection-injury phobia. Psychol Med. 1998;28(5):1129–36.

5. Kleinknecht RA, Lenz J. Blood/injury fear, fainting and avoidance of medically-related situations: a family correspondence study. Behav Res Ther. 1989;27(5):537–47.

6. Öst LG. Blood and injection phobia. Background and cognitive, physiological, and behavioral variables. J Abnorm Psychol. 1992;101(1):68–74.

7. Olatunji BO, Cisler J, McKay D, Phillips ML. Is disgust associated with psychopathology? Emerging research in the anxiety disorders. Psychiatry Res. 2010;175(1–2):1–10.

8. Cook M, Mineka S, Wolkenstein B, Laitsch K. Observational conditioning of snake fear in unrelated rhesus monkeys. J Abnorm Psychol. 1985;94(4):591–610.

9. Mineka S, Davidson M, Cook M, Keir R. Observational conditioning of snake fear in rhesus monkeys. J Abnorm Psychol. 1984;93(4):355–72.

10. Severeijns R, Vlaeyen JW, van den Hout MA, Weber WE. Pain catastrophizing predicts pain intensity, disability, and psychological distress independent of the level of physical impairment. Clin J Pain. 2001;17(2):165–72.

11. Ritz T, Meuret AE, Simon E. Cardiovascular activity in blood-injection-injury phobia during exposure: evidence for diphasic response patterns? Behav Res Ther. 2013;51(8):460–8.

12. Thyer BA, Himle J, Curtis GC. Blood-injury-illness phobia: a review. J Clin Psychol. 1985;41(4):451–9.

13. Öst LG, Sterner U, Lindahl IL. Physiological responses in blood phobics. Behav Res Ther. 1984;22(2):109–17.

14. Vika M, Raadal M, Skaret E, Kvale G. Dental and medical injections: prevalence of self-reported problems among 18-yr-old subjects in Norway. Eur J Oral Sci. 2006;114(2):122–7.

15. Marks I. Blood-injury phobia: a review. Am J Psychiatry. 1988;145(10):1207–13.

16. First MB, Tasman A. DSM-IV-TR diagnosis, etiology & treatment. In: Tasman IMBFA, editor. Anxiety disorders social and specific phobias. Chichester: John Wiley and Sons; 2004. p. 867–95.

17. Oar EL, Farrell LJ, Waters AM, Conlon EG, Ollendick TH. One session treatment for pediatric blood-injection-injury phobia: a controlled multiple baseline trial. Behav Res Ther. 2015;73:131–42.

18. Oar EL, Farrell LJ, Ollendick TH. One session treatment for specific phobias: an adaptation for paediatric blood-injection-injury phobia in youth. Clin Child Fam Psychol Rev. 2015;18(4):370–94.

19. Ollendick TH, Öst LG, Reuterskiold L, Costa N, Cederlund R, Sirbu C, et al. One-session treatment of specific phobias in youth: a randomized clinical trial in the United States and Sweden. J Consult Clin Psychol. 2009;77(3):504–16.

20. Öst LG, Svensson L, Hellström K, Lindwall R. One-session treatment of specific phobias in youths. A randomized clinical trial. J Consult Clin Psychol. 2001;69(5):814–24.

21. Gilchrist PT, McGovern GE, Bekkouche N, Bacon SL, Ditto B. The vasovagal response during confrontation with blood-injury-injection stimuli: the role of perceived control. J Anxiety Disord. 2015;31:43–8.

22. Ritz T, Meuret AE, Ayala ES. The psychophysiology of blood-injection-injury phobia: looking beyond the diphasic response paradigm. Int J Psychophysiol. 2010;78(1):50–67.

23. Olatunji BO, Williams NL, Sawchuk CN, Lohr JM. Disgust, anxiety and fainting symptoms associated with blood-injection-injury fears: a structural model. J Anxiety Disord. 2006;20(1):23–41.

24. Williams NL, Connolly KM, Cisler JM, Elwood LS, Willems JL, Lohr JM. Disgust: a cognitive approach. In: Olatunji BO, McKay D, editors. Disgust and it's disorders. Washington, DC: American Psycological Association; 2009. p. 57–73.

25. Teachman BA, Woody SR, Magee JC. Implicit and explicit appraisals of the importance of intrusive thoughts. Behav Res Ther. 2006;44(6):785–805.

26. Armfield JM. Cognitive vulnerability: a model of the etiology of fear. Clin Psychol Rev. 2006;26(6):746–68.

27. Bar-Haim Y, Lamy D, Pergamin L, Bakermans-Kranenburg MJ, van Ijzendoorn MH. Threat-related attentional bias in anxious and nonanxious individuals: a meta-analytic study. Psychol Bull. 2007;133(1):1–24.

28. Mogg K, Bradley BP, Hallowell N. Attentional bias to threat: roles of trait anxiety, stressful events, and awareness. Q J Exp Psychol A. 1994;47(4):841–64.

29. Sawchuk CN, Lohr JM, Westendorf DH, Meunier SA, Tolin DF. Emotional responding to fearful and disgusting stimuli in specific phobics. Behav Res Ther. 2002;40(9):1031–46.

30. Page AC. The role of disgust in faintness elicited by blood and injection stimuli. J Anxiety Disord. 2003;17(1):45–58.

31. Mathews A, MacLeod C. Cognitive vulnerability to emotional disorders. Annu Rev Clin Psychol. 2005;1:167–95.

32. Williams SL, Kinney PJ, Falbo J. Generalization of therapeutic changes in agoraphobia: the role of perceived self-efficacy. J Consult Clin Psychol. 1989;57(3):436–42.

33. Bernson JM, Elfstrom ML, Berggren U. Self-reported dental coping strategies among fearful adult patients: preliminary enquiry explorations. Eur J Oral Sci. 2007;115(6):484–90.

34. Van Houtem CM, Laine ML, Boomsma DI, Ligthart L, van Wijk AJ, De Jongh A. A review and meta-analysis of the heritability of specific phobia subtypes and corresponding fears. J Anxiety Disord. 2013;27(4):379–88.

35. Association AP. Diagnostic and statistical manual of mental disorders. DMS-5™. 5th ed. Arlington: American Psychiatric Publishing; 2013.

36. LeBeau RT, Glenn D, Liao B, Wittchen HU, Beesdo-Baum K, Ollendick T, et al. Specific phobia: a review of DSM-IV specific phobia and preliminary recommendations for DSM-V. Depress Anxiety. 2010;27(2):148–67.

37. De Jongh A, Bongaarts G, Vermeule I, Visser K, De Vos P, Makkes P. Blood-injury-injection phobia and dental phobia. Behav Res Ther. 1998;36(10):971–82.

38. Locker D, Shapiro D, Liddell A. Overlap between dental anxiety and blood-injury fears: psychological characteristics and response to dental treatment. Behav Res Ther. 1997;35(7):583–90.

39. Poulton R, Thomson WM, Brown RH, Silva PA. Dental fear with and without blood-injection fear: implications for dental health and clinical practice. Behav Res Ther. 1998;36(6):591–7.

40. Oosterink FM, de Jongh A, Aartman IH. What are people afraid of during dental treatment? Anxiety-provoking capacity of 67 stimuli characteristic of the dental setting. Eur J Oral Sci. 2008;116(1):44–51.

41. Skaret E, Raadal M, Berg E, Kvale G. Dental anxiety and dental avoidance among 12 to 18 year olds in Norway. Eur J Oral Sci. 1999;107(6):422–8.

42. Vika M, Skaret E, Raadal M, Ost LG, Kvale G. Fear of blood, injury, and injections, and its relationship to dental anxiety and probability of avoiding dental treatment among 18-year-olds in Norway. Int J Paediatr Dent. 2008;18(3):163–9.

43. Ayala ES, Meuret AE, Ritz T. Treatments for blood-injury-injection phobia: a critical review of current evidence. J Psychiatr Res. 2009;43(15):1235–42.

44. Öst LG, Sterner U. Applied tension. A specific behavioral method for treatment of blood phobia. Behav Res Ther. 1987;25(1):25–9.

Part III

The Voice of Dentally Anxious Patients
Lena Myran

What thoughts and wishes do patients with dental anxiety have, related to dental treatment? These quotes are collected from coping plans (see ▶ Chap. 12), from patients participating in a Norwegian treatment program for dental treatment for sexual abuse survivors (the TADA-project, see ▶ Chap. 22). The most common quotes have been selected.

Here's what I need my dental team to be aware of:

"I've experienced painful dental treatment at a young age – that's why I'm afraid today."

"I haven't been to the dentist in many years."

"I'm so ashamed that I haven't been able to take care of my teeth."

"I have a fear of needles."

"I have a sensitive gag reflex."

"I do not know how to give a stop signal during dental treatment. Setting boundaries is hard for me."

"The waiting room makes my anxiety increase; I don't want my appointment to be delayed."

My catastrophic thoughts and fears:

"I fear that the dentist will not halt treatment at my signal – I might lose control, become helpless or faint in the chair."

"I fear not being heard by the dentist when feeling pain – the dentist asks me "can you manage a bit longer?" I feel helpless."

"My fear might paralyze me, which will make me feel helpless."

"I'm afraid I will lose control – it means that I am a weak person, not good enough."

"My biggest fear is not knowing what is going to happen during treatment, not being prepared for what comes next."

"I fear suffocation – that the dentist will drop instruments or teeth at the back of my throat."

"I fear panic – to lose control, which will cause me to beat wildly around me, getting stuck in the equipment, or make the dentist drill into the nerve or jaw. This will cause shame and embarrassment —I will be the joke of the day"

My triggers:

"Waiting room, sound of the drill, dental office smell, dentist's chair"

My support thoughts:

"I'm the boss of my own body."

"I can't wait to smile again."

"I am in charge of how much discomfort I can tolerate."

Signs that I'm scared, which the dental team can look out for:

"I tense up in the chair."

"My hands are fisted, or I fidget with them."

"I become quiet, 'obedient' and suffer through dental treatment."

"I don't make eye contact."

"I talk a lot to avoid starting dental treatment."

"My voice becomes thick, and I cry silently."

Here is what I need from my dental team when I'm afraid:

"Enough time"

"Don't give me the feeling that we're in a hurry/pressed for time."

"Stop signals are important. Sounds from the throat also mean stop."

"I want the dentist to decide that we take a break for a few minutes."

"Remind me to breathe and to relax."

"I need the dentist to ask questions like 'what are you thinking now?', not 'are you okay?'. Then I will just say 'yes' anyway."

"I wonder what it will be like if I have to stop treatment – explain that to me."

"Speak to me properly and clearly. Don't scold me, patronize me or speak to me like I'm a child."

"I need a little time to recover- or just a few minutes of cheerful small talk."

"Talk to me about how treatment can be as painless as possible."

"Explain what you're going to do, before you do it, including how it's going to feel."

"Make the appointments early in the day (so I won't have to dread it all day) or late (I have difficulty sleeping)."

"Give me a brief description of upcoming sessions so I won't have to wonder and think about what we're going to do next. Write it down — because I forget so easily."

"If I lose my courage and don't show up, it's nice that the assistant calls me."

"Send me a text message appointment reminder because I forget so easily."

Patients with Complex Reactions and Co-morbidity

Contents

People with Mental Disorders in the Dental Clinic

Anne Kristine Bergem

Contents

15.1 Preface

The causes of mental disorders are complex. Genetic factors, adverse childhood experiences, stressful life events, and stress are risk factors.

Schizophrenia, bipolar disorder, anorexia, and post-traumatic stress disorder (PTSD) are some of the diagnoses used to categorize mental disorders. Diagnoses say little to nothing regarding causes or function in daily living but may be useful when it comes to rights, treatments, and financial benefits.

It is useful to have knowledge regarding mental disorders and how the disorders or their symptoms may affect communication and treatment, in order to understand and respond in an effective and professional manner. Post-treatment compliance is of importance to all patients, patients with mental disorders included. Some mental disorders (i.e., depression and schizophrenia) have symptoms that make care for personal hygiene more demanding.

Oral health and mental health are complex topics. Much can be said about oral health literacy, preventive measures, availability of treatments, and financial conditions as factors of importance to the negative correlation between oral health and mental health. In-depth analyses of this will be beyond the scope of this chapter. A short introduction will be given as a backdrop, but the emphasis will be on clinical encounters between dental health professionals and patients.

🎓 Learning Goals

After reading this chapter, you will have
- Learned about how mental health problems can affect oral health.
- Learned how oral health personnel can address topics concerning mental health in a respectful yet direct manner.
- Had the opportunity to challenge your preconceptions on mental disorders.

15.2 Oral Health and Mental Health

People with severe mental disorders have poorer oral health than the rest of the population, with an increased need for dental care [1]. Measures taken to improve dental health in the population have not had the same effect on people with severe mental disorders [2]. Oral health is an important part of somatic health and is correlated with an increase in other diseases like vascular diseases, diabetes, cancer, and respiratory diseases. Poor oral health can also affect eating, speech, and other social and psychological areas of life [3].

The most common oral health problems in people with severe mental disorders have been reported to be dental erosions, caries and periodontal diseases [1, 3], and temporomandibular disorder (TMD) [4]; there are several plausible causes for these problems, more in patients with severe mental disorders:
- Poor nutrition.
- Poor oral hygiene.
- Heavy consumption of carbonated drinks.
- Comorbid substance misuse including tobacco, alcohol, or psychostimulants.
- Dry mouth.
  - Dry mouth is a known side effect of psychotropic medication and is a risk factor for oral health problems.
  - Pathology in the parotid gland is seen in patients with bulimia and may contribute to dry mouth.
- Bruxism may cause attrition.
  - Bruxism is seen in patients with depression.
- Excessive brushing and flossing.
  - In manic phases, people with bipolar disorder can brush and floss in such a manner that dental abrasions and mucosal and gingival lacerations may occur.

In patients with psychotic disorders like schizophrenia, the frequency of decayed teeth and missing teeth is higher than in people without schizophrenia. Schizophrenia is a severe mental disorder, characterized by distortions in thinking, perception, emotions, and sense of self and behavior. Common experiences in people with schizophrenia are hallucinations (hearing voices or seeing things that are not there) and delusions (fixed, private beliefs not shared with the rest of the population) [5].

People who suffer from schizophrenia will, to a greater or lesser degree, struggle with interaction with other people. They may have difficulties understanding social situations and how to handle them. People with schizophrenia also have difficulty with complicated, higher-order cognitive functions, the so-called social cognition. These phenomena mean that patients suffering from schizophrenia may have a reduced ability to understand others' experiences of the world being different from their own. In turn, this means they will have a poorer basis for predicting or understanding other people's intentions in a given social situation. They will, therefore, more easily misunderstand other people and may seem less empathetic in their behavior. It is also common for patients to have problems with attention and memory. Flexibility can also be impaired.

People suffering from schizophrenia themselves will often withdraw from close relationships and live isolated lives. This may be due to the experiences that some people have gone through where thoughts are inflicted on them or stolen or broadcasted. The withdrawal becomes a form of self-protection.

No single symptom is specific or unique to schizophrenia. Similar symptoms may also be seen in other mental disorders. The main and most characteristic symptoms of schizophrenia can be grouped into positive and negative symptoms, with the positive being hallucinations and delusions.

Examples of negative symptoms are loss of motivation, absence of enthusiasm and commitment, or absence of the ability for targeted actions. Another negative symptom is lack of communication of emotions through body language and facial expressions. The patient may appear emotionally flat and uninvolved [6]. The negative symptoms are considered to be of greatest importance when it comes to personal hygiene including oral hygiene [7].

Financial and other factors can be barriers to help-seeking behavior [3]. An episode of schizophrenia can make it extremely difficult, if not impossible, to manage finances well [8]. People with schizophrenia also encounter one of the highest unemployment rates among all vocationally disadvantaged groups [9].

Dental anxiety does not seem to be one among the barriers in people with severe mental disorders like schizophrenia [1]. A Swedish study showed that 81% of people with severe mental disorders respected their dentist's opinion and that satisfaction with the dentist was related to more frequent visits to the dentist.

In many countries, health services are organized in silos, and lack of integration of health services may be of great importance when it comes to oral health. Mental health personnel express ambivalence, reluctance, and lack of training when it comes to raising oral health as a topic in contact with patients, even though they, at the same time, acknowledge the importance of oral health [10]. With the patient's consent, health personnel from different health services are able to communicate and cooperate in the best interest of the patient [11]. Oral health personnel then have the possibility, and the opportunity, to discuss the patient's oral health with the patient's therapist.

Patients with long-term disorders will need specialized care from different health-care services. This can be organized in many ways. In Norway, people with complex and long-term needs are entitled to an individualized plan. Dental health care could, and in many cases should, be a part of health-care plans, which, in turn, should contribute to facilitating collaboration, through commitment, from all participants including the patient.

15.3 Clinical Encounters

Successful treatment in health care, oral health care included, is often accompanied by effective communication between the health-care professional and the person receiving treatment.

Effective communication includes information, oral health education, and motivating patients to comply when it comes to desirable behavioral changes and follow-up after treatment. To be successful as an oral health-care worker regarding these elements, one needs to establish a trustful and reliable relationship with one's patient [12].

Dental health professionals will sometimes have known their patients for years. When somebody you already know develops a mental illness, the situation will be somewhat different than when you do not know anything about the person and meet him or her for the first time.

New patients are a vulnerable population because they are at a high risk of missing subsequent visits or dropping out of care. Some behaviors have the potential to improve the patient's experience. Providing reassurance, telling the patients that it is okay to ask questions, showing them the results and explaining it to them, avoiding judgmental language and behavior, and asking patients what they want at the beginning of a relationship have all shown to be important factors between physicians and patients [13]. There is no reason why the same factors should not be valid in an oral health-care setting. When you meet a patient for the first time, you have little or no knowledge of their medical or oral health history. Both the patient as a person and his or her oral health problems will be unknown to you, and you must figure out both simultaneously.

For individuals with mental health challenges, a consistent and sensitive dentist builds trust and provides continuity of care with individualized approaches. Building rapport takes time, and having a good relationship with a patient puts you in a better position, should this patient develop mental health problems, when trust is already present. In patients you have known for a long time, it may be easier to spot changes in their mental state. You may also rely on former experience regarding communication and treatment.

Whether it is a person known to you or somebody new, when a patient comes to you as a dental health-care professional, it is never a diagnosis or the symptoms of a disorder that enter the office, it is the person! Lists of symptoms of various mental disorders are of little use in everyday life at a dental clinic. The symptoms and signs related to mental disorders mentioned in this chapter are offered as a means of increasing professional confidence in dental health professionals and reducing myths and prejudices toward people with mental disorders.

15.4 Patients, Actions, and Explanations

For the main part, the rest of this chapter consists of clinical examples – stories – followed by actions and explanations as to why a particular action is suggested. There is seldom only one way to act in contact with patients. Examples will nonetheless provide the reader with the opportunity to recognize situations similar to encounters from their own experiences and to reflect on them.

15.4.1 Storytelling as a Method of Learning

Storytelling is an efficient method of learning. Stories are tools through which learners can explore reality [14]. Stories as clinical examples will provide context and meaning to subjects in a manner that other text material will not. Reading textbooks alone will not be sufficient to prepare the reader for clinical work. Stories, on the other hand, will show glimpses of reality. It will also be easier for readers to see the person behind the symptoms and diagnoses through stories. This is especially important when it comes to disorders with a great deal of myths and prejudices [15]. Stories will also challenge readers on prejudices and preconceptions, something that is of vital importance in professional development [16].

Self-consciousness, self-regulation, self-motivation, social consciousness, and social abilities are five skills of vital importance to health workers. The development of these skills happens through emotional engagement [14]. The use of stories may be a contribution, as stories, more than any other written material, appeal to emotions [15].

Stories will put the patient in the center of what is taught and serve to remind the author and the reader about the purpose of learning [15].

15.4.2 Stories

15.4.2.1 Story #1

Mrs. Hansen

Mrs. Hansen has been a regular patient of yours for 10 years. You have an agreement on annually sending her a notice for a consultation. When she enters your consultation room, you can see that she looks different than usual. She is without her usual smile, and she moves like it takes great effort. Her hair is unkempt, and she wears no makeup. You invite her to sit down.

What Do You Do?

Because you know her, you ask how she is today. She recognizes the sincerity in your question and starts crying. She says that she did not remember the appointment today, and, when her daughter came to collect her, she did not want to come. She let her daughter drive her because she did not have the strength to argue. You understand something is going on and sit down next to her. She tells you that her husband of 40 years died of cancer 10 months ago, and she is not coping very well. In fact, she has become depressed. You acknowledge her loss and offer your sympathies along with a tissue. You recognize the effort it took for her to come in for a consultation and praise her for doing so.

After some minutes, she gathers herself and gradually stops crying. You ask if she is getting any help or treatment for her depression and she tells you that her general practitioner (GP) is involved. You then ask if she is undergoing therapy or taking medication or both, and she gives you the name of an antidepressant. You know that this medication may cause dry mouth, and, so, you tell her this. She tells you that dry mouth has become a great problem for her and that she avoids social gatherings because she feels stupid when her upper lip fastens to her teeth and food is difficult to swallow.

You tell her that even though you cannot help with her depression, you can hopefully help with her dry mouth problem. She is happy to talk with you about different measures that can be helpful and lets you to conduct the planned examination.

When she leaves, she seems a bit relieved, and you walk her out to your secretary to make sure that she gets a new appointment in some weeks to check if things are developing as wanted. You also suggest sending a summary of the consultation to the patient's GP, which Mrs. Hansen finds is an excellent idea.

Why?

As a dentist, you are a health professional and bound by professional ethics [17]. You are always to treat patients to the best of your knowledge and with the patient's best interest at heart.

When you see that a patient is troubled, it is within your responsibility to address the situation. You also need to know about any health issues or concerns regarding the patient's health.

Mrs. Hansen's sadness may be a symptom of depression, a suspicion that is supported by her lack of interest in her appearance [18].

Depression is a common mental disorder. It is an illness that can affect how people feel and behave for weeks or months at a time. It is not the same as feeling a bit low. The main symptoms are feeling sad most of the time and losing interest in things one used to enjoy.

In addition, one or more of these symptoms are common: little appetite or more appetite than usual, which can lead to significant weight loss or gain, problems sleeping or sleeping too much, feeling either agitated or sluggish, feeling extremely tired or low in energy, feeling worthless or excessively guilty, finding it hard to think and concentrate, and/or thinking about suicide. It is important to seek medical assistance when depressed. A GP will check that the symptoms are not caused by medicines or other medical conditions. Blood and urine tests will be conducted to rule out these things, and sometimes a computed tomography (CT) scan, a magnetic resonance imaging (MRI), or an electroencephalography (EEG) are required as well. Between 6% and 12% of the adult population will at some point qualify for the diagnosis [19].

It is not within your responsibilities or abilities to treat a patient for his or her depression, which you made clear to Mrs. Hansen, but, as a health professional, you need to make sure that she has contact with her GP or other relevant health services. Her oral health issues are definitely your responsibility, and so is monitoring the situation that has arisen because of her mental health problems and treatment.

You keep the GP informed of what you have done and recommended because it is in the patient's best interest that everybody cooperates. With Mrs. Hansen's consent, you are at liberty to do so.

15.4.2.2   Story #2
Mr. Peterson

This morning, you are receiving a new patient. Mr. Peterson is 45 years old, and you have no prior knowledge about him. He has given his list of medications to your secretary, and, before you collect him from the waiting room, you find his journal in your computer.

His journal says that he takes a lithium preparation. You know of lithium, but, as a quality check, you look it up on the Internet. Lithium is mostly used as a stabilizer for manic episodes as a part of bipolar disorder treatment.

Mr. Peterson tells you that he has booked an appointment with you because he has moved to your area. A friend has recommended you to him. He has had some problems with periodontitis and is adamant to keep the problem under control. The examination goes without any problems, and you are soon finished.

What Do You Do?

You are not sure how to address the medication but choose to ask if he plans to consult you on a regular basis in the future. He confirms.

You then decide to talk a little more and start by saying that he is very welcome as a new patient at the clinic. You also say that you have looked through the information

he had left with your secretary. He nods but does not offer any more information. "You do not use a lot of medication"; you say to him but add that you have noticed the lithium. "I am somewhat familiar with lithium," you continue, "and I know that it is usually prescribed for treating bipolar disorder. I do not know if that is why you are taking it, but I thought I should ask since we are going to keep in touch from now on." He nods and answers that he has not had any manic episodes for the last 7 years.

Why?

It is always important to know a patient's medication, as many substances have side effects that affect oral health. As mentioned in the Preface, people in a manic or depressive phase may exhibit behaviors concerning their mouth or teeth, and knowing about the disorder makes it easier for you to know what to expect and also to give sound advice.

When mentioning both the medication and suggesting a cause for it, you demonstrate to the patient that you are not afraid to talk about mental concerns. To be able to talk freely about mental concerns is a way of showing an absence of prejudice. This may encourage the patient to talk about mental health issues with you at a later time should the need arise.

Between 1% and 2% of the population are affected by some form of bipolar disorder [20]. All people have ups and downs in their moods. In bipolar disorder, mood swings are more extreme and can make life hard. With the right treatments, most people have good life quality. Medication, cognitive therapy, and an everyday life with enough sleep are measures useful to many.

If Mr. Peterson, at some point, would show up at your clinic in a hypomanic or manic phase, it could be because his elevated mood and level of energy made him want to do something about his dental state. It would not be a problem for you to carry out ordinary examinations and treatment if Mr. Peterson wanted you to. You would maybe find him a bit hectic or chaotic in his thoughts and speech. It would be a good idea only to do necessary work and postpone more elaborate work until later. Mr. Peterson's ability to concentrate and cooperate could be somewhat diminished due to the symptoms of mania. Other symptoms of a manic episode are inflated self-esteem or grandiosity, decreased need for sleep, increased activity, and risky activity. Risky activity also includes spending money. If Mr. Peterson wants to start an expensive treatment, it is important to postpone the decision. Agreements made with a person in a manic state is not necessarily binding and may in addition cause the patient financial distress [21].

In a manic phase, Mr. Peterson could very well forget about oral hygiene because of his other activities, but, if he was concerned about his oral health, he might brush and floss vigorously [3]. Because of difficulties with concentration, in a manic state, Mr. Peterson might not be open to elaborate explanations and advice. Telling him to brush with his non-dominant hand and rinse with fluoride may be a practical advice of some importance.

In an actual encounter with Mr. Peterson in a manic state, a calm environment with few stimuli would be good. A close cooperation with Mr. Peterson, his next of kin, GP, and other professional health personnel would be strongly recommended.

15.4.2.3   Story #3

Mrs. Dale

Mrs. Dale is a patient that you have "inherited" from an old dentist in the neighborhood, recently retired. You have not been able to access the old journal system, so you have no previous knowledge about Mrs. Dale. During the encounter, Mrs. Dale starts telling you about her neighbor. She explains to you that her neighbor deliberately troubles her by knocking on the walls at night. According to Mrs. Dale, he also puts toxic gases in the radiators, forcing her to shut them off to avoid poisoning. She is a bit concerned about the cold when winter comes. She also thinks that the toxic gases have caused the loss of several of her fillings. You notice that two fillings are missing from her teeth. Her oral health is otherwise not so bad.

What Do You Do?

You say "It sounds to me like you are having a stressful time at home, Mrs. Dale. I can see that two fillings are gone, and I can help you with replacing them. Do you have anybody supporting you in these stressful times?" After some talking, you learn that Mrs. Dale has a son living not far from her with his family and that she has a GP and services twice a week from the municipality. You suggest to her the need for her GP to know how she is doing and offer to give her a call. Mrs. Dale is a bit skeptical but agrees that she needs help. She cannot take on the neighbor by herself, she comments.

"It is a good thing to accept help when you need it," you assure her.

Why?

Mrs. Dale may have delusions (or she may have a terrible neighbor, one cannot be sure) [22]. Regardless, you should always acknowledge someone's feelings and experiences, even if they seem strange to you. You can acknowledge Mrs. Dale's feeling of being scared and stressed without pretending to believe her reason for feeling so. Mrs. Dale will not recover from her delusions by being told "the truth" from you. Worst-case scenario, you alienate her by pretending to know more about her situation than her or by accusing her of not speaking the truth. In that situation, she may storm out of your clinic and never return. By acknowledging her experience, which is stressful to her no matter what is really happening, she finds you to be trustworthy. Gaining her trust puts you in a situation where you are able to make sure that important information is being passed on to her GP. At the same time, you can continue doing your job, ensuring that her oral health remains good.

Not confronting her with her delusions is not the same as playing along but rather a choice of action. She needs to be treated with respect, and no good comes from confrontations. Her experiences from her apartment are stressful to her, which is something you both can agree on regardless of the cause of the distress.

Delusions are private thoughts or opinions that are not shared with the majority of the population and is a not uncommon in psychotic episodes or disorders. The content is often of persecutory nature. This symptom is often seen in elderly people and may be associated with cognitive impairment [22].

A therapeutic approach to people with delusions is recommended. Empathy and respect are important, and arguing is to be avoided [23].

15.4.2.4   Story #4

Miss Aftani

The first time you met Miss Aftani, she was 17 years old. In her journal, you wrote down a concern for her dental status due to erosions on the palatal side of her teeth and parotid gland swelling. Over the years, Miss Aftani has developed severe bulimia with numerous admissions to a mental health clinic. She is now an inpatient at a district mental health center and is slowly getting better.

After several years without satisfactory oral health care, her oral health status is now pretty bad. She has a lot of pain, particularly when chewing. Clinically, there are extensive erosions on several teeth. You can see old fillings in the middle of new erosions and some molars and premolars with visible red pulpa covered with an extremely thin dentin layer. The cheek mucosa is whiter than normal.

Miss Aftani describes burning sensations in her mouth as well as pain.

She tells you about her attempts at dental care during admissions, without success. There was no cooperation between the psychiatric ward and her dentist. She lost her motivation due to pain and lack of support from the hospital staff, she adds.

What Do You Do?

You have for a long time known the importance of cooperation with her therapist, so, together with Miss Aftani, you have decided on a long-term plan, with small steps at a time.

Today, you start with a thorough examination. There are many findings, but you do not stop until you have the whole picture. When you are done, you describe what you have found to Miss Aftani. You carefully explain what you have found, how the findings correspond with Miss Aftani's pain and other symptoms, and why.

Miss Aftani now knows that vomiting is the cause of teeth decay. The first time you met Miss Aftani, you found it difficult to address your findings. When you look back, it must have been your concern about how she would react that made you hesitate. However, in the end, you decided to tell her. You were respectful and nonjudgmental and told her in a matter-of-fact manner that the erosions most likely came from gastric acid, as gastric acid comes in contact with the teeth during vomiting. She started to cry at the time, but you waited patiently for her to gather herself. She reluctantly admitted to vomiting but did not offer additional information at first. You did not pressure her but continued talking in a calm manner. This first time, you advised her to rinse her mouth with water after throwing up and avoid brushing. You also suggested rinsing with fluoride. She has sporadically been to see you over the years, but it has only been recently that she felt well enough to make plans.

Today, you agree on some temporary treatment to ease her pain – composite on several teeth to avoid biting directly at the dentine covering the pulpa.

You tell Miss Aftani about her options – further work in composite materials or crowns. In both cases, treatment will take time and money. Regardless of which option she chooses, it is important to be in dialogue with her and her team at the mental clinic.

You also suggest a referral to an ear–nose–throat specialist for her parotid glands.

The need for cooperation between all health-care personnel is obvious to you. You know from experience that persons with pain like Miss Aftani prefer soft food to lessen their pain. It is probably a good idea to discuss the situation with both her GP and her therapist at the mental clinic. Maybe even a nutritionist from the hospital could join the team.

It is not possible to reach the therapist by phone while the patient is in your surgery, so you make sure to write the history sheet immediately for the patient to bring with her.

Why?

Changes in the mouth may be among the first physical signs of an eating disorder. An eating disorder is often accompanied by harmful habits and nutritional deficiencies. Such habits can have severe consequences on a person's oral health.

An eating disorder may cause damage to the teeth and mouth [24]. This damage may be temporary but can also be permanent, and early detection of an eating dis-

order is important both for the person's mental and oral health. Oral and dental damage can be tempered. Right information and appropriate guidance from the dentist to the person is vital. The relationship between the dentist and the patient must be strictly confidential to provide a safe environment for sharing concerns about the disorder and oral health problems [25]. Keeping this knowledge in mind, you address the dental damage at the first opportunity even though you are not sure how the patient will respond.

If a person is an inpatient at a mental hospital, your advice would be helpful for the staff in their support of the patient in everyday life at the ward. Neither nurses nor doctors are necessarily educated in oral health. Simple, but important, advice to patients and mental health-care workers can be [25]:

- Patients should swish water in their mouths after vomiting due to the high acidic content in the oral cavity.
- Brushing of the teeth should be halted for an hour to avoid actually scrubbing the stomach acids deeper into the tooth enamel.
- Moisturizing the mouth with water will help keep recurrent decay at a minimum as dry mouth is a risk factor. Dry mouth may be a result of vomiting, poor nutrition, or medication.
- Fluoride rinses may be prescribed as well as desensitizing or remineralizing agents.
- When patients have oral pain, analgesics are not sufficient treatment but may disguise oral problems in need of treatment to avoid further problems.

You may think that as an oral health professional, it is not your job to suggest contact with a nutritionist, but no other health-care professional has your knowledge about how diet can affect oral conditions.

Dietitians have a pivotal role in providing preemptive education and screening of oral health [26]. Malnutrition may, in turn, contribute to deterioration of oral as well as mental health [27].

Helping a patient like Miss Aftani suffering from an eating disorder with his or her oral health, whether it is prevention or recovery, takes time and combined effort. Keeping this in mind, you make sure that both the patient and the cooperating personnel are informed about your assessments and suggestions.

15.4.2.5 Story #5
Miss Potter

Miss Potter has her first appointment today. When she called to make the appointment, she told your receptionist that you had been recommended to her by a friend in an interest group for women with eating disorders. She herself suffers from overeating. The thought of seeking dental care has been far from her mind for many years, but she now has joined the interest group and has recently started therapy. She is an intelligent young woman in her early twenties.

What Do You Do?

When Miss Potter enters your surgery, she is a bit shy, but, nonetheless, she starts out by telling you that she has started a difficult but important process where her goal is to stop feeling ashamed of who she is. She has for many years kept to herself because of her size. She is convinced that she has a lot of cavities due to consuming sweets and a bad oral hygiene. She averts eye contact most of the time and only casts a glance at you when she stops talking.

You tell Miss Potter that she is welcome as a patient and express admiration for her courage. During the examination, you find several cavities. You tell Miss Potter of your findings and come to an agreement on how to proceed. Some cavities you will deal with today, and some next week.

At a point during the treatment, Miss Potter goes limp in the chair, and you notice a glazed look in her eyes. You stop what you are doing and back your chair away from her. "Miss Potter," you softly call, and gently squeeze her hand. Some seconds later, Miss Potter answers. "You were far away for a moment?," you ask. "Yes, I was," she replies, "I don't know what happened."

You straighten the back of her chair to get her in an upright position. You keep your distance from her and carefully ask if maybe she wants to take a break. You offer her a cup of water.

Thinking of her many cavities and what just happened, you start to think that the two things may be connected. You carefully ask her if she maybe has had some bad experiences with laying on her back or getting objects into her mouth. Maybe somebody did something to her before?

She starts to cry when she hears what you are saying. You patiently wait until she gathers herself, offering only a tissue. After a few minutes, she tells you that she was sexually abused when she was in her teens.

Why?

In all, 1 in 20 children and adolescents grow up in surroundings characterized by violence. Among adults, 25% of women and nearly 50% of men report being exposed to violence after the age of 18. In all, 1 in 5 girls and 1 in 14 boys have been exposed to sexual abuse growing up. A total of 9% of all women have experienced rape at some point in their life. Even if the numbers are high in Norway, the prevalence in other countries is even higher. Experience with violence and sexual abuse is unfortunately quite common.

Abuse and maltreatment are the main risk factors for mental health disorders in general [28]. The same can be said for experiencing rape. Almost 40% of rape victims have been found to meet the criteria of current mood or anxiety disorders other than PTSD [29]. Overeating and other eating disorders are seen in people exposed to sexual abuse [30]. Dissociation is not uncommon in people who have survived sexual trauma [31].

Miss Potter's oral health is not good, something that is often the case in people with experiences of sexual violence and abuse. There are strong associations between exposure to childhood adversity and poor dental health [32].

Many people with traumatizing experiences avoid oral health care and have problems with daily hygiene for the same reason. Having a toothbrush in his or her mouth or having toothpaste foaming in the mouth may be triggers of traumatic experiences of sexual abuse.

Several stimuli present in a dental treatment situation may trigger reactions connected to memories of traumatizing events for Miss Potter. Some examples are:

- Lying back in a chair may trigger memories of being defenseless under an attacker or abuser.
- Having one or more persons standing over him or her with no escape route may be a trigger.
- Instruments or fingers inside the oral cavity may trigger memories of oral abuse or rape.
- Being at the mercy of another person may itself be a trigger.

In these situations, Miss Potter may react with hyper- or hypoactivation.

Hyperactivation includes a high degree of strong emotions like anger, fear, shame, and may express itself in the fight–flight range and includes anxiety, unrest, aggressive behavior, etc.

Hypoactivation is a state of avoiding emotions for self-preservation, and it often leaves the person in a "frozen" state or the person may dissociate. That was what happened to Miss Potter on that day.

Dissociation is a form of disconnection from one's surroundings. It may include the experience of detachment or feeling as if one is outside one's body and loss of memory or amnesia. Dissociative disorders are frequently associated with previous experience of trauma. For people in the proximity of a person dissociating, it may seem like the person "disappears" or spaces out like your observation with Miss Potter today. The person can have a glazed look in his or her eyes or may seem to be staring at something far away, like Miss Potter did.

The goal of treatment is to let people stay in their optimal arousal zone where they feel safe, awake, and able to cooperate. In the "window of tolerance" model, this is the state between hyper- and hypoarousal. [33]. The window of tolerance model is explained in detail in ▶ Chap. 2.

Sometimes, oral health care can be planned in cooperation with the person and the therapist/psychologist/psychiatrist and a specialized team. As a health-care professional, you may still meet many patients in your daily work like you did today.

A calming environment, gradual exposure to the examination and treatment, making deals that make sure the patient feels in control and may stop whatever you are doing at any time are all vital. Information and predictability are the key elements.

15.4.2.6   Story #6
Young Mr. Jameson

Young Pete Jameson is 8 years old. He is in for a regular checkup and is accompanied by his mother. When he comes into your surgery, he quickly turns his attention to all the equipment on the counter and starts picking up tools. "What is this," he asks, and without waiting for an answer, he picks up another tool and asks the same question. His mother shrugs apologetically. "He is so curious," she says.

What Do You Do?

It is not the first time that you have had visitors in your surgery with lots of energy and little interest in spending more time sitting down than absolutely necessary. You know that the best solution probably is to let the young man satisfy his curiosity this time and make plans ahead.

You join him at the counter and put forward instruments that he is allowed to touch and make him hold them while you tell him their names.

After some time, you explain to him that you will spend this encounter exploring and preparing so that when he comes back, you will conduct the planned examination and necessary treatment.

He is allowed to try the pedals connected to the chair and fill a cup with water.

His mother smiles at you and is extremely grateful for the way you took the boy seriously.

You tell both the boy and his mother what you are going to do the next time and ask if they have any questions. The boy asks if it will hurt, and you explain the procedure and tell him what might hurt and make a deal on how he can let you know if he wants you to stop.

When they come back after a week, you remind the boy of your deal. You have tidied your surgery, so only the necessary equipment is at hand. He is allowed to fill water in his cup a couple of times, and you take the chair up and down an extra time for his benefit, but, otherwise, you hold him to your deal. You take frequent breaks, as you have planned the examination stepwise. After each break, you tell him what you are going to do next. This time, you do not ask open questions but only questions with possible acceptable answers or questions of a yes/no type. He gets

a little impatient, but you praise him for doing well and are able to finish the examination.

Why?

There are several reasons a child might not be interested in sitting still in a chair in a dental surgery. It is beyond the scope of this chapter to go into all of them. It may be a perfectly natural response to a situation distressing to the child, it may be that the child has had life experiences of an adverse nature, or something different. It may also be that the child meets the criteria for attention-deficit hyperactivity disorder (ADHD).

ADHD is one of the most common disorders of childhood. About 5% of children around the world meet the criteria. The etiology is multifactorial and composed of genetic and environmental factors.

As a child with ADHD, Mr. Jameson will [34]:
- Find it almost impossible to stay still. He will squirm in his seat, fidget, and get up all the time. He never seems to run out of energy. He chatters almost constantly.
- Be impulsive. He does not stop to think before he acts; he seems extremely impatient and is constantly interrupting both his mother and you when you are speaking.
- Touch things he is not supposed to.

The behavior is not Mr. Jameson's fault. Neither his nor his parents' actions are the cause of his ADHD or the symptoms you observe.

The problem with Mr. Jameson is that he is unable to process information in the same manner as other children. He experiences the outside world like a flood of noise and images. It is hard for him to decide what is important and what is not. Therefore, he often gets confused. It can be hard for him to organize and perform daily tasks. In addition, he finds it difficult to concentrate on only one thing at a time.

To be supportive to Mr. Jameson, there are several things that you can do to increase his chance of mastering the situation, and that is what you do the second time the boy comes to your surgery:
- You repeat instructions.
- You break big tasks into smaller tasks and reward each step.
- You keep the environment quiet and calm.
- You do and say one thing at a time.

All the time, you remind yourself that when young Mr. Jameson does not seem to follow your instructions, it is not because he is not listening to what you are saying or does not want to comply. He probably actually cannot hear you. You patiently repeat your instructions after making sure that you have a connection with him.

15.4.2.7 Story #7

Mr. Duffy

"Can you fit Mr. Duffy in as soon as possible?" Your secretary is on the phone. "He has come into the waiting area and I think the other patients are bothered by the way he smells."

Mr. Duffy is a man in his sixties living alone in a cabin at the edge of the woods. He is a loner and is looked upon as the village original. He spends his days collecting bottles from trash cans in public places. You know a little about his story, but he is eloquent in his speech and clearly an intelligent man from what you have observed at earlier encounters.

You ask your secretary to invite Mr. Duffy into the recreational area and offer him a cup of coffee. She frowns but does as asked.

"How are you this afternoon," you ask Mr. Duffy as you welcome him into your surgery. He tells you that he has pain when eating and wants you to help out.

What Do You Do?

You smell that it has been some time since he has had a shower or a fresh pair of clothes. You instinctively put some mentholated ointment under your nose before you put on your face mask. After thinking about it, you decide to be up front with Mr. Duffy. You start by saying that you will accept him as your patient today and will try to be of help. As respectfully as you can, you explain to Mr. Duffy that you are not used to the smell he is bringing with him. You wait anxiously for his response, afraid that he will be cross. At first, he frowns. Then, he laughs heartily. When he sees your surprised face, he tells you that he knows of his smell and is used to people withdrawing from him. He actually values your candor.

You tell about your trick with the mentholatum, and he nods affirmatively.

The examination reveals several teeth in decay. He already has six teeth missing.

You do your best to clean and offer some advice on how to manage oral hygiene under relatively poor living conditions.

Mr. Duffy is in a good mood when he leaves your surgery. He bows to your secretary on his way out and thanks her for the coffee.

Why?

Mr. Duffy does not have a diagnosis of some mental disorder. You may call him a village original, as he certainly has made some original life choices. Truth to be told, you have no way of knowing whether his lifestyle is like it is by choice or if there are some tragic events in Mr. Duffy's life that has resulted in him living like his does.

Not maintaining personal hygiene is an unusual life choice and may arouse prejudice and contempt in other people. Smell and uncleanliness are the opposite of the ideal of being fresh and fit. Nonetheless, it is not illegal per se. On the other hand, in Norway, a case was brought to court some years ago regarding a person who was banned from university because of his smell. He lost when he brought the matter to court. Many years later, when he was admitted to a nursing home, the court made him wash against his will. He did not resist physically but was adamant that the washing was done against his will [35]. The reason for the court's decision was the risk of infection and smell.

When Mr. Duffy appears at your clinic, questions of a legal and ethical nature emerge. Similar questions may arise in other situations if people look, speak, or behave in ways that differ from the norm.

Health-care personnel are, in many countries, legally obligated to provide health care in emergency situations. Ethical rules apply regardless of location, and health personnel have a moral responsibility to provide help, even in cases when they are not legally obligated to do so.

If the degree of emergency is unclear, health-care professionals must examine the patient to find out [36]. An emergency situation means that health care is urgently needed. "Urgently needed" indicates that it takes quite a lot for the duty to occur. In the assessment, emphasis must be placed on whether there is a danger to life or a danger of serious deterioration of a state of health [37].

Oral health problems will seldom be acutely life-threatening but nonetheless is of serious concern. The oral cavity is the entry to both the gastrointestinal tract and the airways. Serious infections in the mouth or teeth may also spread to the blood stream if they are not treated or pus is evacuated properly [38]. In a patient like Mr. Duffy, it is necessary to examine his oral cavity to make sure that severe infections are present. Whether this is urgently needed as stated in the law or not cannot be answered easily. By tending to Mr. Duffy's oral problems, you may have prevented a more serious illness.

If you have decided to reject Mr. Duffy, it would be wise to examine your reasons for doing so. Maybe you were disgusted by his smell and did not want Mr. Duffy in your office. If that was the case, today, you have resisted the urge to send him away.

Unpleasant odors are often caused by illness and poor hygiene. Health personnel may perceive smell as shameful and patients as vulnerable because both are exposed to the disgust of others. Health personnel want to protect patients from shame. The most common action strategies are to remove odors through practical action, avoid showing bodily reactions to odors, and remain silent about odor problems. Silence may intensify the shame and loneliness and, in some cases, contribute to a weakened treatment offer. Patients want more transparency [39]. Your sincerity toward Mr. Duffy strengthened the relationship and made him feel respected.

Not talking about difficult subjects does not make them go away.

As a health-care professional, it is your responsibility to be able to talk to patients about difficult topics, whether it is bad smell or suspicion of an eating disorder or sexual abuse.

15.4.2.8 Story #8

Mr. Rourke

A nurse working in a high-security ward at a mental health-care center nearby has been in touch with you regarding an inpatient at the ward. He has had pain in the oral area and problem opening his mouth for several days, and, even though he took both paracetamol and ibuprofen, he is clearly bothered by the pain.

A high-security unit like this admits patients with severe mental disorders and a potential for violence.

You have, in collaboration with the staff at the ward, made arrangements for the patient to come at the end of the day when there are no other patients in the waiting room.

When Mr. Rourke arrives at your clinic, he is accompanied by two mental health workers that know him very well. This is according to plan. Your surgery is not very big, so it feels a bit cramped in there.

After your examination, you conclude that there is infection around a wisdom tooth.

Mr. Rourke is clearly bothered by the situation, the pain, the confined space, and you literally getting in his face. He starts to swear and shout angrily at nobody in particular.

The two mental health workers remain calm. One of them says "Mr. Rourke, there is no need to shout. We talked about this. If the pain is to go away the dentist must be allowed to help you." "Then help me," Mr. Rourke shouts. He then mumbles something to himself.

What Do You Do?

Reassured by the calmness of the staff, you are encouraged to continue your work. After giving Mr. Rourke a minute, you calmly explain step by step what you are going to do before you do it. You make sure that Mr. Rourke can see you the whole time. You make eye contact but do not stare. You hold your hands as visible as possible the whole time, and when you remove your hands out of Mr. Rourke's sight, you make sure to explain what you are doing. You frequently pause to ask Mr. Rourke if he is okay.

Why?

Psychosis is a condition that affects the way in which a person processes information. During psychosis, a person loses touch with reality. People might see, hear, feel, smell, taste, or believe things that are not real. Psychosis is a symptom not an illness. A mental or physical illness, substance abuse, or extreme stress can cause it. Genetic factors contribute to vulnerability for developing psychosis.

Psychotic disorders, like schizophrenia, involve psychosis. People may have one psychotic episode or several during their lifetime. In all, 25% of people with the diagnosis get well, 50% get better, and 25% are affected throughout their life [40].

People having psychosis are at an increased risk of involvement in violent episodes, but most people with psychosis are not violent [41]. It is not documented that the disorder itself is the reason for the increased risk. It might as well be other factors like substance abuse, exposure to violent environments, and other contextual elements [42].

A patient admitted to a security ward in Norway will be at a risk of violence. The prediction of violent behavior in people with severe mental disorders is done by trained personnel [42]. The risk of violence is a dynamic trait, and the admittance of a person to a security ward does not mean that the person is continuously at a risk of violence. If the health personnel working the patient have decided on taking the patient to dental care, you can be assured a thorough assessment has been made.

The risk factors of concern in a dental setting are:
Related to the patient:
- Persecutory delusions and imperative voices commanding the patient to exercise violence, especially if the patient feels that these symptoms are uncomfortable or stressful and affect him or her emotionally [42].

Treatment with hospitalization and antipsychotic medication will hopefully be of help to Mr. Rourke if he has troublesome symptoms. If Mr. Rourke had seemed troubled by something you did not understand, you could have asked him and acknowledged the stress of having voices telling him unpleasant things if that was his problem.

Related to the physical environment:
- Here, the risk factor is unpredictable behavior by other people and actions interpretable as threats.

To minimize the stress on Mr. Rourke, you keep your distance when possible, explaining what you are doing the whole time. Keeping your hands visible or in touch with Mr. Rourke reduces the possibility of him imagining that you trying to hurt him with hidden objects like weapons.

15.4.2.9 Story #9

Mrs. Johnsen

Mrs. Johnsen is a woman of indeterminate age. Her date of birth says that she is 55, but she looks seventyish. She has had a stressful life. She now lives in public housing and is on disability benefits. She has a long history of various substance abuse including injecting heroine. She drops in at your clinic from time to time, but it is hard for her to keep appointments.

Today, she appears at the reception desk demanding to see you. You can hear her from the surgery because of her loud voice. Your secretary knows her, and soon the voices calm down. Your secretary puts her head in the door and tells you that Mrs. Johnsen has a swollen cheek on the left side of her face and is in a lot of pain.

Mrs. Johnsen needs to be an emergency patient today, so you fit her in between your other appointments. She is angry when she enters the surgery, but you can see tears in her eyes. She throws herself down in the chair as she continues her monologue of profanities.

What Do You Do?

Even though you have a full schedule today and already are behind, you collect yourself and strive to be as polite and patient as you can.

Your calmness transfers to Mrs. Johnsen, who gradually stops talking and looks at you. You ask her what is bothering her today, and she points to her cheek.

She has an abscess.

You tell her what you think is the problem and go on telling her what you need do to relieve the pain. She is not happy with scalpels and tells you so in her own words. The thought of her being afraid of the pain of the incision enters your mind, and you carefully explore the subject. She is terrified of pain. You spend some more time explaining that she will probably feel an instant ease of her current pain when the pressure in the abscess is relieved.

After some discussion, you come to an agreement on how to proceed.

You drain the abscess. Anticipating that she might miss her control appointment, you do as much as you can while having her in the chair. At the same time, you stress the importance of her coming back. During oral examination, you have discovered the reason for the abscess being a carious partly impacted wisdom tooth and that she also has an oral disease with sore and possibly painful mucosa.

The chance of her spending money on medication is slim, so you decide to give her some glucocorticoid liniment to go from your medicine cabinet. You spend some time asking Mrs. Johnsen about her current substance use. After getting an approximate lay of the land, you also give her paracetamol and ibuprofen to help with any pain after the treatment of the abscess.

She would very much like to have some stronger medication from you, but you explain that what you have given her is sufficient if she also treats the candidiasis and takes the antibiotics. She reluctantly accepts. You tell her to come back if she gets worse.

You also tell her that you will send a resumé of the consultation to her GP. She says no at first, but you tell her it is important that all her health-care helpers know about her infection and treatment. She accepts reluctantly.

Why?

Dental problems in people that inject drugs are common, but few receive treatment. Furthermore, those using amphetamines, with poor housing, hygiene, and poor nutrition, are the most at risk [43]. Mrs. Johnsen is certainly a high-priority patient that you should treat when the opportunity arises.

People with drug-related problems have more anxiety toward dental treatment than do others, have access to treatments to a lesser degree than do others, and have sometimes experienced reluctance among some dentists to treat them [44]. The possibility of Mrs. Johnsen having anxiety and bad experiences in addition to her recent pain is likely. Anger and resentment are not uncommon expressions in people that are fearful.

Pain severity is subjective. As the pain tolerance in people with substance abuse problems is often low, pain relief must be administered carefully and sensitively, and establishing a good rapport with the patient is essential [45]. When people with problems with substance addiction ask for analgesics, it may be natural to suspect it being because of their addiction and, hence, refuse to prescribe such medication. The total amount of substances is seldom discussed, and there seems to be a lack of interest in patients with severe substance abuse [46]. As a dental health-care professional, you are legally and ethically obligated to treat the patient to the best of your abilities, regardless of his/her substance abuse. Hence, it is important to include a conversation regarding substance abuse and medications. You realize that you are in no position to take full responsibility of a patient like Mrs. Johnsen, but you can do your part in addition to seeing that the information is shared with others.

15.4.2.10 Story #10
Mr. Bashir

Mr. Bashir is an 18-year-old man and a refugee from Syria. He lives at a refugee reception center, waiting for his application for asylum to come through. He is referred to you by the supervising physician at the reception center due to mouth pain.

He enters your surgery accompanied by an interpreter from the municipality.

You greet them both and ask Mr. Bashir to sit down in the chair. He politely sits down at the edge of the chair, but when you gesture him to take a seat properly, he does as he is told.

You wonder to yourself if Mr. Bashir may have had adverse life experiences that will complicate the examina-

tion and treatment situation and ask him if he is anxious about the examination. When the interpreter has done his job, Mr. Bashir gives you a big smile and shakes his head. He tells you that his uncle in Syria is a dentist. During his childhood, Mr. Bashir loved spending time in his uncle's surgery, and he knows the names of all instruments. If anything, your surgery brings back happy childhood memories.

Reassured by Mr. Bashir's lovely story, you continue your examination and treatment.

You are about to finish when something unexpected happens. Mr. Bashir raises his right hand and moves his index finger up and down while mumbling something that you do not understand. "Mr. Bashir" you call out, but he does not respond. You look at the interpreter who shakes his head. He does not understand what Mr. Bashir is saying either.

What Do You Do?

Since you are done, you pull your chair away and wait. The interpreter says that it seems Mr. Bashir is talking to God. This goes on for a few minutes. Suddenly, Mr. Bashir smiles at you. He seems oblivious to what just happened.

He is awake and seems fine, except he is a bit tired, but you let your secretary stay with him in the waiting room for some more minutes to make sure that he is okay.

You find the incident rather strange and different from what you have experienced before. You make sure to give a detailed description of what happened in Mr. Bashir's journal, of which you send a copy to the supervising physician. To make sure that the physician reads your notice, you call the physician's office and leave a message too. Was it a dissociative episode due to a post-traumatic disorder? Was the patient delusional for a moment or hearing voices? You have many questions.

A couple of weeks later, you receive a letter. Mr. Bashir has given his physician permission to share information with you. After you conveyed your concern about what happened during Mr. Bashir's visit to your surgery, the physician started to investigate.

Mr. Bashir has, amongst other examinations, undergone MRI and EEG, and it has been discovered that he has epilepsy. He is now on medication. It seems Mr. Bashir has had epilepsy since childhood but discontinued his medication when he fled from Syria.

Why?

When working with refugees like Mr. Bashir, it is important to be aware of the possibility of him having experienced torture. It is generally estimated that between 5 and 35% of refugees are torture survivors [47]. In dental health care, it is not necessary to know the details about these experiences, but it is of great importance to know how to meet and treat people with respect and knowledge about trauma-informed dental care [48].

As is the case with many symptoms, it is not always the case that symptoms, which at first glance seem to be of organic origin, actually are the other way around. Mr. Bashir's finger movement and mumbling may have been of a psychological origin but was not. Various mental health disorders are differential diagnoses to epilepsy [49].

Epilepsy is the most common disease of the nervous system and is a collective term for a number of different conditions. The common denominator is recurrent epileptic seizures. One form of seizures is focal seizures with reduced consciousness like the one that Mr. Bashir had. He had a combination of short-term remoteness and pointless, automatic movements for some minutes [50].

The subtleness of Mr. Bashir's symptoms could have contributed to the epilepsy not being discovered had it not been for you. The symptoms could also have been misinterpreted as mental illness, sending Mr. Bashir into mental health care. The epilepsy would probably have been discovered in a situation like that, but an admission to a mental clinic could be a stressful and dramatic situation for a young man.

15.4.2.11 Story #11
Mrs. Gideon

Mrs. Gideon is a woman in her forties. She is the host of a TV show and appears in front of the camera on a regular basis. She smokes and drinks coffee in large amounts, so she regularly comes in to remove discoloration of her teeth. In addition, she always has some other concerns. Today, it is a small mucosal ulcer. As so many times before, she fears cancer. It is not a slight concern, but a strong conviction that she, like her father, has got cancer and will die.

What Do You Do?

You have known Mrs. Gideon for many years. The first few years, her concern made you collect biopsy samples every time to make sure that you did not overlook cancerous changes. Fortunately, they have all been negative. Now, you have more clinical experience yourself in addition to knowing Mrs. Gideon better.

You examine the small ulcer and are satisfied with it certainly being an aphthae.

You acknowledge Mrs. Gideon's fear of cancer and her fear of dying. You then remind her of her tendency to always think the worst and suggest that it may be the case this time too. She questions you a couple of more times whether you are absolutely sure it is not cancer, and you confirm with a twinkle in your eye. "Life is an uncertain project," you say [51], "and that is something that is hard to accept." You remind her of what you have talked about so many times – that her fear of dying inhibits her life.

Why?

Health anxiety affects about 1% of the adult population, and men and women are equally affected. The first symptoms occur at the age of 20–30 years [52].

People affected with health anxiety are convinced that they are seriously ill with a terminal disease. This fear makes people excessively concerned about bodily phenomena. They frequently seek out health-care professionals but are only temporarily reassured by negative findings.

Health anxiety can be understood as an attempt at controlling the uncontrollable.

Health-care personnel must always take a patient and the patient's concerns seriously. Necessary examinations must be performed as usual, but if the patient is known to you and acknowledges his or her health anxiety, then a vital part of the treatment of health anxiety is to accept that it is the fear itself that is the problem. Health-care personnel may help the patient in other ways by interpreting bodily sensations and signs [53].

When you do not take a biopsy of Mrs. Gideon's aphthae, it is because you know that she has health anxiety and that you have an alliance that allows you to take part in her therapeutic work.

> **Take-Home Message**
>
> People with severe mental disorders have worse oral health than the rest of the population and have an increased need for dental care. Poor oral health affects eating, speech, and other social and psychological areas of life. Oral health, therefore, directly impacts mental health and well-being.
>
> Oral health problems in people with mental disorders can be directly associated with the disorder and the symptoms related to it or indirectly through living conditions and economy.
>
> Oral health professionals need to have the communication skills and ability necessary to build trust, in addition to the knowledge needed to examine and treat patients in the dental clinic.
>
> People with mental disorders are different from people without diagnoses. They all have their own lives and histories. Oral health professionals should meet each patient individually, without predisposed opinions or prejudices.
>
> Although health and symptoms can be generalized, people cannot.

References

1. Persson K, Axtelius B, Söderfelt B, Östman M. Monitoring oral health and dental attendance in an outpatient psychiatric population. J Psychiatr Ment Health Nurs. 2009;16:263–71.
2. Høifødt TS, Lund-Stenvold E, Høye A. Ikke glem tennene. Tidsskr Nor Laegeforen. 2018;20.
3. Kisely S. No mental health without oral health. Can J Psychiatr. 2016;61(5):277–82.
4. Velasco-Ortega E, Monsalve-Guil L, Velasco-Ponferrada C, Medel-Soteras R, Segura-Egea JJ. Temporomandibular disorders among schizophrenic patients. A case control study. Med Oral Patol Oral Cir Bucal. 2005;10:315–22.
5. World Health Organization. Schizophrenia [Internet]. WHO 4 Okt 2019. Available from https://www.who.int/news-room/fact-sheets/detail/schizophrenia.
6. Correll CU, Schooler NR. Negative symptoms in schizophrenia: a review and clinical guide for recognition, assessment, and treatment. Neuropsychiatr Dis Treat. 2020;16:519–34.
7. Arnaiz A, Zumárraga M, Díez-Altuna I, Uriarte JJ, Moro J, Pérez-Ansorena MA. Oral health and the symptoms of schizophrenia. Psychiatry Res. 2011;188(1):24–8.
8. Livingwithschizophrenia.org. Staying out of debt. England: Living with schizophrenia; Dec 2015 [cited 2020 Dec 21]. Available from https://livingwithschizophreniauk.org/information-sheets/staying-out-of-debt/.
9. Kilian R, Becker T. Macro-economic indicators and labour force participation of people with schizophrenia. J Ment Health. 2007;16(2):211–22.
10. Scrine C, Durey A, Slack-Smith L. Enhancing oral health for better mental health: exploring the views of mental health professionals. Int J Ment Health Nurs. 2018;27:178–86.
11. The Health Personnel Act 1999. Available from https://lovdata.no/lov/1999-07-02-64/§22.
12. Stenman J, Wennström JL, Abrahamsson KH. Dental hygienists' views on communicative factors and interpersonal processes in prevention and treatment of periodontal disease. Int J Dent Hyg. 2010;8(3):213–8.
13. Dang BN, Westbrook RA, Njue SM, Giordano TP. Building trust and rapport early in the new doctor-patient relationship: a longitudinal qualitative. BMC Med Educ. 2017;17:32.
14. Lehmann J. Teaching professional health care practice: considering the elements of emotions and artistry. Aust Health Rev. 2008;32(1):127–33.
15. Powell S, Scott J, Scott L, Jones D. An online narrative archive of patient experiences to support the education of physiotherapy and social work students in North East England: an evaluation study. Educ Health. 2013;26(1):25–32.
16. Smeby JC, Mausethagen S. Profesjonskvalifisering. In: Smeby JC, Mausethagen S, editors. Kvalifisering til profesjonell yrkesutøvelse. Oslo: Universitetsforlaget; 2017. p. 11–20.
17. Williams J. Dental ethics manual, vol. 133. FDI World Dental Federation; 2007.
18. National Institute of Mental Health. Depression. [Internet]. England: National Institute of Mental Health [updated 2018 Feb; cited 2020 Dec 10]. Available from https://www.nimh.nih.gov/health/topics/depression/index.shtml.
19. The Norwegian Psychological Association. Hva er depresjon? [Internet]. Psykologforeningen; Date or year of publication [updated 2021 Apr 12; cited 2021 Nov 10]. Available from https://www.psykologforeningen.no/publikum/informasjonsvideoer/videoer-om-psykiske-lidelser/hva-er-depresjon.
20. Norwegian Institute of Public Health. Om bipolar lidelse, schizofreni og personlighetsforstyrrelser [Internet]. Folkehelseinstituttet; 2013 Feb 23 [updated 2015 June 10; cited 2020 Dec 14]. Available from https://www.fhi.no/fp/psykiskhelse/psykiskelidelser/om-bipolar-lidelse-schizofreni-og-personlighetsforstyrrelser/.
21. Sperre MdM, Tennfjord VJ, Kvisberg. Avtalerett. JURK (Legal Advice for Women). [Internet]. Norway: JURK; 2018 [cited 2020 Dec 14]. 2018. Available from https://foreninger.uio.no/jurk/brosjyrer/avtalerett.pdf.
22. The Norwegian Directorate of Health. Vrangforestillingslidelse [Internet]. Norway: The Norwegian Health Library; [cited 2020 Dec 15]. Available from https://www.helsebiblioteket.no/

retningslinjer/psykoselidelser/12.hva-er-en-psykose/andre-psykoselidelser/vrangforestillingslidelser.

23. Malt U. Paranoid psykose [Internet]. Store medisinske leksikon on snl.no; 2011 [updated 2019 Oct 19; cited 2020 Dec 15]. Available from https://sml.snl.no/paranoid_psykose.

24. Lo Russo L, Campisi G, Di Fede O, Di Liberto C, Panzarella V, Lo ML. Oral manifestations of eating disorders: a critical review. Oral Dis. 2008;14:479–84.

25. The National Eating Disorders Association (NEDA). Dental complications of eating disorders. [Internet]. New York: National Eating Disorder Organization; 2018 [cited 2020 Dec 15]. Available from https://www.nationaleatingdisorders.org/dental-complications-eating-disorders.

26. Patterson-Norrie T, Ramjan L, Sousa MS, et al. Eating disorders and oral health: a scoping review on the role of dietitians. J Eat Disord. 2020;8:49.

27. Owen L, Corfe B. The role of diet and nutrition on mental health and wellbeing. Proc Nutr Soc. 2017;76(4):425–6.

28. Greger HK, Myhre AK, Lydersen S, Jozefiak T. Previous maltreatment and present mental health in a high-risk adolescent population. Child Abuse Negl. 2015;45:122–34.

29. Littleton H, Breitkopf CR. Coping with the experience of rape. Psychol Women Q. 2006;30:106–16.

30. Thomas R, Siliquini R, Hillegers MH, Jansen PW. The association of adverse life events with children's emotional overeating and restrained eating in a population-based cohort. Int J Eat Disord. 2020;53:1709–18.

31. Johnson DM, Pike JL, Chard KM. Factors predicting PTSD, depression, and dissociative severity in female treatment-seeking childhood sexual abuse survivors. Child Abuse Negl. 2001;25(1):79–198.

32. Ford K, Brocklehurst P, Hughes K, Sharp CA, Bellis MA. Understanding the association between self-reported poor oral health and exposure to adverse childhood experiences: a retrospective study. BMC Oral Health. 2020;20(1):51.

33. Corrigan FM, Fischer JJ, Nutt DJ. Autonomic dysregulation and the window of tolerance model of the effects of complex emotional trauma. J Psychopharmacol. 2011;25(1):17–25.

34. BMJ Best Practice. Attention deficit hyperactivity disorder in children. [Internet]. England: British Medical Journal [cited 2020 Dec 17]. Available from https://bestpractice.bmj.com/topics/en-gb/142/epidemiology.

35. Nrk.no. Hulemannen slipper tvangsflytting [Internet]. Norway: NRK - Norwegian Broadcasting Corporation; 2012 Dec 21 Date or [cited 2020 Dec 17]. Available from https://www.nrk.no/osloogviken/_hulemannen_-slipper-tvangsflytting-1.10849546.

36. The Health Personnel Act 1999. Available from https://lovdata.no/lov/1999-07-02-64/§7.

37. The Norwegian Directorate of Health. Øyeblikkelig hjelp [Internet]. Norway: The Norwegian Directorate of Health 2018 [updated 2018 June 28; cited 2020 Dec 18]. Available from https://www.helsedirektoratet.no/rundskriv/helsepersonelloven-med-kommentarer/krav-til-helsepersonells-yrkesutovelse/-7.oyeblikkelig-hjelp.

38. Gjerde C, Fiehn NE. Kan en tann være livstruende? Aktuel Nordisk Odontologi. 2015;40(1):29–50.

39. Brelevne G, Heggen KM, Bondevik H. Slik håndterer sykepleiere og brukere vond lukt i hjemmet. Sykepleien Forskning. 2018;13:e65987.

40. The Norwegian Health Library. Schizofreni [Internet]. Norway: The Norwegian Health Library; 2019 June 21 [cited 2020 Dec 10]. Available from https://www.helsebiblioteket.no/pasientinformasjon/psykisk-helse/schizofreni.

41. Rasmussen K, Levander S. Schizofreni og vold. Tidsskr Nor Laegeforen. 2002;122:2303–5.

42. The Norwegian Directorate of Health. Voldsrisikoutredning ved alvorlig psykisk lidelse [Internet]. Norway: The Norwegian Directorate of Health; 2018 Apr 28 [updated 2018 Apr 28; cited 2020 Dec 10]. Available from https://www.helsedirektoratet.no/faglige-rad/voldsrisikoutredning-ved-alvorlig-psykisk-lidelse.

43. Laslett AM, Dietze P, Dwyer R. The oral health of street-recruited injecting drug users: prevalence and correlates of problems. Addiction. 2008;103(11):1821–5.

44. Scheutz F. Anxiety and dental fear in a group of parenteral drug addicts. Scand J Dent Res. 1986;94:241–7.

45. Bullok K. Dental care of patients with substance abuse. Dent Clin N Am. 1999;43:513–26.

46. Li R, Undall E, Andenæs R, Nåden D. Smertebehandling av rusmisbrukere innlagt i sykehus. Sykepleien Forskning. 2012;7(3):252–60.

47. Towers R. Recognizing victims of torture in national asylum procedures. Copenhagen: International Rehabilitation Council for Torture Victims (IRCT); 2013.

48. Høyvik AC, Shahnavaz S, Willumsen T. Flyktninger og tannhelse. Aktuel Nordisk Odontologi. 2016;1(41):86–97.

49. The Norwegian Health Library. Pedatriveiledere. Epilepsi [Internet]. Norway: The Norwegian Health Library; 2016 [updated 2016; cited 2021 Jan 8]. Available from https://www.helsebiblioteket.no/pediatriveiledere?key=144642&menuitemkeylev2=5973.

50. Helsenorge. Anfallstyper ved epilepsi[Internet]. Norway: Norsk Helsenett ; 2019 [updated 2019 Jan 3; cited 2021 Jan 8]. Available from https://www.helsenorge.no/sykdom/epilepsi/anfallstyper-ved-epilepsi/#fokale-partielle-anfall.

51. Wilhelmsen I. Livet er et usikkert prosjekt. Pax forlag; 2000. 159p.

52. Norwegian Institute of Public Health. Livet med hypokondri [Internet]. Oslo: The Norwegian Institute of Public Health; 2009 Oct [cited 2020 Dec 12]. 2009. Available from https://www.fhi.no/globalassets/dokumenterfiler/rapporter/2009-og-eldre/livet-med-hypokondri.-erfaringer-fra-mennesker-med-diagnosen.pdf.

53. Norwegian Association for Cognitive Behavioral Therapy [Internet]. Hønefoss: Norwegian Association for Cognitive Behavioral Therapy [cited 2020 Dec 8]. Available from https://www.kognitiv.no/psykisk-helse/ulike-lidelser/angstlidelser/helseangst/.

How to Deal with Gagging

Maren Lillehaug Agdal, Ann Catrin Høyvik,
Marianne Hoås Gudmundsen and Lena Myran

Contents

© The Author(s), under exclusive license to Springer Nature Switzerland AG 2022
T. Willumsen et al. (eds.), *Oral Health Psychology*, Textbooks in Contemporary Dentistry,
https://doi.org/10.1007/978-3-031-04248-5_16

Learning Goals

- To understand what gagging is and why it is a challenge
- To discuss the multifactorial etiology of gagging and the related physiological, psychological, and social factors
- To diagnose and grade the severity of gagging
- To explore the available management options

16.1   Who Are the Patients?

A gag reflex – which is one of several pharyngeal reflexes [1] – is principally a protective mechanism that hinders us from aspirating unwanted objects. For some patients, a sensitive gag reflex is elicited by a gentle touch to the posterior regions of the mouth. If the gag reflex is solely a somatic reaction, then one could expect that patients who gag when a mirror touches the anterior part of the palate also experience gagging in similar nondental settings, for example, when eating with cutlery. Among patients with a severe gag reflex, there may be a high influence of psychological triggers.

Many aspects of dental treatment can trigger a gag reflex. An example from general practice is the patient who struggles with gagging during routine intra-oral X-rays. How should these patients be dealt with? Usually, taking X-rays is a simple task, even for patients who report dental anxiety. It is essential to obtain an understanding of the severity and etiology of gagging. One needs to determine whether the gag problem is due to the size of the sensor and the pressure against the oral tissues or whether the gagging has a more profound psychological etiology. For some patients, gagging may be overcome by regaining a sense of control in the situation, for example, by being allowed to hold the sensor themselves. For other patients, this approach could be just another experience of failure since their gagging problem needs to be met with more psychological knowledge and methodical precision. This example demonstrates why gagging problems require a biopsychosocial understanding – a perspective that may help patients minimize and eventually overcome their gagging difficulties during dental treatment. Helping patients with severe gagging may be extremely difficult, and dental treatment under general anesthesia has often been the treatment of choice [2]. Learning about the complex nature of gagging, and how to handle it, may thus be important to reduce the use of general anesthesia, in addition to enabling patients to carry out their daily oral health-care routine (◘ Fig. 16.1).

◘ **Fig. 16.1**   "The gagging cycle" first presented by Murchie, 2018 [3]

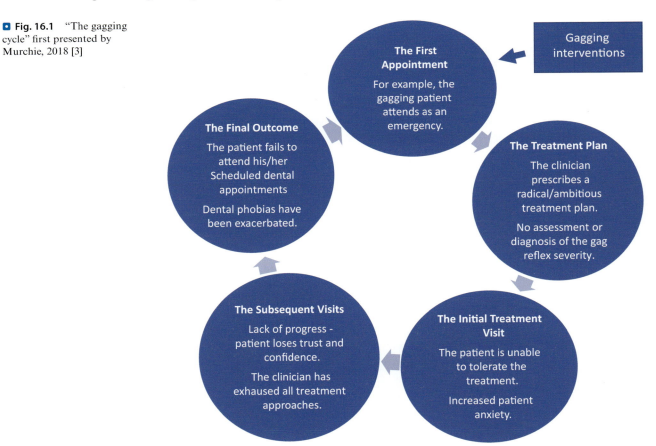

In this chapter, we will describe the elements of a gag response and present management techniques for all severities of gagging problems. This chapter will help the clinician in identifying the patient's problem with gagging and correctly understand its nature and etiology to diagnose and manage a hyperactive gag reflex. A holistic approach is recommended with the aim to understand the physiological, psychological, and social needs of the patient.

16.2 Prevalence and Severity

The prevalence of problematic gagging related to dental treatment has not been widely explored, but 8.2% reported problematic gagging in a population study among Dutch adults [4]. There is great variation in the normal gag reflex, with increased proneness to gagging with age until a peak at around the age of 50 years. Thereafter, the susceptibility to gag decreases. Among the 30% of the population who lack the gag reflex [5], the oldest population is overrepresented [6].

Box 16.1

Dickinson and Fiske [7] have developed an index to help health professionals identify the severity of gagging:

The Gagging Severity Index (GSI)

1. Normal gag reflex: Very mild, sporadic, and controlled by the patient.
2. Mild gagging: The patient struggles to control the gagging and needs reassessment from the dental health team.
3. Moderate gagging: This is persistent gagging that hinders treatment options. Techniques for reducing gagging are usually required.
4. Severe gag reflex: Gagging occurs in all forms of treatment, including single visual gagging. Limited treatment options are available.
5. Very severe gag reflex: This affects the patient's behavior and ability to meet the dentist. The condition makes dentistry impossible to carry out without specific adaptations.

16.3 The Biopsychosocial Model

To understand gagging, the biopsychosocial model is a good place to start. The biopsychosocial model is an interdisciplinary model that looks at the interconnection between biology, psychology, and socioenvironmental factors. The biopsychosocial model suggests that the development of an illness is the result of an interplay of these factors [8]. Biological factors include genetic predispositions, evolutionary vulnerabilities, infective agents, and other biological processes. Psychological factors include behaviors, emotions, and thoughts that influence the onset of a disease (for example, health-related behaviors, the experience of psychosocial stress, beliefs about the disease, and symptom interpretation) and the course of the disease. Social factors refer to socioeconomic challenges, experiences, relationships, and networks. The model was adopted by the World Health Organization in 2002 as a basis for the International Classification of Function (ICF) [9]. In this chapter, we will discuss the biological, psychological, and social perspectives to understand gagging behavior.

16.3.1 The Biological Aspects of Gagging (◘ Fig. 16.2)

16.3.1.1 The Basal Gag Reflex

The basal gag reflex is a biological protective reflex that prevents aspiration of foreign bodies from the upper part of the pharynx to the lungs [5, 11]. This reflex is triggered by touching the soft palate, posterior parts of the tongue, the areas around the tonsils, uvula, and posterior pharyngeal wall. This reflex is controlled from the gagging center in the anterior wall of the fourth ventricle, located in the medulla oblongata. Gagging may be restricted to bilateral contractions of the pharynx but is usually a complicated and reflective interaction with muscular contractions in several muscle groups [6]. During gagging, the mouth is slightly open and the mandible is moved both downward and backward. The tongue is brought up against the pharyngeal wall in the posterior part and down in the anterior part. At the same time, there are powerful contractions of the pharynx, uvula, and the soft palate. Gagging may be extremely unpleasant and distressful, and the patient often feels as if he/she is about to throw up, although this hardly ever happens. On the contrary, gagging, coughing, swallowing, and vomiting are unique reflexes that are rarely triggered in parallel [6].

Even in a patient with a normal and functional gag reflex, gagging may be triggered when, for example, an iatrogenic factor, such as excess impression material or an X-ray sensor, touches the soft palate.

Some children have a hypersensitive gag reflex from an extremely young age. When there is no obvious psychological etiology, the child usually has a hypersensitive biological gag reflex. These children may have trouble with gagging when they brush their teeth, with

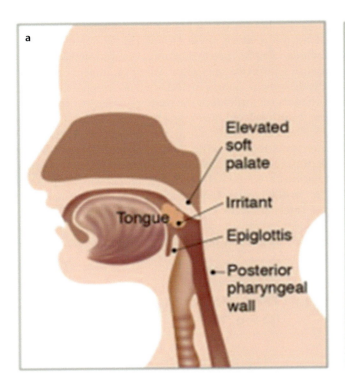

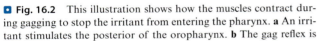

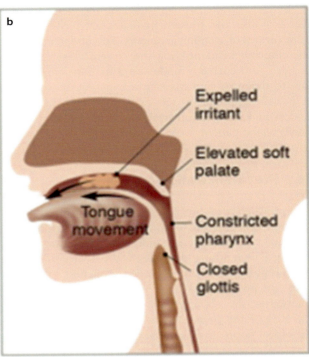

◘ Fig. 16.2 This illustration shows how the muscles contract during gagging to stop the irritant from entering the pharynx. **a** An irritant stimulates the posterior of the oropharynx. **b** The gag reflex is elicited by the irritant. The soft palate is elevated, the glottis is closed by the epiglottis, and the pharyngeal wall contracts to expel the irritant. (First published by Wilson-Pauwels [10])

the risk that the parents become reluctant to brush their child's molars. Consequently, the child perceives that the gagging problem is dealt with by avoidance of situations that trigger the behavior and is not taught to desensitize the spontaneous gag reflex. There is reason to believe that experience with physiological gagging under certain conditions early in life may induce a hypersensitive gag reflex due to psychological conditioning to the situation or stimulus. Early triggers have been researched, and problems with nutrient intake during the first few weeks of life seem to sensitize the reflex [12].

The biological causative factors for gagging are often divided into systemic and local factors.

16.3.1.2 Systemic Factors

Diseases in the gastrointestinal tract, such as reflux, gastric cancer, and medications known to increase nausea such as cytostatics and opioids, may in some cases be the underlying cause of an extreme gag reflex [13, 14]. The case of Mia (73) exemplifies how the gag reflex can be affected by medication and disease:

> ► **Example**
> Mia had visited the dentist regularly her entire life. She had a relatively small mouth and quite an active gag reflex. Nevertheless, she had learned to accept most dental procedures by focusing on her breathing and with the help

of anesthesia. At the age of 72, she was diagnosed with lung cancer and started treatment with chemotherapy. She became quite nauseated by the medication, and her mouth started feeling extremely dry. Some days, even just the thought of putting solid food in her mouth brought about gagging. Halfway through the treatment, she started feeling pain in an upper molar. Considering that infections could be dangerous due to her compromised immune system, she booked a dental appointment despite her poor general condition. When her long-trusted dentist approached her – mirror in hand – it set off an extreme gag reaction, and they both understood that any dental treatment that day was unrealistic. The dentist, who knew the patient's dental history, and suspected a periodontal infection, consulted her cancer specialist who started her on intravenous fluid for 24 h. Following her rehydration, he gave her a good dose of antiemetic medication prior to extraction of the tooth. Six months later, she came back to the dentist for a periodontal follow-up and sat through the dental cleaning with only a few episodes coming near a weak gag. ◄

16.3.1.3 Local Factors

Local physiological factors that may lead to a transient increased gag reflex include chronic dry mouth or conditions that affect the ability to breathe through the nose, such as sinusitis, nasal polyps, and mucus of the upper respiratory tract [14]. In a study among children, a thicker mucosa in the pharynx was suggested to be associated with an absent gag reflex [15].

It has been hypothesized that the number of afferent fibers in the glossopharyngeal nerve may affect the sensitivity of the gag reflex [16]. Moreover, the muscles in and around the pharynx can change the sensitivity to gagging, which will, for example, normally be prevented by swallowing. Thus, the use of the chewing muscles can reduce the tendency to gag probably due to sequential swallowing after chewing [1]. In the dental treatment situation, swallowing is often difficult due to the reclined position of the head and neck. Inadequate habits such as tightening the mental muscle, lifting the back of the tongue, and tightening the muscles in the neck may increase the tendency to gag.

If severe gagging occurs, other nearby brain centers for biological and physiological functions may be activated. Gagging and vomiting are two different reflexes. Both are present in the upper part of the intestinal tract and may occur in the dental situation: gagging to prevent foreign bodies from entering the airways and vomiting usually connected with vasovagal syncope (fainting). From an outside point of view, it may be extremely difficult to separate the two reflexes, especially since gagging may, under certain circumstances, stimulate the vomiting center. Vasovagal syncope occurs as a consequence of activation of the parasympathetic nervous system, with a subsequent drop in blood pressure, usually associated with triggers such as blood and injections. It is commonly preceded by prodromal symptoms of autonomic activation, with sweating, nausea, and vomiting [17]. In patients, gagging may be accompanied by nausea but is not usually associated with cold sweating and dizziness, which are common in vasovagal syncope. At the same time, gagging may stimulate nervous pathways to different areas of the brain, resulting in both psychological and biological activations. Physical triggers like touching the pharynx may result in an increased sympathetic activation and lead to an increased heart rate and blood pressure [18]. Knowledge about the interaction between the different parts of the brain has made us aware that gagging may occur without a physical trigger and may also be generalized to different situations without physical triggers, such as in Mia's case (above), where she started gagging both at home and in the dental office merely by thinking of something entering her mouth.

16.3.2 The Psychological Aspects of Gagging

Gagging is commonly known to have a multifactorial etiology, and the psychological factors are frequently described in the literature [7, 13]. Psychological factors refer to the patient's personality, thinking style, self-esteem, and individual coping skills to handle emotions [8]. Psychological factors influence how individuals perceive and understand their experiences, thereby influencing their interaction with the environment. Having good coping mechanisms or having an optimistic tendency are protective factors that enable individuals to deal with stress more effectively [19]. This is also known as a "buffer." Having poor coping skills or tendencies to become anxious can make a person more vulnerable to developing mental or physical illness [20].

In the science of gagging, psychological factors influence how individuals perceive and think about their gagging behavior and what coping style they are prone to use. For example, a person may have a genetic predisposition to gagging, but he or she must have social factors such as painful experiences with dental treatment or psychological factors such as a proneness for avoidance or anxiety, which all trigger this genetic code for developing severe gagging behavior.

The sympathetic nervous system is often activated when a person gags. Increased blood pressure and heart rate may be associated with the feeling of fear and a desire to avoid the situation. This mechanism may be an early onset of an anxious gag response. Later, the gagging can be triggered by both nontactile stimuli such as visual, auditory, and olfactory stimuli and various situation-triggered emotional stimuli [21].

Although gagging is not always related to dental anxiety, it is often the behavioral part of an anxiety response and therefore is a consequence of psychological activation. Feelings, thoughts, and other bodily reactions linked to gagging vary from person to person. The psychological perspective of gagging should be in focus to gain a deeper understanding of the patient's thoughts, emotions, and actions underlying the gag response. This applies to both children [22] and adults [4, 23], knowing that an increased gag reflex has also been described in individuals with anxious depression and neurotic tendencies [16, 24].

16.3.2.1 Gagging as a Train of Thought

Most people with a gag reflex can relate to the fact that gagging is often caused by their underlying thoughts. In social media, there are many videos showing children and grown-ups gagging when they see, touch, smell, or try to eat something they think negatively about. Then, they suddenly stop gagging when they are informed that it is chocolate not poop or that the soup is made of berries not blood.

Thoughts also have an essential part in the gag reflex of dentally anxious patients. Randall et al. [25] found that patients who have moderate or high severity of gagging reported more dental care-related fear and more negative beliefs about dentistry than did patients who had less dental care-related fear. Scary thoughts and negative beliefs may differ from patient to patient. These thoughts may already start when the patient starts to envision the dental appointment. One patient described this well: "When I think of my experiences with the dentist, the gagging starts already in the car on the way to the dentist. I get scared that I will gag during dentistry, which means that the dentist cannot finish the treatment. Then I must come back over and over again. I am afraid that I will gag during dental treatment, causing the dentist to get annoyed at me and see me as a weak and bad patient." Another patient says: "Then we'll never be finished and always be delayed, that thought makes me even more stressed. Then I have to come back again and start over."

Common Catastrophic Thoughts Related to Gagging

I'm going to lose control over gagging. If I start to gag, I will not be able to stop.

Gagging will prevent the treatment from being finished, and I have to come back over and over again.

The dentist is not going to stop the treatment when I need to gag, making me feel helpless.

The dentist will get annoyed at me and think I am stupid.

My teeth will rot, fall out, and I will need dentures.

16.3.2.2 Losing Control

For many people, anxiety in the dental situation is closely related to the feeling that they lack control, which is a key factor in the etiology of fear [26]. When a major part of a person's anxiety response is gagging, the tendency to gag may be an expression of loss of control in the dentist's chair. In contrast to other anxiety responses, gagging makes the dentist stop immediately. However, many patients also describe that gagging itself gives a terrible feeling of losing control because they are afraid of not being able to stop gagging. What will happen if they keep on gagging? The patients may have negative thoughts concerning the possibility that they may vomit all over themselves or not be able to breathe due to severe gagging. The patient regains control over the situation when the dentist stops. To help the gagging patient, it is therefore important to, in as detailed a manner as possible, understand how patients think about their gagging behavior.

Dental professionals must be aware that patients who have a hypersensitive tendency to gag are often shameful and vulnerable to negative assessment by dental professionals [21]. Negative reactions to excessive gagging can aggravate the patient's shame, contribute to poor coping, and ruin the hope and willingness to undergo dental treatment [27]. Patients may experience a feeling of powerlessness, in that they have no control, and gag despite working hard to avoid it. When they are met with comments about getting along, or comments on the dental procedure's low level of difficulty, the patient may feel both offended and helpless. Patients with an excessive gag reflex often have trouble brushing their own teeth [21]. This may result in the avoidance of tooth brushing and poorer oral hygiene [4]. The patient may have a social embarrassment of breaking down in the presence of others.

Another psychological aspect of gagging is that it can seemingly resemble vomiting. The fear of gagging or vomiting is a common feature of emetophobia (the fear of vomiting). Emetophobia, combined with a sensitive gag reflex, is a demanding condition. To throw up in the presence of others is uncomfortable for most people. Vomiting is often associated with illness, and it is normal to feel a certain aversion to vomiting. Gagging and vomiting originate from different brain centers, and gagging does not normally lead to vomiting [28]. Nevertheless, some patients have experienced such extreme gagging that the center for vomiting is activated [29]. Psychologically, it may elicit strong negative feelings, and an avoidant behavior toward persons who vomit may be biologically reasonable. Other people's gagging or tendency to gag can also arouse emotions. Dental professionals may experience unpleasant feelings such as disgust and have a desire to avoid closeness to the person who is gagging. If the dental staff appear stressed or otherwise show evasion, they can give nonverbal signals that may cause the patients to feel that they are being poorly cared for.

Gagging, stomach ache, and disgust are the generally known common symptoms of being anxious and may be present simultaneously. Persons who have high anxiety for blood–injection–injury (BII) stimuli may feel disgust, [30] and disgust is also highly present in connection with the gag response. Disgust may be triggered by several modalities [31]. Similarly, stomach ache may also be associated with a feeling of nausea. The cognitions that patients associate with emotions are essential for getting them out of the vicious circle (see ▶ Chap. 10). All the different emotions experienced in the dental setting may result in a mixture of subjective feelings like fear due to the risk of danger, lack of control, unpredictability, and disgust [32].

▶ **Example**

An example of a young boy with anxiety-induced gagging that hinders his routine dental checkup:

Tom is a 12-year-old boy, living with his parents and brother in a suburb. He has an appointment for dental checkup at the local dental clinic. It has been 18 months since Tom's last dental visit, and there are no clinical notes regarding problems with gagging. The dental hygienist meets Tom and his mother in the waiting area, and she introduces Tom for taking X-rays. Tom seems calm but refuses to enter the room for X-rays. After talking with Tom and his mother, the dental hygienist understands that Tom has a profound problem with gagging. He tends to gag in situations where he feels anxious. His strategy has been to avoid all situations that involves gagging. The mother informs that he gags in many situations. He is now exempted from making oral presentations at school and has quit football after an increasing tendency to gag before matches. Now, he uses only wide-necked t-shirts and open jackets to avoid feeling suffocated. ◄

16.3.2.3 Gagging as a Coping Strategy to Control Dental Treatment

Being able to stop the dentist is not always easy. Many patients have experienced that despite displaying obvious signs of anxiety, the dentist does not stop drilling or injecting anesthesia. However, when a patient gags, the dentist is forced to stop immediately due to the risk of injuring the patient. Some patients have discovered this and developed a strategy to gag, to stop dental treatment. The strategy might be effective in the short run. Dental treatment stops temporarily. On the other hand, it is not an effective strategy to deal with the underlying problem, i.e., the difficulty in handling dental treatment.

» For some patients, the gag reflex is a strategy to avoid undergoing dental treatment:

"I quickly understood that gagging is a very effective way to make the dentist stop working when I feel discomfort."

"I didn't know how to communicate without being able to talk, so I just gagged."

"All the dentists I've met so far have stopped the dental treatment when I've gagged."

When patients experience relief from their anxiety when the dentist stops, it is a likely outcome that the patients learn, by social learning, that gagging is a protective behavior in a stressful or anxiety-provoking situation.

16.3.3 The Social Aspects of Gagging

A social aspect refers to the patient's previous experiences and cultural, familial, and socioeconomic perspectives [8]. Multiple adverse childhood experiences (ACEs) is a major risk factor for many health conditions [33]. One must keep in mind that all experiences related to the neck and throat, which elicit the fear of not being able to breathe normally, are risk factors for development of an exaggerated gag response. Examples of adverse experiences related to the development of gagging might be violence to the head or neck, bullying, or traumatic experiences during hospitalization (putting a drain in the ear canal, removal of the tonsils, or gastroscopy) [34]. Other common examples are life-threatening events such as torture or accidents. Further scientific research on these connections is required.

Negative life experiences where gagging has been induced, and anxiety associated with feelings of touch and textures in the mouth, may pose a problem in individuals with a hypersensitive gag response. Below, you will find an example highlighting how negative experiences outside the dental situation influence the dental situation:

> ► **Example**
>
> Anna, a well-educated woman of 62, has had a strong gag reflex for as long as she can remember. She relates it to being force-fed porridge in her early childhood. Even now, entering a room smelling of cooked porridge sets off her gagging. Regarding dental consultations, she says: "If I'm having a front-tooth repaired, seeing the dentist doesn't bother me at all. But if I know that the dentist will have to work in the back of my mouth, I often start gagging already in the waiting room." ◄

Anna's case does not describe a patient with dental anxiety but rather anxiety of the physical sensations associated with gagging. Her gagging problem in the dental situation has developed through classical conditioning, where she associates the sensation of having something in the back of her mouth with the feeling of being force-fed. The fear has generalized to an extent that a gag reflex is triggered even by thoughts or smells, and, so, there is a strong psychological component to her gagging problem.

Anna's problems must be addressed with caution. Anna has a sensitivity to gag, and her anxiety for food and textures has been generalized to the dental situation. Her thoughts and assumptions during dental treatment are closely linked to the emotions that she felt when she started gagging as a child. These emotions are usually sympaticus-activated and are strongly related to the wish to flee the situation. Now, during dental treatment, the dentist must know how to address the gag response to avoid a negative situation with increased anxiety and feelings of shame. However, since the gagging physically prevents the dental professional from working within the oral cavity, this is actually a situation of avoidance. When the gag response ceases due to treatment, the patient sometimes experiences an increase in other anxiety responses in the dental situation such as shivering and an overwhelming heart rate. The gag response has previously been an obstacle for dental treatment and dental situations, and, therefore, the patient has not been aware of anxiety related to dental issues, which may now be addressed.

16.3.3.1 Previous Traumatic Events Related to Dentistry

While working with patients with dental anxiety and severe gagging behavior, the dentist often learns their history that led to difficulties in gagging. The most established connection to dental anxiety is experiencing painful dental treatment during childhood while at the same time not experiencing control [35–37]. We assume that the same connection goes for the development of severe gagging behavior related to dental anxiety.

16.3.3.2 Gagging and Sexual Abuse

Studies have indicated that dental fear is more prevalent among sexually abused women than in women in general [38] and, in particular, in women who have experienced sexual abuse involving oral penetration [39]. Uziel et al. (2012) found that sexual abuse was also related to exaggerated gagging in the dental treatment situation [23]. Women who had experienced vaginal penetration during their assault had a higher tendency to gag than did those who had not. The patients were, however, not asked about oral penetration, and there is also a lack of studies involving men who have experienced sexual abuse. To establish the relationship between the different aspects of sexual abuse and gagging problems in the dental treatment situation, more research is needed. We know, however, that an overactive gag reflex is a common sequela of sexual trauma in general [40], and several dentists tell stories similar to the one about Anita [42] who had struggled for years with dental anxiety and mostly avoided dental visits. Her dentist summarizes:

> **► Example**
> Anita (52 yo), a victim of child sexual abuse, had seen her psychologist twice a week for 9 years before she brought up her dental anxiety. She had not seen a dentist for 17 years. When I first met her, in a nonclinical room, she appeared calm and talked rationally about her challenges. The moment we were about to enter the oral surgery, she stopped abruptly and started gagging. The gagging lasted for about a minute, before she managed to stop it using a breathing-and-counting technique that she later told me she had practiced with her psychologist. Then, she was able to proceed into the surgery, and at the end of the session – after two more episodes of gagging – she managed to touch the dental chair. When I got to know her better, I learned that gagging was her typical first reaction to increased anxiety. Now, after learning to trust me, and gaining a sense of control in the dental treatment situation, she seldom gags when I work in her mouth. Still, she almost always has an episode of gagging before we start, before we have gone through the plan for the session. However, she no longer considers herself dentally anxious. She says: "Now I am able to manage the treatment. I'm allowed to breathe, to take breaks, to get scared, and to gag. It passes!" ◄

Patients can experience gagging related to tastes, textures, smells, or the thought of having dentist's fingers or instruments in their mouths. A possible relation might be that the patient experiences a trigger (see ► Chap. 2), leading to disgust or nausea, which again leads to gagging. Disgust is a common emotional reaction to aversive traumas, such as sexual assaults, and has been linked to symptoms of post-traumatic stress disorder (PTSD) [41]. Disgust, therefore, might function as a mediator of gagging in the dental situation for victims of child sexual abuse.

16.4 How to Manage a Severe Gag Reflex in the Dental Setting

16.4.1 What Are the Treatment Goals?

Why do you seek help? What is your dream/goal? Helping a gagging patient manage dental treatment may often be hard, long-lasting, and packed with ups and downs. What the patient has achieved during one consultation may seem almost impossible in the next consultation. The motivation for treatment may vary according to how the treatment gets along. Therefore, the treatment goal must be outspoken, for example, "I want to be able to have a filling in the second mandibular molar" or "My goal is to be able to brush all my teeth without gagging." In some periods, the patients may seem unengaged and reluctant to commit to treatment, and the dentist may have to help them recollect their goals and dreams. The dentist should ask the patients to keep their goals in mind and be open with the patients that the desired results may only be achieved by hard work and endurance. Gagging is sometimes a symptom of dental anxiety and may, in those situations, be parallel to how we treat other anxiety symptoms; we aim to reduce the patients' anxiety to a level where they are comfortable to endure dental treatment. However, compared to symptoms such as rapid heart rate or dizziness, gagging is more visible to everyone in the room. As for other anxiety reactions, extinction of gagging is not realistic for most patients. The goal should be to make the patients experience that they, with self-performed methods, can ameliorate their tendency to gag. Gagging is not a problem if it does not make it impossible to perform dental treatment. As mentioned, gagging can evoke emotional reactions in the dental personnel, and some may be afraid of these reactions. Dental staff should always keep in mind that it is extremely important to be positive toward the patients when they gag to reduce the patients' social embarrassment and feelings of failure.

16.4.2 Exploring the Gagging Problem Clinically

Before commencing treatment, it is necessary to assess all aspects of the patient's gagging problem. Grading the severity of the gag reflex may prove helpful in developing a treatment plan, but it can only be accomplished after a detailed patient history has been recorded. A practical guide to the initial assessment of a gagging dental patient is outlined in ▶ Box 16.2. To explore the problem more structurally, the Gagging Problem Assessment (GPA) questionnaire may be a useful tool (see ▶ Box 16.3). The GPA consists of a patient part that may be filled out prior to the dental appointment and a dentist part that takes approximately 2 min to complete [42].

Box 16.2 Assessment of the Gagging Problem

Gagging problem assessment prior to the clinical examination [3]:

Identify the initiating event

Invite the patient to relate their gagging history. Begin with open-ended questions: "Can you describe your gagging problem?", "Do you remember how it all began?"

Triggers

Ask questions to identify the underlying somatic and/or psychological factors that provoke the patient's gag response.

Clinical features

Ask the patient to describe what happens to her/him when a gag reflex has been triggered. Examples may include sweating, palpitations, fainting, vomiting, and panic attacks.

Dental history

What has been done previously to solve the problem? Has anything been helpful?

Are there some dental procedures that are tolerated?

Relevant patient factors

Are there contributing medical factors?

What are the patient's expectations? Are they realistic?

What type of treatment is the patient willing to consider?

The information gathered can be put into a form – "Gagging coping plan" [43]:

HISTORY OF GAGGING	Name:
	DH number:
Date: –/–/—	D.O.B.

Duration: _____

Onset: _____

Aetiology: Psychogenic ☐ Somatic ☐ Mixed ☐

Triggers: _____
_____

Strategies that have helped: _____
_____
_____

Past methods of coping: _____
_____
_____

Methods of control tried in the past:

Relaxation ☐ Distraction ☐ Desensitisation ☐
Hypnosis ☐ Acupuncture ☐ Oral sedation ☐
RA ☐ IV sedation ☐ GA ☐
Other ☐ _____

Examination possibel: Yes ☐ No ☐

Trigger areas indentified on examination: _____
_____
_____

Gagging severity index: I ☐ II ☐ III ☐ IV ☐ V ☐

Method of control decided on: _____
_____
_____

Gagging prevention index: I ☐ II ☐ III ☐ IV ☐ V ☐

Box 16.3 Gagging Problem Assessment Questionnaire

Gagging Problem Assessment Questionnaire: The Patient Part

The patients are asked to estimate their degree of gagging in the following nine situations. The response alternatives are no, sometimes, often, always, and not applicable.

1. Brushing your teeth
2. Wearing a (partial) prosthesis
3. Lying in the supine position in the dental chair
4. Feeling the mirror in the front of the mouth
5. Feeling the mirror deeper in the mouth
6. Feeling the dental probe in the mouth
7. Feeling the dental probe between the teeth/molars
8. Having an impression taken of the upper jaw
9. Having an impression taken of the lower jaw

Gagging Problem Assessment Questionnaire – The Dentist Part

The patients are asked to indicate their degree of gagging when holding the mirror in the following situations [42]. The response is "yes" if they are unable to perform the action because of the gag response; otherwise, it is "no." The back of the dental chair should be no more than 30° in the upward position.

1. Outside the mouth, in front of the opened mouth
2. In the mouth, at the level of the second molars
3. In the mouth, touching behind the upper incisors
4. In the mouth, touching the transitional area to the soft palate
5. On the inner side of the cheek, at the level of the second molars
6. Touching the maxillary process, at the level of molar 7/8
7. On the back of the tongue, at the level of molar 7/8
8. On the side of the tongue, at the level of the second molars

16.4.3 Relationship Building/ Communication

For all patients who experience difficulties when undergoing dental treatment, a safe clinical relationship is the foundation of the treatment and the key factor for enhancing the chances of a successful treatment [44]. The value of a calm and confident dental professional and the communication between the dental staff and the patient is clearly established [43]. A tailored interview regarding the etiological factors is important to establish a common understanding of the patient's history and maintaining factors for gagging. It is, in this context, extremely important that the dental staff have profound knowledge about the etiological factors. Knowledge substantiates a calm and respectful approach. Research finds that the highest percentage of gagging occurs with the least experienced clinicians [45]. It may also be beneficial for the patient to learn about the mechanisms behind their gagging. For example, it may be explained to them that it is interesting that gagging, a reflex with the purely physical function to prevent aspiration, may become a conditionally learned behavior by association learning. By classical conditioning, a person who gags severly due to water in the back of the mouth due to drilling, may gag due to the sound of the drill at later occasions. Similarly, conditional learning can explain gagging when exposed to specific tastes and smells. Helping patients understand the phenomena contributes to normalizing them.

When negative emotions arise, the brain is designed to concentrate on potential threats, to ensure survival [46]. Individuals who struggle with gagging and anxiety associated with it are, therefore, often good at worrying and escaping from the discomfort. Incorporating new habits is, therefore, a long-term process. On the other hand, once a behavior is learned, it can also be unlearned. The pathway of learning should be visualized for the patients by addressing the cause of gagging in a credible context. This demands an understanding of the etiological factors for each individual patient. What is the underlying problem for this unique patient's gag response? To get to the bottom of this important question, one might address the patient's history of gagging from different angles:

- When did gagging become a problem for you?
- Can you tell me what you think triggered your gag response at the very beginning?
- In what situations do you gag?
- Are you able to recall situations where you gagged without having anything in your mouth?

Some patients experience gagging in many areas of life, and the relation between gagging and triggers in the dental treatment situation is not always apparent. For some patients, the response is mainly physical, but, for many, the psychological aspects are just as explanatory and of high importance [3, 43]. The practitioner must keep in mind that experiences with sexual abuse may be present. Patients might not trust you enough to reveal their reasons for gagging at the early stages of the treatment relationship. However, asking and inviting the patient to tell is still important. By asking, you are signaling that you are interested in cooperating with the patient to help him or her. When you have earned their trust, they might tell you the full story. Whatever reasons patients find plausible for having developed and maintained a hypersensitive gag response, it should be met with interest. Identifying the actual etiological reasons are not crucial to achieving a successful treatment, but the interest shown in the patient is important for establishing mutual respect and trust.

Simultaneously, it is important to help the patient understand that the forthcoming treatment will address and help him/her unlearn a learned behavior. If the patient holds the view that a hypersensitive gag response is solely a biological reflex, then it might be more difficult to engage the patient in the treatment. A sense of hopelessness or denial of the opportunity to influence their own situation is, in these cases, quite common. This places great demands on how therapists respond to patients' subjective issues and how they help them understand their own situations and problems. The techniques used in motivational interviewing (MI) (see ► Chap. 7) may prove useful.

Box 16.4

Many patients state that talking to the dentist is helpful:

"Meeting the dentist and having conversation about possible reasons for my gagging really helped me. Establishing communication and letting him know about my anxiety was a big step."

"By being met with communication I dared to tell my preferences during dental treatment. Now the dentist places the tool in my mouth at a different angle than he did before."

"Because the dentist appreciates my needs, the dentist lets the assistant know that the suction should not rest against my cheek."

"I usually panicked when the dentist placed so many things in my mouth. Now she knows and adjusts the treatment so that I don't have that many objects in my mouth at the same time."

16.4.4 How to Enhance Communication with the Patient During Dental Treatment

It is important that the dentist is aware of the patient's body language. As a dentist, it is important to communicate calmness because anxiety is easily transmit-

ted. The dentist should speak clearly and respectfully to the patient. An honest and open two-way dialogue is preferred. It is essential to have a respectful tone and phasing adjusted for the patient's age. The dentist should explain and prepare the patient for what will happen before, during, and after the dental treatment. For some patients, detailed information about the dental procedures is important to have control in the situation. The dentist should be open and aware of any nonverbal signal that the patient may express, which gives reason to believe that everything is not okay. What you see or hear should be addressed. "I heard you sigh, what are you thinking about?" "Your head turns a bit away from me giving me the impression that you find this exposure difficult. What are you afraid of or afraid will happen if you lean into the exposure?" Open questions must be asked like "What are you experiencing now?", "When you reacted a little, what happened?" The dentist should be careful when asking closed questions like "Are you okay?" or "Should I continue?" seeing that it may be difficult for the patient to say no. It is important to make clear agreements with the patient – and keep them.

Other ways in which dental professionals may contribute to building a relationship are by assuring the patient that they will tolerate the gagging, potential vomiting, or other reactions that can be accommodated and handle any reactions that could occur. The patient must feel that he/she is seen: "No wonder you are afraid of gagging with your experience of being belittled and helpless in the dental situation. Remember that I will never make you responsible for your gag response. That would be as silly as asking your heart to slow down! When you gag, I see a person willing to be exposed and willing to learn. Please, don't focus on controlling the gag response. If you focus on the exercises and thoughts that I will explain to you, the gag response usually ceases over time. By recognizing the patient's efforts (brave for the willingness to address the anxiety, enduring, curious), you also build confidence.

The responsibilities of the dental team must be empathically stated. However, the patients must commit to showing up and spending the time constructively. As the dentist, you should explain that you know that there are many reasons why people struggle with gagging or are afraid of dental treatment. To minimize, or eliminate, the feeling of shame in patients who have not been able to care for their teeth, you should let them understand that this is reasonable given the circumstances.

> It can be difficult to recognize successes during treatment, as it is never gagging or non-gagging, success or defeat. It is degrees of gagging and the tendency of the gagging to get better or worse.

It can be difficult to recognize successes during treatment, as it is never gagging or non-gagging, success or defeat. It is degrees of gagging and the tendency of the gagging to get better or worse. It is therefore important to seek out the small successes during treatment. Some patients describe the successes in thoughts and feelings, others describe them in more specific goals. Examples of the former include "I now understand that I don't have to control everything." Examples of specific goals include "Now I breathe more easily during dentistry," "Now I manage to have the suction in my mouth for several minutes", "Now I manage to have the polishing cup on the tooth further back" or "Now it takes longer time between each time I gag." The dentist should play the role of a detective looking for subgoals that work for each patient and collect the tiny successes, without expecting absolute success right away.

It is important that the dentist does not get annoyed or show frustration when the patient gags. If the dentist becomes impatient or gets irritated, this will be detected by the patient and thus the gag response, and related anxiety, may increase. The dentist should acknowledge the problem, notice it, while not being stressed by it. A useful way to accomplish this is to talk to the patient about the gagging and convey the response as normal and harmless. An explanation will also be useful. You should explain that you understand how unpleasant the gagging is for the patient and that it probably gives thoughts and feelings of a wish to avoid the treatment. However, it is important that the treatment is continued when the gagging subsides to reduce the link between gagging and avoidance of difficult tasks. Talking about this will signal to the patient that the dentist's office is a safe place to experience discomfort – without facing condemnation or rejection. Many patients work hard to avoid gagging, trying intensely to avoid the discomfort of gagging. Some also fear what will happen if they gag: "Maybe the dental treatment needs to be interrupted, maybe I will get water in my throat and suffocate, maybe the dentist will slip the instrument into my mouth and hurt me in some way." It is, therefore, important that the patient dares to check out what happens if gagging occurs and that the dental office may be a safe place to exercise.

When a clinical relationship is built, and the patient can manage dental treatment, it is of utmost importance that the dentist maintains a thorough journal to make sure that the protocol is continued in later appointments. A male dental patient in his fifties, with a recurrent gagging problem explains:

▶ **Example**

On several occasions in life, I have found a dentist who, after working with me for a while, was able to treat my teeth. I gag easily, even when I brush my own teeth. I am, for example, not able to endure taking more than one X-ray per consultation. But, my limits are expanded when I feel safe that the dentist is considerate, and I am often helped by anesthesia. But, repeatedly, it has come down to the same problem: When I come back for a checkup after 6 or 12 months, the dentist has forgotten that I have a gag problem… Then, my trust is lost, and we are back at square one. All those times, I have chosen to find a new dentist, and start over again. ◀

16.4.5 Behavior Modification/Cognitive Behavioral Therapy (CBT)

Patients with a hypersensitive gag reflex, not associated with anxiety, can be treated successfully with the methods described later in this chapter. If, however, the gag response is associated with fear of dental treatment, cognitive behavioral therapy (CBT) may be highly effective [47]. This may be true both when the gagging is a symptom of dental anxiety and when the anxiety is mainly related to the fear of gagging. In the cognitive behavioral approach, it is essential to explore not only the etiology but also, more importantly, the maintaining factors of the fear. What are the patient's thoughts about his/her gagging? What is the patient's answer to the question "What is the worst that can happen when I gag?" To know how to hit the target with exposure therapy, we need to know what the patient's imagined catastrophe is. Does he/she have thoughts or images about getting suffocated? Not being able to breathe? To be rejected or humiliated by the dental personnel? To vomit all over the equipment? Does he/she have visual images about moving his/her head so he/she or the dentist will get seriously injured?

These thoughts are not always immediately present in the patient's mind, and the dentist should spend some time exploring them by asking the patient to visualize the dental setting or looking back at a situation where it happened. When you know the patient's fears, it is easier to give relevant information and education about, for example, the physiology of the mouth, the function of gagging, and planning which steps can be performed in the exposure.

To treat the psychological part of the patient's gag response, there must be a mutual understanding between the dentist and the patient that the psychological factors must be addressed. Normally, patients are aware that triggers other than physical triggers are present. They have different cues, but many have experienced gagging when they enter the waiting room, think about dental treatment, or hear the drill.

The gag response should be addressed in a manner similar to other anxiety responses. The difference is that once the gagging starts, it often interrupts the treatment tremendously. Therefore, it is important to introduce exercises and methods that can render gagging manage-

16

able for the patient like relaxation, habit reversal, systematic desensitization, and distractions to avoid gagging.

16.4.6 Methods Addressing Reflective Muscular Contractions During Gagging

The earliest published studies on gagging in the dental literature are from prostodontics that over time experiences that dental treatment is difficult to achieve with gagging. Mostly, the recommended approach has been different forms of adapted treatments like making prostheses with the small and adjusted palate area and impression materials with a shorter stiffening time [14, 48]. There are a number of methods to address the sensitive gag response, and, in the next sections, we describe how gagging can be treated.

16.4.6.1 Habit Reversal

Gagging is, as per definition, a delicate interplay of muscular contractions. Before gagging becomes conditioned with psychological and social cues, the contractions may be more easily addressed. During the first consultation, the patient should be taught to identify the muscular movements and contractions they have in their neck, throat, and mouth both at rest and when they gag, thus identifying the cascade of contractions. What comes first? Is there high muscular activity in the musculus mentalis or in the neck, which tends to lower the threshold for contractions in the throat? Being aware of muscular contractions is necessary in order to relax. The patient must be asked to contract muscles when gagging and also asked what happens in the back of the mouth. How does the tongue, soft palate, and the upper part of the pharynx work together to close the throat? Is it possible for the patient to gag if he/she simultaneously relaxes? This is the first step in introducing the method of habit reversal, which is a method that focuses on doing opposite movements [49, 50]. The tricky part may be to identify the auxiliary muscles that are part of the gag reflex. Subconsciously controlled the auxiliary muscles may be responsible for starting the reflex, and, once started, it is more difficult to stop it, as opposed to stopping it from the beginning.

The visual differences in the oral gag response are as follows [3]:
1. Open mouth – a normal gap

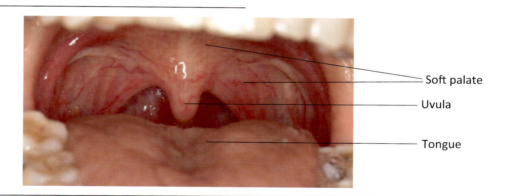

The picture shows the upper part of the throat and tongue at rest. With low muscle tonus in the soft palate, there is a distance from the dorsal wall of the trachea opening the airways to the nose. When the tongue is in a resting position, it comes a bit forward in the mouth, creating an open space to the trachea.
2. Gag response

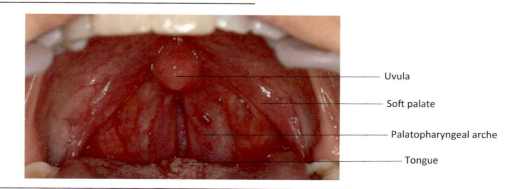

During gagging, the soft palate and the palatopharyngeal arch contract to close the gap between the mouth and the nose. Simultaneously the tongue retracts and pressures towards the posterior wall of oropharynx to close the airways towards the lungs.

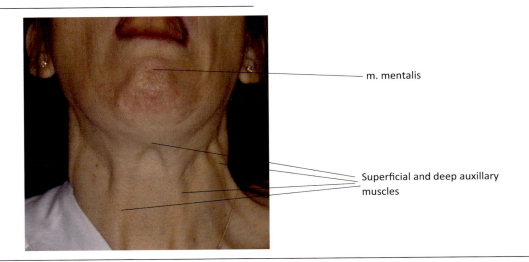

m. mentalis

Superficial and deep auxillary muscles

During gagging, there are a number of auxiliary muscles in the neck that pull the mandible in a posterior direction to facilitate the pressure of the tongue on the posterior wall of the oropharynx.

Coaching a new technique is not always easy. Vocally naming the muscles may help the patient focus on the task. Touching the muscles, like musculus mentalis and musculus masseter, and doing exercises where the patient first contracts and thereafter relaxes the muscles are alternatives that should be tried out. The airways are open during breathing. Therefore, breathing is a good exercise – focus on open airways, feeling the air passing easily from the nose, down the throat, and into the lungs, and then from the lungs, up the throat, and out the nose or mouth. The tongue is relaxed, the mandible falls forward and downward opening the mouth.

> ► Example

Tina is a woman in her mid-forties. In the last year alone, she has had more than 15 appointments with a dentist who practices cognitive behavior therapy, and her dental anxiety has declined. However, she still cannot undergo dental treatment in the back of her mouth, and there is a caries lesion mesially on tooth 26. After all the treatments that she has had, she feels that she is a hopeless case due to her gag reflex.

The new dentist identifies, by looking at Tina, that she has extremely strong and tense muscles in her lower face and in the front of her neck. He asks if Tina notices that she has high muscle tonus and difficulties in relaxing her muscles, which are auxiliary muscles when gagging. She says that she has not been aware of it, but she can feel the difference when the dentist helps her relax by letting the mandible and tongue fall downward and forward. The next step is to be aware of the muscles in the throat. Already on the path to recognizing contractions versus relaxing, Tina is able to identify which muscles she needs to relax to avoid gagging. Already at this point, Tina has become an active part of the treatment and she has a positive attitude toward self-efficacy and being able to undergo dental treatment. ◄

Another habit reversal exercise is to make the patient hum while having instruments or X-rays intraorally. It is reportedly impossible to hum and gag at the same time.

16.4.7   Unlearning the Gag Response by Systematic Desensitization

Systematic desensitization aims to reduce the threshold of gagging progressively to achieve a lasting effect [43]. The marble technique was earlier suggested as a method to habituate patients to having something not eatable in their mouths. The patients started with one marble ball in their mouths and gradually increased the number of marble balls they had in their mouths at the same time [51]. As for the marble technique, the patient should gradually be exposed to different procedures with gradually increased length and difficulty. Over time, the link between the aversive stimuli, which induce gagging, and the feared response will gradually diminish, and the

16

threshold of gagging will be increased. The exposure must be specific, controlled, and gradually more difficult (see ▶ Chap. 12). All exposures must be in cooperation with the patient with a defined start and end. At some point, one could relapse to earlier exposures to make the patient experience how they increase their level of tolerance. This has a major physiological effect on the feeling of success. Dentist communication and attitude to gagging are still important factors to keep in mind. If the patient at any time feels that the dentist is afraid that she/he will gag, the dentist's behavior may stimulate avoidance behavior in the patient. Good communication and collaboration between the dentist and the patient is necessary to find exercises that will produce the best learning effects without triggering a gag reflex. Precise start and stop signals should be defined and rehearsed before the exercise, and the patient may use the stop signal any time. If the patient gags, the dentist needs to stay calm and supportive. The dentist should seek to give feedback, which underlines the understanding that the patient is not responsible for the gag reflex.

While working with desensitization, it is important to keep in mind the relaxation and breathing techniques described earlier. It is impossible to feel both anxiety and relaxation at the same time; therefore, easing the client into deep relaxation helps inhibit the feeling of anxiety. Another important principle while working to reduce gagging is to encourage the patient to "lean into" the exercises. This is also an important principle in treating dental anxiety in general and entails that the patient should be an active part of the exposure. This can be sought for, for example, by asking the patient to open her/his mouth when ready or to approach her/his head with an instrument, ensuring that the patient does not imperceptibly turns her/his head away or apply in other "avoidance maneuvers."

Patients may well be prescribed exercises as homework. Such exercises may consist of holding various dental instruments in their mouths, like a mouth mirror, a suction, or a cotton roll, and manage the exposure at home, keeping a diary of how long they feel comfortable keeping the instruments intraorally. It is extremely important that the patients learn how to expose themselves with gradual and systematic exposure. The exposure may be random, but it should always have a distinct start and stop point. In addition, the patients must be prepared to deal with drawbacks and competitive negative thoughts, which may make the exposures more difficult. By doing this twice a day, the goal is to become less sensitive to the gag reflex. The homework should be personally designed for each patient. An example of homework for a patient whose gag response is triggered when she feels that she cannot breathe is to start practicing breathing through the nose while the mouth is open.

> **► Example: Exposure That Triggers the Gag Response**
>
> Example: Goal – Brushing the buccal surface of tooth 27. Have your toothbrush ready.
>
> 1. Start with touching the buccal surface of the upper left canine with your toothbrush while counting to "1." Relax your muscles and breathe when you start the exposure.
>   - Repeat till you feel confident.
> 2. The same as the previous exposure, but now counting to "5."
>   - Repeat until the exposure feels automated.
> 3. Brush the tooth with small movements while counting to "5."
>   - Repeat
> 4. Involve tooth number 4 and count to "1."
>   - Repeat and expand the time of the exercise. Always decide in advance what to count to. If the task triggers gagging, withdraw by decreasing the number you count to.
> 5. Repeat exercise number 1. Feel the change!
> 6. The same as exercise number 4, but involve a new tooth. Start counting to "1."
>   - Make several repetitions before you expand to "5."
>   - Remember to do your job. Focus on relaxing your muscles and feel the air filling your lungs.
> 7. Could you now include teeth 26 and 27 or do you need more repetitions? ◄

This is a basic desensitization program, which can be expanded to all areas of the mouth. One must begin near the lips. It is important to do the exercises in a gradual, systematic, and controlled manner and to be specific about the start and stop of every step. We advise that the patient performs this exercise at least two times a day, in relation to the daily oral hygiene. One can also do additional practice for faster progression. One can choose to agree on a specific time interval, e.g., 5 min two times a day. Many patients find it motivating to reach a specific goal, so one can also practice until the goal is reached. The quality of the exposure is more important than the duration of the task.

> **Tip: What to Say to Patient**
>
> Remember that gagging is a natural response. If you gag, it is not a sign of failure. You should deal with gagging with questions like "Ok, I gagged, what where my thoughts?" "How can I improve the quality of the exposures?" "Did I do the job, focusing on the air floating down my open throat, relaxed chest, jaw, tongue and soft palate?"
>
> In every exposure, you should focus on the task that you are doing. You should not look ahead, thinking about exposures that you are not ready for, not even in your thoughts.
>
> You should motivate yourself for an exposure that triggers the gag response. This is your goal for the day.

Our experience is that for many patients, it can be challenging to conduct the exercises correctly at home. One pitfall is that the patient induces gagging and thereby reinforces the fear and gets the feeling of a step back or hopelessness. These issues should be prepared for and talked through in advance.

16.4.8 Distraction

It is challenging when patients' thoughts are the triggers for gagging because, contrary to physical triggers, they are not visible to the dentist. Dentists should address patients' negative and triggering thoughts to make them aware of how thoughts and behaviors are closely linked. Only when patients are able to differentiate which thoughts are linked to gagging, can their thoughts be addressed and altered over time. Since gagging during treatment makes treatment difficult, a change in focus and thoughts may often be the easiest way to achieve a change in behavior. When the gag reflex has decreased to a level that allows longer exposure durations, the patient may need methods to distract from triggering thoughts. Distraction is best achieved by doing physical movements such as raising the legs or drawing numbers in the air with the feet. If there are elements of heaviness or difficulty in doing the exercise correctly, the exercises seem to distract the most. Moreover, the dentist may help the patient focus on the physical distraction by sequentially naming the body parts that are in focus "Feel how you have open and relaxed airways. The air easily floats down your windpipe, your tongue, throat and jaw are relaxed. Giving space for the air to flow. The air fills your lungs and you now feel the air going from your lungs to your nose." This form of distraction technique is useful in two ways since it has a relaxing effect in addition to distracting the patient. Distraction can, however, be a doubled-edged sword. It is important that the patient focuses on tasks that have the potential to reduce the learned behavior and anxiety. If the distraction techniques are used to withstand and overcome the exposures, then patients are at risk of developing safety behaviors, behaviors that take the patients' focus off the "task at hand," and instead increase self-focused attention [52].

Distraction may be used to address difficulties due to competing thoughts. Standing on one foot with the other foot 45° to the side is an exercise that can be done simultaneously with desensitization exercises.

16.4.9 Adjustments/Facilitations

The first-choice approach to gagging is behavior modification. However, we need to take into consideration the whole life situation and health of the patient. Some will have psychiatric comorbidities or life circumstances that make it too demanding/difficult to go through such treatment at this point of time. A flexible dentist with an ability to find alternative ways to carry out difficult dental procedures will bring the patient closer to his/her goal of achieving dental treatment. If graded exposure has been attempted, but the patient for some reason or the other is not able to follow through, it is advisable to explore adjustments of the dental situation to help the patient manage it. This way, the patient may feel some mastery and can be ready for behavioral therapy at another point of time. Gagging may even decrease as the patient gets a sense of control and feels confident about the dentist. Thus, making adjustments may be the start of a virtuous cycle.

Some patients experience variations in their gag reflex depending on the time of the day. Therefore, it is advisable to schedule appointments at the best time of the day for each patient. In line with a trauma-sensitive treatment approach, the patient's triggers should be explored and alternative ways of conducting the procedures should also be explored. For example, many patients feel that it helps sitting in a more upright position in the dentist's chair. Some patients feel that using a smaller X-ray sensor triggers less gagging, and some dentists use the thumb of a latex glove around the sensor instead of the usual plastic cover, to touch the palate less. In some cases, it may be possible for patients to hold the sensor themselves, which increases their sense of control. For some patients, it will be helpful to reduce the palatial extension of prosthesis. All adjustments that make procedures go faster are usually welcomed, like using fast set, non-flowable impression materials and bulk fill restoratives. Application of a rubber dam may be helpful to stop water from entering the oral cavity and throat. Which adjustments to choose is best decided in collaboration with the patient and will depend on which triggers and catastrophic thoughts the patient holds. Moreover, the patient should be asked whether he/she has found certain routines for avoiding the gag response, like drinking cold water, using salt on the tongue, etc.

Case Study

The case of a woman in her fifties who had experienced childhood sexual abuse:

After a few sessions of graded exposure, it suddenly appeared to me that the patient only started gagging when I used the metallic impression tray, not the one in plastic. When I asked her what she thought about this, she said: "When I think about it, I also prefer eating with plastic cutlery. Metal in my mouth tends to set off reactions... especially if it touches the palate." In practicing a trauma-sensitive approach, I was aware that she was a CSA survivor, but we had never talked about the details. Now she told me that her abuser on several occasions had held a gun in her mouth. Due to her complex PTSD, her psychologist is of the opinion that it will take years of cognitive therapy to overcome this challenge. In the meantime, making the proper adjustments has helped her survive the needed dental treatment without re-traumatization.

16.4.10 Pharmacological/Technical Interventions

Treatments to reduce a gag response are highly demanding and tough for patients, who must have high motivation to deal with them. Some patients want dental treatment and are not motivated for treatments addressing gagging. Others are skeptical about the effect of behavioral approaches. They may often have the opinion that there is nothing that they can do to change the gag response. For these patients, and for patients with an acute need for dental treatment, we recommend the use of sedative medication.

Gagging is a symptom of anxiety when it is triggered by smell, taste, thoughts, and previous experiences. Sedation reduces the psychogenic part of the gag problem [53, 54]. Benzodiazepines, with midazolam as the first choice due to its short half-life, is effective [55]. Midazolam may be taken as pills. For children who cannot take pills, the bad taste of midazolam may trigger gagging. In these circumstances, a nose spray may be easier to use. Nitrous oxide is a sedative gas without odor and taste that gives a quick onset and can be removed quickly if needed. In addition, nitrous oxide causes the mucous membranes to have a certain numbness and thus become less sensitive to touch, which may also reduce the gag reflex. The disadvantage of nitrous oxide is that good patient cooperation is required to be able to use the nitrous oxide mask. If patients are sensitive to clothing near their faces, such as neck serviettes, or if they react to the dentist's hand close to their faces, then there is a chance that the mask is too difficult to wear. In severe cases, a combination of midazolam and nitrous oxide may be the treatment of choice because nitrous oxide may be titrated to its optimal concentration and reduced when the most gag-eliciting procedures are conducted. Experience has shown that the effect of sedation against gagging is good when the patient is medicated, but there seems to be a low learning effect in later consultations. Both the patient and dentist should keep this in mind to reduce expectations of reduced gagging when sedation is not used during later appointments.

Anesthesia may be used to reduce patients' sensory trigger for gagging [56]. Both superficial anesthesia and injected alternatives may have positive effects. The surface mucosa may be numbed with anesthesia such as a xylocaine spray or different forms of gels. Areas in the back of the mouth, especially the uvula and pharynx area, render the oral cavity less sensitive to stimuli [57]. The advantage of superficial anesthesia is that it is easy to use and is usually easy for patients to accept. When the patient needs dental treatment, the mandibular block and distal palatal infiltration are commonly used. The less common glossopharyngeal nerve block is also effective in reducing the gag reflex [58], though this technique is less used among dentists.

Medications with indication for nausea and vomiting show some, but not significant, reduction in the gag response [59]. The effect may be related to the emotional association between nausea and gagging. Whether the drugs directly affect cells in the gagging center is unknown to us. Examples of such drugs are metoclopramide hydrochloride (Afipran) and scopolamine (Scopoderm).

Always, when medication is used, there is a question of whether the method only enables the patient to endure treatment, in contrast to learning to manage it. With focus on a good clinical relation, trust, and control in the situation, the patient may have positive experiences that are important for the patient–dentist cooperation to overcome the problematic gagging during dentistry.

ASSESSMENT SEVERITY AND CAUSES OF GAGGING

SEVERITY OF GAGGING	MILD AND MODERAT GAGGING		SEVERE GAGGING		
NEED FOR (URGENT) DENTAL TREATMENT	YES	NO	YES		NO
TREATMENT OF CHOISE	RELATIONSHIP BUILDING	RELATIONSHIP BUILDING	RELATIONSHIP BUILDING		RELATIONSHIP BUILDING
	BEHAVIOUR MODIFICATION TECNIQUES	BEHAVIOUR MODIFICATION TECNIQUES	↓	BEHAVIOUR MODIFICATION TECNIQUES	BEHAVIOUR MODIFICATION TECNIQUES
	SEDATION		GENERAL ANASTHESIA	SEDATION	
	ADJUSTMENT/ FACILITATIONS	ADJUSTMENT/ FACILITATIONS	ADJUSTMENT/ FACILITATIONS	ADJUSTMENT/ FACILITATIONS	ADJUSTMENT/ FACILITATIONS
			PHARMA-COLOGICAL INTERVENTIONS	PHARMA-COLOGICAL INTERVENTIONS	PHARMA-COLOGICAL INTERVENTIONS

Summary

Gagging is a divergent problem, affecting a heterogeneous group of patients. Since it has the potential to be difficult to treat, any early signs of gagging in the dental clinic should be taken seriously and addressed. As for dental anxiety at large, techniques to address anxiety must be based on delicate teamwork with emphasis on trust and control. Psychology plays an important role in the development of gagging problems. The dentist must be positive and respectful and meet the patient's tendency to gag with knowledge about the biological source and sustaining psychological and social factors. It seems that feeling safe and calm is essential to overcome the gagging problem. Thus, every intervention should aim at reducing stress and leading the patient toward feeling more relaxed.

16

References

1. Miller AJ. Oral and pharyngeal reflexes in the mammalian nervous system: their diverse range in complexity and the pivotal role of the tongue. Crit Rev Oral Biol Med. 2002;13(5):409–25.
2. Yoshida H, Ayuse T, Ishizaka S, Ishitobi S, Nogami T, Oi K. Management of exaggerated gag reflex using intravenous sedation in prosthodontic treatment. Tohoku J Exp Med. 2007;212(4):373–8.
3. Murchie BD. Gagging – bringing up an old problem part 1: aetiology and diagnosis. Dent Update. 2018;45:609–16.
4. van Houtem CM, van Wijk AJ, Boomsma DI, Ligthart L, Visscher CM, de Jongh A. Self-reported gagging in dentistry: prevalence, psycho-social correlates and oral health. J Oral Rehabil. 2015;42(7):487–94.
5. Davies AE, Kidd D, Stone SP, MacMahon J. Pharyngeal sensation and gag reflex in healthy subjects. Lancet. 1995;345(8948):487–8.
6. Leder SB. Gag reflex and dysphagia. Head Neck. 1996; 18(2):138–41.
7. Dickinson CM, Fiske J. A review of gagging problems in dentistry: I. Aetiology and classification. Dent Update. 2005;32(1):26–8, 31–2.
8. Engel GL. The need for a new medical model: a challenge for biomedicine. Science. 1977;196(4286):129–36.
9. Hopwood V. Current context: neurological rehabilitation and neurological physiotherapy. In: Livingstone C, editor. Acupuncture in neurological conditions; 2010. p. 39–51.
10. Wilson-Pauwels L. Cranial Nerves Vagus X. https://bmc.utm. utoronto.ca/cranialnerves/vagus.html: Utoronto ca; 2013 [3rd].
11. Roberts MW, Tylenda CA, Sonies BC, Elin RJ. Dysphagia in bulimia nervosa. Dysphagia. 1989;4(2):106–11.
12. Nichols H. Gag reflex and disgust sensitivity in selective eaters: Western Washington University; 2018.
13. Bassi GS, Humphris GM, Longman LP. The etiology and management of gagging: a review of the literature. J Prosthet Dent. 2004;91(5):459–67.
14. Conny DJ, Tedesco LA. The gagging problem in prosthodontic treatment. Part II: Patient management. J Prosthet Dent. 1983;49(6):757–61.
15. Tubbs RS, Webb D, Smyth MD, Oakes WJ. Magnetic resonance imaging evidence of posterior pharynx denervation in pediatric patients with Chiari I malformation and absent gag reflex. J Neurosurg. 2004;101(1 Suppl):21–4.
16. Wright SM. An examination of factors associated with retching in dental patients. J Dent. 1979;7(3):194–207.
17. Brignole M, Moya A, de Lange FJ, Deharo J-C, Elliott PM, Fanciulli A, et al. 2018 ESC Guidelines for the diagnosis and management of syncope. Eur Heart J. 2018;39(21):1883–948.

18. Muller MD, Mast JL, Cui J, Heffernan MJ, McQuillan PM, Sinoway LI. Tactile stimulation of the oropharynx elicits sympathoexcitation in conscious humans. J Appl Physiol (1985). 2013;115(1):71–7.

19. Gartland D, Riggs E, Muyeen S, Giallo R, Afifi TO, MacMillan H, et al. What factors are associated with resilient outcomes in children exposed to social adversity? A systematic review. BMJ Open. 2019;9(4):e024870.

20. Taylor SE, Stanton AL. Coping resources, coping processes, and mental health. Annu Rev Clin Psychol. 2007;3:377–401.

21. Hainsworth JM, Hill KB, Rice A, Fairbrother KJ. Psychosocial characteristics of adults who experience difficulties with retching. J Dent. 2008;36(7):494–9.

22. Katsouda M, Tollili C, Coolidge T, Simos G, Kotsanos N, Arapostathis KN. Gagging prevalence and its association with dental fear in 4–12-year-old children in a dental setting. Int J Paediatr Dent. 2019;29(2):169–76.

23. Uziel N, Bronner G, Elran E, Eli I. Sexual correlates of gagging and dental anxiety. Community Dent Health. 2012;29(3): 243–7.

24. van Houtem CMHH. Anxiety, fainting and gagging in dentistry: Separate or overlapping constructs? Amsterdam: University of Amsterdam; 2016.

25. Randall CL, Shulman GP, Crout RJ, McNeil DW. Gagging and its associations with dental care-related fear, fear of pain and beliefs about treatment. J Am Dent Assoc. 2014;145(5):452–8.

26. Armfield JM. Cognitive vulnerability: a model of the etiology of fear. Clin Psychol Rev. 2006;26(6):746–68.

27. Moore R, Brodsgaard I, Rosenberg N. The contribution of embarrassment to phobic dental anxiety: a qualitative research study. BMC Psychiatry. 2004;4:10.

28. Miller AJ. In: Sleisenger MH, editor. The handbook of nausea and vomiting. United States: Caduceus Medical Publishers, Inc.; 1993.

29. Logemann JA. Swallowing physiology and pathophysiology. Otolaryngol Clin N Am. 1988;21(4):613–23.

30. Teachman BA, Saporito J. I am going to gag: disgust cognitions in spider and blood-injury-injection fears. Cogn Emot. 2009;23(2):399–414.

31. Toronchuk JA, Ellis GFR. Disgust: sensory affect or primary emotional system? Cognit Emot. 2007;21(8):1799–818.

32. Armfield JM, Mattiske JK. Vulnerability representation: the role of perceived dangerousness, uncontrollability, unpredictability and disgustingness in spider fear. Behav Res Ther. 1996;34(11–12):899–909.

33. Felitti VJ, Anda RF, Nordenberg D, Williamson DF, Spitz AM, Edwards V, et al. Relationship of childhood abuse and household dysfunction to many of the leading causes of death in adults. The Adverse Childhood Experiences (ACE) Study. Am J Prev Med. 1998;14(4):245–58.

34. Kvist T, Annerbäck EM, Sahlqvist L, Flodmark O, Dahllöf G. Association between adolescents' self-perceived oral health and self-reported experiences of abuse. Eur J Oral Sci. 2013;121(6):594–9.

35. Berggren U, Meynert G. Dental fear and avoidance: causes, symptoms, and consequences. J Am Dent Assoc. 1984;109(2): 247–51.

36. Raadal M, Strand GV, Amarante EC, Kvale G. Relationship between caries prevalence at 5 years of age and dental anxiety at 10. Eur J Paediatr Dent. 2002;3(1):22–6.

37. Skaret E, Raadal M, Berg E, Kvale G. Dental anxiety among 18-yr-olds in Norway. Prevalence and related factors. Eur J Oral Sci. 1998;106(4):835–43.

38. Leeners B, Stiller R, Block E, Gorres G, Imthurn B, Rath W. Consequences of childhood sexual abuse experiences on dental care. J Psychosom Res. 2007;62(5):581–8.

39. Willumsen T. Dental fear in sexually abused women. Eur J Oral Sci. 2001;109(5):291–6.

40. Spiegel J. Sexual abuse of males: the SAM model of theory and practice. New York: Brunner-Routledge; 2003.

41. Jones AC, Brake CA, Badour CL. Disgust in PTSD. In: Tull MT, Kimbrel NA, editors. Emotion in posttraumatic stress disorder. Academic Press; 2020. p. 117–43.

42. van Linden van den Heuvell GF, de Boer B, Ter Pelkwijk BJ, Bildt MM, Stegenga B. Gagging problem assessment: a re-evaluation. J Oral Rehabil. 2015;42(7):495–502.

43. Dickinson CM, Fiske J. A review of gagging problems in dentistry: 2. Clinical assessment and management. Dent Update. 2005;32(2):74–6, 8–80.

44. Faigenblum MJ. Retching, its causes and management in prosthetic practice. Br Dent J. 1968;125:485–90.

45. Sewerin I. Gagging in dental radiology. Oral Surg. 1984;58: 725–8.

46. Nesse RM. Evolutionary explanations of emotions. Hum Nat. 1990;1(3):261–89.

47. Haukebø K, Skaret E, Ost LG, Raadal M, Berg E, Sundberg H, et al. One- vs. five-session treatment of dental phobia: a randomized controlled study. J Behav Ther Exp Psychiatry. 2008;39(3):381–90.

48. Ansari IH. Management for maxillary removable partial denture patients who gag. J Prosthet Dent. 1994;72(4):448.

49. Azrin NH, Nunn RG. Habit-reversal: a method of eliminating nervous habits and tics. Behav Res Ther. 1973;11(4): 619–28.

50. Himle MB, Woods DW, Piacentini JC, Walkup JT. Brief review of habit reversal training for Tourette syndrome. J Child Neurol. 2006;21(8):719–25.

51. Singer IL. The marble technique: a method for treating the "hopeless gagger" for complete dentures. J Prosthet Dent. 1973;29(2):146–50.

52. Blakey SM, Abramowitz JS, Buchholz JL, Jessup SC, Jacoby RJ, Reuman L, et al. A randomized controlled trial of the judicious use of safety behaviors during exposure therapy. Behav Res Ther. 2019;112:28–35.

53. Kaufman E, Weinstein P, Sommers EE, Soltero DJ. An experimental study of the control of the gag reflex with nitrous oxide. Anesth Prog. 1988;35(4):155–7.

54. Robb ND, Crothers AJ. Sedation in dentistry. Part 2: Management of the gagging patient. Dent Update. 1996; 23(5):182–6.

55. Malkoc MA, Demir N, Ileri Z, Erdur A, Apiliogullari S. Intranasal midazolam may prevent gagging reflex: a case report. J Oral Maxillofac Res. 2013;4(3):e5.

56. Soweid AM, Yaghi SR, Jamali FR, Kobeissy EE, Mallat ME, Hussein R, et al. Posterior lingual lidocaine: a novel method to improve tolerance in upper gastrointestinal endoscopy. World J Gastroenterol. 2011;17(14):5191–6.

57. al-Ashiry MK, Salah MA. The effect of visco-anaesthetic medicament on tactile gag reflex control. Egypt Dent J. 1993;39(3):457–60.

58. Garg R, Singhal A, Agrawal K, Agrawal N. Managing endodontic patients with severe gag reflex by glossopharyngeal nerve block technique. J Endod. 2014;40(9):1498–500.

59. Barenboim SF, Dvoyris V, Kaufman E. Does granisetron eliminate the gag reflex? A crossover, double-blind, placebo-controlled pilot study. Anesth Prog. 2009;56(1):3–8.

Child Sexual Abuse and Oral Health Challenges

Tiril Willumsen, Therese V. Fredriksen, Siri Søftestad and Vibeke Kranstad

Contents

Learning Goals
- To increase knowledge of how oral health is affected in people exposed to child sexual abuse
- To gain a deeper understanding of how people exposed to sexual abuse in childhood experience daily dental care and dental treatment
- To increase knowledge about relevant adjustments to be used in daily dental practice

17.1 Introduction

Several studies have found associations between a history of child sexual abuse and/or domestic violence, daily dental care habits and high dental anxiety [1–4]. As the sequela from CSA include both a psychological and a social component in addition to behavioural aspects of dental treatment, the authors of this chapter conducted a multidisciplinary qualitative study among female and male CSA survivors, about half of them attended dental treatment regularly. The overall aim was to explore their oral care challenges from three different professional perspectives: social, psychological and dental. The authors have different professions, but all have clinical experiences from treatment of CSA survivors, one social worker (SS), one psychologist (TVF) and two dentists (VK and TW). This chapter is based upon three published papers from this study, as well as clinical experiences and literature reviews [5–7].

Most sexual abuse situations include violence, feelings of being held down or trapped in combinations with pain. It is easy to imagine that these issues may resemble elements of a dental treatment situation. Especially vulnerable is children who in the middle of a sexual abuse period (a secret they can't tell anybody) meet a dentist or dental hygienist without proper knowledge and skills. It is a sad but based upon clinical experience to confirm that almost every patient with CSA background tells about such meetings with dental personnel. Being exposed to forced oral sex make oral care particularly difficult. The mouth may be the most intimidating part of the body during abuse, as a result of the abuser's hand in front of mouth and nose to keep the victim from screaming, forced kissing or forced oral sex. Willumsen [1] found in her study that 85% with this kind of experience had very high dental anxiety. This is quite logical. If someone is forcing something into the mouth that is painful and also prevents free breathing, it is extremely potent as a life-threatening event, and consequently provokes both anxiety and trauma reactions. However, there have been relatively few research reports addressing these associations. This may have several reasons. First, it may raise difficult ethical concerns to investigate issues this intimate and difficult psychologically. Another reason may be that

the person him/ herself does not associate the reactions during dental care with former trauma situations. Often decades pass before being sexual abused is admitted to oneself and even longer before one is capable of telling about it [8]. Some barriers identified in the studies of disclosure are shame, self-blame and anticipation of unsupportive responses [9–13]. A Swedish world-famous athlete who won gold medal in world championships and Olympic games in the 1980s is giving an example of the reasons for delayed disclosure in a book he wrote at the age of 46. The book revealed his big secret, that his coach and stepfather sexually abused him from the age of 11. He had kept this secret from everybody, including his mother and his wife [14]. After his athletic career he like many other sexual abused men in periods had turned to substance abuse. It is interesting to note that boys and men seem to have even more difficulties than women admitting and talking about sexual abuse [15, 16]. Thus, it is reasons to have attention to both genders.

The present chapter will describe issues of specific importance for dental health professionals when giving help and advises in prevention and treatment of oral diseases. First, we will describe typical reactions that may be seen before, during and after dental treatment. These reactions may be subtle and therefore difficult to perceive, or they may be powerfully acted out and difficult for the dentist to understand and handle. This section will be guided by CSA survivors' experiences with dental treatment. Then we will give examples of how deeply oral health-related problems may have impact on a CSA survivor's daily life as well as understanding of self. These insights urge us to improve and facilitate dental treatment practice to prevent re-victimization and trauma reactions as well as to make dental treatment possible for these patients. Therefore, we will end the chapter by sharing the idea of using trauma-sensitive care in dental treatment. A range of practical advises will be presented and discussed.

17.2 Possible Trauma Reactions Before, During and After Treatment

A typical reaction of a CSA survivor is to avoid, consciously or unconsciously, similar situations and sensory impressions experienced during abuse. Also, being reminded of abuse causes strong negative emotions and represents a risk of reliving one's childhood trauma.

Reminders of traumatic memories are triggered by modalities, such as sights, sounds, smells, taste, tactile stimuli, body positions, words or scenes of the original trauma. The reaction involves a very strong physiological response that produces the feeling of being in danger and the need to fight, flee or freeze to survive.

Multiple impressions are perceived during traumatic events. What determines what is later re-experienced? Patients have reported re-experiencing brief moments from the trauma, such as "hearing the abuser breathe" or "hearing footsteps behind me". Ehlers et al. [17] analysis indicated that these kinds of sensory impressions represented signals of the onset of the trauma or the onset of its worst moments. In that perspective the intrusions had functional significance in that they represented stimuli that predicted the worst moments of trauma and had thus acquired the status of warning signals [18].

Posttraumatic flashbacks consist of intrusive reliving of traumatic experiences in the present. Most dramatically, people lose all contact with current reality and respond as if the trauma is happening at that moment. Intrusion of mental pictures or "a movie" of the event is often part of the reactions. Bodily sensations may be re-experienced, and elements of the trauma in repetitive nightmares. Posttraumatic rumination characterizes that the person is thinking of and bothered by the traumatic events but lacking the sensory re-experiencing and is oriented of time and place [19]. To meet necessary trauma-sensitive adjustments, it is important to assess whether the patient experiences flashbacks or rumination during dental treatment/care.

17.2.1 Consciousness Level – Dissociation

Disconnecting your thoughts and feelings from a present situation is a normal shift in consciousness level. For instance, to think of other things during automatized activity, such as driving or brushing your teeth. You are somewhat mentally distant and simultaneously fully aware of your presence in the situation. This flexibility is even a marker for mental health [20]. The ability to intentionally divert yourself from a stressful situation by disconnecting is an adaptive strategy to regulating emotions, for instance, when a patient finds a dental treatment challenging.

Dissociation is defined by disruption and fragmentation of the usually integrated functions of consciousness, memory, identity, body awareness and perception of the self and the environment [21]. If the process of disruption and fragmentation is clearly related to traumatizing events, it is considered a symptom of pathological dissociation. Pathological dissociation is not well controlled [22]. The bad things that have been done to you is in a sense automatically disconnected from your consciousness and stored in sensory fragments ("keeping my mouth open over time", "the taste and smell of rubber"). Dissociation may start to occur during the abuse ("I saw myself being abused from a distance", "I know my childhood was bad, but I don't remember much specific from my childhood"). Even though the

abuses have ended, dissociation often continues to occur in everyday life, especially when similar feelings as when abused are activated.

Memories of sexual abuse are body related and may lead to withdrawal or rejection of the body, possibly leading to reduced contact with the body. Therefore, traumatized individuals often find it difficult to attend to inner sensations and perceptions, and sometimes even deny any somatic awareness [23]. "I am not afraid of pain at the dentist. Pain helps me disappear". "I just stop breathing and can't feel my legs when I am at the dentist".

This aspect of dissociation and body experience is rarely addressed in the literature. In our clinical practice, a central element in CSA dental patients is their lack of body ownership. The experience of the body as "my body" is acquired in early development and is based on physical experiences accompanying with clear definitions of boundaries between self and others. A body image may be severely impaired by threats to the physical integrity and/or violations of body.

In a psychological perspective, when abuse is not happening anymore, dissociation serves a purpose of avoiding extreme unpleasant emotions when triggered or even displace memories of abuse.

> **A No Win Situation – The CSA Patients' Possible Dilemma**
>
> If the CSA patient forces himself to receive needed dental treatment, he runs the risk of dissociation partially or completely from the dental situation.
>
> If the CSA patient is present (avoid dissociation), he runs the risk of reliving the terrifying experience and feelings of being abused, during dental care/treatment.
>
> If the CSA patient refrains from necessary dental treatment to avoid the psychological consequences above, toothache and other oral health issues are inevitable.
>
> By failing to acknowledge and address these dilemmas in treatment, the CSA patients most likely will continue to avoid dental care and treatment until the toothache is unbearable and extraction is the only option.

In other words, dissociation was a protective solution during abuse, but becomes part of the problem during dental care/treatment. When patients dissociate during dental care/treatment, the sensory apparatus fails to process what is really going on, namely dental care/treatment. To be present enables the patient to integrate what is really going on (dental treatment), and at the same time distinguish sensations of dental treatment from past experiences of abuse. From our experience, this is essential in trauma-sensitive dental care.

17.2.2   **Triggers**

To give the best framework for dental treatment, it is essential to know what to look for to understand the link between the patient's reactions in present and traumatic events possibly experienced in the past.

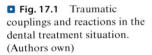 Figure 17.1 presents some examples from the study concerning reminders of abuse triggered in the dental treatment situation and some possible physical reactions.

The dental treatment situation is challenging for both the patient and dental staff because, to be able to provide high quality dental treatment, it is often not possible for the dental staff to avoid triggering the patients' traumatic hot spots. A key factor in our experience is to make the relationship between the dentist and patient equal. By saying to the patient, for instance, "I am an expert on dental treatment and know a lot about usual reactions in the dental treatment situation for patients with a history of CSA. But equal important is that you are the expert on how different elements of dental treatment are perceived and experienced internally by you", you communicate the wish for an equal relationship which is absent in a relationship of abuse.

It may be useful to encourage the patient to describe his or her reactions in the dental chair in advance of any dental procedures. In this way the dentist may explain known reactions described in this section and the patients may recognize reactions in themselves. In this manner you build together a platform of possible adjustments to avoid overwhelming the patient and for the patient to be able to separate what they experience in the present and what is echoes from traumatic experiences in the past. A self-instruction during dental treatment might be "What I am experiencing know is me receiving health care. That is why I am opening my mouth, experiencing things inside my mouth while laying on my back". Also, when the dentist is saying "You open your mouth when you are ready", is a statement signalling to the patient that he or she invites the dentist over their personal boundary instead of being invaded.

17.2.3   **How CSA Survivors Experience Dental Treatment**

Dental anxiety in CSA survivors is trauma driven and possibly one of the long-term effects of child sexual abuse [5, 24]. Trauma-driven dental anxiety is different from a simple dental phobia. In contrast to a simple dental phobia issues connected to interpersonal relations and closeness of dental staff are even more important

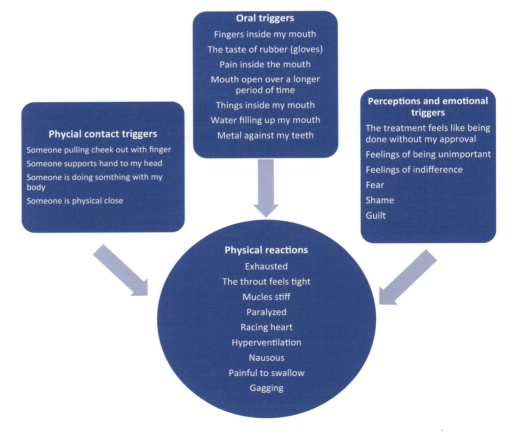

Fig. 17.1 Traumatic couplings and reactions in the dental treatment situation. (Authors own)

Oral triggers
Fingers inside my mouth
The taste of rubber (gloves)
Pain inside the mouth
Mouth open over a longer period of time
Things inside my mouth
Water filling up my mouth
Metal against my teeth

Phycial contact triggers
Someone pulling cheek out with finger
Someone supports hand to my head
Someone is doing somthing with my body
Someone is physical close

Perceptions and emotional triggers
The treatment feels like being done without my approval
Feelings of being unimportant
Feelings of indifference
Fear
Shame
Guilt

Physical reactions
Exhausted
The throut feels tight
Mucles stiff
Paralyzed
Racing heart
Hyperventilation
Nausous
Painful to swallow
Gagging

17

[25]. Both simple dental phobia and dental phobia in CSA survivors have complex aetiology and it is important to have in mind the overlap between the two. In common with simple dental phobia, the perception of having control is important.

To be successful with trauma-sensitive dental care a deeper understanding and empathy from dental health workers is essential. To be able to build empathy, an understanding of how CSA survivors think and feel about dental care is essential. However, this kind of knowledge is not easy to accomplish. Qualitative analyses are best suited for this kind of deeper insight into emotions and subjective experiences. However, there are still few studies on this topic.

Thus, in the qualitative study analyses from the same study population as Søftestad et al. [7]. (16 persons, 12 women and 4 men) it was aimed to focus upon the informants' experiences, like thoughts, emotions, physical sensations and reactions of dental treatment.

Analyses were performed with focus upon the psychological processes in association with dental care. During the analysis negative experiences associated with someone putting something inside my mouth' emerged as the main concern. The problem was "someone" and it was described as a struggle to make that "someone" into a caring dentist or dental hygienist and not an abuser in the patients mind and thoughts. The informants explained the struggle in preparing for the treatment as well as the complex reactions after dental treatment.

> ### Preparing for an attack and recovering from the battle

In the study the informants described how they prepared for dental treatment by using mental resources to cope with expected danger. In similarity to patients with dental phobia, treatment is something CSA survivors begin to dread long before the appointment.

» Is it going to be a torment in slow motion?

They struggle with memories of negative feelings from earlier dental treatment. As a clinician meeting adult patients exposed to CSA it is heart breaking when patients tell stories about their experiences of dental treatment in a period of extreme vulnerability when they were children and lived a "secret" life with regular sexual abuse. This makes it very relevant to reflect upon the importance of proper paediatric dental care (see ► Chap. 9). In this context it is also easy to understand that it may be difficult to have trust in dentists, or people in general.

All the way through dental treatment the CSA patients expect danger. These expectations as well as direct experiences may all be indirectly coupled to abuse situations. Such traumatic coupling refers to how traumatized persons may unconsciously couple their experiences (feelings, sensations or reactions, and generate emotional or physical responses) in the present to traumatic memories. Overwhelming expectations and experiences during dental care may in this way be stored as sensory experience without words and thoughts [26].

Many perceptions trigger these expectations. The sound of breathing from the dental staff may be coupled with an abuser's heavy breath. To be laying back with the mouth open may resemble an abuse situation. The smells associated with dental treatment are many and couplings may be, for instance, the smell of the dentist may resemble the smell of the abuser; the smell of rubber gloves or rubber dam may couple to the smell of condoms or the smell of disinfectant alcohol reminds of the abuser breath's smell of alcohol.

To overcome these expectations of danger CSA survivors, report a mental fight to mobilize enough willpower to do the opposite of what the body dictated, which often led to postponing or cancelling appointments, and not being able to complete the dental treatment by returning several times to finish.

» ... just being laid back and the mouth kept open ... I find it ... I don't know, but that's what I have been afraid of. Not the pain.

I hate to get things around my neck. So, getting that paper napkin around my neck is just terrible. ...

Likewise, when you are sitting in the dentist's chair and are being tilted backwards... and they are coming ... ah, that feeling of the dental staff leaning over you ... and, no! ... You feel you have no chance. I believe I almost had the same feelings there [at the dentist's] as I had during the abuse.

During the treatment many reported to relive the abuse. This is from clinical experience most often associated with being either in a freeze state (hypoactivated and immobilized without tools to stabilize oneself back into the window of tolerance), often with flashbacks or hypoactivated (feeling numb and disappearing into a state of dissociation).

» ... when I am laying there, no, I just shut everything out in a way and only feel stressed and scared to death, and that I am not able to breathe.

... you arrive [at the dentist's] and then the sweating, itching... begins

... when the dentist is groping in the back of the mouth, fingers are coming, ... I freeze... yes, yes, stiffen, yes...

I just disappeared in a way out of my body, ...

... when the dentist is doing something in the back of my mouth, along with fingers coming, then..., then..., then I freeze... not in the sense of being cold... but stiffen.

I seem very calm and secure to others, but personally it is chaos internally.... No one understands my dental anxiety...

I do not remember... then... I completely disconnect... I am not present

The struggle between keeping oneself present in the present and reliving the abuse situations in flashbacks is a challenge to many

» I get so many pictures of granddad when I have... or when I was at the dentist then.

... when I see the face of [name of the dentist], it resembles that of my uncle. It is almost as though he is also in the room.

I feel as if I am being abused again

I try to stay within my body, I think. But when the pictures [from abuse] come up [during dental treatment], I must talk to myself: 'I'm an adult now, right ... You are here. You are here and now.'

After dental treatment almost all CSA survivors feel exhausted and they need to rest. It is important to instruct the patients to take this feeling seriously and make room for safe and calm surroundings after dental treatment.

» I went straight back home to sleep. My body was exhausted. All my muscles were battered. Just as if I had been in a fight.

Some may experience difficult feelings and bodily sensations. If emotions and reactions are held back during treatment, they may come back as delayed reactions. These reactions may be very challenging. As a dentist it is very important to address the possibility for these kinds of reactions and discuss with the patients whether it would be beneficial to discuss these reactions in a consultation following a dental treatment with an adequate person, like a psychologist or psychiatrist.

» But like, when you are tense and in abuse situation much of the time, you are alerted and when you get away from the situation, sort of safe on the ground, then the emotional reactions emerge in the aftermath.

'It was difficult afterwards ... you do not know what she has done inside there [the mouth] ...'

'I am no longer able to speak for myself. So, people get to do as they please, and then I cope with it afterwards.'

... just being laid back and the mouth kept open ... I find it ... I don't know, but that's what I have been afraid of. Not the pain.

I hate to get things around my neck. So, getting that paper napkin around my neck is just terrible. ...

When dental staff understand the elements of trauma-driven anxiety reactions, the complexity of the reactions and the complexity associated by talking about the reactions, they will have better basis for taking an adequate empathic perspective.

17.3 Oral Health-Related Problems Invade Deeply into the Lives of CSA Survivors

In a qualitative study among 16 persons (12 women and four men) exposed to CSA, the impact of oral health-related problems were described in seven areas: Causing serious oral health symptoms, triggering trauma reactions, increasing emotional distress, shaping the understanding of self, intruding daily life practices, restraining social interactions and generating financial problems [7]. The following quotations in ▶ Sect. 17.3 are taken from this study.

17.3.1 Causing Serious Oral Health Symptoms

CSA exposed persons have increased risk of almost every disease through mechanisms described the conceptual model in ACE pyramid [27]. As shown in ◘ Fig. 17.2a, b, based upon the ACE pyramid, we have constructed a modified version focusing specifically on oral health.

From clinical experience it is observed that many CSA survivors have very poor oral health. The mechanisms or steps in the pyramid of oral diseases are comparable to other diseases. Being exposed to sexual abuse gives social, emotional and cognitive difficulties that often include little focus on, knowledge of and skills in oral health prevention strategies, like tooth cleaning, diet and adequate use of fluorides. This leads to increased risk of dental caries, and in association with dental anxiety and/or comorbidity/economic difficulties, teeth are infected and eventually lost.

17.3.2 Triggering Trauma Reactions in Everyday Life

Many CSA survivors report gagging reflexes and avoidance of having instruments, like a toothbrush, toothpaste or dental instruments in the mouth. Clinical experiences show a clear connection between forced oral sex, flashbacks and gagging. This may be illustrated with a question from the first author's practice:

» Lisa (39): I cannot use toothpaste, both the foam and taste give me flashbacks, do you know any tooth paste without foam or taste?

a

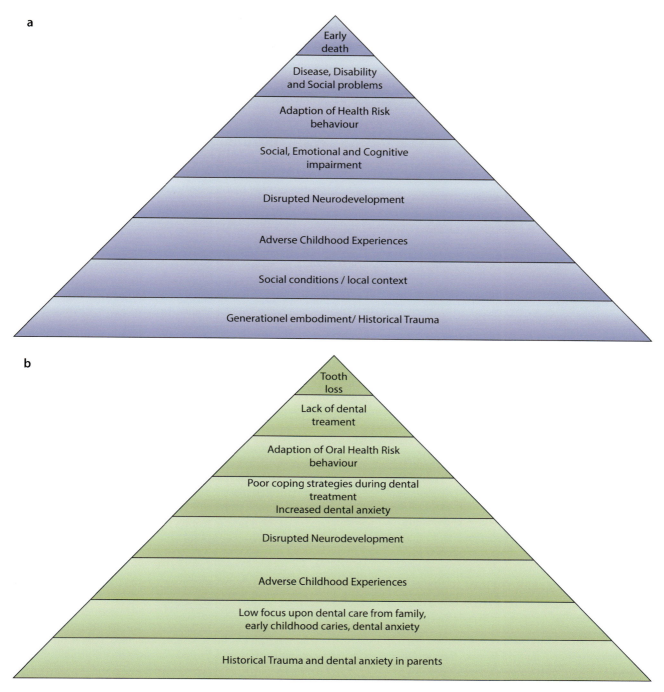

○ **Fig. 17.2** **a** The conceptual model of general health effects from CSA [28]. **b** A modified conceptual model of oral health effects from CSA. (Authors own)

17.3.3 Increasing Emotional Distress

Challenges associated with dental treatment may lead to emotional distress in a broader extent in life than just in oral care situations. The shame and constant struggle between the wish for doing the "right" things, like brush-ing your teeth or going to the dentist, and the avoidance behaviour driven by anxiety [29] as well as distrust of people in general, including dentists [1], enhance emo-tional distress, especially feelings of shame. Shame is a major element in CSA survivors [30, 31], and many experiences the oral cavity to be particularly shameful.

In this context meeting new dental personal is a very vulnerable situation. In Andy's situation, this has rather significant consequences:

» I moved abroad, and when something was wrong with my teeth, I travelled all the way back to my dentist because I wouldn't dare to consult a new one. Consequently, I commuted even if I had to drive for nine hours since I didn't have the courage to go to a new dentist.

17.3.4 Shaping the Understanding of Self

As most people have expectations for themselves to take care of their oral health by during daily oral care and regular dental treatment, the failure in doing so many CSA survivors experience it triggers shame, including negative impressions, like bad conscience, powerlessness and low self-esteem. In a longer time perspective this may integrate in the understanding of self. As oral issues may be triggered several times each day (brushing teeth, eating, pain, etc.) it will act as a constant reminder of "myself as a person without abilities to take care of essential matters in life". When in a dental treatment situation, a person with this kind of understanding of self is vulnerable for getting the feeling that the dentist treats them as an object and not as a human being, as well as vulnerable during treatment with dentists that actually act in such ways. Examples may be dentists who fail in building relation, do not communicate properly (e.g. using the four habits model) or fail to treat the patient with respect despite their poor dental condition. The patients may feel they are unimportant, and their feelings are not taken seriously, but unfortunately most often they are not able to express these feelings [5]. These experiences amplify an already negative feeling of self-guilt. An example in contrast to this is Henry when he describes how a trusted dentist treated him like a fellow human being:

» Interviewer: – The preparations are helpful?
Henry: – Yes
Interviewer: – Making you feel more secure, or...?
Henry: – Yes, I feel more secure and that I'm being treated with respect.... He treats me like a human being capable of listening to information. Compared with an abuse situation, he is ... the way he behaves is significantly different to an abuse situation.

As CSA survivors often do not talk about their abuse, or do not dare to express negative feeling in a dental treatment situation, it may be important to address whether the patient feels safe. A method dentist may use is to check out the alliance by asking: "It is important to me to make you feel safe that we are working as a team, have you any thoughts about whether I succeed in this?" Read more about this in ▶ Sect. 19.4 as well as in ▶ Chaps. 4 and 13.

17.3.5 Intruding Daily Life Practices

Oral health problems may affect everyday life. These problems may involve both physiological pain from teeth or gums, in addition to psychological struggles as, for instance, intrusive memories, nightmares and hypervigilance. As known from literature, numerous CSA survivors suffer from complex trauma and symptom complexity [32, 33]. As many CSA survivors have comorbidity it is likely to assume that dry mouth may be a problem that may affect both speaking (try to speak when you are nervous), eating (you have to have ca. 1.5 mL saliva to process food and swallow) and sleep (wakening up several times at night). In addition, muscle tensions from the jaw, in the tongue or oral muscles or grinding may be substantial negative parts of everyday life.

17.3.6 Restraining Social Interactions

Poor oral health is stigmatizing in many societies and numerous CSA survivors who struggle with oral care suffer from this condition. Poor oral health may be a huge problem for all patients, but in many cases, it is even more complex to handle for CSA survivors. It may affect not only intimate relationships and social arrangements but also professional life. Two examples are as follows:

» George: – I used to work in a hotel, and I made efforts to have a friendly appearance, even when I didn't smile. But, when I got a new boss: 'You have to smile, you cannot have such a serious face when you stand in front of ...'. So, I have been told, but I'm acting politely and correctly. 'Yes, but you have to smile.' That is the feedback from the bosses, and so on.
Interviewer: – You were told directly and... pretty direct. What do you think of it?
George: – It hurts, and I think they commented like that because of my teeth.
Henry: – In intimate situations or in my private life, it has ... yes, it has reinforced the need to keep people at a distance.... It is due to shame, I think; you don't feel worthy, or ... well, you come close and as I see it ... bad teeth and bad breath ... Bad breath is so disgusting.

17

17.3.7 Generating Financial Difficulties

CSA survivors have a number of challenges, including lower educational level [34] and higher financial strains [35]. As dental treatment in adults is based upon a high degree of private financing in most countries, this is a barrier without tools to handle too many CSA survivors. Gina reported like this:

» I cannot work, so I do not have the ability to pay, really, so … the dentist understood, and reduced the bill pretty much, and then … in the end she said: 'Just pay for the materials. It was like I had won the National Lottery!

This challenge may be solved by pro bono work from a dentist as shown in this case. However, if sexual abuse and oral health should be taken seriously as a health problem, we recommend that economical support for dental treatment should be in the same economical systems as other health problems.

17.4 Trauma-Sensitive Dental Treatment of CSA Survivors

In a study among 99 women exposed to CSA 82% reported indecent intercourse and 44% reported forced oral sex. The majority of these women had never told a dentist about their CSA. The main reasons given were "because the abuse incidents have been repressed during certain periods, I have not always been aware of the relationship" and "I have had problems in dental treatment situations, but I have never thought about whether this could be related to having being sexually abused" [1]. Considering the Swedish athlete's and many other CSA survivors' stories of their long-term denying of CSA it is quite obvious that dentists sometimes treat CSA survivors without knowing. Thus, a trauma-sensitive approach to all patients is essential (see ▶ Chaps. 2 and 6).

If the dentist or dental hygienist observes reactions that cause suspicion of CSA, it may be difficult to decide what to do. As a main rule the dentist does not need to do anything, just observe, respect and make adequate adjustments during treatment. If assessed useful exploring further, it should never be done by confrontation with the dentist's suspicions. One possibility is to ask something like *"I can see that you react quite strong being laid back in the chair (a concrete situation), this kind of reaction is natural and often has its origin in negative experiences inflicted in a person usually as a child or adolescent. These sorts of experiences may be of different kinds, such as negative situations at the dentist or more complex trauma related situations like neglect, violence, abuse or bullying. Do you think this is something that may be relevant to you? If so, I don't need to know any details but if you want to talk about anything you think may be relevant for dental treatment it may be beneficial to make dental treatment best possible for you".*

If the patient expresses the need to tell details of abuse, try to stop him/her from giving details not relevant for the dental treatment situation. Headlines are OK but exploring and analysing trauma reactions should be done in a context with adequate professional competence. If the patient has no such help available, dentists should have knowledge about local possibilities for achieving such help and offer to the patient to help them seek care. Either way, it is important to clarify with the patient if he/she is being abused or if the abuse has stopped, and if the perpetrator(s) still is a possible threat to the patient.

> **Box**
>
> Dentists do not need to know details about the sexual abuse, but they must know that this may explain physical or psychological reactions.
>
> The dentist needs to know the patient's individual difficulties concerning oral care, to understand the complexity in the difficulties and to have a set of tools to help the patient overcome the difficulties.

All patients have the right to best possible health care and it is important to have in mind that dental treatment always may include a risk of re-traumatization of CSA survivors, meaning that dental treatment may increase the patients dental as well as general trauma-related symptoms. Thus, it should be mandatory for dental personnel meeting patients with complex traumatic backgrounds, like CSA, to consider cooperating with competent health professionals, like doctors, psychologists, etc. Likewise, the goal for the treatment output in the dental office should be assessed. If the patients seeks out help to overcome their trauma-driven anxiety, it may be beneficial to refer to specialist care (special dental fear clinic) or it may be a good solution to arrange for interdisciplinary treatment in cooperation with a mental health worker.

» Karen, a young woman 24 years of age, contacts the dental clinic, she is suffering from trauma driven dental anxiety as one of several post-traumatic symptoms and she has been diagnosed with a personality disorder (unsecure). At the first visit in the dental clinic she brings her boyfriend. It is decided that she should talk to her psychologist and ask if he has the opportunity for a meeting, Karen, the psychologist and the dentist have a consultation where a tentative treatment plan is made for Karen. The day after each treatment session in the dental office she is offered a session with the therapist. This arrangement works very well for Karen. Her boyfriend still follows her to the consultations but waits in the waiting area. She gradually manages dental treatment and she discusses reactions emerged during dental treatment with her psychologist the next day.

In the qualitative study the informants who attended a general dental practitioner emphasized the importance of a good and safe alliance. Thus, having the above-mentioned considerations in mind, a general dental practitioner with adequate skills may approach the treatment situation alone. The dentist should test out the treatment situation with a trauma-sensitive approach and give special notice to elements discussed in this chapter. Use of sedation should also be a possibility in cases where the CSA survivor does not have problems with being sedated (some have experienced to be sedated in association with abuse) or feel that being sedated would reduce their control. If the dentist and the dental team follow these treatment options, it should represent a minor chance of re-traumatization. But the possibilities for re-traumatization should always be contemplated, and if in doubt interdisciplinary cooperation should be considered.

Based on the findings from the qualitative analyses by Kranstad et al. [6] six elements of dental treatment assessed as decisive for success when treating CSA survivors in general practice is presented.

17.4.1 Offering a Good Start

As CSA survivors often start the process with preparing for dental treatment long time in advance it is important to make individual arrangements for scheduling treatment sessions. CSA survivors have individual needs, e.g. some like to book an appointment 6 months in advance but others prefer very short notice. The dental nurse or receptionist has an essential role in this phase. To meet the patient with a warm and friendly attitude, to explore details about best possible way to schedule a treatment session (to schedule long time in advance, to give a call the week or day before, early in the morning or late in the afternoon etc.) and if it is perceived difficult to sit in the waiting area, it may be planned for the patient to wait outside and give him/her a call when the dentist is ready.

As a rule, if the patient signalizes that he/she has dental anxiety of any kind, he/she should be offered at least one non-treatment pre-visit without any dental treatment done. Such a visit could be a very good investment as it is effective in building an alliance, making a proper treatment plan and in the end making treatment possible. From an economical point of view it should also be considered as a beneficial investment as it is

more likely to keep the patient within his/her window of tolerance and thus be able to make adequate plans for treatment adjustments, treatment progression and financial arrangements.

> » They would not have to do much treatment but having the opportunity to use a visit or two on getting to know each other! Because I think that is very important, being familiar with the persons (dental personnel).

17.4.2 Being Competent

As discussed in the former section, an understanding of sequela in dental care situations for CSA survivors is essential for all members of the dental team. Many of the reactions are unexpected and difficult to understand for the patient. If dental personnel has adequate knowledge and an open attitude for acceptance of the complexity in reactions, they may be able to communicate that this is "normal reactions" evoking from earlier "unnormal situations", and that science shows these reactions to be very individual and the reasons for them may be unconscious. The non-verbal element of communication is essential to signal competence and a safe atmosphere. However, it is important to remember that CSA survivors often have problems expressing themselves. Start signal is a must ("tell me when you are ready") and all stop signals must be rehearsed. A trained dentist may be able to read the patient's signals.

> » I know I just have to look at her, and she will understand that I need a break

However, it is easy to miss these signals. Signals to stop using body language may be safer and work better than verbal expressions.

> » It's not easy for me to say 'May I have five minutes break?'. I can't manage to express myself in the situation. But it works when we have agreed upon and tested out me raising my arm to say "stop".

It is also important to inhibit good clinical skills. A dentist who seems uncertain and slow working increase risk of the patient to feel insecure. Thus, it may be a good idea for a young and inexperienced student or dentist to prepare properly before treatment sessions and if possible, get supervision from an older colleague.

> » And to know that the dentist is familiar with the reasons for … removes many of the difficulties and emotional obstacles, and things like that.
>
> He was very competent too. When I sat in the chair, the phone rang and I overheard how a dentist asked him for advice, so I became aware of his competence. In addition, he had a calming effect on me.

In this context it is also relevant to mention that many of CSA patients who have difficulties with oral care have quite complicated oral health problems. For clinical experience on general practice, it is well known that sometimes the patient due to his confidence in the dentist (or his anxiety for a new) tries to make the general practitioners perform treatment he/she usually refers to specialists. This may not always be a good idea. A better solution would be to prepare the patient and the specialist by making a specific coping plan for the specialist treatment (e.g. endodontics or surgery) to share with the specialist. If the patient gets a good experience with the specialist, it is very beneficial for his/her coping in general and reduces safety seeking behaviour.

» It is me who manage to cope with this situation, not my very special and kind dentist.

17.4.3 Being Aware of the Influence of Staff Behaviour

As trauma-driven dental anxiety most often is closely connected to the relation and the closeness to dental personnel there are several issues to be taken into consideration.

The gender of the dentist. Some CSA survivors seem to be neutral to the dentist's gender, while others prefer the dentist to have opposite gender than of the abuser. This should be discussed with the patient.

» I prefer a female dentist. That feels safer because I hate male professionals, I don't trust men.

It the dentist has the same gender as the abuser it may be more challenging to the patient, but on the other hand, if it provides a positive experience, it may have a beneficial effect on relationships to this gender in general. To bring a supporting friend or family member may make gender less important.

Tips

- Create a good and safe alliance.
- The atmosphere between the dental staff is essential.
- Do not work behind the patient's back.
- Be competent.
- Consider cooperating with competent health professionals, like doctors, psychologists, etc.

The atmosphere between the dental staff is essential. Many CSA survivors have many adverse life experiences, including physical and psychological violence,

and as a result they are sensitive in picking up a tense or hostile atmosphere. The same goes with stress. If the atmosphere signals stress, it is easier for the patient to feel overlooked and thereby objectified. It is important to remember that when a patient is at the top of his window of tolerance, "better safe than sorry" assessment of situations is normal. This means that if there is a small sign that a lion is hungry, the patient will act like "it is very hungry and run". If there is any small sign that the dental staff are stressed out, the patient will think "they will treat you as an object, concentrate on trying to get it over with or run".

The dental personnel should try to establish a warm and welcoming atmosphere where the patient is at the centre. A light atmosphere has a positive effect, but the dental staff should be aware of differences in humour, for instance, if the wrong kind of jokes is prominent, the patients' issues could feel overlooked and less heeded.

Do not work behind the patient's back. CSA survivors are often vulnerable towards people taking "secret" actions outside their view or hearing. Thus, all tasks should be done visible to the patient and all conversation between the dentist and the dental nurse should be made in a language and with explanations understandable to the patient. For instance, try to have all necessary equipment ready and placed within the view of the patient before the treatment session starts. And try not to do tasks behind the patient (e.g. getting instruments from a drawer), but if it is needed, prepare the patient: *I will need some more equipment for making this filling, the nurse will collect this in the drawers behind me, is it OK to do that now?*

17.4.4 Building a Safe Relationship

To counteract the tendency to confuse the dentist with the abuser, it is important to act as a fellow man, be a person who wants to strive to help the patient in a best possible way.

» Yes, she is not really a dentist; she is a more of a fellow human. 'I will take care of you, even though I'm doing this'.

In this context it may be a good definition of a fellow human to be personal, not private. As many CSA survivors have difficult histories and strong reactions it is important to balance the role as an empathic caring person as well as a dental professional in a way that takes care of the patient, but also the dental professionals.

❯ In Kranstad et al.'s study [6] the importance of a long-term patient–dentist relationship was highlighted.

❯ The patients underlined their wish to be given the opportunity to be treated by the same dental team in a long-term perspective. In a dental clinic it is important to make several people well known to the patient to make the long-term aspect more robust. If the dentist is quitting, the dental nurse may secure the safe relationship and vice versa. At the same time, it is important to avoid the patient to become totally dependent on his or her dental professional. To enhance development of the patient's own robustness, self-management increases the patient's ability to trust different healthcare professionals.

❯ It may also be beneficial to bring a support person who knows the patient well.

Together with the dental personnel's trauma-sensitive approach this may help the patient to feel more relaxed and protected. A clinical observation from treating CSA survivors is how easy it is for a dentist to oversee signs of dissociation/hypoactivation as described happening to the patient Eric at the end of ► Chap. 2. In Eric's case he recovers fast, but dissociation may be more serious, and as described earlier in this chapter the patient may be in dissociation the rest of the treatment and further on if not handled properly. Thus, a support person who know the patient's reactions may be of invaluable help to detect signs of hyper- or hypoactivation and if so, help the patient give stop signal to the dentist and regulate back into the window of tolerance. The support person should be someone the patient trust and who knows him/her well, for instance, a mental health worker, a friend or a family member.

Finally, it should be noted that the relationship between a CSA survivor and a dentist is fragile. As a dental professional it is important always to inform and make agreements with the patients on how to perform treatment. Even the best dentist may on occasions unintentionally forget these understandings, but usually it is possible to mend the relationship by apologizing and correcting the unfortunate incident for the future. However, in the fragile situation for CSA survivors it may be devastating for the relationship to forget this. Thus, as a dental professional it is important to evaluate whether a change of dentist may be beneficial if the relationship becomes challenging.

17.4.5 Exploring and Coping with Individual Triggers

A general rule when treating CSA survivors is to start out with the patient in a regular chair for a pre-clinical discussion about the planned treatment as well as thoughts about individual triggers and how to cope with them. At the beginning of treatment, it is beneficial to discuss and make a coping plan (see example ◻ Fig. 17.3).

At the start of successive treatment sessions, it may be beneficial to go through reactions after the last visit, the coping plan and discuss if there are any revisions to be made to further improve the treatment situation.

Situations and actions that triggers trauma-related reactions are highly individual, but there are some typical situations many CSA survivors find difficult.

To be pulled back in the dental chair makes many CSA survivors feel vulnerable and exposed. The action is out of their control.

» To be pulled back (in the dental chair). Imagine the feeling. You have no control.

One alternative is to lower the back of the chair before the patient is asked to sit down and then he/she can lay back in his/her own tempo and consequently experience total control. To be lying on your back in a horizontal position may be very challenging and may increase the feeling of being under the command of somebody. It is important to explore the chair's position together with the patient. For some patients, a flexible dentist who may also work standing up will be a good start. The patient will often feel more in control (including vision) in a more upright position and when a more secure relation is established, it will be easier to find a more horizontally working position in collaboration with the patient.

Explaining the smell of dental equipment and materials can counteract negative sensations of the distinct dentistry smell.

» Everybody knows the dental odour. And I associate dentists with something frightening – a frightening odour is taking me back to the abuse. Thus, it is just another warning sign starting to flash.

17.4.6 Reducing Possible Perceptions of Being Trapped

One of the similarities between an abuse situation and being in a dental treatment situation is the feeling of being trapped.

» You are really exposed in the dental chair, with the tray right over your stomach, and things like that. The possibilities to escape are minimal, with armrests on both sides too.

Many CSA survivors have experiences from being restrained during abuse situations, but unfortunately it is not unusual to have experiences from been held down physically as a child in the dental chair as well. In the treatment situation it is important to address this issue and suggest action that may increase control and ability to escape. First, it should be stressed that it is important to make use of stop signals and take a break when the feeling of being trapped increases. The tray with equipment should be placed at a convenient distance for the patient. It is all right to give a signal and stand out of the dental chair or maybe just sit up or have something to drink. It is essential that the patient understands that this is not adjustments to be used when treatment is intolerable, but necessary arrangements when anxiety starts to rise to make treatment work (see ▶ Chap. 12). As giving signals to stop often are difficult to CSA survivors these actions should be tested out practically and it should be discussed whether the patient finds it difficult to stop the treatment. *"We know that many patients find it very difficult to signal a stop, how do you think this will be for you?"* In the process of learning the patient to give adequate stop signals it is important that the dental nurse or support person reminds him/her during treat-

◘ **Fig. 17.3** Coping plan for Anna, a woman with a sexual abuse history and dental anxiety

Coping plan Anna

The aim of the coping plan is to facilitate a best possible treatment situation during dental treatment.

WHAT the dentist/dental hygienist/dental nurse needs to know about me

(background, cause of fear, special needs, triggers):

1. I need to feel safe and have predictability (clarify what will happen + how long it will take)

- *A calm atmosphere without stress*
- *To start out with a conversation about this sessionv's treatment*
- *Help me to give sign to stop when you see signs that it's needed*
- *I need breaks to regulate into my window of tolerance if something gets difficult*
- *Sit down in the chair after it has been adjusted to "working" position*
- *I don't like to have lots of things or big cotton rolls in my mouth*
- *I've been a victim of sexual abuse*

My catastrophe thoughts/ what I'm most afraid of:

- *Getting stuck in the dentist's chair, and not be able to get up. Most afraid that I'm going to get stuck in the chair, that dental professionals will either leave me there at the dentist's office and that I'll be there alone overnight, or that they're going to abuse me*

What increases my anxiety

- *Sitting in the dental chair. To feel that I have no control, that things are being done to me that I do not want and feel that I am left alone/hopeless. When it gets quiet. When the dentist or others are behind me*

What do I do if I feel the anxiety rises (my coping strategies)?

- *First, I get nauseous, dizzy and tense – I catch my breath all the way up my throat and get upset in*
- *Body. Eventually, if I can't stabilize myself, I'll take a bit of a look at myself and feel like I'm stuck, I feel like I can't move my body*
- *My coping strategy will be to give stop signal (I may need help with that) to stop the treatment and use time to regulate my activation*

My bodily reactions when anxiety rises (to be observed by the dentist/dental hygienist/dental health secretary):

- *I stop breathing/or I breathe only in the upper part of the chest*
- *I start to get upset and fiddle with my hands, avoiding eyecontact, before getting 'stuck' in the dental care chair and before I switch off contact*
- *Before I switch off contact, I'll be distant in my gaze and others make little contact with me*

Relevant adaptions

(breaks, quality of dialogue, explanation, counting during treatment, etc.):

Fig. 17.3 (continued)

- *I need the dental team to have an eye on my body language and help me to stabilize me when I get upset and starts fiddling with my hands*
- *I need the dental team to help me taking initiatives for breaks*
- *During breaks I may need to get out of the dental chair to stand or walk (If possible)*
- *I need help to activate my body while I'm sitting in the chair to prevent being dissociation*
- *To activate I need to be spoken to all the time and to be oriented for time and place*
- *I need the dental team to ask me how it's going*

Stop signals:

- *I will lift my left hand – I need to experience that it is respected*

Routine   in case of cancellations/no show:

- *I always show up, but in case I don't it's nice to contacted if I don't show up for treatment…*

ment. It is also relevant to check out after treatment: *"Was it at any point during treatment you felt for giving a stop signal but did not do it?"*

A very simple concrete action that has been shown effective is to tell the patient to have one foot on the floor during treatment. In this way the body is grounded to the floor and at the same time the body is prepared for a quick "withdrawal from the war zone".

Other concrete actions may be to offer the patient to bring a personal object that increases the feeling of safety, for instance, laying under a blanket may reduce the feeling of being exposed.

Finding solutions to mouth-related obstacles can help overcoming problems with opening the mouth and having fingers or dental equipment put inside it.

» Putting things in the mouth. My mouth is the problem, sort of, yes, it was there everything was going on; it was in the mouth he (the abuser) was active.

Many CSA survivors have problems when "someone is putting something inside my mouth". The symptoms may be retching, vomiting or panic attacks. Many patients benefit from being shown the dentist's instruments and explained how they work. It may be discussed whether it is better to use instruments, like the mirror, to hold back the cheek rather than a finger. Or it may be a solution to ask the patient him-/herself to hold back the cheek with his/her own finger. Generally, it should be aimed to have as few instruments and fingers as possible inside the mouth.

The use of rubber dam may be an adequate solution, but it is dependent upon how this alternative is presented to the patient. If you say *"I suggest putting on a rubber dam. I will place a clamp on some of your teeth and the dam will cover your mouth, it is important that we place the dam in a way that it don't interfere with your nose breathing"*, it is likely that the patient will feel

trapped and be very aware that breathing may be difficult. It is better to focus on the positive consequences of rubber dam and say *"I suggest putting on a rubber dam. In this way it is only the teeth that we are working on that are available for me, they are in a way outside the mouth, and instruments, water and materials will not have access to the rest of your mouth"*.

The most important attitude for the dentist to hold is to be creative, flexible and try to make the patient feel "in the driver's seat" during treatment. Being attentive and considerate, discussing and making individual adaptions will in addition help building a trustful alliance.

17.4.7 Strategies to Regulate Trauma-Driven Anxiety in CSA Survivors

Both strategies for reducing and increasing tension as well as to be present in the presence are relevant (see ▶ Chap. 12). It is important to keep the patient within his/her window of tolerance. If the patient has tendency to disappear, dissociate or go into hypoactivation the main goal will be to find strategies to "wake up" the patient.

Grounding techniques are strategies that seek to keep the patient present in the presence.

Focus upon perceptions that may work is to focus upon feeling the material of the chair, or holding on to something, like a stress ball, a key holder or another personal item. Focusing upon these items prevents the typical feelings of numbness in the hands associated with dissociation. The same purpose may go with clapping the hands against the shoulders, rubbing the hands against one's thighs, standing up and walk around in the room or stomping with the feet on the floor.

Body scanning may be useful, but as relaxation may be the opposite of what the patient needs, focus should be on the difference between tightening, stretching and relaxation in the muscles. *"Curl and stretch your toes, tighten the muscles in your legs and buttocks- and relax"* (see body scanning ▶ Chap. 12).

Focus may also be placed at trying to make the patients concentrate on neutral items he/she observes: *"Can you find three red items in this room?"*

To be given the possibility to use a blanket may reduce the feeling of being exposed, and the patient is allowed to have his/her own private zone under the blanket.

Talking the patient to the present *"Can you tell date and time today? You are at the dentist's office. We are here to help you with your teeth"* will help the patient stay here and now.

Summary

Specific issues are of importance for dental health professionals when giving help and advises in prevention and treatment of oral diseases to CSA survivors. Trauma-driven dental anxiety is different from a simple dental phobia. Reminders of traumatic memories are triggered by modalities, such as sights, sounds, smells, taste, tactile stimuli, body positions, words or scenes of the original trauma. The experience of being attacked with threatening stimulus, frightening emotions and perhaps memories, involves very strong physiological responses that might lead to some level of dissociation and even memory loss from the dental visit. In common with simple dental phobia, the feeling of control and predictability is important. To succeed in offering trauma-sensitive dental care a deeper understanding and empathy from dental health workers is essential. Some of these patients expose reactions that may be subtle and difficult to perceive, and therefore, a profound sense of awareness from the dental staff is required. Others may disclose reactions powerfully acted out and thereby difficult for the dental personnel to understand and handle. To give dental staff and patients the best framework, it is essential to understand how child sexual abused survivors prepare – battle during and recover after dental treatment. The resemblance between the patient's experiences in the present and traumatic events possibly experienced in the past is most relevant.

It is important to have in mind that dental treatment always include a risk of re-traumatization of CSA survivors. This fact urges for a specific preparation and practice. A good and safe alliance with the dental staff is essential. The dentist should test out the treatment situation with a trauma-sensitive approach and give special notice to the following elements presented in this chapter: offering a good start, being competent, being aware of the influence of staff behaviour, arranging a secure treatment situation, exploring and coping with individual triggers, reducing possible perceptions of being trapped and using strategies to regulate trauma-driven anxiety.

Failing to help CSA survivors with oral health-related problems may lead to severe difficulties. CSA survivors struggle with dental treatment as well as daily oral care situations. The impact of oral health-related problems is recognized as causing serious oral health symptoms, triggering trauma reactions, increasing emotional distress, shaping the understanding of self, intruding daily life practices, restraining social interactions and generating financial problems.

In conclusion, to increase a trauma-sensitive approach in dental treatment for CSA survivors, dentists should be utmost considerate every step of the way, building long-term solid relationships, discuss and test out coping strategies individually adapted to the specific needs of the CSA survivors, in a safe environment.

References

1. Willumsen T. Dental fear in sexually abused women. Eur J Oral Sci. 2001;109(5):291–6. https://doi.org/10.1034/j.1600-0722.2001.00069.x.
2. Leeners B, Stiller R, Block E, Görres G, Imthurn B, Rath W. Consequences of childhood sexual abuse experiences on dental care. J Psychosom Res. 2007;62(5):581–8.
3. Humphris G, King K. The prevalence of dental anxiety across previous distressing experiences. J Anxiety Disord. 2011;25(2):232–6.
4. Bright MA, Alford SM, Hinojosa MS, Knapp C, Fernandez-Baca DE. Adverse childhood experiences and dental health in children and adolescents. Community Dent Oral Epidemiol. 2015;43(3):193–9. https://doi.org/10.1111/cdoe.12137.
5. Fredriksen TV, Søftestad S, Kranstad V, Willumsen T. Preparing for attack and recovering from battle: understanding child sexual abuse survivors' experiences of dental treatment. Community Dent Oral Epidemiol. 2020;48:317–27.
6. Kranstad V, Søftestad S, Fredriksen TV, Willumsen T. Being considerate every step of the way: a qualitative study analysing trauma-sensitive dental treatment for childhood sexual abuse survivors. Eur J Oral Sci. 2019;127(6):539–46.
7. Søftestad S, Kranstad V, Fredriksen TV, Willumsen T. Invading deeply into self and everyday life: how oral health-related problems affect the lives of child sexual abuse survivors. J Child Sex Abus. 2020;29(1):62–78.
8. Steine IM, Winje D, Nordhus IH, Milde AM, Bjorvatn B, Grønli J, Pallesen S. Langvarig taushet om seksuelle overgrep: Prediktorer og korrelater hos voksne som opplevde seksuelle overgrep som barn. [Prolonged silence about sexual abuse: predictors and correlates in adults who experienced sexual abuse as children.]. Tidsskr Nor Psykologforen. 2016;53:889–99.

9. Gilligan P, Akhtar S. Cultural barriers to the disclosure of child sexual abuse in Asian communities: listening to what women say. Br J Soc Work. 2006;36(8):1361–77.

10. Jonzon E, Lindblad F. Disclosure, reactions, and social support: findings from a sample of adult victims of child sexual abuse. Child Maltreat. 2004;9(2):190–200.

11. Jonzon E, Lindblad F. Adult female victims of child sexual abuse (CSA): multitype maltreatment and disclosure characteristics related to subjective health. J Interpers Violence. 2005;20(6):651–66.

12. Ruggiero KJ, Smith DW, Hanson RF, Resnick HS, Saunders DE, Kilpatrick DG, Best CL. Is disclosure of childhood rape associated with mental health outcome? Results from the National Women's Study. Child Maltreat. 2004;9(1):62–77.

13. Staller KM, Nelson-Gardell D. "A burden in your heart": lessons of disclosure from female preadolescent and adolescent survivors of sexual abuse. Child Abuse Negl. 2005;29(12):1415–32.

14. Sjöberg P, Lutteman M. Det du inte såg. [What you did not see.]. Stockholm: Norstedts; 2011. 412 s.

15. Easton SD, Saltzman LY, Willis DG. "Would you tell under circumstances like that?": barriers to disclosure of child sexual abuse for men. Psychol Men Masculinity. 2014;15(4):460.

16. Evensen MH, Fluge SS, Kjoberg TS, Bye HH. Menns opplevelse av å bli utsatt for seksuelt overgrep i voksen alder. En kvalitativ metasyntese. [Adult male survivors of sexual abuse– A qualitative metasynthesis of their experiences.]. Tidsskr No Psykologforen. 2019;56(4):246–64.

17. Ehlers A, Hackmann A, Steil R, Clohessy S, Wenninger K, Winter H. The nature of intrusive memories after trauma: the warning signal hypothesis. Behav Res Ther. 2002;40:1021–8.

18. Ehler A. Understanding and treating unwanted trauma memories in posttraumatic stress disorder. Z Psychol/J Psychol. 2010;218(2):141–5. https://doi.org/10.1027/a000001.

19. Bækkelund H, Berg AO. Kartlegging og diagnostisering av traumerelaterte lidelser. I: Anstorp T, Benum K. red. Traumebehandling. Komplekse traumelidelser og dissosiasjon. Oslo: Universitetsforlaget; 2014. s.78–99.

20. Anstorp T, Nupen Å, Willumsen T. Traumesensitiv tannbehandling – hva trengs? I: Willumsen T, Myran L, Lein JPA. red. Odontologisk psykologi. Oslo: Gyldendal Norsk Forlag AS; 2018. s. 227–248.

21. Lanius RA, Brand B, Vermetten E, Frewen PA, Spiegel D. The dissociative subtype of posttraumatic stress disorder: rationale, clinical and neurobiological evidence, and implications. Depress Anxiety. 2012;29(8):701–8.

22. Nijenhuis ERS, Van der Hart O, Steele K. Traumerelatert strukturell dissosiasjon av personligheten. Teoretisk forståelse og begrepsavklaring. I: Anstorp T, Benum K, Jakobsen M. red.

Dissosiasjon og relasjonstraumer – integrering av det splittede jeg. Oslo: Universitetsforlaget; 2006. s. 73–88.

23. Scheffers M, Hoek M, Bosscher RJ, van Duijn MAJ, Schoevers RA, van Busschbach JT. Negative body experience in women with early childhood trauma: associations with trauma severity and dissociation. Eur J Psychotraumatol. 2017;8:1,1322892. https://doi.org/10.1080/20008198.2017.1322892.

24. De Jongh A, Fransen J, Oosterink-Wubbe F, Aartman I. Psychological trauma exposure and trauma symptoms among individuals with high and low levels of dental anxiety. Eur J Oral Sci. 2006;114:286–92.

25. Willumsen T. The impact of childhood sexual abuse on dental fear. Community Dent Oral Epidemiol. 2004;32(1):73–9.

26. Levine PA. Waking the tiger – healing trauma. Berkely: North Atlantic Books; 1997.

27. Felitti VJ, Anda RF, Nordenberg D, Williamson DF, Spitz AM, Edwards V, Marks JS. Relationship of childhood abuse and household dysfunction to many of the leading causes of death in adults: the adverse childhood experience (ACE) study. Am J Prev Med. 1998;14:245–58. https://doi.org/10.1016/S0749-3797(98)00017-8.

28. Centres of disease control and prevention [Internet] [2020; 2021 May 10]. Available from: https://www.cdc.gov/violenceprevention/aces/about.html.

29. Berggren U, Meynert G. Dental fear and avoidance: causes, symptoms, and consequences. J Am Dent Assoc (1939). 1984;109(2):247–51.

30. MacGinley M, Breckenridge J, Mowll J. A scoping review of adult survivors' experiences of shame following sexual abuse in childhood. Health Soc Care Community. 2019;27(5):1135–46. https://doi.org/10.1111/hsc.12771.

31. Dorahy MJ, Clearwater K. Shame and guilt in men exposed to childhood sexual abuse: a qualitative investigation. J Child Sex Abus. 2012;21(2):155–75. https://doi.org/10.1080/10538712.2012.659803.

32. Briere J, Kaltman S, Green BL. Accumulated childhood trauma and symptom complexity. J Trauma Stress. 2008;21(2):223–6. https://doi.org/10.1002/jts.20317.

33. Cloitre M, Stolbach BC, Herman J, van der Kolk B, Pynoos R, Wang J, Petrova E. A developmental approach to complex PTSD: childhood and adult cumulative trauma as predictors of symptom complexity. J Trauma Stress. 2009;22(5):399–408. https://doi.org/10.1002/jts.20444.

34. Daignaut I, Hebert M. Profiles of school adaption: social, behavioural and academic functioning in sexually abused girls. Child Abuse Negl. 2009;33(2):102–11.

35. Eslami B, Viitasara E, Macassa G, et al. The prevalence of lifetime abuse among older adults in seven European countries. Int J Public Health. 2016;61(8):891–901. https://doi.org/10.1007/s00038-016-0816-x.

17

Providing Dental Care to Torture Survivors

Ann Catrin Høyvik and Marit Irene Woldstad

Contents

Use of torture is increasing worldwide, and many survivors of torture are refugees or asylum seekers. Torture and imprisonment in inhumane conditions often result in physical injuries and ailments of the oral cavity. Therefore, many torture survivors have a need for comprehensive dental treatment. In addition, the psychological impact of torture may influence when or if help is sought, as well as the ability to endure dental treatment. In this chapter, we will address what dental professionals need to know to provide adequate dental care to victims of torture.

Learning Goals
- Know what torture entails
- Know about identifying and documenting torture
- Understand the oral consequences of torture
- Understand the physical and psychological late effects of torture
- Understand why receiving dental treatment may be a challenge to torture survivors
- Become familiar with how dental professionals may tailor their treatment approach to facilitate dental treatment of torture victims.

18.1 What Is Torture?

United Nations defines torture as "...any act by which severe pain or suffering, whether physical or mental, is intentionally inflicted on a person for such purposes as obtaining from him or a third person information or a confession, punishing him for an act he or a third person has committed or is suspected of having committed, or intimidating or coercing him or a third person, or for any reason based on discrimination of any kind..." [1].

United Nations Torture Convention Article 1.1

For the purposes of this Convention, the term "torture" means any act by which severe pain or suffering, whether physical or mental, is intentionally inflicted on a person for such purposes as obtaining from him or a third-person information or a confession, punishing him for an act he or a third person has committed or is suspected of having committed, or intimidating or coercing him or a third person, or for any reason based on discrimination of any kind, when such pain or suffering is inflicted by or at the instigation of or with the consent or acquiescence of a public official or other person acting in an official capacity. It does not include pain or suffering arising only from inherent in or incidental to lawful sanctions.

Torture is intentional and executed for a purpose, for example, to force forth information and to break down the victim physically and psychologically. Furthermore, torture is inflicted by public authorities or by someone acting on behalf of public authorities. Countries that have ratified the United Nations Convention of Torture, thereby support the total ban against torture, and the rights of torture survivors to rehabilitation and redress.

Healthcare workers may come in contact with torture survivors at their workplace without realizing it. As the purpose of torture is to destroy the victim's trust in other people, one cannot expect torture victims to talk openly about their experiences. Despite the fact that most countries lack a functioning system for documenting torture or following up on torture survivors, health care personnel still have the ultimate responsibility to diagnose, document, and treat torture injuries. Thus, it is important to be familiar with the existing guidelines and protocols, the most important being the Istanbul Protocol [2].

18.2 Investigation and Documentation of Torture Injuries

Torture injuries are often complex and require a thorough diagnosis. The Istanbul Protocol is a useful resource and starting point, especially when the patient is in need of a health declaration. Such health declarations may be required to get the necessary health care and rehabilitation, and may contribute to compensation through the legal system.

The Istanbul Protocol consists of a general section in addition to sections intended for somatic and psychological diagnostics and documentation. Dental health personnel should be especially conscious to document and integrate the following in the total report:
- Gender, age, and country of origin
- Type of violence toward the orofacial area (teeth, mouth, and/or face)
- Lesions and scars on the oral mucosa, lips, and face
- Clinical examination: caries, tooth fractures, tooth wear, periodontal status, symptoms of temporomandibular dysfunction (TMD: collective designation of inflammatory conditions, symptoms and dysfunctions related to the temporomandibular joint)
- X-rays: OPG and BW of all patients, if necessary supplemented with apical X-rays
- If possible, to retrieve journals from earlier dental visits [3].

An oral cavity free for pathology does not rule out that oral torture has occurred, but it makes the objective documentation more difficult. As many torture survivors are refugees, there is often a high degree of oral pathology. Therefore, it may be difficult to decide which oral injuries are caused by torture.

18.2.1 Where Does Torture Occur?

Torture occurs practically all over the world, and the use of torture is unfortunately increasing. Amnesty International [4] has estimated that torture is practiced in one-third of all countries. How, where and when torture is carried out depends on the degree to which the torturers attempt to hide the abuse, and what the purpose of the torture is in the particular instance. However, prisoners are especially at risk to be tortured, as it is often used to force out information or confessions. Various studies have shown the prevalence of torture experience among refugees to be from 5% to 57% depending on country of origin and how and where the studies are conducted [5]. There is a degree of uncertainty around this prevalence, and possibly large dark numbers, as not all of those interviewed are familiar with the definition of torture and a certain proportion are unwilling or incapable of talking about their experiences.

18.2.2 Who Are the Torture Survivors?

In all conflicts causing people to seek refuge, the use of torture exists. Therefore, there are many torture survivors among refugees and asylum seekers. However, as torture occurs in most part of the world, and even in countries not at war, other groups of people may also have been subjected to torture. For example, war veterans or others who have been imprisoned in countries that are known to practice torture are at risk. Still, it can be noted that among asylum seekers and refugees an especially high proportion have experienced torture.

Asylum seekers and refugees also experience challenges related to other factors than torture. Thus, it may be difficult to determine the etiology of potential psychological ailments, and a challenge to find the right treatment for these patients.

18.2.3 Trauma Following War and Refuge

Refugees often have recurrent experiences of loss in their lives. They may have lived in difficult conditions, having to deal with poverty, hunger, poor conditions, and escape. Many have personal war experiences, and may have lost friends or family members. Some have witnessed others being killed, raped, or tortured. A proportion of refugees and asylum seekers are child survivors of abuse or neglect, which may increase their vulnerability to develop mental problems. At the same time, many refugees and asylum seekers have significant psychological, social, or professional resources that they wish to use and which the receiving countries should support. With this in mind, it is important for health professionals not to focus solely on identifying psychological trauma or other mental issues in the meeting with these groups of patients.

18.3 Torture Against Teeth and Facial Area

Torture can be psychological or physical, and both forms can lead to serious consequences to the subjected individual. Physical injuries may be comprehensive, and chronic pain is common in the aftermath of torture. There is a correlation between type of torture and the resulting physical injuries. At the same time, the torturers often strive to conceal the torture so that it does not result in obvious signs of physical injury. Long-term imprisonment in inhumane conditions may cause physical and psychological after effects that health care workers not immediately understand or interpret as consequences of torture. This may for example be related to lack of food or malnutrition, sense deprivation, lack of possibility to personal hygiene or to be forced to take on certain body positions over time.

This part of the chapter mainly pertains to physical torture against teeth, mouth, and the facial area, and the consequences of torture to the oral cavity.

Common physical torture methods to the teeth and facial area are:

- Strokes or kicks, with or without the use of tools such as gunstocks
- Loosening or extraction of teeth without the purpose of treating
- Grinding or filing down teeth
- Electric shocks
- Other electric tortures, such as electrodes connected to the lips, gingiva, or tongue, electrodes from the mouth to genitals or electrodes connected to the jaw joint area to cause painful muscle contractions
- Burns
- Acid attacks
- Exposure to strong light
- Suffocation techniques, including water torture such as "waterboarding" or "submarino"
- Sexual torture including oral–sexual rape
- Being forced to drink urine or eat feces
- Non-hygienic conditions which can lead to unhealthiness and disease, including lack of possibility to maintain oral hygiene [3, 5, 6].

18.3.1   Oral Consequences of Torture

The mouth and face are sensitive areas, and therefore preferred targets for torturers who have the intention to downgrade and inflict pain. Studies have shown a high need for general dental treatment among torture survivors, not only due to direct dental torture, but also because it often takes years of rehabilitation before a torture victim has the possibility to, or is capable of seeking and receiving dental treatment [7, 8].

> ► **Example**
>
> Somalian Noor (29) has survived strokes to her face, burning, and sexual torture. She has comprehensive oral health problems, but wishes to postpone having dental treatment. Her description illustrates why many refugees and asylum seekers choose not to prioritize dental health in a life phase where other problems are deemed more important:
>
> » I feel I fight an equivalent war in Norway as I have in Somalia. I have suffered hardship my entire life. I do not know if the father of my children is alive… Initially, my asylum application was rejected. One time the police came and took my children away as I was supposed to be deported. Now, we have finally received residency. We will move out of the reception center, and my son needs to change schools again. He has experienced going to new schools many times as we needed to move to new reception centers. He has experienced a lot of social exclusion. My teeth are bad-looking, and sometimes very painful. But I need to think about my children first… ◄

The most common physical consequence of torture is pain, which may be acute or chronic [5, 9]. To someone who has been tortured, such continual episodes of pain represent a constant reminder of the experienced torture. Furthermore, quite a few talks about problems with eating and sleeping due to toothache or other oral complaints, and about pain that may influence their ability to partake in social events and to perform daily chores. Oral pain is often caused by fractured teeth or carious lesions with exposed dental pulp, loose teeth, untreated gum disease, or infection or damage to the mucous membranes. Symptoms from the jaw joint are also common, and may result from strokes or electric torture, or from psychological after effects involving chronic teeth grinding (bruxism) or tooth clenching. Many torture survivors also complain of chronic headaches, a common consequence of repeated strokes and kicks to the head, and the torture method termed "telefono"—simultaneous strokes against both ears, often results in chronic dizziness and loss of hearing.

Lack of teeth, or discolored or fractured teeth in visible areas, is a common reason that many torture survivors avoid smiling or showing their teeth. This can lead to full or partial avoidance of social interaction, and can negatively influence the integration of refugees and asylum seekers. Some also reveal that the sensation of missing teeth with the tongue may set of traumatic reactions.

Scars from electrical shocks, burn marks, or acid etches are other examples of consequences after torture in the oral facial area.

Dental health professionals often have an important role in the complete rehabilitation of torture survivors in terms of providing pain relief, treatment of infections, and functional and esthetic rehabilitation of the oral cavity.

18.4   Late Effects of Torture

18.4.1   Psychological Consequences

As the torture is targeting to do harm, and to force or subdue, it leaves the victim with little or no sense of control. To be exposed to torture is about being hurt and degraded, and often under the threat of being killed. The victim is left in a state of stress that may persist for a long time after the acute danger is over. Torture is often executed to cause permanent damage, to ensure total submission and degradation of the individual. Torture is performed or staged by human beings. As a consequence, the victim's ability to trust in other people, and engage in interpersonal relationships may be seriously impaired. An example is the typical torturer who consciously shifts between being nice and forthcoming, and to breaking down and injuring the victim. Such behavior can cause the victim to expect that other individuals who are nice and good to them can suddenly change and expose them to violence and degradation. Hence, torture brings with it a fundamental feeling of insecurity, a feeling that may be present even when the victim is cognitively aware that he is currently safe.

Torture is often intended to hurt not only the subjected individuals but also their families. Targets may also be social, ethnic, or political groups. In this way, torture and the risk of torture are used to gain control over different groups of people. Thus, when we talk about psychological consequences, as well as consequences for the individual torture survivor, we also mean consequences for the victim's family, friends, and society.

Survival of torture is a strong predictor to developing post-traumatic stress disorder (PTSD). In addition to PTSD being a frequent consequence of torture, researchers have found that certain conditions during the torture situation result in a higher risk of developing trauma disorders like PTSD. Experiencing loss of control is a significant factor. Furthermore, it has been shown that the risk for PTSD is increased if the torture included factors such as deprivation of basic needs, sexual torture, exposure to extreme temperatures, isolation, and being forced to take different physical positions over a long time, as compared to other physical methods of torture [10].

PTSD is thoroughly presented in the chapter on trauma sensitive dental treatment (see ▶ Chap. 2). Briefly summarized, in order to diagnose PTSD, the following symptoms need to be present: intrusion symptoms (e.g., flashbacks, nightmares, or physical reactivity to traumatic reminders), avoidance of trauma-related stimuli, negative alterations in cognitions and mood (e.g., depression or concentration problems), and trauma-related alterations in arousal and reactivity [11].

A trigger, or traumatic reminder, for a trauma patient is any form of stimuli which can provoke (trigger) a stress response, flashbacks, or other psychological symptoms. For instance, a torture survivor may react with discomfort and pain to cold temperature if the individual was held under freezing conditions during torture or imprisonment. For many torture victims, pain functions as a trigger: Anesthetic injections during dental treatment may trigger memories of extreme pain experienced during torture. Triggers may also be internal feelings or sensations, such as hunger or happiness. For torture survivors, triggers can be particularly central in the post-traumatic stress disorder, due to the frequent use of triggers as a part of the torture—to optimize the feeling of distress, unsafety, alertness, and fear. For example, torture may be executed to beautiful music, with the result that such music may set off traumatic reactions in the victim even long after the torture has ended. In that manner, the torturer secures his power over the victim. As dental health professionals, we must be aware that reactions to triggers are a major challenge for torture survivors, and that focusing on reducing stress caused by triggers is an important part of the treatment.

18.4.2 Pain as a Consequence of Torture

As mentioned earlier, pain is the most frequent physical ailment after torture, and may be a consequence of specific or chronic physical injuries. Pain may also result from the psychological consequences of having been subjected to pain [12]. Health professionals working with torture survivors should therefore pay special attention to pain assessment and treatment of any pain (see ▶ Chap. 3).

It is often difficult for a patient to explain where the pain is coming from. This may be attributed to several conditions. Nuances in language and individual and/or cultural explanatory models for pain are possible contributors. However, this may also be due to conditions related to the experienced torture, to shame and taboos, dissociative amnesia, or alienation. It may also be that the torture survivor was exposed to sensory deprivation, for example, by blindfolding, or was unconscious during part of the torture and therefore unaware of what he had gone through. Furthermore, the fear of pain and the anxiety associated with it will increase the pain experience [13]. On the other hand, it is common for torture survivors not to express their pain, as it was important during torture not to show signs of weakness to avoid being killed or tortured further.

Factors like method of torture, inflicted injury, magnitude, and duration of torture may also increase the victim's future expectations of pain. Patients who have survived torture may be especially sensitive to pain, and hold expectations that pain will occur, or be inflicted on them, during dental treatment.

18.5 Torture and Dental Anxiety

People who have been subjected to torture will mostly try to avoid anything that may possibly remind them of their traumatic experiences. Torture may be inflicted under the presence of doctors or other health professionals. This may be to ensure that the victim does not die during the torture, but health personnel may also be directly involved in the torture. Therefore, some torture survivors endure a lot of pain or other health problems before seeking medical or dental treatment. They often have a difficult time trusting health personnel or the health care system. Many torture victims and others who have been refugees or imprisoned under difficult conditions have experienced painful dental treatment under primitive conditions, for example tooth extractions and drilling without anesthesia. Such experiences may well give rise to dental anxiety [8].

Many aspects of the dental visit may trigger memories of torture experiences, and hence constitute a risk or re-traumatizing the torture victim. The dental treatment situation in itself may provoke anxiety: feeling trapped in the dental chair, lying almost underneath the dentist, in the sharp operating light, and mouth filled with cotton and instruments.

Unnecessary waiting time may set off anxiety reactions that can easily destroy trust built over time. Other possible triggers that dental personnel should be aware of are other patients who are crying, uncompassionate or unfriendly staff members, rooms without windows, needles, sharp instruments, certain electronic devices, and strong lights. Individuals who have experienced water torture may have difficulties with being reclined in the dental chair, especially if the dentist uses instruments with water spray. In addition, many torture survivors find it uncomfortable to be exposed to questioning. Prisoners are interrogated during torture and their revelations are used to inflict harm on them or on others. Thus, recording the medical history may bear strong resemblance to the interrogation experienced during torture. Torture survivors may become scared of what could happen, and uncertain of what the information will be used for, and thus we may end up not receiving the information we need to do a good job.

In other words, the dental treatment situation as a whole, or specific parts of the treatment procedure or necessary instruments may set in motion traumatic reactions. This is not just relevant for dental personnel who work with adult patients. Even small children can be affected by having witnessed or heard the sound of torture. Younger children may be more traumatized than older children, who are capable of putting into words what they have experienced and of expressing their fears [5].

> **► Example**
> When Ahmad, a 45-year-old man from Syria, was asked what he thought about going to the dentist, he answered that he did not have any problems with it. He had visited the dentist quite often in his home country, and had a few fillings and crowns placed. When the Norwegian dentist directed the light toward Ahmad, and approached his mouth with the dental mirror, he began to shiver and shortly after fainted. It became clear that it was his first dental visit following his traumatic experiences in prison, and he was not prepared for such mental interconnections. ◄

As illustrated in the example with Ahmad, we should be aware that patients who have survived torture do not always understand or are prepared for what may trigger a reaction.

Triggers in dental treatment can activate strong emotional reactions connected with earlier trauma. This is known as re-traumatization and it may cause flashbacks, fear, anger, or panic, which in turn may lead to avoidance of dental visits or failure to follow the advice and recommendations given by dental professionals.

18.5.1 Adapting the Dental Treatment

To be able to safeguard the dental patient, and ensure that adequate treatment is provided, the dental practitioner needs to be informed if the patient was previ-

ously exposed to psychological trauma. However, it is not necessary for the dental professional to know every detail of the patient's trauma history (see ► Chap. 2). For a patient who is not psychologically rehabilitated, a detailed go-through of the history might set in motion a mental reliving of the trauma (flashbacks) and thus cause re-traumatization. It is, however, important that the dental personnel take the time to listen to what information the patient wants to share, and no matter how unbelievable the story seems, it is of utmost importance not to show doubt or denial [5].

It may feel uncomfortable, or even frightening, for health professionals to ask patients about their trauma history, and in some cases, it may be tempting to just avoid asking. It is therefore important to be aware that by asking questions, we can contribute to breaking the evil circle of unfairness that torture victims are subjected to. By further referral, to for example psychologists, medical doctors, social workers, or physical therapists, we may contribute to a more complete rehabilitation. In addition, the dental treatment usually proceeds more effectively when the background history is known.

18.5.1.1 Identifying Triggers
Identifying triggers is important in diagnosing and treating torture survivors. It is therefore important that the dental health professionals build a good relationship with the patient, in such a manner that the patient is able and ready to reflect on what may trigger a reaction. Examples of triggers are described in the section on torture and dental anxiety.

18.5.1.2 Use of Interpreters
Many torture survivors are refugees or asylum seekers and not fluent in the native language of the country in which they are resettled, and thus the use of professional interpreters should be considered. Even patients who appear to master the new language may have difficulties with understanding medical terms or discussing complex topics. A good advice may be: If you are in doubt whether to use an interpreter—use an interpreter!

Interpreting clinical conversations require specific qualifications, and family members, especially children, should never be used as translators. When communicating through a professional interpreter, some useful guidelines are:
- Turn to the patient while talking
- Express yourself as clear and concise as possible
- Avoid complicated medical terms
- Give the interpreter time to translate
- Keep eye-contact with the patient.

In-person interpreters may not always be available, and phone or screen interpreters may be easier to access and more cost efficient. When working with torture survivors, it is especially important to be aware of their difficulties with trusting other people. As an example, Nathanael from Ethiopia preferred to stutter with broken English rather than using the interpreter present. He was suspicious that the interpreter could be a spy for the organization he had fled from. In such instances, a more anonymous telephone interpreter may be a good alternative.

The use of interpreters may be challenging and time consuming, but in the majority of cases the advantages of building trust and mutually agreeing on the treatment plan will outweigh the disadvantages.

18.5.1.3 Cultural Understanding and Culture-Sensitive Approach

How well we communicate with each other is not just influenced by language. Cultural background can influence how we experience symptoms, how we describe and communicate our difficulties, when and how we seek help and the relation between the health professional and the patient. Cultural background is a lot more than originating country or language spoken. Asylum seekers and refugees must be seen for their individual needs, and not as representatives for a group or culture. To achieve this, we need to bear our own culture in mind in the meeting of others: The health personnel's own attitudes, experiences, traditions and interpretations affect the patient meeting to the same degree as the patient's cultural baggage.

To prepare for good patient meetings, independent of the patient's background, we should:

- Identify the patient's background, for example, country of origin, ethnicity, language, medical history, refugee history, and residential status
- Explore the patient's individual capacity for understanding, ways of expression, resources, and needs
- Understand how our own culture may limit or facilitate both the treatment relations and the clinical work.

18.5.1.4 Building Trust and Sense of Control

As breaking down trust is a fundamental element in torture, effort is required from health personnel to re-build trust. Following are some practical advice on how to develop trust and build a good relationship to a torture survivor:

- Put aside enough time for the first visit
- Take your time to explain and discuss
- Use an interpreter if necessary
- The first meeting should preferably take place in a non-clinical environment, and never with the torture victim placed in the dental chair.

Useful questions in the first consultation are for example: "Before we start, is there anything more you think I should know?", or "What can I do to make you more comfortable?".

> **Box**
> If the patient reveals traumatic experiences, a possible response may be:
> - "I am very sorry that this happened to you. How are you doing now?"
> - "It is good you are telling me about this. Is there anything I can do, as your dentist, to make it better for you?"
> - "I appreciate that you are telling me this. No one deserves to experience what you have told me…"
> - "Do you think this affects you today? If so, would you like me to refer you to someone you can talk to about this?"

Sense of control is extremely important for traumatized patients. The general principles to increase the sense of control are described in ► Chap. 6, and are equally relevant when working with torture survivors.

When health professionals become aware that a patient has been subjected to torture, it is crucial to avoid situations that bear resemblance to torture and interrogation, and delays should be avoided if possible. If the patient has experienced electrical torture, it is recommended to steer clear of ultrasound cleaning and electrical sensitivity tests. Be aware that many torture survivors may have problems with memory and concentration, and therefore have difficulties with remembering new information [9]. This emphasizes the importance of having enough time available for the first consultation. It may prove useful to write down for the patient what was agreed upon, both the treatment plan and the patient's responsibilities in connection with the treatment. If an interpreter is used, he or she can write down the information in the patient's preferred language. Be aware that problems with learning new information, both new languages and practical skills, is a common symptom of PTSD [5]. Thus, the need for an interpreter may be present even though a torture survivor has been resettled for many years.

For some patients, the oral treatment needs are so comprehensive that treatment under general anesthesia is relevant to consider. For many torture survivors, this may be a useful and adequate solution. It is, however, important to consider each individual patient's history, and to acknowledge that for people who have been exposed to abuse/torture involving the mouth, being sedated may increase or bring back their feeling of losing control.

► **Example**

A 35-year-old woman described:

» Waking up from the sedation, my mouth felt completely different. The safety I had built up through the countless hours at the psychologist crumbled down in a few seconds. Once again, someone had done something to my mouth without me having control over it... ◄

18.6 Choice of Dental Treatment

Some basic guidelines for dental treatment of torture survivors may be:

- Establish trust
- Inform carefully about procedures and treatments
- Avoid waiting time
- Avoid situations that may remind about torture and interrogation
- Agree on a treatment plan with individual considerations and room for flexibility [14]

Missing teeth, or visible discolored or fractured teeth may bring forth reminders of torture every time a survivor looks in the mirror, or feels the teeth with the tongue. Furthermore, many torture victims live with chronic oral or dental pain. Consequently, oral rehabilitation may represent an important part of the total rehabilitation of a torture survivor.

When deciding on a dental treatment plan, it should be taken into consideration that further removal of teeth may be experienced both as a parallel to the torture, and as a direct consequence of the torture. Thus, to safeguard the patient's mental health, it is sensible to conserve and retain as many teeth as possible [6]. Many torture survivors reveal that they have problems with wearing removable dentures, as these may also be a constant reminder of torture experiences. Regardless of the choice of treatment, it is important that the diagnoses and treatment alternatives are thoroughly discussed with the patient, and that the final decision is made with informed consent (see ► Chap. 6).

The mouth and face are sensitive areas, which often are targets for torture. As a consequence, torture survivors often suffer from pain in the orofacial region, in addition to esthetical ailments. Oral health-related complaints have a significant impact on quality of life in torture survivors. Still, quite a few find it difficult to seek and undergo dental treatment.

Torture survivors often have complex physical and psychological difficulties. Chronic pain or increased sensitivity to pain is a common late effect of torture, in addition to psychological consequences such as lack of trust and symptoms of posttraumatic stress disorder (PTSD). Several aspects of the dental treatment situation may trigger traumatic reactions related to torture experiences, and some torture survivors are highly dentally anxious. Dental health personnel should know the principles for trauma-informed dental treatment, and focus on developing a relationship of trust and giving the patient the sense of control. It is important to strive to avoid delays and situations that may remind the patient of torture and interrogation. Patients should be carefully informed about procedures and treatments, and the dental treatment must be planned with individual adjustments. In many cases, the rehabilitation of oral health is an important part of the torture survivor's total rehabilitation.

References

1. United Nations. UN convention against torture and other cruel, inhuman or degrading treatment or punishment. United Nations; 1984. [cited 2020 Nov 1]. Available from: https://www.refworld.org/docid/3ae6b3a94.html.
2. UN. Istanbul protocol. Manual on the effective investigation and documentation of torture and other cruel, inhuman or degrading treatment or punishment. United Nations, New York and Geneva: United Nations High Commissioner for Human Rights; 2004. Available from: http://www.ohchr.org/Documents/Publications/training8Rev1en.pdf.
3. Arge SO, Hansen SH, Lynnerup N. Forensic odontological examinations of alleged torture victims at the University of Copenhagen 1997-2011. Torture. 2014;24(1):17–24.
4. Amnesty International. Stop torture: Amnesty International; 2021. Available from: https://www.amnesty.org/en/get-involved/stop-torture.
5. Rabin M, Willard C. Torture and refugees. In: Annamalai A, editor. Refugee health care: an essential medical guide. New York: Springer; 2014. p. 181–92.
6. Jerlang P. Odontological treatment of torture victims. Torture J. 1992;(suppl. 1.9):38–40.
7. Singh HK, Scott TE, Henshaw MM, Cote SE, Grodin MA, Piwowarczyk LA. Oral health status of refugee torture survivors seeking care in the United States. Am J Public Health. 2008;98(12):2181–2.
8. Høyvik AC, Lie B, Willumsen T. Dental anxiety in relation to torture experiences and symptoms of post-traumatic stress disorder. Eur J Oral Sci. 2019;127(1):65–71.

18

Summary

To be exposed to serious physical or psychological pain or suffering is defined as torture in the case that it is inflicted by a public person, with the purpose to punish, break down, discriminate, or force forth a confession. Torture is exercised in up to every third country, and may result in physical and psychological ailments with significance for oral health. Torture survivors often have problems in trusting health professionals, and they often find it difficult to talk about their torture experiences.

9. Quiroga J, Jaranson JM. Politically-motivated torture and its survivors: a desk study review of the literature. Torture. 2005;15(2–3):1–111.

10. Başoğlu M. A multivariate contextual analysis of torture and cruel, inhuman, and degrading treatments: implications for an evidence-based definition of torture. Am J Orthopsychiatry. 2009;79(2):135–45.

11. American Psychiatric Association. Diagnostic and statistical manual of mental disorders, 5th edition: DSM-5. Arlington: American Psychiatric Association; 2013.

12. Sveaass N. Destroying minds: psychological pain and the crime of torture. NY City L Rev. 2008;11(2):303–24.

13. Keefe FJ, Rumble ME, Scipio CD, Giordano LA, Perri LM. Psychological aspects of persistent pain: current state of the science. J Pain. 2004;5(4):195–211.

14. Bøjholm S, Jørring L, Bakke M. Torturoverlevere - generelle og odontologiske aspekter (torture survivors – general and odontological aspects). Tandlaegebladet. 1995;99(18):910–2.

The Psychosocial Impacts of Orofacial Features: With Examples from Orthognathic Surgery

Paula Frid, Sarah R. Baker and Jan-Are Kolset Johnsen

Contents

The objectives for orthognathic surgery are clear in most cases, in that it seeks to improve function and aesthetics in individuals with orofacial/dentofacial deformities. However, the term *deformity* or *anomaly* is viewed by many as having a negative connotation (as a "deviation") and, as such, the term maxillo-mandibular discrepancies will be used throughout this chapter. Despite the clear objectives of orthognathic surgery, the surgical results do not necessarily harmonize with patient motivation or satisfaction. In this chapter, the psychosocial impacts of orthognathic surgery will be highlighted, and the objectives for different orthognathic surgery procedures will be described. A case report will provide further insights into the complexity that orthognathic surgery might constitute for patients. It is important to have in mind that different oral health conditions such as missing teeth, severe orthodontic malocclusions, and teeth with inherited disorders such as Amelogenesis imperfecta will have similar psychosocial challenges as orthognathic surgery.

🔖 Learning Goals
- To learn about the psychosocial relevance of orofacial features
- To learn about body dysmorphic disorder
- To learn about the objectives of different orthognathic surgery procedures
- To learn about the psychosocial outcomes of dental interventions with alteration of orofacial features such as orthognathic surgery

19.1   The Psychosocial Relevance of Orofacial Features

The way we appear to ourselves and others has profound psychological and social impacts [1, 2]; however, the role of the mouth, teeth, and jaws (i.e. orofacial features) in research on appearance has perhaps received less attention than other facial aesthetic features, for instance, facial symmetry [3]. A poignant example of the importance of appearance taken from Nancy Etcoff's popular science book on the science of beauty encapsulates the essence of this topic [4]. Here she refers to the work of Donald Giddon and colleagues [5] where research participants would manipulate the facial features of an image of a person in profile, and where minute changes – down to a few millimetres – could change the perception of a face profile as either attractive or unattractive.

Judgments of attractiveness, albeit seemingly superficial, are known to have real-life consequences both on an interpersonal and intrapersonal level. For instance, attractiveness judgements influence how we regard others, choose friends or romantic partners, and how we view ourselves (for an overview, see [1, 6, 7]). From an evolutionary perspective, perceptions concerning facial appearance could have relevance as markers of the quality of a potential mate, for instance giving indirect information about the health status of an individual [8–10], and interestingly perceptions of facial attractiveness has been shown to predict longevity [11]. As for the individual's own judgments and perceptions, however orofacial areas – and the mouth in particular – could be argued to constitute a hierarchy of needs that includes both biological and social elements, which range from survival, via socialization, to self-actualization [12]. Thus, the importance of the orofacial areas in human life reaches beyond concepts such as "beauty" and "attractiveness". The lower levels of this hierarchy address the fundamental biological needs, most prominently perhaps the acquiring of sustenance. These aspects are readily accepted as important to oral health professionals, since it is a clear link between functionality and health behaviours, for instance that tooth loss among the elderly prevents eating behaviours [13]. Also, more fundamental social functions, for instance related to non-verbal communication of emotional states as well as verbal communication, are related to orofacial functioning or perception of orofacial elements [14, 15]. At the higher levels of this hierarchy, however, one will find psychological concepts such as an individual's experience of self-esteem and self-worth, both which are closely related to perceptions of both general quality of life and health-related quality of life [16–18]. These increasingly abstract concepts can perhaps be difficult to apply in oral health care settings, due to biomedical thinking or lack of time or tools to assess these states. In line with this, some authors have argued that self-evaluation processes such as self-esteem should be regarded as both a protective factor and a potential risk factor related to physical and mental health, and that self-esteem should be specifically targeted in development of health promotion programs [19]. Although self-esteem is not exclusively tied to one domain such as appearance or attractiveness [18], it nevertheless becomes highly relevant to view orofacial areas and functional aspects as part of a broader picture of general health and well-being. This also ties in with the modern definition of oral health as outlined in ▶ Chap. 5.

Thus, any surgical efforts to alter or manipulate orofacial areas, whether it is for aesthetic or functional reasons, should be viewed also in light of their psychosocial impacts. One example of such a surgical effort is in orthognathic surgery.

> **Box**
> Important: Alterations of orofacial features in orthognathic surgery may influence not only function and aesthetics but also general health and well-being!

19.2 Body Dysmorphic Disorder (BDD)

Body Dysmorphic Disorder (BDD) also known as dysmorphophobia, is an disorder that encompasses excessive preoccupation with physical appearance [20]. While other psychiatric diagnoses might involve distorted evaluation of physical appearance (for example, anorexia nervosa), BDD appears to be specifically sensitive to the individual's own facial appearance [21]. Explanations of BDD range from psychosocial risk factors [22] to abnormalities in visual processing and perception, in particularly related to the face [23]. Concerning oral health, BDD has been linked to requests for orthognathic surgery since patients suffering from the disorder could be more likely to seek out physical and aesthetic procedures aimed at alleviating their symptoms [24, 25] rather than addressing other aspects of the disorders (for example, psychological treatment). A recent systematic review has indicated that the prevalence of BDD within the population of orthognathic patients is between 5% and 13% [25], and even outside the diagnostic criteria of BDD, a high percentage of patients appear overly and excessively concerned with their appearance [26]. Based on this, there has been increased attention on psychological assessment of patients referred to orthognathic surgery [24] and to increase the clinical competence among oral health professionals with regards to this topic [27]. Also, it is worth noting that patients referred to orthognathic surgery may have other psychological problems, notably symptoms of depression, OCD, and anxiety [28–30], which may merit consideration among oral health professionals.

19.3 Orthognathic Surgery

Orthognathic surgery, i.e. corrective surgery of the facial skeleton, aims to improve both the functionality and aesthetics [31]. The term orthognathics means "straight jaws" coming from the Greek language (orthos = straight, gnathos = jaws).

There are different types of maxillo-mandibular discrepancies such as (1) *mandibular prognathia / hyperplasia* (■ Fig. 19.1); increased anterior–posterior growth of the mandible, (2) *mandibular rethrognathia / hypoplasia* (■ Fig. 19.2); reduced anterior–posterior growth of

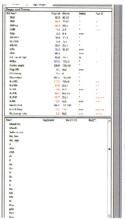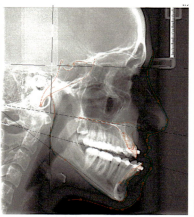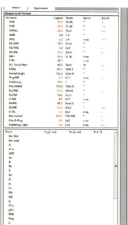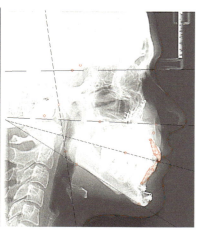

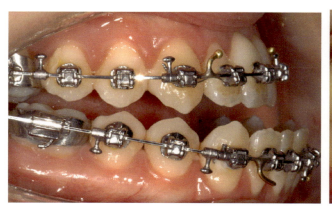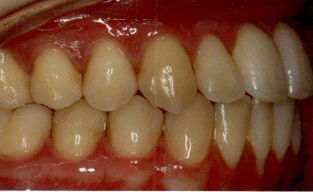

■ **Fig. 19.1**   Cephalograms and photos of mandibular prognathia treated with bimaxillary orthognathic surgery and genioplasty. (Photos permission granted by the patient)

the mandible, (3) *maxillary prognathia / hyperplasia* (■ Fig. 19.3); increased anterior–posterior growth of the maxilla, (4) *maxillary rethrognatia / hypoplasia* (■ Fig. 19.4); reduced anterior–posterior growth of the maxilla, (5) *Apertognathia* (■ Fig. 19.5); reduced vertical growth of the posterior part of the mandible and increased growth of the posterior part of the maxilla resulting in an anterior open bite, and (6) *mandibular asymmetry* (■ Fig. 19.6); asymmetric growth of the mandible.

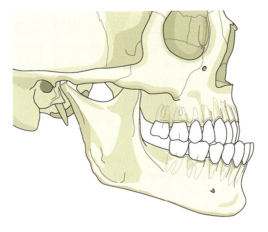

■ **Fig. 19.4**   Maxillary rethrognatia. (Copyright by AO Foundation, Switzerland. Source: AO Surgery Reference, ► www.aosurgery.org)

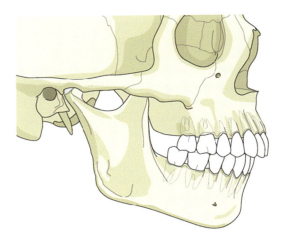

■ **Fig. 19.2**   Mandibular rethrognathia. (Copyright by AO Foundation, Switzerland. Source: AO Surgery Reference, ► www.aosurgery.org)

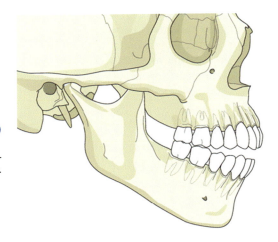

■ **Fig. 19.5**   Apertognathia. (Copyright by AO Foundation, Switzerland. Source: AO Surgery Reference, ► www.aosurgery.org)

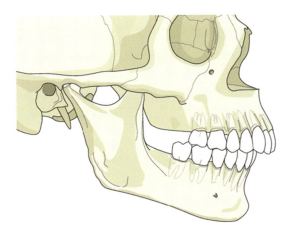

■ **Fig. 19.3**   Maxillary prognathia. (Copyright by AO Foundation, Switzerland. Source: AO Surgery Reference, ► www.aosurgery.org)

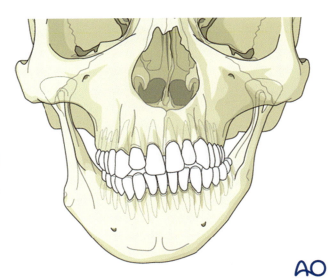

■ **Fig. 19.6**   Mandibular asymmetry. (Copyright by AO Foundation, Switzerland. Source: AO Surgery Reference, ► www.aosurgery.org)

> **Box**
>
> Examples of maxillo-mandibular discrepancies:
> 1. Mandibular prognathia/hyperplasia
> 2. Mandibular rethrognathia/hypoplasia
> 3. Maxillary prognathia/hyperplasia
> 4. Maxillary rethrognatia/hypoplasia
> 5. Apertognathia
> 6. Mandibular asymmetry

19.3.1 Prevalence

In the Scandinavian countries Norway and Sweden with 15 million inhabitants, approximately 1300 patients undergo orthognathic surgery annually at the different University Hospital clinics and some County Hospitals [32, 33]. In USA, 10345 patients were hospitalized in 2008 [34] and in England and Wales, 2600–2900 patients undergo these treatments annually [73].

19.3.2 Treatment *Strategies*

Malpositioned teeth caused by maxillo-mandibular discrepancies may be treated by three different strategies [31]: (1) Growth modification by orthopaedic appliance (how much growth may be altered is a controversial topic) (2) orthodontic camouflage by orthodontics alone (mild maxillo-mandibular discrepancies) and (3) orthognathic surgery combined with orthodontics is often required in severe maxillo-mandibular discrepancies.

19.3.3 Indications for Surgery

Most patients going through orthognathic surgery are healthy individuals with a maxillo-mandibular discrepancy (sagittal, vertical, transversal) affecting orofacial function. Impaired orofacial function may lead to problems with chewing, mouth opening, phonetics, and maintenance of optimal oral hygiene. Mouth breathing may be the result of lip incompetence (inability to fully seal the lips) due to excessive vertical growth of the maxilla. There are also psychosocial impacts to address, and these can affect the patient's quality of life (QoL) [24, 35, 36].

However, some patients have growth related maxillo-mandibular discrepancies associated to sleep apnoea [37], airway defects and soft tissue discrepancies such as cleft-lip-and palate deformities [38] and also discrepancies associated with temporomandibular growth disturbances [39]. Further, patients with syndromes such as Crouzon, Apert, and Treacher Collins often have maxillo-mandibular discrepancies [40]. Therefore, the goal for treatment is to normalize the chewing and phonetic function, to improve the airway space and to improve the psychosocial function [31].

19.3.4 Evaluation of the Facial Morphology

Analyses of lateral X-rays (cepahlograms) of sagittal and vertical discrepancies are evaluated by the orthodontist. The goal of cephalometrics is to compare the patient (or victim in forensic investigations) with a normal reference group [41]. Facial morphology depends on different factors such as gender, ethnicity, race, and genetic constitution. The normal reference group may therefore differ between different groups [42]. In cases with asymmetry and a tilted occlusal plane, evaluation of frontal X-rays and CT scans are performed, and the soft tissue is evaluated. The profile is divided into a convex, concave or a straight profile. The nasolabial angle is measured and also how much of the teeth are present in a relaxed position and in a smile position is calculated.

19.3.5 Orthognathic Surgery Osteotomies

Different osteotomies are described in the literature such as the Vertical Ramus Osteotomy (VRO), the Bilateral sagittal split osteotomy (BSSO), the Le Fort I osteotomy, the Genioplasty, and the Bimaxillary osteotomy [31]. Together with conventional orthognathic surgery, there is also the distraction osteogenesis osteotomy [43].

19.3.5.1 Vertical Ramus Osteotomy

This procedure is used for correction of a class III relation and an open bite. It may be performed either with an extraoral (EVRO) or an intraoral (IVRO) approach with osteosynthesis or intermaxillary fixation, respectively (◘ Fig. 19.7). The osteotomy is performed between the incisura of the ramus and vertically down to the posterior border of the ramus. Skeletal relapse is reported to be 17% for EVRO [44] and 12–26% for IVRO [45, 46] 6–12 months after surgery. With the EVRO procedure there will be a 2.5-cm-long scar behind the jaw angle but the majority (97%) of the patients are satisfied after surgery [44]. The risk of facial nerve damage is low. With the IVRO procedure, there is no facial scar but a small risk of sensory damage of 9% [47].

19.3.5.2 Bilateral Sagittal Split Osteotomy

Bilateral sagittal split osteotomy (BSSO) is the most common osteotomy in orthognathic surgery, first introduced by Hugo Obwegeser in 1957 [48]. Through this osteotomy, it is possible to move the mandible in all

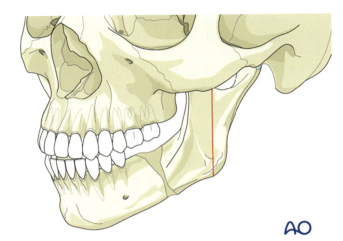

Fig. 19.7 Vertical ramus osteotomy (VRO). (Copyright by AO Foundation, Switzerland. Source: AO Surgery Reference, ▶ www.aosurgery.org)

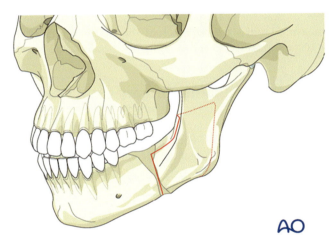

Fig. 19.8 Bilateral sagittal split osteotomy (BSSO). (Copyright by AO Foundation, Switzerland. Source: AO Surgery Reference, ▶ www.aosurgery.org)

directions, i.e. mandibular prognathism, mandibular retrognathism, mandibular asymmetry and apertognathia (open bite) (▶ Fig. 19.8).

With a BSSO a sagittal osteotomy in the ramus and the body of the mandible is performed with preserved bony contacts between lateral and medial sites. Between these bony fragments the inferior alveolar nerve is situated and can be damaged during surgery. Osteosynthesis with bicortical screws or plates are used.

Approximately 50% of the patients have changed sensibility in their lower lip and chin after the BSSO osteotomy [44, 47], and the risk is increased above the age of 35. However, most of these patients are not so bothered by this.

The relapse is 17% for a mandibular setback [44] and 33% when the mandible is moved forward [49].

Most (95%) of the patients are satisfied after a BSSO osteotomy and mandibular setback [44] and 84% of the patients are satisfied after moving the mandible forward [33].

19.3.5.3 Le Fort I Osteotomy

In 1901, the French doctor Renè LeFort dropped skulls of cadavers to study the fracture pattern. The Le Fort fractures I, II and III were introduced. Indications for a Le Fort I osteotomy are maxillary rethrognathia/hypoplasia, maxillary asymmetry, apertognathia, and maxillary hyperplasia / gummy smile (a lot of exposed gingiva when smiling). The Le Fort 1 osteotomy [50] is performed 5 mm superior from the apices of the teeth through the lateral part of the front wall of the maxilla and superior from the nasal floor [31] (▶ Fig. 19.9). The osteotomy separates the pterygoid plates from the maxilla. Fixation is performed by osteosynthesis plates, and it is possible to perform 1, 2, and 3 piece segmental maxilla. Few complications are seen after a Le Fort I osteotomy and relapse is 18% of the movement [51] and most patients are satisfied after this osteotomy [33].

19.3.5.4 Genioplasty

A genioplasty is indicated when the patient has a retruded, asymmetric or a very prominent chin. A horizontal osteotomy is performed of the anterior part of the chin and moved to the desired position and fixed with osteosynthesis plates (▶ Fig. 19.10). It is also possible to transplant bone into the osteotomy or remove bone depending on the desired movement. Instead of a bony osteotomy, it is also possible to adapt a silicon or a polyethylene implant directly on the chin [52]. Some patients may have changed sensibility after the proce-

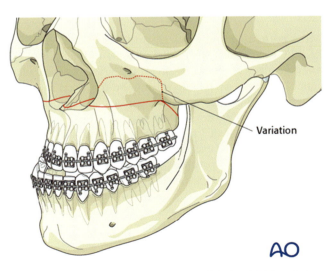

Fig. 19.9 Le Fort I osteotomy. (Copyright by AO Foundation, Switzerland. Source: AO Surgery Reference, ▶ www.aosurgery.org)

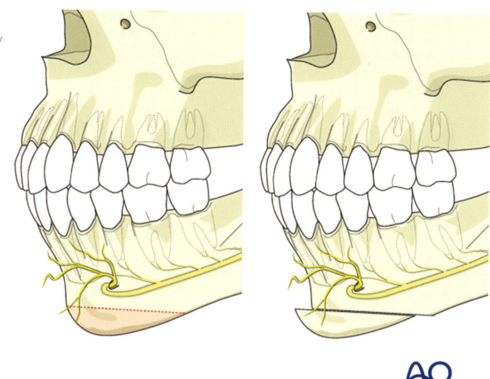

Fig. 19.10 Genioplasty. (Copyright by AO Foundation, Switzerland. Source: AO Surgery Reference, ► www.aosurgery. org)

dure and skeletal relapse is approximately 8% of the movement forward [53]. A sliding genioplasty forward is very predictable and most patients are satisfied with this procedure.

19.3.5.5 Bimaxillary Orthognathic Surgery

When the total movement is large, the orthognathic procedure is often distributed on both jaws due to aesthetic reasons and also not to compromise the posterior airway space with a too large setback movement in the lower jaw (■ Fig. 19.11).

19.3.5.6 Distraction Osteogenesis

In cases with a large movement, especially in patients with a severe rethrognathic mandible and high-angle cases, distraction osteogenesis may be more stable over time compared to conventional orthognathic surgery [39, 43] (■ Fig. 19.12).

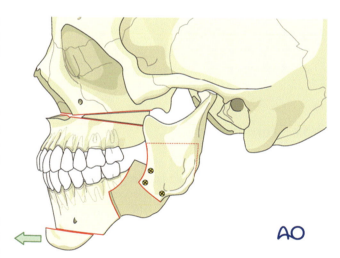

Fig. 19.11 Bimaxillary orthognathic osteotomies. (Copyright by AO Foundation, Switzerland. Source: AO Surgery Reference, ► www.aosurgery.org)

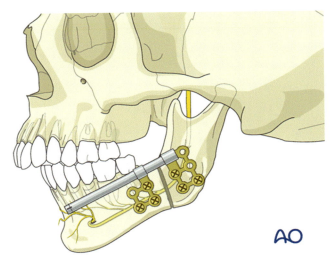

□ **Fig. 19.12** Mandibular osteotomy with the distraction device. (Copyright by AO Foundation, Switzerland. Source: AO Surgery Reference, ► www.aosurgery.org)

Box
Examples of orthognathic surgery osteotomies:
- Vertical ramus osteotomy
- Bilateral sagittal split osteotomy
- Le Fort I osteotomy
- Genioplasty
- Bimaxillary orthognathic surgery
- Distraction osteogenesis

19.3.6   Terminology

The terminology often used in relation to orthognathic surgery treatment need, for instance, "dentofacial deformity" or "anomaly", refers to a comparison with normal standards [41]. Based on these standards, nearly 30% of the general population present with malocclusions determined to be in need of orthodontic treatment, and 5% with dentofacial deformities in need of orthognathic surgery [54]. However, since ideas about aesthetics and normality could be argued to be somewhat malleable and flexible [55, 56], the validity of the normal standards for orthognathic surgery can perhaps also be debated [42]. Recently, the appropriateness of the terminology "dentofacial deformity" has been specifically questioned, not only in light of issues concerning accuracy [57], but also in light of the social implications of this particular term [58]. Alternative terms, such as maxillo-mandibular discrepancy, has been suggested [58]. While it is important that terminol-

ogy is clear and consistent in the research literature and within a clinical discipline, it is also important to acknowledge that the terminology and language used in healthcare settings matters and could be a contributing factor in the dehumanization of patients [59, 60]. Development of terminology that is consistent and accurate, while remaining neutral and respectful of the patient's perspective, should be encouraged, perhaps along the lines suggested for the media with regards to how to address visual differences [61].

19.3.7   Case Report

Most patients report satisfaction after going through orthognathic surgery [33, 35], and orthognathic surgery has shown to have a positive impact on the QoL of patients with maxillo-mandibular discrepancies [62]. However, the current case will provide an example where the patient at first was not satisfied with the result after orthognathic surgery.

A 20-year-old woman was referred to the Department of Oral and Maxillofacial Surgery at the University Hospital North Norway and Public Dental Service Competence Centre of North Norway (TkNN), Tromsø, for evaluation and treatment of her maxillo-mandibular discrepancy. She had problems with her bite/occlusion and phonetics and was diagnosed with a skeletal class III relation and an open bite. Treatment suggestion was a bimaxillary orthognathic surgical procedure together with a sliding genioplasty, which was accepted by the patient. The patient went through the procedure without any medical complications. A sliding genioplasty was however not performed during this first surgery, but was planned as a second procedure after asking the patient about her thoughts about it. After the first surgery, the patient was not satisfied. She told the surgeons that she thought her face had become much shorter and that she felt depressed because of this. In response, a second procedure with a sliding genioplasty with anterior and inferior advancement was planned for, but the patient wanted to talk to a psychologist before proceeding with another surgery. Together with her depression, she also developed a myalgia in her muscles of mastication and was therefore treated with Botulinum Toxin (Botox®).

Psychological assessment and psychometric testing were done by a psychologist working with dental phobia at TkNN, and the results indicated that the patient suffered from severe depression and had massive challenges with regards to accepting her appearance and adjusting to her new, post-operative life situation. Her symptoms had marked impact on her daily activities and life in general. For instance, she experienced social withdrawal relating to friends and social gatherings, loss of interest in activities that had been important to her and difficulties with motivation concerning important life decisions, such as choice of education and ideas about future vocation. Negative thoughts and self-evaluation featured prominently and appeared across many different situations.

From the psychological consultations, some key themes emerged. Concerning the motivation for treatment, it became clear that the patient had been aware of considerable external expectations for orthognathic surgery during her childhood and adolescence, and that her own motivation for surgery appeared in large parts tied to these external expectations. Although she noted negative experiences with functional aspects of her bite, and some notable experiences of being bullied or teased (for example, she had been given a derogatory nickname), she expressed that she had been quite content with her facial aesthetics, and that the functional aspects in her eyes were minor. Overall, she appeared to be relatively unprepared for both the physiological and psychosocial consequences of surgery; for instance, the experience of waking up after surgery with her jaws locked, and the marked change of her appearance. Furthermore, her depression and problems adjusting to her "new appearance" showed signs of being tied to the loss of her own personal identity, also related to her entry into young adulthood with heightened expectations related to life choices and identity formation. Also, since all external agents that were important to her and that had been involved in the decision to undergo surgery (friends, family) appeared to be positive about her undergoing orthognathic surgery, as well as about the results, she had little opportunities to express her displeasure about the outcome and the process. At some point, the psychological consultations perhaps became more about providing her an emotional outlet than about specific psychological treatment, although elements of cognitive therapy were implemented throughout the sessions. The patient was scheduled for in total 27 appointments with the psychologist after surgery. Four years after the first surgical procedure, she completed the genioplasty and expressed that she was satisfied with the result after this. Finally, the decision regarding accepting genioplasty should be regarded not merely as an attempt not only to regain some of her former orofacial characteristics, but also as a definite and mature decision of her own choosing, which can be viewed as a contrast to her former experiences regarding surgery.

This case report highlights the potential negative psychological impact of orthognathic surgery, and in particular the insight that measurements that might be interpreted as an objective need for invasive procedures

does not necessarily mirror the patient's motivational mindset or guarantee success. Case reports and patient narratives related to orthognathic surgery are rare, most often addressing surgical outcomes in relation to specific pre-existing conditions or diagnoses. The current report describing the experiences of a unique, young individual, nevertheless mirror others' experiences, for instance the importance related to the patient's pre-surgical "true motivation" for surgery [63]. Also, the case report provides support to former research that indicates that motivation and satisfaction with surgical outcome often have strong ties to aesthetic judgements [64, 65], and that satisfaction can be impacted by unexpected post-surgical events [66]. As a result of this case report, inclusion of a psychologist in the team of orthognathic surgery now is a standard care at the Department of Oral and Maxillofacial Surgery at the University Hospital North Norway and Public Dental Service Competence Centre of North Norway (TkNN) in Tromsø, Norway. All patients going through orthognathic surgery assessment are offered a pre- and post-evaluation by a psychologist.

> **Box**
>
> Practical guidelines: Inclusion of a psychologist in the team of orthognathic surgery and other dental interventions where the orofacial features will be changed may be an important support in pre- and post-evaluation of the patient. Careful consideration should be made with regards to the patient's true motivation for surgery, and steps should be taken to prepare patients for the physiological and psychosocial consequences that may follow. For patients in need of psychological support, such efforts should preferably be initiated pre-surgery and followed up post-surgery.

19.4 Psychosocial Outcomes of Orthognathic Surgery

As outlined in the previous section, orthognathic treatment can impact on individuals in a number of ways, including oral function, psychosocial well-being and wider quality of life (QoL). This section will provide an overview of the psychosocial outcomes of orthognathic surgery, reflect on the limitations of the evidence base so far, and suggest future avenues for research in the area.

Since the 1980s, when the first paper in the area was published, there have been a plethora of articles on the psychosocial outcomes of orthognathic surgery. Given the large and ever-growing evidence-base, we will focus this section only on published reviews, primarily systematic reviews. This is because well-conducted systematic reviews attempt to identify, appraise and synthesize all empirical evidence that meets pre-specified eligibility criteria and as such are considered to be the highest levels of evidence reviews (when including randomized controlled trials).

In the first systematic review in the area, Hunt and colleagues (2001) identified 29 studies published between 1984 and 2000 [67]. Nearly all studies that were included in the review concluded that there were beneficial psychosocial effects resulting from orthognathic surgery. Benefits included improvements to body image, personality, self-esteem, social and interpersonal functioning, and overall mood. However, most of the studies were deemed to be of low quality with nearly all including no control group (28 out of the 29 studies). In addition, there was a lack of consistency in how psychosocial status was measured across studies (the 29 studies included 30 different questionnaires!), with few of these measures having been validated. There were also very few longitudinal studies (17 of the 29 studies), which would allow for an assessment of pre- to post-surgery changes in psychosocial outcomes. As a result, the authors of the systematic review suggested that any psychosocial benefits should be interpreted with caution.

In a more recent (non-systematic) review, conducted by one of the authors of this chapter (SB) and her colleagues (Liddle et al. 2015) [36], 38 new articles were identified between 2001 and 2013. These studies were conducted in many countries around the world including Europe, USA, China, Brazil, Japan, and Scandinavia. The studies reported improvements in areas such as satisfaction with facial appearance, self-confidence, self-esteem, body image, anxiety and social functioning. Findings in relation to, for example, facial appearance, showed that patient-rated improvements varied across studies but were high (57–97%). As we noted in our review, the lowest percentages were most likely due to when patients were asked to rate their appearance; that is, shortly after surgery (4–6 weeks) when recovery was not yet complete, and patients may still have been experiencing post-surgery discomfort. Interestingly, very few studies explicitly asked patients about dissatisfaction. It is therefore difficult to know whether those that did not rate being satisfied were actively dissatisfied or neutral.

Gains in self-concept and more specifically self-esteem, self-confidence and body image were reported in a number of studies. For example, several studies have reported improved confidence ratings for between 58% and 85% of participants. Unfortunately, many of these studies report percentage increases post-surgery, with no statistical (or indeed clinical) significance provided. As such, it is difficult to assess whether patients do have higher scores at follow-up than control patients.

Social functioning has received much less attention in the literature. In the 38 studies included in the review, those that had subscales related to social functioning reported improvements in social interactions, and communication and social relations. For example, some studies reported that participants felt orthognathic treatment had a positive impact on relationships with family, friends and colleagues (20% of participants; although it is worth noting that 44% felt there was no effect). Others have found participants were more comfortable eating in front of others (54% of participants), positive influence on relationships with the opposite sex (49%), social activities (54%), and their "personal lifestyle" (49%).

Most of the 38 studies included in the review incorporated a measure of patient satisfaction with treatment outcome. Levels of satisfaction tended to be high, ranging from 73% to 100%. Interestingly, the percentage of patients who would choose to have orthognathic treatment again ranged from 61% to 88%, and between 70% and 90% would recommend the treatment to others. Reasons for dissatisfaction were often not explicitly explored in studies, although rates of dissatisfaction ranged from 4% to 8%. It may be that patient dissatisfaction was linked to treatment outcomes (e.g. changes to facial appearance, post-surgery complications), expectations (e.g. unrealistic expectations may be linked to more dissatisfaction), or motives for surgery (e.g. aesthetic or functional reasons).

Liddle and colleagues (2015) [36] noted that 13 years on from the earlier systematic review by Hunt et al. (2001) [67], there was still limited use of validated measures and often confusion and inconsistency about the concepts under study. The wide variation in how concepts were defined and measured meant that comparisons across studies remained difficult. Interestingly, Liddle and colleagues found more consistency in the areas of mental health and QoL [36]. These studies indicated that mental health appeared to worsen in the immediate post-surgery phase but that this improved by 6 months post-surgery – or there was a return to pre-surgery levels of functioning. Again, this was difficult to untangle as there were few longitudinal studies that included a measure of mental health at baseline (i.e. pre-surgery) alongside a matched control group. Indeed, of the 38 studies included in the review, only two were of a prospective design with a control group. A further 18 (of 38 studies) were longitudinal allowing some assessment of psychosocial outcomes over time but few followed patients beyond 2 years after surgery. Although these studies suggest that there may be significant gains in self-concept, social functioning, emotional and interpersonal relationships, mental health, QoL and satisfaction which are sustained, caution is needed without non-patient (or waiting list) matched comparison groups and studies with longer post-surgery follow-up periods.

Given the methodological limitations of the studies conducted between 1984 and 2013 and included in the reviews by Hunt et al. (2001) and Liddle et al. (2015), it remains difficult to answer, with any degree of certainty, the question *'Do patients show psychosocial benefits from orthognathic surgery?'* [36, 67]. In a recent systematic review in the area, Broers and colleagues (2017) attempted to definitively answer this question in order to help inform dental health professionals and oral surgeons in treatment planning and decisions for individual patients [68]. To do this, they conducted a systematic review that was based on very rigorously defined criteria; including only prospective studies with a minimal follow-up of 6 months, a parallel control group, and measures of psychosocial functioning and/or patient satisfaction. With such tightly defined criteria, it is perhaps not surprising that the review only included nine studies. In addition, the authors concluded that all nine studies were at high risk of bias. Risk of bias was assessed by whether there was selection bias (randomization, concealment), information bias (blinding), or completeness of data (complete description of all patients included). The authors concluded that there were no valid studies to support the claim that orthognathic surgery for adults leads to benefits in patient satisfaction and psychosocial functioning. They went further and stated "we would recommend for practitioners to explain to patients >17 years of age, who consider elective orthognathic surgery, that there is no evidence for the benefit of this surgical intervention for adults, in terms of psychosocial functioning and patient satisfaction" and "it is not clear whether patients will gain sufficient and sustainable benefit from this rather invasive procedure" (p. 417). As with the two earlier reviews described above, Broers et al. (2017) drew attention to the poor methodological quality in the area – despite the large and ever-growing number of studies [68].

Hot-off the press, the very latest recently published systematic review by Meger and colleagues (2021) also included the first meta-analysis of studies in the area [62]. This review was focused specifically on quality of life, for which they used the World Health Organization's (1995) definition; 'the individuals perception of their position in life in the context of the culture and value systems, in which they live and in relation to their goals, expectations, standards and concerns'. Although a far broader concept than psychosocial functioning, the topics of this current section, the two are very much linked, with psychosocial status a key determinant of an individual's QoL.

The authors included very clear criteria for study inclusion; only observational cohort studies with pre- and post-surgery QoL, which used either of two validated measures; the oral health impact profile (OHIP-14) and the orthognathic quality of life questionnaire (OLQL). There were 12 studies that met the criteria. All had small sample sizes between 14 and 74 patients, and a follow-up between 3 and 12 months. Of the 12 studies, 11 reported improvements in oral health and/or orthognathic specific quality of life as a result of surgery. As was reported in the previous systematic review, the authors found that in terms of the risk of bias, four studies were at high risk, eight at moderate risk, and none at low risk.

For the meta-analysis, Meger and colleagues (2021) included only those studies that had a 6-month follow-up and which were of moderate risk of bias ($n = 7$) [62]. For the OHIP-14, three studies were included with a mean pre-post surgery difference of 7.63 (1.62–13.65 95% CI). This difference was significant indicating that orthognathic surgery had a positive impact on oral-health related quality of life. For orthognathic specific quality of life (OLQL), six studies were included with a mean difference of 20.53 (14.27–26.79 95% CI). Again, the difference was statistically significant indicating a positive effect of surgery. Although this study reports a positive benefit of orthognathic surgery, as in previous reviews, the authors' note that the studies were not of high methodological quality, none of the studies were at low risk of bias, and given the small sample sizes, with no sample size calculation reported, more well-designed studies are needed.

Summary

Consistent positive psychosocial outcomes have been reported as a result of orthognathic treatment. Yet, despite the plethora of and seemingly ever-increasing number of studies in the area, there is a need to develop more well-designed studies which incorporate pre- and post-surgery assessments of a range of psychosocial outcomes, utilizing standardized and validated measures, with adequate sample sizes. The small sample sizes in studies to date limit the statistical power of the analysis and few studies in the area have reported effect sizes. In other areas of oral and dental research, we have increasingly seen treatment centers collaborate and this is helpful to enable more appropriate samples. Additionally, multi-site studies may help to facilitate recruitment of a wider representation of participants in terms of for example, sex, ethnicity and age group – this will enable us to understand more about how psychosocial outcomes of surgery potentially vary on key socio-demographics for example, between men and women.

With regard to outcome measures, future research in the area needs to ensure consistency in measures used to evaluate psychosocial status. There have been some interesting developments in measures developed and validated specifically for orthognathic patients, and these are to be welcomed to ensure consistency (and thus comparisons) across studies. For example, the Orthognathic Quality of Life Questionnaire (OQLQ; Cunningham et al. 2000) which assesses oral functioning, facial aesthetics, social functioning and awareness of dentofacial appearance [69]. Although not specific to orthognathic patients, or to the orofacial region, the Derriford Appearance Scale (DAS-59; Carr et al. 2000) measures distress and dysfunction resulting from body image disturbance [70]. A further suggestion would be to develop a Core Outcome Set (COS), which could be used in all future studies evaluating orthognathic treatment. Such an approach has been advocated by the COMET Initiative (Core Outcome Measures in Effectiveness Trials) (▶ https://www.comet-initiative.org/) and a number of COS have been developed in relation to oral and dental conditions (e.g. Ni Riordain et al. 2020) [71].

Future studies also need to ensure the use of suitable matched control groups, and consistency in follow-up points. At present, follow-up time points have varied considerably, have been unclearly specified and often do not go beyond 6 months. It may well be that for some psychosocial outcomes of interest, 6 months or less may not be sufficient time for changes in self-concept, body image and improvement in interpersonal and emotional functioning.

Aside from methodological issues, in terms of the focus of future research, further exploration is required of processes underpinning adjustment to facial change, the role of psychological support during treatment and the decision-making process. There have been some interesting qualitative studies in recent years which have served to provide more detail from an idiothetic perspective on orthognathic surgery, together with research on decision-making (e.g. Paul et al. 2021) [72]. These studies enable us to begin to understand the complexity of patient experiences during the lengthy treatment process, as well as the factors, which play a role in decision- making. A recent study by one of the authors of this chapter (SB) and her colleagues (Paul et al. 2021) [72], for example, provided a detailed exploration on the role of dental professionals in decision making. The study included face-to-face interviews with 22 patients in the UK of which 12 were 6- to 8-week post-surgery, four were 1–2 years post-surgery, and six were in the decision-making phase. Data were also collected from online forums and blogs to supplement the understanding of processes involved in decision making for orthognathic treatment. There were six themes related to decision making; awareness about their underlying dentofacial problems and the treatment options available, information available about treatment, the timeline of when surgery would occur, patients' motivations and expectations, social support available, and fear of the surgery itself, of hospitalization and the possibility of disliking their new face. As part of this study, we concluded that clinicians needed to be informed about the importance of their role in the decision-making process (being far from a neutral observer) and on how they could improve the patient experience.

Regarding practical guidelines for interventions altering orofacial features, such as orthognathic surgery, a multidisciplinary approach should be taken with regards to the planning and follow-up of surgical procedures. This should include psychological assessment prior to surgery, and psychological follow-up after surgery, which would warrant the inclusion of a mental health professional in the team of clinicians.

Psychological Implications of Complex Dentistry Affecting Appearance

Dr. Nicola M Stock

Senior Research Psychologist

Centre for Appearance Research, University of the West of England, Bristol, UK

As a Research Psychologist, my role is to understand the psychological impact of appearance-altering conditions, and to trial interventions to reduce psychological distress in those affected. Complex conditions, such as cleft lip and palate, often result in a visibly different appearance, and involve long-term multidisciplinary intervention to improve facial appearance as well as function. Those requiring complex dentistry may be up to five times more likely to experience intrusive questions, staring, and teasing as a result of their appearance. These experiences can have a long-term impact on emotional wellbeing, relationships, and academic performance.

Improving appearance through dental work can have a positive impact on psychological health, but the process needs to be carefully managed. Dental professionals can support this process by learning more from the patient/parent about the origin of the problem and what other interventions (e.g. counselling, other specialist treatment) are being implemented. Understanding a patient's motivations for treatment can determine whether their expectations of the outcome are realistic. Further, not all patients are concerned about their appearance, and treatment specifically to improve appearance may therefore not be necessary.

Appearance is a sensitive topic, and both patients and health professionals can worry about how to raise it. Screening/decision-making tools can be helpful in assessing the degree of appearance concern, and beginning a beneficial dialogue about the patient's goals for dental work. Using neutral language (such as 'condition'), rather than stigmatising medical terminology (such as 'disfigurement' or 'deformity') is important for building rapport. Helping the patient to feel informed and empowered to make their own decisions based on what is right for them at that time is one of the most important opportunities a health professional can offer. If more serious concerns about appearance, teasing, or emotional wellbeing are flagged, dental professionals can refer patients to a psychological specialist, and signpost them to reliable local/national support services.

Acknowledgements We would like to acknowledge psychologist Silja Sundsfjord for contributions to the case report.

References

1. Zebrowitz LA, Montepare JM. Social psychological face perception: why appearance matters. Soc Personal Psychol Compass. 2008;2(3):1497.
2. Little AC, Jones BC, DeBruine LM. Facial attractiveness: evolutionary based research. Philos Trans R Soc B. 2011;366:1638–59.
3. Rhodes G, Proffitt F, Grady JM, Sumich A. Facial symmetry and the perception of beauty. Psychon Bull Rev. 1998;5(4):659–69.
4. Etcoff N. Survival of the prettiest: the science of beauty. Second ed. London: Abacus; 2000.
5. Giddon DB, Bernier DL, Evans CA, Kinchen JA. Comparison of two computer-animated imaging programs for quantifying facial profile preference. Percept Mot Skills. 1996;82:1251–64.
6. Bull R, Rumsey N. The social psychology of facial appearance. New York: Springer; 1988.
7. Klages U, Zentner A. Dentofacial aesthetics and quality of life. Semin Orthod. 2007;13(2):104–15.
8. Rhodes G. The evolutionary psychology of facial beauty. Annu Rev Psychol. 2006;57:199–226.
9. Johnston VS. Mate choice decisions: the role of facial beauty. Trends Cogn Sci. 2006;10(1):9–13.
10. Ward R, Scott NJ. Cues to mental health from men's facial appearance. J Res Pers. 2018;75:26–36.
11. Henderson JJA, Anglin JM. Facial attractiveness predicts longevity. Evol Hum Behav. 2003;24(5):351–6.
12. Giddon DB. Orthodontic applications of psychological and perceptual studies of facial esthetics. Semin Orthod. 1995;1(2):82–93.
13. Rodriguez HL Jr, Scelza MFZ, Boaventura GT, Custódio SM, Moreira EAM, Oliveria DL. Relation between oral health and nutritional condition in the elderly. J Appl Oral Sci. 2012;20(1):38–44.
14. Diego-Mas JA, Fuentes-Hurtado F, Naranjo V, Alcañiz M. The influence of each facial feature on how we perceive and interpret human faces. i-Perception. 2020;11(5):1–18.
15. Adams RB Jr, Garrido CO, Albohn DN, Hess U, Kleck RE. What facial appearance reveals over time: when perceived expressions in neutral faces reveal stable emotion dispositions. Front Psychol. 2016;7:986.
16. Kermode S, MacLean D. A study of the relationship between quality of life, health, and self-esteem. Aust J Adv Nurs. 2001;19(2):33–40.
17. Mikkelsen HT, Haraldstad K, Helseth S, Skarstein S, Småstuen MC, Rohde G. Health-related quality of life is strongly associated with self-efficacy, self-esteem, loneliness, and stress in 14–15-year-old adolescents: a cross-sectional study. Health Qual Life Outcomes. 2020;18:352.
18. Crocker J, Wolfe CT. Contingencies of self-worth. Psychol Rev. 2001;108(3):593–623.
19. Mann M, Hosman CMH, Schaalma HP, de Vries NK. Self-esteem in a broad-spectrum approach for mental health promotion. Health Educ Res. 2004;19(4):357–72.
20. Rosen JC. The nature of body dysmorphic disorder and treatment with cognitive behaviour therapy. Cogn Behav Pract. 1995;2(1):143–66.

21. Moody T, Shen VW, Hutcheson NL, Henretty JR, Sheen CL, Strober M, et al. Appearance evaluation of others' faces and bodies in anorexia nervosa and body dysmorphic disorder. Int J Eat Disord. 2017;50(2):127–38.

22. Mallinger G, Weiler A. Psychosocial risk and body dysmorphic disorder: A systematic review. J Hum Behav Soc Environ. 2020;30(8):1030–44.

23. Beilharz F, Castle DJ, Grace S, Rossell SL. A systematic review of visual processing and associated treatments in body dysmorphic disorder. Acta Psychiatr Scand. 2017;136(1):16–36.

24. Cunningham SJ, Feinmann C. Psychological assessment of patients requesting orthognathic surgery and the relevance of body dysmorphic disorder. Br J Orthod. 1998;25(4):293–8.

25. Dons F, Mulier D, Maleux O, Shaheen E, Politis C. Body dysmorphic disorder (BDD) in the orthodontic and orthognathic setting: a systematic review. J Stomatol Oral Maxillofac Surg. 2021.

26. Vulink NCC, Rosenberg A, Plooij JM, Bergé SJ, Denys D. Body dysmorphic disorder screening in maxillofacial outpatients presenting for orthognathic surgery. Int J Oral Maxillofac Surg. 2008;37(11):985–91.

27. Sinnot PM, Hunt N, Shute J, Cunningham S. Psychological support for orthognathic patients: who is doing what? J Orthod. 2020;47(3):205–12.

28. Collins B, Gonzalez D, Gaudilliere DK, Shrestha P, Girod S. Body dysmorphic disorder and psychological distress in orthognathic surgery patients. J Oral Maxillofac Surg. 2014;72(8):1553–8.

29. Häberle A, Alkofahi H, Qiao J, Safer DL, Mittermiller PA, Menorca R, et al. Body image disturbance and obsessive-compulsive disorder symptoms improve after orthognathic surgery. J Oral Maxillofac Surg. 2020;78(11):2054–60.

30. Alanko OME, Svedström-Oristo A-L, Tuomisto MT. Patients' perceptions of orthognathic treatment, well-being, and psychological or psychiatric status: a systematic review. Acta Odontol Scand. 2010;68(5):249–60.

31. Reyneke JP. Essentials of orthognathic surgery. 2nd ed. Hanover Park: Quintessence Pub; 2010. viii, 272 p.

32. Andrup M, Elenius J, Ramirez E, Sjöström M. Indications and Frequency of Orthognathic Surgery in Sweden - A Questionnaire Survey. Int J Oral Dent Health. 2015;1:019. https://doi.org/10.23937/2469-5734/1510019.

33. Espeland L, Høgevold HE, Stenvik A. A 3-year patient-centred follow-up of 516 consecutively treated orthognathic surgery patients. Eur J Orthod. 2008;30(1):24–30.

34. Venugoplan SR, Nanda V, Turkistani K, Desai S, Allareddy V. Discharge patterns of orthognathic surgeries in the United States. J Oral Maxillofac Surg. 2012;70(1):e77–86.

35. Schilbred Eriksen E, Moen K, Wisth PJ, Løes S, Klock KS. Patient satisfaction and oral health-related quality of life 10-15 years after orthodontic-surgical treatment of mandibular prognathism. Int J Oral Maxillofac Surg. 2018;47(8):1015–21.

36. Liddle MJ, Baker SR, Smith KG, Thompson AR. Psychosocial outcomes in orthognathic surgery: a review of the literature. Cleft Palate Craniofac J. 2015;52(4):458–70.

37. Prinsell JR. Maxillomandibular advancement surgery in a site-specific treatment approach for obstructive sleep apnea in 50 consecutive patients. Chest. 1999;116(6):1519–29.

38. Kloukos D, Fudalej P, Sequeira-Byron P, Katsaros C. Maxillary distraction osteogenesis versus orthognathic surgery for cleft lip and palate patients. Cochrane Database Syst Rev. 2018;8:CD010403.

39. Frid P, Resnick C, Abramowicz S, Stoustrup P, Norholt SE, Temporomandibular Joint Juvenile Arthritis Work Group T. Surgical correction of dentofacial deformities in juvenile idiopathic arthritis: a systematic literature review. Int J Oral Maxillofac Surg. 2019;48(8):1032–42.

40. Stavropoulos D, Tarnow P, Mohlin B, Kahnberg KE, Hagberg C. Comparing patients with Apert and Crouzon syndromes – clinical features and cranio-maxillofacial surgical reconstruction. Swed Dent J. 2012;36(1):25–34.

41. el-Batouti A, Ogaard B, Bishara SE. Longitudinal cephalometric standards for Norwegians between the ages of 6 and 18 years. Eur J Orthod. 1994;16(6):501–9.

42. Pogrel MA. What are normal esthetic values? J Oral Maxillofac Surg. 1991;49(9):963–9.

43. Norholt SE, Pedersen TK, Herlin T. Functional changes following distraction osteogenesis treatment of asymmetric mandibular growth deviation in unilateral juvenile idiopathic arthritis: a prospective study with long-term follow-up. Int J Oral Maxillofac Surg. 2013;42(3):329–36.

44. Hågensli N, Stenvik A, Espeland L. Extraoral vertical subcondylar osteotomy with rigid fixation for correction of mandibular prognathism. Comparison with bilateral sagittal split osteotomy and surgical technique. J Craniomaxillofac Surg. 2013;41(3):212–8.

45. Mobarak KA, Krogstad O, Espeland L, Lyberg T. Stability of extraoral vertical ramus osteotomy: plate fixation versus maxillomandibular/skeletal suspension wire fixation. Int J Adult Orthodon Orthognath Surg. 2000;15(2):97–113.

46. Schilbred Eriksen E, Wisth PJ, Løes S, Moen K. Skeletal and dental stability after intraoral vertical ramus osteotomy: a long-term follow-up. Int J Oral Maxillofac Surg. 2017;46(1):72–9.

47. Westermark A, Bystedt H, von Konow L. Inferior alveolar nerve function after mandibular osteotomies. Br J Oral Maxillofac Surg. 1998;36(6):425–8.

48. Trauner R, Obwegeser H. The surgical correction of mandibular prognathism and retrognathia with consideration of genioplasty. I. Surgical procedures to correct mandibular prognathism and reshaping of the chin. Oral Surg Oral Med Oral Pathol. 1957;10(7):677–89; contd.

49. Mobarak KA, Espeland L, Krogstad O, Lyberg T. Soft tissue profile changes following mandibular advancement surgery: predictability and long-term outcome. Am J Orthod Dentofac Orthop. 2001;119(4):353–67.

50. Tessier P. The classic reprint: experimental study of fractures of the upper jaw. 3. René Le Fort, M.D., Lille, France. Plast Reconstr Surg. 1972;50(6):600–7.

51. Dowling PA, Espeland L, Sandvik L, Mobarak KA, Hogevold HE. LeFort I maxillary advancement: 3-year stability and risk factors for relapse. Am J Orthod Dentofac Orthop. 2005;128(5):560–7. quiz 669

52. Kahnberg KE, Holmstrom H. Augmentation of a retrognathic chin. I. Use of HTR-polymer implants in a long-term prospective clinical and radiographic study. Scand J Plast Reconstr Surg Hand Surg. 2002;36(2):65–70.

53. Shaughnessy S, Mobarak KA, Høgevold HE, Espeland L. Long-term skeletal and soft-tissue responses after advancement genioplasty. Am J Orthod Dentofac Orthop. 2006;130(1):8–17.

54. Borzabadi-Farahani A. An insight into four orthodontic treatment need indices. Prog Orthod. 2011;12(2):132–42.

55. Naini FB, Moss JP, Gill DS. The enigma of facial beauty: esthetics, proportions, deformity, and controversy. Am J Orthod Dentofac Orthop. 2006;130(3):277–82.

56. Jacobsen T. Beauty and the brain: culture, history and individual differences in aesthetic appreciation. J Anat. 2010;216(2):184–91.

19

57. Beshkar M. Dentofacial deformity is not an appropriate term. J Craniofac Surg. 2013;24(6):2221.

58. Beshkar M. Malformation, deformity, and discrepancy. J Craniofac Surg. 2014;25(5):1928.

59. Dawson J. Medically optimised: healthcare language and dehumanisation. The British journal of general practice : the journal of the Royal College of General Practitioners. 2021; 71(706):224. https://doi.org/10.3399/bjgp21X715829.

60. Haque OS, Waytz A. Dehumanization in medicine: causes, solutions, and functions. Perspect Psychol Sci. 2012;7(2): 176–86.

61. Changing Faces. Media guidelines. London: Changing Faces; 2021. Available from: https://www.changingfaces.org.uk/for-the-media/media-guidelines-disfigurement/.

62. Meger MN, Fatturi AL, Gerber JT, Weiss SG, Rocha JS, Scariot R, et al. Impact of orthognathic surgery on quality of life of patients with dentofacial deformity: a systematic review and meta-analysis. Br J Oral Maxillofac Surg. 2021;59(3):265–71.

63. Pavone I, Rispoli A, Acocella A, Scott AA, Nardi P. Psychological impact of self-image dissatisfaction after orthognathic surgery: a case report. World J Orthod. 2005;6(2): 141–8.

64. Lazaridou-Terzoudi T, Kiyak HA, Moore R, Athanasios AE, Melsen B. Long-term assessment of psychologic outcomes of orthognathic surgery. J Oral Maxillofac Surg. 2003;61(5): 545–52.

65. Zhou YH, Hägg U, Rabie AB. Concerns and motivations of skeletal class III patients receiving orthodontic-surgical correction. Int J Adult Orthodon Orthognath Surg. 2001;16(1):7–17.

66. Türker N, Varol A, Ögel K, Basa S. Perceptions of preoperative expectations and postoperative outcomes from orthognathic surgery: part I: Turkish female patients. Int J Oral Maxillofac Surg. 2008;37(8):710–5.

67. Hunt OT, Johnston CD, Hepper PG, Burden DJ. The psychosocial impact of orthognathic surgery: a systematic review. Am J Orthod Dentofac Orthop. 2001;120(5):490–7.

68. Broers DLM, van der Heijden GJMG, Rozema FR, de Jongh A. Do patients benefit from orthognathic surgery? A systematic review on the effects of elective orthognathic surgery on psychosocial functioning and patient satisfaction. Eur J Oral Sci. 2017;125(6):411–8.

69. Cunningham SJ, Garratt AM, Hunt NP. Development of a condition-specific quality of life measure for patients with dentofacial deformity: I. Reliability of the instrument. Community Dent Oral Epidemiol. 2000;28(3):195–201.

70. Carr T, Moss T, Harris D. The DAS24: a short form of the Derriford Appearance Scale DAS59 to measure individual responses to living with problems of appearance. Br J Health Psychol. 2005;10(Pt 2):285–98.

71. Ni Riordain R, Glick M, Al Mashhadani SSA, Aravamudhan K, Barrow J, Cole D, et al. Developing a standard set of patient-centred outcomes for adult oral health - an international, cross-disciplinary consensus. Int Dent J. 2021;71(1):40–52.

72. Paul NR, Baker SR, Gibson BJ. Decision making from the experience of orthognathic surgery patients: a grounded theory approach. JDR Clin Trans Res. 2021:23800844211014440.

73. Royal College of Surgeons of England. Commissioning guide: orthognathic procedures. London: RCS; 2013.

Part IV

The Voice of CSA Survivors
Lena Myran and Vibeke Kranstad

What do patients who have been sexually abused think about dental treatment, and what wishes and needs do they have regarding facilitation? The quotations below are collected from a Norwegian treatment program for dental treatment for sexual abuse survivors (the TADA-project, see ► Chap. 22). User organizations have been given an opportunity to comment on the statements to ensure that the content is in line with their experiences.

About Dental Treatment
"The dental situation sometimes reminds me of the abuse."

"I feel disgusting at the dentist. I feel sorry for the dentist who has to treat me. This can make it difficult to go back to the same dentist."

"Once the dentist started on the second tooth, which we had agreed he would not work on today. It made me very uncomfortable. I had just started to trust him."

"I did not understand why going to the dentist was so difficult, until long after I finished the treatment."

"I did not tell the dentist about the abuse in the beginning. It took a while before I knew if I could trust her."

"Stopping on time was the most important thing the dentist taught me through dental treatment."

About the Communication Between Dentist and Patient
"I want the dentist to know that I have been abused. It's better that he knows, then I won't have to hide it."

"I think it's strange that no dentist has asked me if I have been abused. I want them to dare to ask."

"I can't bear to talk about the abuse with the dentist as well, but I do want her to know about it so she can deal with it."

"I understand that the dentist cannot be my psychologist. When I tell my story, the dentist can say, 'You can talk to your psychologist about this'."

"Give me the opportunity to stop the treatment if the discomfort becomes too overwhelming. Explain to me what happens if we stop."

"Don't ask, 'Are you okay?' Then I just answer 'yes' regardless of whether I am or not. Instead, ask, "What did you experience now?"

"Ask me how I'm feeling, so that we can adjust the plan if I don't feel so good."

About Facilitations During Dental Treatment
"I would like to meet everyone who will be in the room during the treatment in advance. I don't like when people I've not met come in while I'm undergoing treatment." (*)

"I do not want people surrounding the chair, especially not on both sides of me. (*)

"Accommodating my needs -such as leaving the door ajar, or letting me hold some of the equipment myself, such as the X-ray film holder and saliva suction tube, and even letting me take it out when needed – is important to me."

"Learn of my challenges with closeness and touch, to avoid standing directly behind me or accidentally pulling my hair."

"Explain to me what is going to happen and how it may feel, such as water splashes or saliva suction."

"Give explanations in advance of movements such as a supporting hand against my cheek: avoid sudden unforeseen movements."

"To be able to bring a support person who knows me well into the treatment room. This person can help me set boundaries, and also helps me to be able to attend appointments."

"A conversation before and after treatment can ease discomfort."

"Agreeing on a stop signal with me is one of the most important things a dentist can do. The stop signals that work for me are checked out in advance, so that I feel in control of the situation."

"If I dissociate, the dentist can invite me into the conversation again, help me by talking about things in the room. I may need to get out of the chair, feel my feet against the floor to help me get out of the difficult feeling more easily."

"Make deals with me – and stick to it. It calms me down."

"Plan the next session, so I don't have to wonder what we'll do next. Write down the plan, since I forget so easily."

(*) It is not always possible to carry out this facilitation. It is advisable that the dentist and the patient discuss this point, clarify expectations between them and find a solution that takes into account both the patient's experience of feeling safe and the dentist's ability to carry out the work.

After Treatment

"I will not ask for help even if I know my rights."

"Refer me to someone else if you see that I need more than you are able to facilitate."

"Inform about the possibility of the exemption card or that my therapist can write a declaration that gives rights within the National Insurance Scheme."

Professionalism

Contents

Dental Professionalism and Professional Behaviour in Practice and Education

Sandra Zijlstra-Shaw and Ronald C. Gorter

Contents

Learning Goals
- To learn about the various descriptions and definitions of professionalism
- To learn about the importance of professionalism for health care, including dentistry
- To learn about a (conceptual) model of professionalism in which four themes are described
- To learn about the importance of reflection for the development of professionalism
- To learn about education and assessment of professionalism

20.1 General Features of Professionalism

Professionalism as a term dates back to 1856, and is defined as the body of qualities or features characteristic of a profession [37]. This circular definition therefore requires definitions for professions and the qualities which make them a distinctive form of occupation.

Professions as a social form have their roots in the mediaeval guilds [1], who acquired the responsibility for the registration and training of specific, highly valued occupations. Attempts to study the professions systematically, however, did not occur until the twentieth century. This occurred at a time of increased interest in the social sciences and follows the development of the professions in the nineteenth century into a form that can be recognised today [1].

Professions are distinctive not only because their members are highly skilled but also because the profession itself controls and develops its knowledge base, and the training of its "members".

Features of professionalism are variable, individual-based and include both normative and ideological aspects. These in turn include responsibility, accountability, trust and discretion (especially in client/practitioner relations) and risk analysis and expert judgement (often seen as a part of professional competence). All of these factors are assimilated by training and socialisation via a professional culture into the identity of the professional practitioner and then used for both public benefit and that of the individual client.

Professionalism can, therefore, be seen to be the aspects of an occupation which are demonstrated not especially by what is done or produced, but more by how decisions are made and work prescribed. These aspects cover the areas of responsibility, accountability and justification. Thus, professionalism can be seen as the ability of the individual member of a profession to demonstrate their acceptance of their professional responsibility and accountability by being able to justify their actions to the patient (or client), their profession, the society in which they work, and themselves.

> In short, professionalism is the organised autonomy to carry out work which requires specific expertise, and which is justified by accountability.

Reflection is described as the means through which professionals decide the manner in which they carry out other competences such as communication and technical procedures [46]. The presence of reflection amongst the qualities inherent to professionalism therefore implies that professionalism is a second-order skill, one which is demonstrated by the way tasks are carried out and is thus one which can only be demonstrated when, as Evans [15] has stated, doing something. Verkerk et al. [53] described it as follows: Professionalism must be conceived as a second-order competence—a reflective and evaluative competence which can be expressed only via the performance of other competences.

The performance of (medical or dental) practice involving the discretionary use of expertise in situations where the outcome is uncertain often places the practitioner in a dilemma. Perhaps the key to professionalism that it is the ability to be motivated by the everyday challenge presented by having to balance uncertainty with responsibility when making decisions about the right thing, in the right way, at the right time for the right patient, and then being able to account for the actions taken. This is also expressed by Verkerk et al. [53] when they write that: A professional is someone who can explain why in this case, for this patient, the professional's behaviour or decision was appropriate. Professionalism here does not mean clinging to absolute norms or values, but implies that one is prepared to be accountable in the light of public, professional and personal norms and values.

The study of professionalism within health care provides a context in which professionalism can be elicited. The act of diagnosis, prescribing and then carrying out treatment can all be carried out in both a professional or unprofessional manner. It is the "do" which Evans [15] states is necessary for professionalism. The fact that medical expertise is not in or of itself professional, but requires to be carried out in order to demonstrate professionalism confirms professionalism as a second-order competence. Moreover, the expression of this competence depends on the autonomy given by society to professionals, who in turn must demonstrate accountability in order to maintain public trust [19, 44]. In other words, accountability lies at the heart of professionalism.

An interesting framework to categorise professionalism is described by Irby and Hamstra [24], who distinguish virtue and behaviour based on professionalism and identity formation.

Virtue-based professionalism has a focus on moral character, moral reasoning, and humanism. Appropriate action is a result of internalising the right values and ethical principles until habits are created. Behaviour-based professionalism has a focus on behaviours, milestones, and competencies. Appropriate actions are a result of clear expectations, feedback on performance, and reinforcement from external stimuli. Professional identity formation is about evolving and changing identities. Appropriate action results from the development of a professional identity by socialisation into a community of practice.

20.2 Importance of Professionalism to Health Care and Dentistry

Professionalism has become increasingly important as a core competency to practice dentistry. Throughout health care there has been a shift towards a patient-centred approach with higher expectations of health care professionals as the norm [26, 45, 49, 50].

Professionalism is consistently agreed to be an integral part of the competencies required to practice dentistry. Brown, Manogue and Rohlin [10] point out that professional attitudes are an important feature of professional life, ensuring that dental students and dentists are safe professionals who satisfy society's demands for accountability and control. The Association for Dental Education in Europe (ADEE) describes professionalism as one of its domains of competence required to practice dentistry [33].

Professionalism has become increasingly important as a core competency to practice dentistry.

Professionalism is also a sociological phenomenon, since professional status is granted by society [26]. Professionals have, therefore, an obligation to meet the requirements of the society in which they practice and as these requirements change so do the obligations.

Such professional changes in response to societal changes are clearly evident. Over the last 25 years, emphasis on professionalism has made it an increasingly important aspect of medical and dental practice. This is thought to be the result of broad societal changes that include media attention to health care, especially in respect to high-profile cases, the increased availability of information via the internet, changes in the philosophy of patient care, especially with respect to teamwork, and changes to regulatory bodies brought about by governmental pressures [26, 45, 49].

For example, patient–clinician relationships have moved from authoritarian to a more democratic patient-centred approach. Medical professionals can no longer expect passive acceptance by the public of their autonomy and authority. This has a profound effect on the relationship between health care professionals and patients [2, 25, 40]. Professional standards are increasingly questioned [11], especially with the increase in public expectations of the quality of patient care and service delivery, often led by health consumer groups [2].

The type of care provided is itself changing with the greater complexity of care needed, especially in an ageing population, and rapid expansion of medical knowledge and skills [45].

There are changes too in the philosophy of patient care with a movement away from an individual doctor/patient relationship to multidisciplinary teamwork and shared care [43]. As was already pointed at, there is also a movement towards a patient-centred approach [5]. Moreover, health care providers themselves are changing; more women are entering the professions and part-time practice is more common, along with questions about work/life balance [29], leading to the questioning of the values of self-sacrifice seen within the more traditional concepts of professionalism.

These changes have led to calls for revised regulation and challenges to professional self-regulation [26, 43]. Internal and external criticism of regulatory bodies has focussed on lack of transparency and accountability, the emergence of a stronger sense of consumerism in health care, and media coverage of a number of high-profile cases of substandard care and abuse [28]. All of these have been accompanied by greater central control within, for example, the National Health Service, with performance targets for consultants, more emphasis on clinical governance and audit, and the compilation of national treatment guidelines [43].

Within medicine a number of working parties, reports, and recommendations, whilst based on traditional values, called for more transparency, more patient involvement, an increased emphasis on reflection and an increased role for the teaching and assessment of professionalism within medical education [3, 29, 45]. These changes resulted in the publication of "Good Medical Practice" (2006b) and "Tomorrow's Doctors" (2009) by the (British) General Medical Council.

Consequently, the increased attention given to professional standards, not only by the professions themselves, but also as a response to government and general public pressure, has given rise to the current emphasis on professionalism, which in turn requires dental educators to understand precisely what is meant by "professionalism" in relation to dentistry in order to both teach and assess it. At the end of this chapter attention will be given to these educational aspects.

20.3 Dentistry as a Profession

Many of the descriptions of professionalism within dentistry are of North American origin. Within this literature the conflict between dentistry as a profession and dentistry as a commercial operation is a central theme [13, 32, 36, 54–56]. Ozar and Sokol [38], whilst describing both a commercial and a normative model of professionalism, explain that dentists have professional obligations which arise due to the obligations of the profession as a whole to the community at large. The obligation to the community is also seen in Welie's definition [54]:

> A profession is a collective of expert service providers who have jointly and publicly committed to always give priority to the existential needs and interests of the public they serve above their own interests, and in turn are trusted by the public to do so.

This conflict between dentistry as a profession and dentistry as a commercial operation is seen less in European literature. The Association for Dental Education in Europe (ADEE) describes professionalism as follows [33]:

> Professionalism is a commitment to a set of values, behaviours, and relationships, which underpin the trust that the public hold in dental care professionals.

Professional behaviour, in their view, includes appropriate behaviour towards patients, appropriate behaviour towards all the members of the dental team, knowledge of the social and psychological issues relevant to the care of patients, ability to manage and maintain a safe working environment, and knowledge and awareness of the impact of the dentist's own health on the ability to practice dentistry, alongside the need for continued professional development and education.

20.4 Themes Within Dental Professionalism

Professionalism is an essential competence to practice dentistry. However, as Shaw [47] points out, dentists may also be unprofessional in any of the areas of competence. For instance, it is possible to communicate both professionally and unprofessionally.

An overview of the health care literature on professionalism leads to the conclusion that there is no single clear discrete definition of this essential competence. However, many themes recur consistently within the descriptions of professionalism found throughout the literature. These can be divided into those seen in the traditional view of professionalism and those that appear in more contemporary views of professionalism.

Box. Themes Within Dental Professionalism

— **Theme**
  - Altruism
  - Accountability
  - Autonomy
  - Compassion
  - Excellence
  - Honesty and integrity
  - Knowledge of ethical standards
  - Moral reasoning
  - Reflection
  - Respect
  - Self-awareness
  - Self-motivation, particularly with respect to lifelong learning
  - Social responsibility
  - Trustworthiness
  - Working with others

Box. Comparison of Traditional and Contemporary Professionalism [51]

Traditional professionalism	Contemporary professionalism
Accountable to oneself	Accountable to others
Solo, individual	Partnership model, teamwork
Decision made by doctor	Shared decision making
Experience-based practice	Evidence-based practice
Attention to professional development lacking	Continuous professional development mandatory
Internal quality control	External quality control
Very gradual increase in knowledge and information	Knowledge and information overload
Cure	Care

20.5 Empirical Research and Dental Professionalism

Historically, the qualities characteristic of a profession can be summarised as the organised autonomy to carry out work, which requires specific expertise, in the interests of the common good [1, 18, 21, 34, 39].

More recently, there has been an emphasis on individual accountability and transparency [11, 16, 26, 45, 49, 50].

However, professionalism cannot be judged by behaviour alone; knowledge of the reasoning behind the action is also required [20]. In this way, professionalism is a reflective or evaluative second-order competence; in other words whilst knowledge about professionalism can be tested in written examinations, professionalism can only be demonstrated when doing something [15, 52, 53].

Therefore, whilst based on norms and core values, professionalism requires accountability for decisions taken and actions performed rather than adhering to rigid protocols. This description also explains why it is very difficult to produce a well-circumscribed description of professionalism and why it is so context dependent [4, 27, 48] as it incorporates the reasoning and motivations behind students' actions [20]. This facet of professionalism is also echoed by Hilton and Slotnik [23] who state that professionalism is learnt as a meta-skill. The fact that expertise is not in or of itself professional, but requires to be carried out in order to demonstrate professionalism further confirms professionalism as a second-order competence.

> Professionalism can be seen, therefore, as the ability of the individual member of a profession to demonstrate their acceptance of their professional responsibility and accountability by being able to justify their actions to the patient (or client), their profession, the society in which they work, and themselves. In short, professionalism is the organised autonomy to carry out work which requires specific expertise, and which is justified by accountability. Professionalism is thus both a complex construct and a second-order competence.

A qualitative study conceptualising professionalism in dentistry [57] concluded that its core is the manner in which one reflects on and reconciles different aspects of professional practice, and which demonstrates acceptance of professional responsibility and accountability. It is manifested in the manner in which work is carried out. The balance of the various aspects varies with and is appropriate to the context. Accountability means that the professional is expected to be able to justify his/her actions to the patient, the profession, the society in which they work, and themselves. Their analysis revealed

that professionalism in dentistry is conceptualised within four main themes:

- Professionalism as a second-order competence
- The expression of professionalism as dependent on context
- Professionalism encompasses personal aspects which are both tacit and overt
- Reflection as a necessary component.

These themes were then combined into a conceptual model (◘ Fig. 20.1).

The data were consistent with the construct being both multifactorial and context dependent. Furthermore, professionalism was seen as a complex construct which, in addition to being multifactorial, vague, and variable, encompassed both attitudes and behaviour.

The data confirmed professionalism as a second-order competence when it was described in relation to carrying out other competences, such as technical and communication competences. This is also seen in the work of Evans [15] where she states that professionalism can only be demonstrated when doing something.

This second-order nature of professionalism partly explains its vague nature. Not only is professionalism linked to actions, but it is also the reasoning behind those actions. This echoes the work of Verkerk et al. [53] who require professionals to be able to account for their actions, in order to reveal this second-order aspect.

20.6 Professionalism in Context

The context-dependent nature of the manifestation of professionalism was seen in many ways within the data, where professionals were described as adaptable, flexible, and responsive to the many variable needs of their patients. Professionalism was seen to vary over time, with outdated modes of professionalism being contrasted with current practice. This variation was also seen in relation to dress and professional image. Finally, the influence of both culture and institution arose in the data, with examples of the influence of colleagues and contrasts in the manifestation of professionalism by practitioners native to the UK and those of other countries. This influence and interaction of external factors relating to context is again seen as a recurring theme in the literature [22, 23, 35].

The importance of the context is also seen in the descriptions of the interface between professionalism and aspects of "Fitness to practise", i.e. rules and regu-

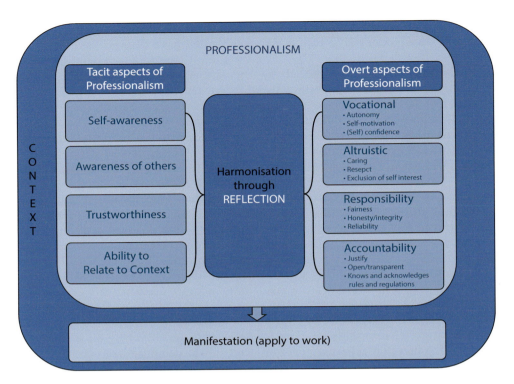

Fig. 20.1 Conceptualising dental professionalism [57]

lations, and ethics, where the resulting relationship amongst the three is described in both the data and by Shaw [47] as neither simple nor clear cut. This can be explained by seeing the "Fitness to practise" aspects as part of the external context in which professionalism is manifested.

20.7 Professionalism as a Personal Quality

The difficulties of clearly describing personal professional qualities derive from them being both tacit and overt. Trustworthiness, self-awareness, awareness of others, and the ability to relate to context are seen as being tacit in a similar manner to "tacit knowledge"; Polanyi [41] suggested that we know more than we can say. In other words, these aspects are used without conscious awareness, which makes them more difficult to transfer to another person by means of words or symbols and thus they usually require extensive personal contact along with joint or shared activities to be imparted from one person to another. Again, this observation reveals the cultural aspect of context dependence and has important consequences for dental educators as this must be taken into consideration when designing curricula.

The overt aspects of professionalism include personal qualities such as altruism and a sense of vocation, alongside autonomy, responsibility, and accountability.

These are more easily explained in verbal terms and relate to more readily interpretable behaviours.

20.8 Reflection as a Core Component

The importance of reflection as a component of professionalism is both a central theme of the data and within the literature [6–9, 14, 42, 46]. Reflection occurs as an overarching theme, an "awareness" and way of thinking that allows the practitioner to harmonise the many other factors involved in any given situation. Reflection is also seen as a means of improving professional performance by encouraging the professional to *recognise where your shortcomings actually are and to act on them"*, concurring with the literature [9, 14, 46], but in an essentially practical manner.

The application of personal qualities to a context requires harmonisation of the internal and external factors. This arises from the data as a process of reflective harmonisation, thus confirming reflection as an essential element of professionalism and leading to the definition of professionalism as the manner in which one reflects on and reconciles different aspects of professional practice and which demonstrates acceptance of professional responsibility and accountability. It is manifested in the manner in which work is carried out. The balance of the various aspects varies with and is appropriate to the context. Accountability means that the professional is expected to be able to justify his/her actions to the patient, the profession, the society in which they work, and themselves.

In order to expect from a professional to be skilled to reflect on one's behaviour, reflection should be an essential part of education. Intensified focusing on teaching reflection skills, both for teachers and students, is necessary in order to discuss professional behaviour [30]. The importance of educating and assessing professionalism will be discussed in the next paragraph.

20.9 A Word on Teaching and Assessment of Professionalism

The Association for Dental Education in Europe (ADEE), in their "Profile and Competences of a Dentist", [17], describes the domains of professionalism as follows:

> *On graduation, a dentist must be competent in a wide range of skills, including research, investigative, analytical, problem solving, planning, communication, presentation, team building and leadership skills and has to demonstrate a contemporary knowledge and understanding of the broader issues of dental practice.*

This was subsequently updated to [33]:

> *Professionalism is a commitment to a set of values, behaviours and relationships, which underpin the trust that the public hold in dental care professionals.*

In a report also published by the ADEE, the following conclusions were summarised concerning professionalism in the dental curriculum [12].

Professionalism was generally seen as being developed through observation and reflection. Assessing professionalism is challenging and the use of multiple methods and tools is encouraged for evidencing professional development, including workplace-based assessments and measures that are longitudinal and provide a better view of professionalism. Feedback and refection can strengthen the value of assessment.

Although formal curricula for professionalism have been defined, teaching and assessing professionalism is recognised as complex. Alongside the formal curriculum, mentoring, and reflective practice, role modelling and the hidden curriculum play a notable part in the development of professionalism. No one approach is most effective or successful for teaching professionalism, and thus multiple approaches are encouraged.

In a recent dissertation on how to identify, classify, and respond to unprofessional behaviour in medical students, Mak - Van der Vossen [31] summarised the current state of affairs when it comes to the teaching and assessment of professionalism in medical school, which also exemplifies very well the situation within dental education. Her summary is further summarised below.

Generally, professionalism is not thought of as an innate trait, but as a quality that can be learned and must be taught, starting in medical (or dental) school. Professionalism must be made practical and applicable in the undergraduate curriculum. Outcomes that will stimulate students' professional development include interpersonal skills, understanding of roles, capacity for teamwork, cultural competence, collegiality, respect for patients and colleagues, and ethical conduct.

To achieve these outcomes, the teaching must comprise different aspects: a cognitive basis of professionalism has to be taught, describing expectations; and by practicing, receiving feedback, and reflection, students will be stimulated to develop professionalism skills and values.

During the course of the curriculum, teaching shifts from mainly explicit addressing values, truths, and meaning, to more implicit through role playing. Practical courses, simulated and real patient contacts offer the opportunity offer students the possibility of subjectively experiencing primary events, which contribute to becoming a professional care giver. It also shows the student that becoming a professional is a process.

The influence of what is called the "hidden curriculum" is highly important in this process of professional development. The informal messages of educators, peers, and other role models, either positive or negative, influence students and will have an impact on their professional development.

When it comes to assessment of professionalism, observation is a core method. By providing feedback as formative assessment (meaning mid-course), the student is enabled to reflect on what is needed to improve and how to do this. Summative assessment (at the end of the course) can confirm that the student has reached the desired goal. Multiple methods, and multiple moments, multiple settings, and multiple assessors are essential in order to develop professional growth. Amongst the methods one may think of rating forms, Objective Structured Clinical Examinations (OSCEs), moral reasoning assessments, behavioural assessments, peer rating, etc.

When it comes to apparent unprofessional behaviour shown by a student, the phenomenon of "failure to fail" is well known. It refers to the difficulty teachers experience to fail a student, with the underlying connotation that the teacher may feel he or she has failed to teach, motivate, or create a learning environment in an effective manner for a particular student. Educators' reluctance to fail a student is unfortunate, because when underperforming students are not identified, they cannot be offered assistance to help improve their performance.

20.10 Remediation

Professionalism lapses are viewed as acts of inappropriate behaviour and reflect a lack of skill in negotiating conflict-prone situations. Irby and Hamstra [24] describe the most common professionalism lapses as follows:
1. Lapses in responsibility (e.g. late or absent, unreliable)
2. Lapses related to the health care environment (e.g. cheating, falsifying data, disrespecting other members of the team)
3. Lapses related to diminished capacity for self-improvement (e.g. arrogance, defensiveness)
4. Lapses around impaired relationships with patients (e.g. poor rapport).

Remediation strategies in educational situations often involve a system to identify lapses, meeting with the student when a lapse is observed, developing a remediation plan, and monitoring compliance with the plan. Other frequently used strategies for remediation include mandated mental health evaluation/treatment, completion of a professionalism assignment, mandated professionalism mentor, and counselling for stress or anger management.

20.11 Conclusion

In conclusion, professionalism is an essential competence required by all dental professionals. ADEE states that [33]:

> *Professional behaviour can be understood as the manner in which one reflects on and reconciles different aspects of professional practice, demonstrating acceptance of professional responsibility and account- ability. It is an overarching competence which must permeate all aspects of good dental practice and is manifested in the manner in which high-quality oral health care is provided.*

Professionalism is also a never ending, adaptive competence which is both essential and aspirational. It is essential in order to provide safe, effective patient-centred care and aspirational in that it encourages all dental care professionals to practice with a view to excellence. Finally, it is continually changing as it involves a com-

mitment to social justice which also changes with the demands of society.

Whilst what we perceive as professionalism is indeed also a reflection of changes in society and culturally influenced, at the same time the core of professionalism is as ancient as the days of Hippocrates. By declaring to obey to the Hippocratic oath the graduating dentist symbolises that patients can put their trust in him or her.

References

1. Abbott A. The system of professions. London: University of Chicago Press; 1988.
2. Allsop J. Regaining trust in medicine professional and state strategies. Curr Sociol. 2006;54(4):621–36.
3. American Board of Internal Medicine. ABIM project professionalism. Philadelphia: American Board of Internal Medicine; 1995.
4. Arnold L. Assessing professional behaviour: yesterday, today, and tomorrow. Acad Med. 2002;77:502–15.
5. Askham J, Chisholm A. Patient-Centred medical professionalism: towards an agenda for research and action. Oxford; 2006. Picker Institute
6. Atkins S, Murphy K. Reflection: a review of the literature. J Adv Nurs. 1993;18(8):1188–92.
7. Aukes L. Personal reflection in medical education. Academic thesis. University of Groningen, The Netherlands. 2008.
8. Boenink AD. Teaching and learning reflection on medical professionalism. PhD free University of Amsterdam. 2006.
9. Boud D, Keogh R, Walker D. Reflection: turning experience into learning. London: Kegan Page; 1985.
10. Brown G, Manogue M, Rohlin M. Assessing attitudes in dental education: is it worthwhile? Br Dent J. 2002;193:703–7.
11. Calman K. The profession of medicine. Br Med J. 1994;309:1140.
12. Cowpe, J., Bullock, A., Gilmour, A., et al. Professionalism: a mixed-methods research study. Report. Association for Dental Education in Europe. 2020. Available through: www.adee.org.
13. Dharamsi S, Pratt DD, MacEntee MI. How dentists account for social responsibility: economic imperatives and professional obligations. J Dent Educ. 2007;71(12):1583–92.
14. Eraut M. Developing professional knowledge and competence. London: Falmer; 1994.
15. Evans L. Professionalism, professionality and the development of educational professionals. Br J Educ Stud. 2008;56:20–38.
16. Evetts J. The sociological analysis of professionalism: occupational change in the modern world. Int Sociol. 2003;18:395–415.
17. Field JC, Cowpe JG, Walmsley AG. The graduating European dentist: a new undergraduate curriculum framework. Eur J Dent Educ. 2017;21(Suppl. 1):2–10.
18. Freidson E. Professionalism the third logic. Cambridge: Polity Press; 2001.
19. General Medical Council. Good medical practice. London: General Medical Council; 2006.
20. Ginsburg S, Regehr G, Lingard L. Basing the evaluation of professionalism on observable behaviors: a cautionary tale. Acad Med. 2004;79:S1–4.
21. Greenwood E. Attributes of a profession. Social Work. 1957;II:45–50.
22. Hafferty FW, Castellani B. A sociological framing of medicine's modern-day professionalism movement. Med Educ. 2009;43:826–8.

23. Hilton SR, Slotnick HB. Proto-professionalism: how professionalisation occurs across the continuum of medical education. Med Educ. 2005;39:58–65.

24. Irby DM, Hamstra SJ. Parting the clouds: three professionalism frameworks in medical education. Acad Med. 2016;91:1606–11.

25. Irvine D, Hafferty F. Every patient should have a good doctor. In: Bridgewater B, Cooper G, Livesey S, Kinsman R, on behalf of the Society for Cardiothoracic Surgery in Great Britain & Ireland, editors. Maintaining patients' trust: modern medical professionalism. Henley-on-Thames: Dendrite Clinical Systems Ltd; 2011. p. 64–70.

26. Irvine D. The performance of doctors. I: professionalism and self-regulation in a changing world. Br Med J. 1997;314(7093):1540–2.

27. Jha V, Bekker HL, Duffy SRG, Roberts TE. Perceptions of professionalism in medicine: a qualitative study. Med Educ. 2006;40:1027–36.

28. King's Fund. Professional regulation – briefing. London: King's Fund; 2007.

29. Levenson R, Dewar S, Shepherd S. Understanding doctors harnessing professionalism. London: King's Fund; 2008.

30. van Luijk SJ, Gorter RC, van Mook WNKA. Promoting professional behaviour in undergraduate medical, dental, and veterinary medical curricula in the Netherlands: evaluation of a joined effort. Med Teach. 2010;32:733–9.

31. Mak – Van der Vossen M. Learning from lapses. Academic thesis. Amsterdam, The Netherlands: VU University. 2019.

32. Masella RS. Renewing professionalism in dental education: overcoming the market environment. J Dent Educ. 2007;70(2):205–16.

33. McLoughlin J, Zijlstra-Shaw S, Davies JR, Field JC. the graduating european dentist—domain I: professionalism. Eur J Dental Educ. 2017;21(Suppl. 1):11–3.

34. Millerson G. *The qualifying associations*. London: Routledge and Kegan Paul Ltd.; 1964.

35. Monrouxe LV, Rees CE, Hu W. Differences in medical students' explicit discourses of professionalism: acting, representing, becoming. Med Educ. 2011;45:585–602.

36. Nash DA. On ethics in the profession of dentistry and dental education. Eur J Dent Educ. 2007;11:64–74.

37. Oxford English Dictionaries. The New Shorter Oxford English Dictionary. Oxford: Clarendon Press; 1993.

38. Ozar DT, Sokol DJ. Dental ethics at chairside, professional principles and practical applications. Washington, D.C.: Georgetown University Press; 2002.

39. Parsons T. The social system. London: Routledge and Kegan Paul Ltd.; 1951.

40. Pfadenhauer M. Crisis or decline? Problems of legitimation and loss of Trust in Modern Professionalism. Curr Sociol. 2006;54(4):565–78.

41. Polanyi M. The Tacit dimension. Reprinted University of Chicago Press 2009. New York: Anchor Books; 1967.

42. Rest JR. Research on moral development: implications for training counselling psychologists. Counsel Psychol. 1984;12:19–29.

43. Rosen R, Dewar S. On being a doctor; redefining medical professionalism for better patient care. London: King's Fund; 2004.

44. Royal College of Physicians and Surgeons of Canada. The CanMEDS physician competency framework. Ottawa: The Royal College of Physicians and Surgeons of Canada; 2006.

45. Royal College of Physicians of London. Doctors in society: medical professionalism in a changing world. Report of a Working Party of the Royal College of Physicians of London. London: Royal College of Physicians of London; 2005.

46. Schön D. The reflective practitioner how professional think in action. New York: Basic Books; 1983.

47. Shaw D. Ethics, professionalism and fitness to practise: three concepts, not one. Br Dent J. 2009;207(2):59–62.

48. Van de Camp K, Vernooij-Dassen M, Grol R, Bottema B. How to conceptualise professionalism: a qualitative study. Med Teach. 2004;6(8):696–702.

49. Van Mook WNKA, de Grave WS, Wass V, O'Sullivan H, Zwaveling JH, Schuwirth LWT, van der Vleuten CPM. Professionalism: evolution of the concept. Eur J Intern Med. 2009a;20:e81–4.

50. Van Mook WNKA, van Luijk SJ, O'Sullivan H, Wass V, Zwaveling JH, Schuwirth LWT, van der Vleuten CPM. The concepts of professionalism and professional behaviour: conflicts in both definition and learning outcomes. Eur J Intern Med. 2009b;20: e85–9.

51. Van Mook WNKA. Teaching and assessing professional behaviour: an overview and a Dutch perspective. Centre for Excellence in Developing Professionalism symposium held in Liverpool; 2010.

52. Verkerk MA, de Bree M, Jaspers F. Reflectieve professionalisering. Naar een invulling van het CCMS-competentiegebied 'Professionalisering'. Tijdschrift voor Medisch Onderwijs. 2005;24:162–7.

53. Verkerk MA, de Bree MJ, Mourits MJE. Reflective professionalism: interpreting CanMEDS' "professionalism". J Med Ethics. 2007;33:663–6.

54. Welie JVM. Is dentistry a profession? Part 1. Professionalism defined. J Can Dent Assoc. 2004;70(8):529–32.

55. Welie JVM. Is dentistry a profession? Part 2. The hallmarks of professionalism. J Can Dent Assoc. 2004;70(9):599–602.

56. Welie JVM. Is dentistry a profession? Part 3. Future challenges. J Can Dent Assoc. 2004;70(10):675–8.

57. Zijlstra-Shaw S, Robinson PG, Roberts TE. Perceptions of professionalism in dentistry – a qualitative study. Br Dent J. 2013;215:E1.

Living in a Golden Cage? Work Stress, Burnout Risk, and Engagement in Dental Practice: Background and Prevention

Ronald C. Gorter, Lena Myran and Tiril Willumsen

Contents

Note – Parts of this chapter have been published in:
D.I. Mostofsky, F. Fortune (Eds). Behavioral Dentistry (2nd ed). John Wiley & Sons. Inc., 2014.

Learning Goals

- To understand the concept of stress and how it may affect work and health
- To understand what burnout is, and how it may be experienced by dentists and dental students
- To understand how job resources may help create positive engagement in work
- To learn how to prevent burnout and how to accommodate when experiencing burnout

21.1 Introduction

The most common definition of dental erosion is "loss of the tooth's hard tissue by a chemical process that does not involve the influence of bacteria" [37]. This implies that erosion, unlike caries, occurs on a tooth surface that does not have bacterial coating. Acid attacks while there is a lack of saturation of hydroxyl and fluorapatite in saliva, causing dental substance to be lost – layer by layer – and an erosion injury occurs.

Just as we have dental erosion injuries, we can also talk about psychological erosion injuries, which occur due to small daily drips that hit us that in the same place, day after day, and can cause loss in the "hard tissue" of the psyche: empathy. For dental professionals, working under demanding situations, being exposed to patients' strong emotions, the psyche is under constant attack, causing psychological erosion – layer by layer – with loss of empathy and emotional exhaustion as a possible result.

Does work cause illness? In most publications on work and health, the emphasis is on health risks as caused by work and work circumstances. The literature on work-related illness is abundant and describes nearly every imaginable kind of physical, psychological, or social malfunctioning as explained by work-related factors. So, it is plausible to state that work does cause illness indeed.

On the other hand, awareness grows that work also provides for a positive influence on a person's life [4, 33]. There is a growing stream of literature in which the health effects of "structured, goal directed activities, of a compulsory kind" (also known as: work) are described. Occupational therapy, for instance, is a widely used means for recovery. Even more so, from studies on unemployment, we know that loss of work may lead to serious health problems, including suicide risk. Therefore, the proper conclusion is that work contains both health-threatening and health-provoking aspects.

In many people's eyes, dentists have a wonderful professional life: good income, fascinating clinical work, challenging technical developments, etc. Still, there is plenty evidence that dentists often feel "caged" in their profession. Would it be right to speak of a dental career as of a "golden cage"? It looks so attractive from the outside, but from within one feels the burden?

This chapter is divided into two parts: background and prevention. In Part I: "Background" both the health-threatening and the health-promoting aspects of working as a dentist will be described, focusing on mental health. In particular, the interplay between work stress and burnout, and work resources and positive engagement, will be discussed, using the Job Demands – Resources Model as a frame [3]. Also, some remarks on dental student stress will be given. In Part II: "Prevention" advices for burnout prevention will be given. The focus will be both on work environment and on intrapersonal processes, and how these may help to experience resilience and become less vulnerable for the demands that are put on working as a dentist.

21.2 Part I: Background

21.2.1 Stress and Work

In its original meaning, stress refers to a condition in physics where pressure is put upon tissue, to the extent that the structure of the tissue is about to be irreversibly changed (☐ Fig. 21.1).

In psychology, stress refers to the variables that influence one's well-being. This is usually meant in a negative way, distress would be the correct word, whereas it is also recognized that a certain amount of stress – eustress – is needed in order to be stimulated and achieve results. Work stress usually refers to the demanding aspects of

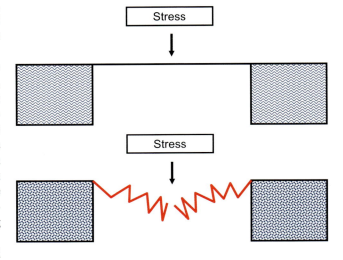

☐ **Fig. 21.1**   Stress. (Adapted from: Gibbons and Newton [12])

Living in a Golden Cage? Work Stress, Burnout Risk, and Engagement in Dental Practice: Background…

317   **21**

work that make a person feel to be "under stress." This illustrates the somewhat confusing way the word stress is used in everyday language; it is both used as a causal factor and as a result of things.

A common approach to work stress emphasizes the interaction between an individual and the work environment [24]. When an individual evaluates the (work) situation as being threatening and does not know how to deal with the threat, then stress is likely to occur. The demands of working as a dentist, such as work contents, circumstances, terms of employment, and professional relations, in combination with one's individual perception of predictability, controllability, and social support, can make identical work a nuisance for one dentist, while a joy for another [15].

Thus, one may perceive one's work and the work environment to be demanding, and yet feel perfectly able to deal with the circumstances (coping). Work pressure is not only to be found in an overload of work, it can also be the result of a lack of fit between one's personal capacities or ambitions. Things become difficult when one no longer feels capable of managing them, for instance, as a result of lack of energy. In other words, there is an interaction between the demands one is confronted with and the available resources one has. The perception of this interaction is highly subjective; one's personal interpretation of demands and resources is decisive for one's well-being. Demands and resources may be in or out of balance (◘ Fig. 21.2).

As stated above, one performs best with a certain amount of tension or stress. Too little challenge can also be experienced as stressful. Having to deal with a chronic overload or a chronic lack of challenge may result in health complaints; physical complaints, negative thoughts, mood problems, changes in social relations or changing behavior are symptoms that often coincide with being under chronic stress.

21.2.2 The Job Demands–Resources Model

An often used model to describe the interplay between demands and resources in the work setting is the Job Demands–Resources model [3, 32]. At the starting point of the Job Demands – Resources model is the assumption that, regardless of the type of job, psychosocial work characteristics can be categorized into two groups: job resources and job demands. Job demands refer to those aspects of a job that require sustained physical and/or psychological effort and are therefore associated with certain physiological and/or psychological costs. Job resources refer to the physical, psychological, social, or organizational aspects of a job that: (a) may reduce the negative effects of job demands, (b) are functional in achieving work goals, and (c) stimulate personal growth, learning, and development [22].

The interplay between job demands and resources may result in either health impairment, or motivation, to a certain extent (◘ Fig. 21.3). Prolonged experience of job demands, without sufficient buffering work resources, may result in professional burnout, which is to be described below. Alternatively, when job demands are dealt with adequately, and work resources are plenty, positive engagement may be the result. Engagement will also be further described below. It is also understood that demands and resources have cross-over effects on engagement and burnout.

21.2.3 Burnout

A possible reaction to chronic work stress is burnout [25]. Burnout is defined as:
(a) A state of emotional exhaustion
(b) In which one becomes cynical about one's recipients of care
(c) Feels less is accomplished in work

The Maslach definition has been leading in burnout research ever since its introduction in the early 80s, but very recently, a promising renewed conceptualization of burnout was developed by Schaufeli and colleagues [34]. Four core dimensions were described, three of which refer to the inability to invest energy (i.e., exhaustion,

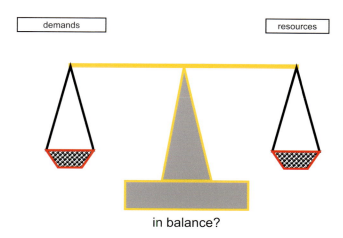

◘ Fig. 21.2 Balance between demands and resources

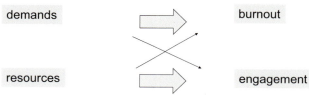

◘ Fig. 21.3 The Job Demands–Resources model

cognitive, and emotional impairment) and one referring to the unwillingness to invest energy (i.e., mental distance). Moreover, three atypical secondary dimensions were distinguished that often co-occur with the core symptoms (i.e., depressed mood, psychological distress, and psychosomatic complaints). This clustering into core and secondary dimensions is unique in the sense that the previous literature usually focused on burnout as either mere exhaustion or as a syndrome consisting of two or three dimensions. Parallel to this new conceptualization, a new burnout measure was developed, the Burnout Assessment Tool (BAT). While the most commonly used burnout instrument – the Maslach Burnout Inventory (MBI) – suffers from certain methodological flaws, the BAT may very well appear to become the standard instrument for burnout measurement in the future.

Burnout should be considered as a process; it is not so much a state of being burned out or not. Metaphorically speaking, burnout is like trail leading downhill of which one realizes he or she is upon it when already quite a distance going down. In another metaphor, one could speak of a battery still providing energy for light, but not receiving any input, and therefore running empty. In essence, burnout occurs to those dedicated to their job, willing to give much, and often not realizing or ignoring the fact that "the candle burns at both ends." The dedicated professional realizes that all energy is used when this already is a fact. One is used to a pattern of demanding so much of oneself that the thought of postponing things or restrict oneself otherwise never occurs, or is ignored.

21.2.4 Positive Engagement

In recent years, research is also focusing on what is called positive psychology of work, in addition to a long history of studying health-threatening aspects of work. Work engagement is described as a multidimensional construct, defined as a positive, fulfilling, work-related state of mind that is by vigor, dedication, and absorption [32].

1. Vigor is characterized by high levels of energy and mental resilience while working, the willingness to invest effort in one's work, and persistence even in the face of difficulties.
2. Dedication is characterized by a sense of significance, enthusiasm, inspiration, pride, and challenge.
3. Absorption is characterized by being fully concentrated and deeply engrossed in one's work, whereby time passes quickly and one has difficulties with detaching oneself from work.

Although conceptually apparently the opposite of burnout – also consisting of three underlying dimensions – research indicates that burnout and engagement can be present in a professional at the same time to a certain degree [13].

21.2.5 How Do These Processes Appear Among Dentists?

To illustrate the process of a dedicated professional in dentistry turning into a burnout victim, the dentist's story in ▶ Box 21.1 is illustrative.

Box 21.1   A Dentist's Story

I graduated when I was 24, so now I have been a dentist for 15 years. As a student, I was already used to working quick and efficiently. When I graduated, the banks were all too keen to loan me money so I could start a brand new practice.

From the moment I started in my practice, I had one focus: all attention is for the patient. I did not pay much attention to creating a nice atmosphere for my staff, since I thought that everything that was not focused upon the patients' needs was of secondary importance.

When patients had to wait, I felt stressed because I kept them waiting. And with pain it was even worse; in this profession you cannot avoid to sometimes cause pain. But, it was as if I felt that pain myself. That's the strange thing in our profession: you are a "good" dentist when you haven't hurt the patient, even when that means your treatment wasn't optimal.

It's in my nature to want to do everything myself. If I had others do things, I always had to check it myself and

do it over anyway, so I was used to doing it myself straight away. Especially so in my solo practice of course. But also in my private life I tend to be the first person that stands up when something has to be done. I am active in several community organizations, and also there I feel responsible that everything is done well.

At home I become more and more irritated. When I woke up, I already felt tired. Because I have to look in patients' mouths in a concentrated way, I got eye problems. In the evening I could not stand watching TV after work. When we went on holidays as a family, it always took me days and days before I was used to big wide open space around me. And at the end of the holidays, when I was finally relaxed, I hated it that I had return to all these little mouths.

I had had a slight pain on my chest before. My physician advised me to slow down, but you know, our clinic agenda is always full. And I was used to being harsh to myself, I have always been. No staying home when you

Living in a Golden Cage? Work Stress, Burnout Risk, and Engagement in Dental Practice: Background...

319

21

have the flu for me, you just take a pill. When others called sick, I always thought they were not suited to be a dentist. So I continued in the same way.

I must say my social environment did warn. My family, some friends. They saw me running and running. And also noticed my changing mood. I got angry outbursts more often, was irritated more easily. But I denied their remarks.

Then, one day, I broke. It was in busy time before the end of the year, after which some health insurance policies would change. So many patients wanted to have something fixed under the old policies. One patient called by telephone with a simple question about this insurance

change. And I went mad! I kicked at the wall, shouted to the patient through the phone, yelled at my assistant! And then I broke out in tears, and I went home...

I had given everything I had for my patients for 15 years. And now I could no longer. That was so emotional. I have been out of practice for more than half a tear. I had professional therapists counseling, and I used some medication. Then I slowly started to start working on a therapeutic basis. Together with my wife I am trying to work out changes in our life pattern. My life has been out of balance for so long, I cannot get that back in balance at once. I am happy we had professional help, this is something you cannot fix yourself.

21.2.6 Burnout Profiles

One could raise the question whether the burned out dentist is characterized in one typical way, or that a variety of profiles of burned out dentists exists. From a series of interviews with dentists suffering from burnout-related complaints, rather than one typical type of "the" burned out dentist, five typical profiles could be derived [14]. The dentist as portrayed in ▶ Box 21.2 would be a typical example of the "frantic runner."

Box 21.2 Burnout Profiles of Dentists

The Treadmill Walker

This dentist is caught in the daily, repetitive routine of dental practice. He can see no way out and is resigned to his fate. He can see few career options and he feels that his professional development is at an end.

The Crushed Idealist

The crushed idealist is the disillusioned dentist. His image of dental practice has been crushed by the reality of clinical practice and can see no way forward in his career.

The Frantic Runner

This type of dentist tries to pack more and more into an already busy schedule. He has the tendency to become physically and emotionally exhausted.

The Disgusted Dentist

This dentist has come to dislike every aspect of dental practice. He realized at an early stage in his career that he had chosen the wrong profession. He finds it difficult to interact with his patients and yearns for retirement.

The Depressed Dentist

This type of dentist is miserable and unhappy. He finds no rest from his depressed state whether at home or at work. He neglects his family, colleagues, and patients and finds little satisfaction in any aspect of his lifestyle.

21.2.7 Demanding Work Aspects in Dentistry

There is a steady line of research on job demands in dentistry throughout the last decades (e.g., [7, 9, 10, 15]). And although specific aspects may differ by country, certain factors of the dental work environment appear to be identified so regularly that they can be considered at the core of job demands for dentists (▶ Table 21.1).

Table 21.1 Work demands in dental practice

Practical management	Working solitarily
Difficult patients	Lack of recognition
Physical pressure	Lack of career perspective
Routine	Time pressure
Changes (micro/macro)	Restrictions to free-entrepreneurship
Fear of lawsuit	

Again, the list in ◲ Table 21.1 is not exhaustive. Some of these factors have shown to be relevant in explaining burnout among dentists. Lack of career perspective, difficult patient contacts, and general work pressure appeared to be strongly related to a high burnout risk among dentists. Also unfulfilled expectations one had at the start of a career explained differences in burnout among dentists to a high degree. On the other hand, research also showed that the more specialized dentists are, the lower the burnout levels found [10, 20].

21.2.8   Burnout and Health Complaints

Research among dentists shows that there is a strong and significant relation between burnout and physical complaints. Although no clear cause and effect can be determined, given the cross-sectional design of most research, the correlations between physical and psychological conditions are univocal. Dentists who were identified with a high burnout risk reported statistically significant more (physical) health complaints than their colleagues with a low burnout risk [17].

In many cases, when one becomes mentally exhausted, bodily tensions are felt more intensely. On the other hand, when one suffers from a growing number of physical complaints, it costs more mental energy to continue what one is doing. Therefore, the causal relation is difficult to determine. Nonetheless, both processes seem to play a role among dentists with a burnout risk.

The dental profession is known for its demanding character with regard to physical aspects. Every dentist will know by experience how often patient treatment is done while keeping one's body in unnatural postures. Working on the upper front teeth with indirect sight is just one example of this. In addition to this, generally speaking, the lack of sufficient attention for ergonomics in the dental curricula, and the ingredients are there for a career in which one's body is gradually undermined. Even though dentists can be regarded as a relatively healthy professional group, when compared to professions with a lower socio-economic status, musculoskeletal and cardiovascular complaints are widespread among the profession [6]. Also ear and eye complaints are common among dentists. Given the high correlation between physical complaints and burnout risk, increasing attention for the prevention of physical discomfort may also be useful in burnout prevention.

21.2.9   Job Resources

Just as work demands show a correlation with burnout, the Job Demands – Resources model assumes that stim-

◲ **Table 21.2**   Job resources in dental practice

Seeing good results	Grateful patients
Succesful diagnose and treatment	Completing interesting restaurations
Relieving patients' pain	Gaining patients' trust
High quality of work	Working with head, hands and heart
Fixing problems	Seeing patients laugh again

ulating aspects from the work environment, also labeled job resources, show a correlation with engagement. Job resources have been investigated among dentists, and factors such as immediate and long-term results of work, aesthetics, and working with patients do show strong relations with engagement [16, 21] (◲ Table 21.2).

21.2.10   The Job Demands–Resources Model Among Dentists

As was already indicated above, lack of career perspective, difficult patient contacts, and general work pressure are among the major job demands that explain differences in burnout levels among dentists. Also certain job resources appeared to explain differences in engagement levels among dentists; engagement was influenced by treatment results, doing well toward patients, and the joy of manual – technical work [18].

Dentists reporting to do their work with a certain idealism show higher engagement levels. It is acknowledged that there is an overlap between terms such as idealism and, for instance, dedication, which may partly explain this relation. Experiencing satisfaction from the results of their work is a strong job resource among male dentists which explains higher engagement, whereas the same goes for female dentists with regard to receiving satisfaction from patient care. Aspects such as entrepreneurship and material benefits show a relatively low correlation with engagement among dentists.

A lack of career perspective, which was among the job demands list, showed a strong predictive value for burnout risk. From a different perspective, it shows that those dentists not characterized by a lack of career perspective show higher engagement levels (and lower burnout levels) [10, 18].

When mean levels are discussed, it is always important to underline that individual differences may not be neglected. What is seen as a burden for one dentist may be a joy for another one. Take for example patient contacts, which may be troublesome for some, and can be the core of satisfaction in work for others. The same

21

Living in a Golden Cage? Work Stress, Burnout Risk, and Engagement in Dental Practice: Background...

321

21

goes for entrepreneurship, which may be exciting and challenging for some, but a real worry for others.

There is evidence that burnout levels among dentists differ between males and females [15]. While among male dentists, the middle-aged group (roughly ages 40–55) shows highest mean scores, among females the first 10 years of practice (roughly ages 25–35) appear most vulnerable. Depending on the situational context, a certain selection mechanism plays a role in explaining this difference. In many countries, the male dentist is the principal family cost winner, which leaves little opportunity for diminishing one's working hours. Female dentists often combine work with family responsibilities, and choose to work less hours when children are still young. Those females who succeed in organizing work and private life best are usually not the ones with burnout risk.

In many countries, there is a shift in percentages of females working as a dentist, in the sense that more females will graduate as a dentist than males. Also the traditional gender roles with regard to principal cost winner and family care are shifting. This will affect the way in which dentistry is practiced, organization wise, with probably more people working part time. As a result, this will also affect burnout outcomes among dentists in the near future.

21.2.11 Person Environment Fit

At the beginning of this chapter, it was already pointed out that individual differences are decisive when it comes to describing burnout risk. A common term in organizational psychology to refer to this is the person environment fit. When there is no fit between an individual professional, such as a dentist, and the working environment, one speaks of a "mismatch." This mismatch is a subjectively experienced matter, as a situation of chronic imbalance in which the job demands outweigh the dentist's ability to function satisfactorily and provides less satisfaction than a dentist needs [26]. Instead of a single root cause for burnout, such as emotional overload, six types of person–job mismatches are considered to be potential sources of burnout:

1. Work overload (one has to do too much in too little time with too few resources)
2. Lack of control (no opportunities to make choices and decisions or to use solving problem abilities)
3. Lack of reward (inadequate job resources)
4. Lack of community (a loose and unsupportive social fabric, social isolation, and chronic and unresolved problems)
5. Lack of fairness (employees are inequitably treated and respect and self-worth are not confirmed)
6. Value conflict (the requirements of the job do not agree with personal principles)

21.2.12 Dental Students and Stress

Stress among dental students has been topic of study frequently during the last decades (e.g., [1, 11, 30]). Most studies show that the dental school environment is particularly demanding for students with regard to examinations, clinical requirements, patients, financial problems, lack of time for relaxation, and faculty feedback or criticism. These dental school-related demands appear to be stable in time and region, since they have been reported by dental students since the 80s until very recently, regardless of geographical position. Some studies indicate a difference in experienced stress between preclinical and clinical years, whereas also sex differences are reported. These differences may vary per region or period.

A few studies have also picked up dental students' burnout risk [8, 19, 23, 29]. From these studies, it can be learned that while still at dental school, burnout risk is a serious phenomenon. From year one to graduation, there is a growing percentage of students that suffer from burnout risk. Some students try to cope with study stress by consuming cigarettes, alcohol, or drugs in alarming quantities. Even while at the relatively young age of a student, experienced stress was strongly related to physical complaints.

An important aspect with regard to dental student stress concerns its possible relation with future professional stress as a dentist. In fact, how one copes with stress at dental school may be indicative for how one copes with stress in dental practice. Studies that examine these relations are, however, scarce. Neither is much known about successful stress prevention or intervention at dental school. Rather than another examination of perceived stress factors during dental education, future research should focus on these relatively unexplored fields.

21.3 Part II: Prevention

21.3.1 Warning Signs of Exhaustion

A day in the dental office is busy with many consultations, demanding dental procedures while constantly looking after the patients' perspective and needs. Earlier in this chapter, the link between burnout, adverse health habits and poor health in dentists was described [17], it can also be pointed at that symptoms can start early in dentists' professional careers [35]. The experience of being delayed, causing discomfort/pain to patients, having high workload pressures, waiting for patients who arrive too late, treating patients who are anxious/afraid and doing treatment on patients that are difficult to communicate with are all factors that contributed greatly to the stress among dentists [27]. In a Norwegian study, it was found that performing preservative dental treatment on young children was stressful, especially in younger dentists [31].

It is therefore of great importance to have knowledge of symptoms and signs of exhaustion. It is important to focus on how this can be avoided throughout one's professional life. Working with people in a real, empathetic, and accepting way will make dental staff both affected and emotionally activated. The question therefore is not *whether* one is affected, but *how* one is affected and what to do about it. The stronger the patient's feelings are, the stronger the transference to the dentist. This, in turn, gives stronger countertransference to the patient. It is close to imagine that the more stressed and tired the dentist is, the greater the effect of the transference. The intensity of emotions can become a problem if they become too strong for the dental professional.

Zachrisson [36] describes how this can be expressed in a psychotherapeutical situation, which may also be illustrative for the dental context:

- The therapist dreads to the hours, is unusually concerned with the patient between hours, begins to argue with the patient in the appointments or is emotionally wounded by the patient's criticism.
- The therapist makes mistakes with appointments, times, or feels anxious about making mistakes.
- The therapist is overwhelmed by fatigue, helplessness, or a feeling of powerlessness.
- The therapist has difficulty finishing hours or is too "kind" to the patient.

► **Example**

Nils is a caring dentist who is employed at a large dental clinic. He has a lot to do and has a good reputation for being calm and good with patients with dental anxiety. He fells a pressure towards how many patients he treats and how much money this generates. He has two daughters of 15 and 17 years. For a period of time, he receives many patients referred from an abuse center in the municipality. He finds this rewarding but also tiring and it takes a lot of time. The employer is referring to increasing his earnings, which he finds difficult when working with this patient group. He receives signs of burnout and describes how the process evolved from early strain to congestion. "I realized afterwards that it all started with the job getting a little too close to my everyday life. I had even started having daughters at the age that my patients (who had been raped), were in. I worked longer and longer days, there was less time for exercise and pleasant activities. I no longer managed "small talk" with new people (thought signs). I slept badly, could wake up with nightmares (physiological signs). Drank more often wine to fall asleep in the evening. Eventually I started to feel stings in my chest and became worried about whether I had heart disease- something my GP could debunk (physiological signs). I eventually also had to consult a physiotherapist for a lock in the neck (physiological signs). I realized I should talk to someone about this but was ashamed of not being able to handle it myself - I didn't want anyone to know I couldn't handle the work (emotional impact). Eventually, me and my GP decided I needed a sick leave, I could not go to work anymore". ◄

When talking about burnout prevention, one always has to realize two things. Firstly, there is usually no clarity about cause and effect; is the dentist exhausted because he/she always faces a full waiting room, or is this dentist already exhausted and therefore experiences his/her full waiting room to be a burden? Any adaptation should therefore be aimed at both the person and his environment. Secondly, there is no guaranteed success formula to extinct work stress. On the other hand, if a dentist structurally neglects obvious precautions, he or she should not be surprised to find himself seriously exhausted at some point in his or her career (► Box 21.3).

Box 21.3   Stress and Burnout Prevention Measures

Identification and acknowledgement of work demands. Although possibly too obvious, this is the starting point for stress prevention. Too often family, friends, or even colleagues have given warning signs that a dentist appears to be under stress, that have been denied. All starts with the realization that work is too much demanding. Unfortunately, the professional culture in dentistry seems to take it for granted that always something extra should and will done by the professional, and is not inviting for a dentist to openly express his worries about his own functioning.

Learning to relax. When a dentist is under pressure, his balance between demands and resources is disturbed, both physically, mentally, and often also socially. Learning to relax both inside and outside the work situation can bring great relief. In a physical sense, attention for one's posture while at work may reveal that one tends to structurally keep his muscles tight of fixate one's neck. Mentally, a change in interpretation of events can be very helpful; when a patient does not show up for an appointment it usually frustrates a dentist, whereas this also can be embraced as a welcome moment to spend some time on

Living in a Golden Cage? Work Stress, Burnout Risk, and Engagement in Dental Practice: Background…

323   **21**

other things, such as administration or a cup of coffee. And socially, in a busy practice, patient needs are prevailing, naturally. But paying attention to and taking measures for a good team spirit is equally necessary in order to function well (and prevent early staff drop-out).

Time management and organization of work. In most dental curricula, traditionally, little to no time was reserved for practice management. In modern curricula, this aspect is getting some attention, although it will never be more than "an introduction to." Difficulty with practice management-related aspects of work is one of the key causes for experiencing work pressure among dentists. The positive side of this notion is that practice management difficulties are well solvable, if paid attention.

Realistic professional expectations. Some dentists, keen on being a free-entrepreneur, have become disappointed because of all the rules and regulations that exist in health care. Others, with the aim to help others in need, have become disillusioned because often patients do not show their gratitude, but instead, take all efforts for granted, or worse, are difficult when it comes to paying the bill. Working in a patient's mouth is different from tinkering in a hobby room. While perfectionism is a characteristic strongly present among dentists, in a dental practice the perfect solution is often not the realistic one, frustratingly. Once again, attention for career expectations is highly underdeveloped in most dental curricula.

Social skills. Most modern curricula pay attention to dentist – patient communication skills. Ideally, this is done not only theoretically, but in communication skills practice courses where students receive professional feedback on their performance. Since dentistry is a profession in which communicating with – sometimes emotionally vulnerable – patients play such an important role, also for graduated dentists, training one's skills is highly useful. And apart from the patient aspect, staff communication skills are also on the basis of good practice management.

Healthy lifestyle. Nothing is as an overworked subject as healthy life style, when looking at stress prevention advice. But, nothing may be as effective either. Eating and drinking habits, physical exercise, nightly rest, breathing fresh air, taking time off, occasional change of routine, etc. Any of these aspects, and more, do make a difference when it comes to balancing demands and resources.

Collegial contacts. In many practices around the world, dentists act alone, only supported by an assistant. Feedback from a colleague upon one's achievement is often missed. Patients may take excellent work for granted and will only respond when they have a complaint. Reflections upon how one plans his practice and his career, his future expectations, or how to deal with a patient, or staff member, are not shared by others. Especially younger, starting dentists would benefit from a regular consult with an experienced colleague, as a mentor providing feedback.

Dental schools. It was mentioned above a few times already, but dental curricula can play an important role in burnout prevention. Paying attention to student stress while still at dental school may help an individual student learn how to cope with stressful situations. Practice management and patient communication skills are some aspects already mentioned that are decisive when it comes to being prepared for practice. Schools may also focus on these topics in their program for postgraduate education.

21.3.2 How to Take Care of Yourself as a Dental Professional

It is safe to assume that dental professionals are less likely to experience greater emotional strains than health professionals who work closely with violence practitioners, abuse victims, or in child protection services. However, it is appropriate that dental professionals know of risk factors for overload, so that one can prevent experiencing it. It is also important to recognize warning signals so that action can be taken at an early stage and thus avoid persistent and unnecessary late side effects.

There are several known risk factors for the development of a "worn out" state. If a dentist repeatedly hears stories of violence and abuse and work independently without guidance, he or she can be more vulnerable. If one's work involves an empathetic presence to the patient's painful history and one works with people who behave offensively, there is an increased risk. If one has a recurrent feeling of inadequacy, that one does not reach the standard (high requirements for your own work), one may be at risk.

What measures are most appropriate depends entirely on the cause of the overload as well, as how **charged** one is. In any case, the following measures can be useful to know, and act as both preventive and therapeutic measures if you experience a persistent strain:

21.3.2.1 Putting Words on Thoughts and Feelings

Putting into words the feelings that pop up and think out loud with someone one trusts is the most important strategy to prevent emotional **exhaustion**. To handle one's own reactions, it is important to recognize them. Many health workers struggle with their reactions alone and are reluctant to talk to anyone about their thoughts and feelings. Often one goes to great lengths to bury the doubt that one does not **do** it. Recognizing one's own feelings of shame, helplessness and inadequacy can be liberating to the person in question [5]. When one is most burdened and in doubt, the thoughts inside one's head sound convincing. If, on the other hand, one is challenged to say the thoughts out loud, many immediately become aware of the incongruity of the content.

Many health care workers also express how liberating it is to hear about each other's experiences, fallibility, and experience of vulnerability. The advice may sound simple, but how does one really start talking about what is difficult? The thing to do is finding someone one trusts think along without ridiculing or condemning. An opening line might be: "It's something I need to help understand" or "It's something I wonder so badly about that bothers me." The earlier one manages to give words to one's feelings the better it is.

21.3.2.2 Seeking Guidance

One may want to seek guidance from management or seek support from experienced colleagues. Through guidance, one has the opportunity to develop knowledge and become more confident in working on difficult issues. In order to prevent exhaustion, it is important to get guidance not only on both case and process, that is, both case/solution, but also on what the patient does to you as a professional. Examples of process may include putting words on transference and countertransference (see Chap. 4), experience of being inadequate or helpless. It is important to break out the **insulation**, break with the taboo of being clever. It is not only perfectly normal to make mistakes, but also a necessary **prerequisite** for being in development and learning. The earlier one seeks guidance, the better it is. Eriksen and Sæthre (2012) describe good questions to get to know their own reactions and personal vulnerability:

— "How do you notice that a patient you're working with overwhelms you?"
— "In what way do you think your colleagues can feel it on you?"
— "What do you need from your colleagues when you feel like that?"

21.3.2.3 Increasing Your Knowledge

Strengthening one's own theoretical and clinical knowledge makes someone better equipped to understand and manage both patient and own reactions and will be one of the best ways to protect yourself from exhaustion. Increased knowledge can prevent helplessness.

21.3.2.4 Sources to Gain Powers

"The best advice we give to our colleagues regarding their privacy is to have one" ([28] p.166). Art, culture, practical work, and socializing, all activities that seem immersive and make one forget about work are general recommendations that provide opportunities for replenishment and vitalization. Another source of gaining power is to ensure basic needs for sleep, food, and physical activity. The body's needs are downgraded when living under stress and are the first to slip through prolonged strain. Good questions one can ask oneself can be:
— "What is my source of energy and excess?"
— When was the last time to forget about time and place?"

21.3.2.5 Reducing Exposure

Another strategy deals with reducing exposure to what drains one of power. This may be having fewer patients that put you emotionally out of action, ask one's boss for varied tasks, or take the hardest patients at the best possible time for. Think of it as a mastery plan and fill in the section "my arrangements" – to ensure that one's needs are taken care of in the working life.

► **Example**

Nils who we met in the previous paragraph can tell that he would not be besides the overload. "'I've now relaxed about meeting *the wall, I can't die from it! I have realized that I had normal reactions to abnormal loads. I'm not crazy or weak, I'm completely normal. I now know what my limits are so that I can prevent so that I don't get a kink like last time. The importance of getting guidance* has *been great, I have now* become good at *sorting in what is about* me and what is *not. The most important thing I bring into my everyday life now is talking to others every time I burn inside with something that bothers me. I'll take the heaviest patients Tuesday morning, not Friday afternoon like I did before. I often pat myself on the shoulder and think "yes, you've done a little bit, more you don't get done this time."* ◄

21.3.3 Enrichment and Traumatic Growth: Implications

Challenging patient treatment and periods of stress can also give rise to good coping experiences for the dentist. This is called traumatic growth. Most patients will be easy to collaborate with and give an experience of mastery and satisfaction. At the same time, the **outgoing** treatment sequences can also provide positive personal changes for those who are processing. The changes can have an impact on increased personal strength, better relationships with other people, new priorities, and increased spiritual awareness. Arnold [2] found that practitioners who worked with trauma victims reported experience of increased sensitivity, insight, tolerance, and empathy. Some may experience an appreciation of what oneself has in life, others describe a deeper recognition of man's strength and resilience.

The paradoxal effect of learning about psychological trauma and trauma-sensitive care is that one will develop a new set of glasses, and one will start seeing the world and one's traumatized patients in a trauma-sensitive way, making one vulnerable for powerful impressions and strong impacts. The difficult patient becomes the scared patient. The troublesome patient becomes the traumatized patient.

Conclusion

As it appears, there are many factors in the dental environment that may provoke a feeling of being trapped in a "cage." From the outside, it may look shiny and golden, but from the inside one experiences being caught, with little possibilities to open the door. Still, dental work offers many possibilities to create a fitting match between what one hopes to find in professional life and how it actually looks like. The crucial element is that one has to actively work on achieving this right balance between expectations and reality. Even from dental school onwards, every dentist will benefit from evaluating on a regular basis to what extent personal needs are met in professional life, and what is needed. In this chapter, a wide variety of points of attention are given that may be of help. The "golden cage" may have more doors that can be opened than one thinks.

Box 21.4

by Roslyn McMullan, retired orthodontist at NHS. It was 11 am and the dentist was just emerging from the surgery in search of some human interaction, a seat by the window and a coffee. It had been a successful morning so far. All patients had turned up on time and, despite patient's and dentist's anxiety, a first-stage RCT had gone well.

As she opened the door, she heard a commotion at the reception. It was a patient loudly and aggressively telling the receptionist that the practice was most unhelpful in suiting her need for an immediate routine check-up appointment. The coffee and seat were all behind the reception desk. "Oh well, never mind," she thinks as she quietly retreats back into the surgery, hoping she wasn't noticed, leaving the receptionist to placate the patient.

A number of months ago, at a practice meeting, it had been suggested that they would benefit from a Mental Wellbeing Lead. "We are all getting quite stressed these days" was the chorus. "Let's build wellbeing into our daily routines." One of the dental nurses expressed an interest and she had just completed her Mental Health Awareness and First Aid training. She was due to do a 4-h structured training on suicide prevention in 4 weeks' time.

She too heard the commotion, but instead of hiding away until it was all over, she had learnt to recognize the patient's distress. She came and stood alongside and quietly asked, "Mrs Smith, are you all right?". "I'm fine," came the snapped retort. She quietly asked again, "Mrs Smith, are you all right?", and this time the patient turned with tears in her eyes and gave no reply. The nurse said, "Let's go and get a cup of coffee while the receptionist finds a space for you in the appointment book, and we can have a chat."

So it was the mental wellbeing lead and the patient who had human interaction and a cup of coffee beside the window, and as a result the patient made an appointment to visit her doctor and a long overdue phone call to relate.

References

1. Alzahem AM, van der Molen HT, Alaujan AH, Schmidt HG, Zamakhshary MH. Stress amongst dental students: a systematic review. Eur J Dent Educ. 2011;15:8–18.
2. Arnold D, Calhoun LG, Tedeschi R, Cann A. Vicarious posttraumatic growth in psychotherapy. J Humanist Psychol. 2005;45(2):239–63.
3. Bakker AB, Demerouti E. The job demands-resources model: state of the art. J Manag Psychol. 2007;22:309–28.
4. Bakker AB, Schaufeli WB, Leiter MP, Taris TW. Work engagement: an emerging concept in occupational health psychology. Work & Stress. 2008;22:187–200.
5. Berge T. Secondary traumatization, temporary traumatizing and caring stress. Journal of Norsk Psycologists' association 2005;42(2):125–7.
6. Burke FJT, Main JR, Freeman R. The practice of dentistry: an assessment for premature retirement. Br Dent J. 1997;182:250–4.
7. Collin V, Toon M, O'Selmo E, et al. A survey of stress, burnout and well-being in UK dentists. Br Dent J. 2019;226:40–9. https://doi.org/10.1038/sj.bdj.2019.6.
8. Collin V, O'Selmo E, Whitehead P. Stress, psychological distress, burnout and perfectionism in UK dental students. Br Dent J. 2020;229:605–14. https://doi.org/10.1038/s41415-020-2281-4.
9. Cooper CL. Job satisfaction, mental health, and job stressors among general dental practitioners in the UK. Br Dent J. 1987;162:77–81.

10. Denton DA, Newton JT, Bower EJ. Occupational burnout and work engagement; a national survey of dentists in the United Kingdom. Br Dent J. 2008;205(7):E13.

11. Garbee WH Jr, Zucker SB, Selby GR. Perceived sources of stress among dental students. J Am Dent Assoc. 1980;100:853–7.

12. Gibbons D, Newton T. Stress solutions for the overstretched. London, UK: British Dental Journal; 1998.

13. González-Romá V, Schaufeli WB, Bakker AB, Lloret S. Burnout and work engagement: independent factors or opposite poles? J Vocat Behav. 2006;68:165–74.

14. Gorter RC. Burnout among dentists; identification and prevention. Academic thesis. Amsterdam: University of Amsterdam; 2000.

15. Gorter RC, Albrecht G, Hoogstraten J, Eijkman MAJ. Work place characteristics, work stress and burnout among Dutch dentists. Eur J Oral Sci. 1998;106:999–1005.

16. Gorter RC, te Brake JHM, Hoogstraten J, Eijkman MAJ. Positive engagement and job resources in dental practice. Community Dentistry Oral Epidemiol. 2008;36:47–54.

17. Gorter RC, Eijkman MA, Hoogstraten J. Burnout and health among Dutch dentists. Eur J Oral Sci. 2000;108:261–7.

18. Gorter RC, Freeman R. Burnout and engagement in relation with job demands and resources among dental staff in Northern Ireland. Community Dentistry Oral Epidemiol. 2011;39:87–95.

19. Gorter R, Freeman R, Hammen S, Murtomaa H, Blinkhorn A, Humphris G. Psychological stress and health in undergraduate dental students: fifth year outcomes compared with first year baseline results from five European dental schools. Eur J Dent Educ. 2008;12:61–8.

20. Gorter RC, Jacobs BL, Allard RH. Low burnout risk and high engagement levels among oral and maxillofacial surgeons. Eur J Oral Sci. 2012;120:69–74.

21. Hakanen JJ, Bakker AB, Demerouti E. How dentists cope with their job demands and stay engaged: the moderating role of job resources. Eur J Oral Sci. 2005;113:479–87.

22. Hakanen JJ, Schaufeli WB, Ahola K. The Job Demands-Resources model: a three-year cross-lagged study of burnout, depression, commitment, and work engagement. Work & Stress. 2008;22:224–41.

23. Humphris G, Blinkhorn A, Freeman R, Gorter R, Hoad-Reddick G, Murtooma H, O'Sullivan R, Splieth C. Psychological stress in undergraduate dental students: baseline results from seven European dental schools. Eur J Dent Educ. 2002;6:22–9.

24. Lazarus RS. Theoretical perspectives in occupational stress research. In: Crandall R, Perrewé PL, editors. Occupational stress: a handbook. Washington, DC: Taylor & Francis; 1995. p. 3–14.

25. Maslach C, Jackson SE, Leiter MP. Maslach burnout inventory manual. 3rd ed. Palo Alto: Consulting Psychologists Press, Inc.; 1996.

26. Maslach C, Leiter MP. The truth about burnout. How organizations cause personal stress and what to do about it. San Francisco: Jossey-Bass Publishers; 1997.

27. Moore R, Brødsgaard I. Dentists' perceived stress and its relation to perceptions about anxious patients. Community Dent Oral Epidemiol. 2001;29(1):73–80.

28. Pearlman LA, Saakvitne KW. Trauma and the therapist: countertransference and vicarious traumatization in psychotherapy with incest survivors. WW Norton & Co; 1995.

29. Pohlmann K, Jonas I, Ruf S, Harzer W. Stress, burnout and health in the clinical period of dental education. Eur J Dent Educ. 2005;9:78–84.

30. Polychronopoulou A, Divaris K. Perceived sources of stress among Greek dental students. J Dent Educ. 2005;69:687–92.

31. Rønneberg A, Strøm K, Skaare AB, Willumsen T, Espelid I. Dentists' self-perceived stress and difficulties when performing restorative treatment in children. Eur Arch Paediatr Dent. 2015;16(4):341–7. https://doi.org/10.1007/s40368-014-0168-2.

32. Schaufeli WB, Bakker AB. Job demands, job resources, and their relationship with burnout and engagement; a multi-sample study. J Organ Behav. 2004;25:293–315.

33. Schaufeli WB, Bakker AB, Salanova M. The measurement of work engagement with a short questionnaire. A cross-sectional study. Educ Psychol Meas. 2006;66:701–16.

34. Schaufeli WB, Desart S, De Witte H. Burnout assessment tool (BAT) - development, validity, and reliability. Int Environ Res Public Health. 2020;17:9495. https://doi.org/10.3390/ijerph17249495.

35. Singh P, Aulak DS, Mangat SS, Aulak MS. Systematic review: factors contributing to burnout in dentistry. Occup Med. 2016;66(1):27–31. https://doi.org/10.1093/occmed/kqv119.

36. Zachrisson A. Motoverføring og endringer i synet på den psykoanalytiske relasjonen. Tidsskrift for Norsk psykologforening. 2008;45(8):939–48.

37. Zipkin J, McClure FJ. Salivary citrate and dental erosion. J Dent Res. 1949;28:613–26.

Working in Partnership for Better Oral Health Care

Benefits and Challenges in Interdisciplinary Work in Oral Health Care

Lena Myran, Jostein Paul Årøen Lein, Margrethe Elin Vika, Ulla Wide, and Wendy Knibbe

Contents

Learning Goals

- Knowing how psychologists and dental health care workers can enhance each other's work
- Knowing when to incorporate a psychologist in dental treatment
- Be aware of the benefits and challenges of interdisciplinary work

22.1 Introduction

The foregoing chapters have demonstrated the applicability of psychological theory and practice to dentistry, together with examples from clinical practice. Collaboration between dental health care professionals and psychologists has a long and successful history. The application of psychological insights to the practice of dentistry has led to improvements in the oral care of patients and at the same time there is a beneficial synergy for the discipline of psychology in working with dentistry. In the field of specific phobia, for example, the study of dental phobia has furthered the understanding of the development, maintenance, and management of specific phobias in general. The treatment of dental phobia in return is enhanced by knowledge from the field of exposure therapy (a psychological treatment that help people confront their fears). Similarly, the science of behaviour change has adopted dental behaviours such as flossing and toothbrushing as examples of common habitual and volitional behaviours for the development of behaviour change theory and interventions, while knowledge from behavioural sciences is used to develop programmes to improve oral health behaviours. In this chapter, we will discuss benefits and challenges of collaboration between dental health care professionals and psychologists. In the last part of the chapter, we will illustrate how different countries have integrated psychologists within dental teams (◘ Fig. 22.1).

22.2 The Biopsychosocial Approach

The biopsychosocial model suggests that the development and experience of illness is the result of an interplay of biological, psychological, and social factors [1]. The biological factors include genetic pre-dispositions, evolutionary vulnerabilities, infective agents, and other biological processes. The psychological factors include behaviours, emotions, and thoughts (cognitions) that influence the onset of disease (for example, health-related behaviours, the experience of psychosocial stress, beliefs about disease, and symptom interpretation) and the course of the disease. The social factors are socio-economic challenges, relationships, and network. Whilst both psychologists and members of the dental team will have experience of, and training in, the assessment and appraisal of aspects of the patient's experience of illness, each has expertise which they can bring to assessment and treatment planning. The dental team is often trained in the understanding of the impact of disruption of biological systems brought about by dental disease. The psychologists can complement this with their understanding of the impact that thoughts and emotions have on patients' perceptions of their health, disease, and oral health-related behaviour, and how psychological illnesses and earlier life experiences may give rise to difficulties in undergoing dental treatment.

The biopsychosocial model of illness provides an important background to understanding why a collaborating partnership between the dental team and the psychologists is beneficial to the patients and will improve treatment outcome.

◘ **Fig. 22.1** The Biopsychosocial model. (Photo Courtesy: Brett Guise)

Psychology symbol

The story of the psychology symbol involves some mythology and the strange evolution of the term "psi" (ψ). It's the twenty-third letter in the Greek alphabet, and at some point, the Romans transliterated it to form the word psyche.

Dentistry symbol

The Greek letters Delta (Δ) and Omicron (O) represent dentistry and "odont" ("having teeth"), respectively.

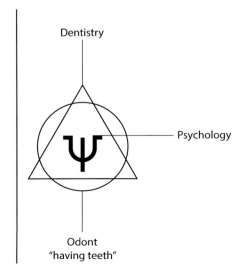

22.3 Benefits of Collaboration

In this part of the chapter, we will discuss some of the benefits of having psychologists in the dental team based on the experience of the chapters' authors. We hope the benefits for the psychologists, the dental health care professionals, and the patients can serve as an inspiration for more collaboration between dental health professionals and psychologists.

22.3.1 Communication

> **Key Point**
> Communication is central to all healthcare and a vital part of a successful dental treatment.

Communication is central to all healthcare and a vital part of a successful dental treatment. The dental surgery sets challenges which are rarely found in other healthcare settings and can get in the way of adequate communication with the patient. Here, the emphasis is on treatment, rather than on conversing about treatment. The dentist is expected to perform the required treatment on the patient, often under time constraints. Finally, whilst treatment is taking place in the oral cavity, the patient is excluded from any meaningful verbal communication. This anxiety may influence the quality and quantity of communication taking place in the dental surgery.

Dental treatment takes place in the mouth, and as such affects many important functions, making it an emotionally charged subject for many patients. Some are especially concerned about the aesthetic effects of dental prostheses, others suffer because of the effects on speech, while still others have difficulty eating as a result of dental problems. People may have experiences of being judged because of the appearance of their mouth or may even remain indoors to prevent others from seeing them. Perceived failure to acknowledge and empathize will affect the relationship and can as a result negatively influence treatment outcome. Taking the time to talk to the patient about their experiences, expectations and emotions can contribute to effective and successful treatment.

Psychologists can work with dental teams to identify and train effective communication strategies. Working together in a multidisciplinary team can make dental professionals more aware of these issues and more confident about dealing with them effectively. We refer the reader to ▶ Chap. 10 to read more about its importance and how to establish effective communication.

22.3.2 Psychological Illnesses

22.3.2.1 Dental Phobia

The most common psychological illness creating problems in the dental office is dental phobia. Previous chapters have explored the nature and management of anxiety presenting in the dental setting. Psychologists working with the dental team can both explore the patient's anxiety and assist in the treatment of anxiety, from an increasing dental anxiety to a manifest dental phobia.

Screening/Intake

The management of dental anxiety should be proportionate to the degree of anxiety experienced by the individual. Psychologists can play a role at several levels of the stepped care approach as suggested by Newton [2]. This is summarized in ◘ Fig. 22.2.

The foundation of the stepped care model lies in the assessment of dental anxiety. If the patient has a high degree of dental anxiety, a psychologist may help the dental health care professional. Note that the main focus is to treat the anxiety. Many of our dental phobia cognitive behaviour therapy (CBT) patients first undergo adapted treatment due to urgent dental treatment need, before CBT. When urgent dental treatment needs are met, CBT has main priority (◘ Fig. 22.3).

Working together with a psychologist in intake and screening will also help the dentist in understanding other possible psychological illnesses or psychiatric disorders making dental treatment difficult and causing dental anxiety. Several of these disorders or illnesses may affect the patients' experience with dental treatment, cause a more general anxiety in the dental office,

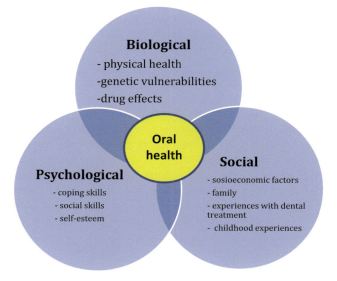

◘ **Fig. 22.2** Engels "Biopsychosocial model"

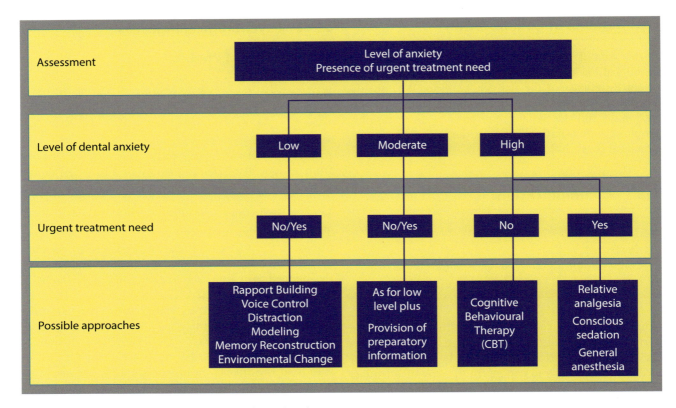

■ **Fig. 22.3**   Proportionate management model of dental anxiety

or give rise to difficulties in treatment. Understanding this will make it easier to establish a holistic treatment plan that incorporates the patients psychological and psychiatric difficulties. ▶ Chapter 15 describes these different illnesses and how they will affect the treatment more in detail.

❯ Dentists working with anxious patients often make it a habit to ask all patients if they are afraid of dental treatment or have a history of sexual abuse. Common feedback from these dentists is that surprisingly many patients confirm.

Many dentists are afraid to ask questions regarding dental anxiety, afraid they will end up in a situation they do not know how to handle or afraid they will harm their patients unnecessary. For some dentists, it is easier to ask these questions if they know that they can discuss the answers afterwards with a psychologist. Or in some cases invite the psychologist into the office if the patients have a reaction to the questions. It could also be helpful if a psychologist on the team addresses these fears with the dentist and coaches them so they become more confident to ask this type of question.

Treatment

By working with psychologists, dentist may learn to recognize mild and moderately fearful patients more easily, as well as become skilled in a range of techniques to address the anxiety. Working with patients with dental anxiety includes implementing sensitive practice into their ordinary clinic. The dentist thus gets to accommodate these patients at an early stage, offering adjustments during dental treatment. This prevents the patient from developing stronger fear that might lead to odontophobia or absence from further dental treatment. This is time saving in the long run and saves the patient pain and anxiety.

❯ The psychologist is trained to distinguish between those patients who need a push into anxiety-provoking conditions and those patients who need to be held back.

However, considering the specialized nature of dental treatment, exposure to the real thing, the dental treatment can only be performed by the dental health care workers themselves. Other dental health care professionals will therefore prefer to be trained in theory and practice of exposure therapy to be able to perform the treatment themselves. Which path is chosen differs in different countries, or organizations, or even between dentists. The choice that is made has implications for the way teams treating dental phobia are set up. In each case, close collaboration between dentists and psychologists is essential.

22.3.2.2 Other Mental Health Problems

While dentists, in collaboration with psychologists, can treat dental phobia, they can also see patients with a range of mental health problems needing dental treatment (See ► Chap. 15). Eating disorders, with vomiting or refusal to eat, can lead to reduced oral health. Persons with psychotic disorders and mood disorders have periods where they are unable to organize their oral hygiene. Blood and injection phobia often lead to avoidance of dental treatment because the anaesthesia appears frightening. Use of psychotropic drugs can cause dry mouth and make one more vulnerable to caries development. Child abuse and neglect can give children poor skills in taking care of their oral health or boundary setting. Mental health problems may impair the patient's ability to undergo treatment, cause dental health problems, be a source of inadequate treatment wishes or cause problems in the interaction between dentist and patients. All psychiatric diagnoses associated with anxiety and depression are associated with greater tooth decay and loss of teeth [3].

Most patients will at one point in their lifetime meet the criteria for a psychiatric diagnosis, but some diagnoses are harder to handle then others. The patients' psychiatric problems may therefore cause difficulties for the dental professional. For example, working with borderline personality disorder, schizophrenia, or the more common counter-transference issues (see ► Chap. 4) can make great disturbances in the dental treatment. If the dentist is striving in the relationship or senses that the patient is struggling with mental issues, the psychologist may contribute. The psychologist may help the dental professional to understand what is going on, both intra-psychological (personally) and inter-psychological (between people). Dental health personnel can also contact a psychologist when they become uncertain about further progress in the treatment or acute assessments of mental health are needed.

> ❯ All psychiatric diagnoses associated with anxiety and depression are associated with greater tooth decay and loss of teeth.

In all these situations, patient care is improved when dental health care professionals work together with psychologists. Psychologists can help assess the influence of the specific psychopathology on the patient's ability to undergo treatment, work with dentists and patients to develop ways to make dental treatment possible and advise dentists on how to approach patients with severe psychopathology. When psychopathology influences behaviour to the extent that patient's behaviour is harmful to their health (like for example in anorexia), psychologists can work with dentists to cope with these patients and their own emotional response to this behaviour. Psychologists can coach dentists to be not only empathic and understanding but also professional in their treatment. Finally, psychological assessment can be essential in treatment planning for patients whose treatment wishes are guided by psychopathology, rather than realistic treatment wishes, as can be seen in patients with body dysmorphic disorder.

22.3.2.3 Working with Specific Patient Groups

Patient groups such as patients with intellectual disabilities, physical disabilities, birth defects, dementia, and so on, each pose their own challenges to dentists. Some of these challenges lie in the interaction with the patient. Psychologists, or other behaviour specialists, can coach and educate dentists to help the interaction proceed as smoothly as possible. When working with these patients, it is important to consider a multidisciplinary approach at an early stage. When a psychologist only becomes involved once treatment progress is hampered, it is often too late. At that point patients may not feel like their complaints are taken seriously, but rather that they are dumped at the psychologists' because the dentist does not know what to do anymore. Therefore, in specialized settings, it is important that a psychologist is involved early on in the process. This can for example be done by incorporating routine pre-treatment screening or scheduling more time for the first meeting with the patient, to make room for an extensive biopsychosocial history. Based on this, the psychologist can consider possible challenges in the treatment process and possible obstacles for building an alliance, making the dental team aware of the challenges that may arise. Then the dental team together with the psychologist can devise a multidisciplinary treatment plan to prevent or overcome these challenges.

In a regular dental practice, routinely including a psychologist for intake and/or screening would be ineffective. However, the dentist can consider using general screening questionnaires for specific groups to assess specific treatment needs and decide if this can be provided at the practice. This may, for example, include brief screeners for dental phobia for patients who present with anxiety, or screening questionnaires like those that are included in the DC/TMD Axis II for patients presenting with non-dental orofacial pain complaints.

22.3.2.4 Temporomandibular Disorders, Adaptation to Dental Prosthetics, and Gagging Reflexes

While all health, mental and physical is determined by biopsychosocial factors, in those conditions that are known to be influenced strongly by psychosocial factors, such as temporomandibular disorders, adaptation problems in (partially) edentulous patients, and excessive gagging reflexes, this is especially relevant. When patients present with these problems, psychological screening before the patient's first visit can be an important tool. In a specialized dental office, screening can help determine who should be present for the first visit (dentist, psychologist), whether referral for additional psychological treatment is desirable, and identify possible factors affecting treatment success. At a regular practice, screening questionnaires can be used as a tool when deciding whether or not the patient needs to be referred to a specialized dentist.

Treatment for these problems is often multidisciplinary, with dentist, psychologists, and/or physiotherapist each adding treatment in their own field of expertise, but all guided by a shared conceptualization of the patients presenting problem. The role of the psychologist often lies both in treatment (for example, psychoeducation, exposure and response prevention, habit reversal, stress management, treating psychological trauma) and in helping the team steer away from unnecessary, at times invasive, dental procedures.

22.3.2.5 Orthognathic Surgery

A specific patient group is those referred for or asking for jaw-surgery. Both before and after surgery, psychological assessment and guidance can play an important role. As discussed above, patients can have a range of reasons for wanting a specific treatment to be performed. When they are somehow misguided in their beliefs about what surgery can and cannot solve, bigger problems will follow after surgery than existed before. Pre-surgery assessment of both patient expectations and mental health, combined with extensive education about the procedure, its effects and the recovery period can help prevent these problems. Generally, psychological complaints need to be treated by a psychologist and are not solved by surgery. The same goes for a long history of adaptation problems: if time after time dentists, specialized dentists such as implantologists, or oral surgeons have done their utmost to perform adequate dental treatment and for no clear reasons, the patient's complaints persisted, surgery is unlikely to solve the problem and psychological treatment focussed on adaptation and acceptance, and often stopping a range of oral behaviours such as clenching, grinding, and tongue pressure is a better choice. (For more information about psychological challenges working with orthognathic surgery, see ▶ Chap. 16.)

On the other hand, dentists may also be confronted with patients after orthognathic surgery who have gotten stuck in recovery, often with enduring pain problems as a result, but at times also struggling with their altered appearance. Psychologists, and at times physiotherapists, are generally the most appropriate professionals to help patients overcome these problems. They can also help dentists avoid the trap of trying to solve these issues with more invasive treatments, which will generally aggravate the problems, rather than relieve them.

22.3.2.6 Children

Based on the knowledge regarding the aetiology of dental anxiety and dental phobia, it is very important that the Public Dental Service are building competence in respect to both prevention and treatment of dental anxiety in children and adolescents. The mean onset of dental anxiety is reported to be around the age of 12 [4]. Consequently, the Public Dental Service must manage both prevention and treatment of these conditions. This means that the dental staff must have competence at two different levels: (1) All members of Public Dental Service must have a minimum level of knowledge regarding both prevention of dental anxiety and phobia, and how to detect and treat a dawning anxiety. Furthermore, it is also important that the staff have a realistic understanding of their competence in this specific area, so that they can refer the patients in need for more competence, to a level (2) Pedodontist or specially trained dental staff. Pedodontist may have skills regarding the treatment of children and adolescents with severe dental anxiety or phobia. To ensure that a Pedodontist, a dentist or a dental hygienist specially trained in phobia treatment, involving of psychologist is strongly recommended.

To involve psychologist's on both a systemic level to facilitate the overall theoretical and clinical knowledge in dentistry, regarding both prevention and treatment of dental anxiety or phobia is required. In our opinion, the treatment of dental anxiety is a perfect and significant crossing point between dentistry and psychology. Some children and adolescents have adverse childhood experiences (e.g. sexual abuse, violence, neglect) and experience indicates that some of these children may experience dental treatment as retraumatizing due to the dental staffs lack of theoretical and clinical skills. The same can be said for medical treatment. Although they are intended to help the child and do not necessarily constitute an adverse event as such, they can be experienced as traumatic by children. For those children, dental treatment can also be experienced as retraumatizing. Detecting children that may go in submissive state or understand why some are reacting with aggression or being rude may be decisive for these children, not only regarding dentistry, but also in respect to their psychological future. Furthermore, there is also a need for a broader expertise in the treatment of children diagnosed with numerous conditions and syndromes (e.g. ADHD, Autism, Asperger Syndrome, severe learning disabilities). To offer the best possible dental treatment and to give all children the best possible experience with dentistry, including psychologist in the Public Dental Health Care may be required in respect to the children but also advantageous for the dental staff. Working with psychologist may also clarify when it is indicated to offer exposure therapy or were it is indicated to offer a more adapted dental treatment. This interdisciplinary teamwork may also be helpful in the assessment process according to whether to contact the patient's parents, doctors, teachers, the school health services, the psychiatric health services etc., to be able to help the patients.

22.3.3 Understanding Patient Behaviour

Dentists are basically good human connoisseurs, or eager to learn. We say this by experience. By working with psychologists though, learning basic principles of a psychological approach, dentists gain a theoretical foundation, thus confirming their practice to be right, or helping them adopt more effective practices.

> ❯❯ I have sometimes thought that I have said exactly what the psychologist says to the patient, but the psychologist has a different way of talking and comes up with a slightly different angle that makes the patient turn around and happily try to implement something she has previously said is completely impossible to achieve.

If the dentist is lost in translation with a patient, it might help to include a psychologist. (See quote). The psychologist may also join during the therapeutic process in the dental office if the process stagnates or is locking. A pair of new and psychological "glasses" may discover the ongoing dynamic and give advice how to modify further therapy.

Dentists report that they experience greater personal resilience and can to a greater extent talk to all their patients, when collaborating with psychologists. This is due to psychology being the science of human behaviour, including the behaviour of both young and adults, scared and not scared.

22.3.4 Ripple Effect

The treatment with help from a psychologist has great potential for "transfer value" or "ripple effect". Quite frequently, histories of the transfer value/ the ripple effects of dental anxiety treatment, are heard: The woman who now dares to stay in the checkout line without constantly letting other customers go ahead of her. The man who dared to talk to the boss about awkward working conditions. The woman who finally fulfilled the dream of buying a caffe macchiato and defied the fear of taking up the baristas time. The man who stopped taking Valium when he visited his overbearing parents. The transfer value is a bonus; the patients understand their psychological functioning better and learning tools they may implement in the many arenas of life.

> ❯ The transfer value is a nice side-effect after treatment. The patients understand their psychological functioning better and learning tools they may implement in the many arenas of life.

22.3.5 Economy

The research concerning the economic benefits for the collaboration between dental care professionals and psychologist is limited. What is known is that the consequences of chronic untreated oral diseases are often severe and can include unremitting pain, sepsis, reduced quality of life, lost school days, disruption to family life, and decreased work productivity. The costs of treating oral diseases impose large economic burdens to the dental health care system. [5]. Across the European Union, this has been estimated to increase from €54 Billion in 2000 to €93 Billion in 2020. This is greater than the costs for stroke and dementia combined [6]. Equally, the human cost is significant; 34,205 children under 10 years of age required treatment in a hospital in England due to tooth decay between April 2016 and March 2017, compared to 19, 584 children requiring treatment for asthma [7].

Adding psychologists to the dental team can help prevent some of these costs by aiding treatment in several areas. The basis for a healthy dentition is laid in early childhood. For most children regular dental visits and oral hygiene instruction for parents are enough. However sometimes it proves difficult to maintain a healthy mouth already for very young children. When fear, developmental disorders, psychological problems or difficult circumstances in the family play a role, child psychologists can play a role to assist the child, parents, or caregivers and dentists in establishing proper oral care. In adulthood, dental fear can be a factor involved in deteriorating oral health. Treating dental fear, in the collaboration between psychologists and dental care professional, will help the vulnerable patient to regularly attend dental appointments, and hence reduce cost of the mentioned consequences. Once teeth are lost, (partial) dental prosthetics are generally made; however, some patients have difficulty adjusting to these. While the solution to adjustment problems generally lies in behaviour and psychology, within dentistry, patients and oral health care providers tend to mostly seek for solutions in dentistry. Often to no avail. Early involvement of psychologists can reduce costs immensely. Finally chronic orofacial pain, dental and other, can be a debilitating problem that is most effectively treated in a multidisciplinary team, including a psychologist.

22.3.6 Increasing Dental Team Resilience

Becoming an experienced dentist treating patients with dental anxiety or special needs might become a disadvantage to some dentists. The portfolio of patients requiring special care can get disproportionately high. This is due to the patient's desire to stay with the good dentist, feeling the dentist is the only one able to help them. Colleagues often see that the sensitive dentists are successful with their patients. Since patients with dental anxiety and with special needs are sometimes considered time consuming and tend to create a feeling of insecurity for the less experienced dentist, these patients might get transferred from colleagues to the more sensitive dentist. Since these patient groups are demanding to work with, the sensitive dentist might feel burdened and even burn out the empathy for these patients. To reduce the chance of work-related burnout in these sensitive and experienced dentists, it may be beneficial to work with a psychologist. Both for increased understanding of the processes involved in the treatment, and what working with anxious and perhaps traumatized patients might do to you as a health care professional when you are not working.

22.4 Challenges

22.4.1 Identifying the Members of the Team

The success of multidisciplinary treatment is very much determined by making the right choices about which members of the multidisciplinary team to involve at what stage of treatment. Our experience is that if a psychologist only becomes involved once treatment progress is hampered, it is often too late. Especially when treating children, patients with a dental phobia, and patients with an excessive gagging reflex a combined intake with a dentist and a psychologist may be advisable. In addition, psychological screening can be useful for treatment planning and identifying possible factors affecting treatment success. At the same time, using the psychologist for all patients will likely be unnecessary. It is important

that a framework for collaboration with joint expectations from both the dental team and the psychologists is established. We recommend that different professionals meet on a regular basis.

22.4.2 Perspectives

Dental practitioners and psychologists may have different perspectives on both the goals of treatment and the time frame for successful treatment. Dentists are used to completing treatment in a relatively brief time, often within one treatment session. Failing to achieve this, for example, with the anxious patients can be exasperating. Psychologists are aware that completely succeeding in treatment is not always possible. Patients' characteristics, motivation, life circumstances, and life events influence whether one succeeds or not. Partial success can then be considered a big win. When working together with patients, it may be advisable to discuss perspectives on what can be considered a successful treatment and how to tolerate a less than perfect treatment outcome.

22.4.3 The Lack of a Common Culture and a Shared "Language"

This notion that dentists and psychologists may have different perspectives, might be exacerbated by the lack of a shared technical language. Each profession converses in its own jargon which may be hard to understand for other professional groups. It can take time to learn and integrate these "tribe languages". For example, the goal of phobia management for the dental team may be the successful completion of dental treatment – particularly if the treatment is urgent. However, for the psychologist, the goal of cognitive behavioural therapy for dental phobia is for the patient to overcome their anxiety and be able to attend regularly for primary dental care for the rest of their lives.

The tribal languages often share the same words, but with different semantics. The word treatment and trauma mean dental treatment and dental trauma for the dentists, and psychological treatment and psychological trauma for the psychologists. This may result in misunderstandings until the languages are calibrated.

22.4.4 Time Pressures

Dental treatment on patients with psychological issues can be not only challenging but also time consuming. Offering adjustments and extra sensitive dental treatment takes time that often cannot be charged for.

22

Therefore, treating these patients can be costly for the dentist. Dentists are paid for the procedures completed, so their focus will be on getting this work done.

Psychological treatment takes place in a different timeframe, with sessions taking 45 min at least and treatment taking place over a period of months and sometimes years. Treatment is financed accordingly, where psychologists are being paid for the time rather than the procedures completed. From this perspective, a specific phobia is a disorder that with adequate treatment can show great progression after just a few sessions. When working together, dentist and psychologist will have to communicate about how they will deal with this subject, considering both the dental and the psychological needs of each patient, and the practical limitations of each profession.

22.4.5 Availability of Psychologists

Although working together with a psychologist could be helpful in many situations, there are not sufficient psychologists working in dentistry to ensure that even large centres have a team of psychologists they can call on. To provide the best possible care to all patients, an important challenge is ensuring sufficient members in all professions required in a multidisciplinary dental team. Through training and encouraging placements in dentistry as part of the training of psychologists this may be achieved.

22.5 Future Perspectives

We think that there is a great potential to improve dental care by including more psychologists, both for dental anxiety treatment and in other clinical areas, to provide more effective treatment. While in primary health care there has been a successful development including multiple professionals, such as psychologists and physiotherapists, this has not happened in dentistry. A future direction could be for dentistry to become more and more a part of the general primary care health field and work together structurally with other disciplines.

Next, collaboration between psychologists and dentists can create an environment in which new methods, treatment measures, and tools can see the light of day. For example, virtual technology for dental treatment (Virtual Reality Exposure Therapy, VRET), handbooks, e-learning programs, and APPS have been developed in interdisciplinary cooperation.

Finally, the main contributing factors to poor dental health are poor eating habits like high sugar con-

sumption and high intake of soda with acid, and lack of good health habits like brushing teeth. Dentists and oral hygienists are routinely reminding their patients about this, hoping that informing patients will lead to behaviour change. Evidence from the social sciences tell us, this approach generally does not work. Dentists and oral hygienist know this, but often lack the knowledge and skills to implement a different approach. Several ways can be envisioned in which psychologists' knowledge about promoting behaviour change can be incorporated in efforts to promote oral health. One way would be by working together with a psychologist who can apply behaviour change interventions to help the patient establish good health habits. This approach is becoming increasingly common. Another approach is to develop campaigns aimed at specific population groups, using scientific knowledge about behaviour change. In the Netherlands, a comprehensive program aimed at oral health in children has been developed in this way [8]. Finally, dentists can be trained in applying interventions and communication skills aimed at promoting behaviour change. Courses training dentists to do this could be taught by psychologists and included in the curriculum in dental schools, and in courses in further education. To some extent, this is already happening in several countries, but not yet to such an extent that dentists feel confident to apply these strategies structurally.

Summary

In this chapter, we have discussed our insights into approaches that maximizes the benefits of collaboration while acknowledging the pit falls. We hope this chapter has made you more prone to contact a psychologist when you anticipate that treatment of a patient may be challenging, now knowing how a collaboration can enhance the oral health care for your patient. We hope you feel more ready for handling situations to come when our professions work together.

Collaboration between dental health care professionals and psychologists has a long and successful history. Still, we have much to learn from each other, and many countries have yet to develop interdisciplinary collaborations. We hope this chapter can inspire you to find a way for improving our collaboration, for a better oral health care.

As psychologists working with dental teams, we are familiar with these challenges. Our experience is that being aware of the challenges is important. By being aware of them, you as an interdisciplinary team, should make room to discuss the possible disagreements, and listen to each other's perspectives. You should also be open-minded and respect that the different professions have different backgrounds that is important to allow in the collaboration. With communication and respect these challenges may, together with the benefits, give the patients a better oral treatment.

In the following pages, we will give you a description of already established interdisciplinary partnerships that form the basis for the insights in this chapter.

22.6 Descriptions from Interdisciplinary Work

In the first two parts of the chapter, we have provided some benefits and challenges in working together in partnership. A lot of that insight is derived from our own experiences as psychologists working with health care professionals. In this last part of the chapter, we want to give you some descriptions and our perspectives on how four different countries have established this partnership and how this partnership is organized. This might be for inspiration if you as a reader is interested in how you can contribute to a partnership in your own clinic, or if you would like to see how an already established relationship may be broadened.

United Kingdom: Tim Newton
Netherlands: Wendy Knibbe
Norway: Margrethe Elin Vika
Sweden: Ulla Wide

22.6.1 Psychology and Oral Health Psychology in the United Kingdom

22.6.1.1 History

Prior to 1992, the main interactions between psychologists and members of the dental team centred on the management and treatment of individuals with dental phobia. Given the high prevalence of dental phobia, psychologists were often presented with instances of individuals with such phobias who had delayed treatment and required support to receive much needed dental treatment. While the primary focus of psychological approaches was the rehabilitation of the dental phobia and enabling the individual with a dental phobia to engage with dental treatment with a reduced state of anxiety, there was synergy with the dental team who had the focus on ensuring that urgent dental treatment was completed.

In the early 1990s in the United Kingdom, the General Dental Council reviewed the curriculum for the training of dentists and extended the course to a full 5-year degree. As a result of the increased time, several new topics were included in the core curriculum, including the social and behavioural sciences. A small group of academic dentists and psychologists working in the field of medicine produced a book detailing guidance on the scope of the new curriculum, which highlighted four main areas of teaching in the area of psychology:

- Communication skills
- Managing dental anxiety
- The role of behaviour in disease and behaviour change
- Pain management

The guidance also emphasized the important role that psychologists could play in research and service provision, though this was not the primary focus of the initiative.

The introduction of the social and behavioural sciences to dental training in this manner led to the creation of specific posts for psychologists to work with dental teams, either embedded within the dental schools or seconded from Medical schools (which in the UK are a separate degree). As a result, there was burgeoning interest in the field.

Currently, the contribution of psychologists to the dental field in the United Kingdom and internationally is widespread. Within my own institution we have nine psychologists embedded within dentistry, three who are full-time academics/researchers, and six on the service provision team. In addition, there are numerous doctoral and post-doctoral research students employed under limited term contracts. The contributions of the team can be grouped into four main areas:

- Education
- Research
- Healthcare services
- Policy development and influence on health service provision

I shall provide a brief overview of each in turn.

22.6.1.2 Education

All training for members of the dental team at the undergraduate level now requires the teaching, practice, and assessment of applied psychology. This includes the development of all dental healthcare professionals including dental nurses, dental hygienists, dental therapists, dental technicians, and dental practitioners. This teaching largely focuses on the core topics originally described in the original curriculum review, though this has since been updated with the direct involvement of psychologists in the field who contributed to the General Dental Council core curricula. There have been extensive developments in the teaching of communication skills, and across the UK, psychologists involved in such training have standardized on a modified version of the Calgary Cambridge model as the foundation of their training. The assessment of communication has become a core component of the teaching and training of dental healthcare professionals with psychologists developing new and innovative approaches to teaching and assessing such skills. At my own dental school, communication skill is a stand-alone examination for the Final award of the Dental degree.

Several textbooks have been written for the undergraduate market, including one from my own institution in 2016.

Scambler S, Scott SE & Asimakopoulou K. *Sociology & Psychology for the Dental Team.* Cambridge, Polity Press.

In addition, advanced training and education is provided for postgraduate specialist courses.

22.6.1.3 Research

Research into the application of psychological theory in dentistry has burgeoned over the last 30 years, with the growth in personnel involved in this area. Within my own Institution, our focus can be categorized into the following area:

- Theory-based interventions to enhance oral health to enhance oral health-related behaviour.
- Theory-based interventions to enhance early recognition of cancers
- Interventions to reduce anxiety in individuals attending for dental treatment
- Third-wave CBT-based interventions for chronic pain

Since 1992 our academic team have published over 350 academic peer reviewed papers in this area and received grant funding in excess of US$6,000,000.

Two UK-based psychologists have been recipients of the International Association of Dental Research, Distinguished Scientist Award in the field of Behavioural, Epidemiological, and Health Services Research – Professor Sarah Baker and Professor Tim Newton.

22.6.1.4 Healthcare Services

Psychologists provide direct healthcare services for people with issues that relate to their oral and dental health. Within the United Kingdom, there are a range of services including

- Routine opportunistic screening of all dental patients within our institution for undiagnosed psychological difficulties. Given the prevalence of mental health problems is about 10% of the general population, we have encouraged the use of screening questionnaires to identify those patients attending for dental treatment who might otherwise not have their problems identified. This can then form the basis of an appropriate referral for management. In this way, we hope to give patients a more holistic and patient-centred dental experience.
- The provision of CBT-based interventions for individuals with dental phobia. The first dedicated service delivering CBT for individuals with dental phobia in the United Kingdom was set up at my institution and drew on the successful models in the United States and Sweden. This service was recommended as a model of excellence in service delivery by our government in 1999, and as a result many similar services have been set up across the UK.
- The provision of support for individuals with chronic orofacial pain, TMJ pain and altered sensation. We have adopted a model of the use of compassion focussed therapy and acceptance and commitment therapy in the management of long-term chronic pain. This is delivered both on an individual basis and within groups.
- Screening of individuals attending for major facial surgery for potential issues such as body dysmorphic disorder and difficulties in coping with the impact of surgery. This has also allowed us to develop a programme to help patients prepare for their surgery.
- Interventions for individuals who have a hypersensitive gag reflex that interferes with their quality of life and/or ability to engage with dental treatment.
- Support and assistance in behaviour change in relation to oral health – using theory-based, empirically tested interventions to enhance oral health behaviour, including brief motivational interviewing, and the creation of implementation Intentions.

22.6.1.5 Policy Development and Influence on Health Service Provision

With the increasing identification of the relevance and importance of psychology in the dental field, this has led to the opportunity for psychologists to be involved in the development of national policy regarding the delivery and development of dental healthcare. For example, Professor Tim Newton is an Honorary Consultant Adviser to the government body that oversees dentistry in the UK – the Office of the Chief Dental Officer. This has provided the opportunity to contribute to the implementation of preventive care, particularly within the limitations of dental practice imposed by COVID-19.

The Alliance for a Cavity Free Future is a global group of collaborators led by a team comprising dentists and psychologists to support the mission of improving the oral health of all individuals across the globe (▶ www.acffglobal.org).

22.6.2 Psychology and Oral Health Psychology in The Netherlands

22.6.2.1 History

In the Netherlands, most psychological treatment related to dentistry takes place in specialized centres for Centrum Bijzondere Tandheelkunde (CBT). There are 30 such centres in the Netherlands, mostly located in general or academic hospitals; however, not all centres employ psychologists. The largest centre for special care dentistry is Stichting voor Bijzondere Tandheelkunde (SBT), an independent organization in Amsterdam, providing care for all patients who cannot be seen in regular dentistry practices due to, for example, dental phobia, physical disability, intellectual disability, or psychiatric disorders. Specialized departments focus on gerodontology, pedodontology, maxillofacial prosthetics, temporomandibular disorders, anxiety, and disabilities. Psychologists at these centres are involved in treatment planning, individual psychological treatment, and support dentists in patient management. Group educational sessions can also be given by psychologists.

To a lesser extent, dentists across the country refer to psychologists when they feel psychological treatment could benefit the outcomes of the work of the dentists, for example, when psychological distress or negative life events appear to be of influence on the problem the patient is presenting with. Overall, dentists mostly tend to refer to a cognitive behavioural therapy (CBT) when they feel treatment cannot be accomplished in their practice, including when psychological intervention is needed.

Research and development in dentistry takes place at the three dentistry faculties at universities in Amsterdam, Groningen and Nijmegen. At these faculties research aimed at the intersection between dentistry and the social sciences focuses mostly on preventative dentistry, dental phobias, dental pain, and the mental health and wellbeing of the dentist. Research is carried out by scientists with a range of backgrounds, including dentistry and social sciences. Also, at these faculties, departments specializing in areas of dentistry, such as orofacial pain and periodontology, focus on the role of psychosocial factors in these specific dental health problems in their research. Some of these departments also employ or work together with psychologists.

When it comes to treating patients, psychologists contribute in several ways, as is described below:

22.6.2.2 Dental Phobia

Although there are clinics specializing in providing dental treatment under general anaesthesia to, among others, patients with dental phobia, the consensus in the treatment of dental phobia is to focus on treating the fear rather than focusing on dentistry. As such, CBT's employ specialized dentists working systematically towards reducing fear by applying the principles of cognitive behavioural therapy, especially exposure-based treatments. Psychologists provide pre-treatment psychological screening, work together with dentists in joined intakes and treatment planning, and provide individual psychotherapy to those patients for whom more intensive treatment is needed. Especially when a history of negative experiences with dentistry prevents the patient from profiting from exposure therapy, psychologists are often involved in treatment. A preferred treatment for psychological trauma related to dentistry is eye movement desensitization and reprocessing (EMDR). After one or more EMDR sessions, depending on the nature, and number of traumatic events and progress of EMDR treatment, the patient returns to the specialized dentist to start or continue exposure therapy.

From the outset of treatment, it is discussed with the patient that treatment at the centre is temporary and the goal of treatment is to reduce the fear to such an extent that the patient can be referred back to a general dental practice for regular care.

22.6.2.3 Psychiatric Disorders, Intellectual Disabilities, and Gerodontology

Although the general aim is to have patients treated in general dental practices, for some patients in these groups this is not a realistic goal. These patients remain patients at a centre for special dental care. Psychologists can be consulted to help dentists find the best way to work with a patient. They can also work with patients individually to help them increase their ability to undergo treatment by a dentist. This often means working on psychological trauma resulting from negative experiences related to dentistry, or other negative events that can affect a patient's response to dental treatment. This can include negative experiences with medical treatment, abuse, sexual abuse, maltreatment, etc. If a patient is severely traumatized, he or she will be referred to a mental healthcare organization for psychological treatment.

22.6.2.4 Maxillofacial Prosthetics and Temporomandibular Disorders

Together with dentists, psychologists work on improvement in the physical complaint the patient presents with. They also help patients cope with complaints that may not improve and at times work on coming to terms with the (orofacial) consequences of a medical condition or accident. Chronic pain, excessive gagging reflexes, and problems adapting to dental prostheses are the most common complaints psychologists work with in these patient groups. However, at times patients with congenital malformations are also referred to a psychologist, mostly because of the psychological impact of the malformation or distress related to negative (childhood) experiences related to the malformation.

As with other patient groups, involvement of the psychologist starts with psychological screening. In these groups, screening is aimed to assess whether it is likely that psychosocial factors play a role in the presenting complaint or can hamper treatment progress. After screening a patient can be referred to a psychologist after intake, or a joined intake session can be planned. In some centres, depending on screening outcome, orofacial pain intakes are done by a physiotherapist and/or a psychologist rather than a dentist.

Patients with chronic pain, an excessive gagging reflex or chronic problems with their prostheses often expect that a dentist will work on a physical solution for their problems. They do not generally expect to be helped by a psychologist. Education about the specific complaint and the role psychosocial factors can play in this specific situation is therefore an important ingredient of these treatments. After educating the patient and coming to an agreement that psychological interventions may indeed help the patient, a treatment plan is made that can contain a range of psychological interventions, depending on the nature of the problem being tackled. Possible psychological trauma related to the presenting complaint, either by location or in time, is assessed as unresolved trauma can be a maintaining factor for a range of complaints. Cognitive behavioural treatment, pain education, behaviour modification, trauma-focused treatment, and stress management can for example be part of the treatment offered to these patient groups.

22.6.3 Psychology and Oral Health Psychology in Norway

22.6.3.1 History

In 1979–1980, two dentists, one at the University in Oslo and one at the University in Bergen completed course (Jönköping in Sweden) in the use of nitrous oxide (NOX) to facilitate dental treatment in patients with severe dental anxiety. Relatively short after introducing NOX not only for children but also for an emerging number of adults, the shortcomings of NOX appeared. The idea of co-operation with psychologists was born. In 1991, a formalized partnership was established between dentists and psychologist for the treatment of both children and adults suffering from different anxiety disorders that complicated dental treatment. This interdisciplinary collaboration between the Faculty of Psychology and the Faculty of Odontology also included the Public Dental Health Service from 1992.

22.6.3.2 Clinical Work

The anxiety disorders that complicate dental treatment has, from the start, primarily been focused to dental phobia and BII-phobia in both children and adults. However, a large proportion of the dental patients have other anxiety disorders, e.g. general anxiety disorder, panic disorder, OCD, etc. Furthermore, a relatively large proportion of the dental phobic may be more complex to treat due to sexual abuse, severe care failure, torture, PTSD, etc. Successful dental treatment of complex cases demands a well-established interdisciplinary teamwork. In 2012, this cooperation expanded extensively, due to the formation of the nationwide TADA-project (torture, abuse, dental anxiety project), with TADA-teams specially trained for treating these three groups (Dentists, oral hygienists, dental secretaries, and psychologists).

When a TADA patient is referred to a TADA-team, the patients' course will in general be as follows: The secretary fulfils a short telephone interview with the patient to explore how the patients master dental treatment now, and to convey relevant information about the TADA-project as well. Thereafter, all patients undergo a comprehensive interview performed by the psychologist: Brief information about the TADA-project, a short general anamnesis, exploring background for problems related to receiving dental treatment, a diagnostic interview related to their possible rights related to TADA.

After the interview, the patients will be set up for either CBT or a more trauma-sensitive approach to manage necessary dental treatment, or a combination of these. In most cases, the approach is openly discussed with the patients.

For patients diagnosed with DP or strong DA as main cause for not managing dental treatment, background, triggering stimulus, catastrophic thoughts, panic-related symptoms of it are thoroughly explored. It is important to evaluate both the benefit of and the patient's motivation to participate in CBT. Finally, psychoeducation and extensive information about the principles of CBT are given. The patients must understand the importance of their own contribution in relation to CBT, and that they are well educated in the rational of CBT. The significance of their understanding of rationale for treatment, motivation, obligation, the necessity of avoiding using safety behaviours and so on are stressed. Undergoing CBT is definitely hard work for the patients, on the other hand it may give them an opportunity to master dental treatment in a lifetime perspective.

Most of the CBT related to DP/DA patients are performed by the dentist or oral hygienist. The dental staff is specially educated and trained in exposure treatment of dental phobia. In case of non-respondence and/or patients with severe comorbidity, the psychologists are consulted and take a more active part in the treatment process. One of the main focuses of the pure-bred treatment is to give the patients knowledge, understanding and experience regarding how to face and master their anxiety. Some patients are not adequately motivated for hard core CBT, resulting in a mix between CBT and facilitated treatment, where we have focus on a decreased anxiety as the motivating element.

Patients labelled as complex cases, e.g. having severe comorbidity and/or where it is difficult or impossible to perform a normal therapeutic process and conversation, due to a severe degree of dissociative disturbances, massive flashbacks, pervasive relational problems, they may nevertheless, benefit from a more adapted trauma-sensitive approach in managing necessary dental treatment. In the treatment of complex cases, the psychologist has a more active role depending on how experienced the dental staff is. Some key points for the psychologist intervention are stabilization, more customized psycho-education, and suggesting and testing suitable exercises (see ▶ Chaps. 12 and 13).

Innovation

The process of establishing the TOO-project (TADA-project) has made many new innovations see the day of light, including an app, textbook, handbook, virtual reality (VR) technology and interdisciplinary treatment for children.

The app "Tannskrekk" (dental fear) was published in 2017. It contains an overview of the facilitations dentally anxious patients can ask at the dentist office. Examples of facilitations can be the stop signal, trauma-sensitive arrangements and explanations.

A handbook for dentally anxious patients has been developed and given to patients included in the TOO-project (TADA-project). The handbook contains information on dental phobia, trauma theory, clinical reasons for developing dental anxiety, facilitations and a coping plan.

A handbook for clinicians working with dentally anxious patients has also been made, holding information of dental anxiety, trauma-sensitive treatment and clinical examples from the interdisciplinary work with anxious patients.

The textbook "Odontologisk psykologi" (odontological psychology) was published in Norway in 2018. It contained contributions from experienced psychologists, dental care professionals and researchers. The textbook was the precursor for the book you are now reading.

Virtual reality (VR) is technology where people can explore a virtual world inside a headset. A VR scenario for dentally anxious patient is developed, and the patients can explore the dental office virtually. Examples of scenarios to explore are the dental office, the dentist, the syringe and the drill.

After developing interdisciplinary treatment for adults with dental anxiety, a project with children, Tbit (safe children in dental treatment) has been put to life and is establishing several places in Norway.

These as some of the newest innovations that has come to life during since the beginning of the interdisciplinary work between dentist and psychologists in Norway.

Research and Innovation

Research in dentistry has primarily taken place at three of the universities in Norway; Oslo, Tromsø and Bergen. During the last decades, a large proportion of the research in the area of dental phobia has been performed in collaboration between dentists and psychologists. Since 2012 all the six health regions in Norway established Oral Health Centres of Expertise. Research and developing clinical expertise in the field of odontological psychology has been carried out in these centres, and all of them have psychologist present in the staff. There has been both qualitative and quantitative studies related to the different groups in the TADA-project, including patients that have experienced torture or that have been sexually abused. Research and developing more clinical experience related to anxiety in the dental situation in both children and adolescents is also carried out. There are also ongoing studies that explore the effect of using digital platforms and apps related to fear and anxiety of dentistry.

22.6.4 Psychology and Oral Health Psychology in Sweden

22.6.4.1 History

In the early 1970s, dentists in Gothenburg, Sweden, based in the Public Dental Service and the Faculty of Odontology, initiated a collaboration with psychologists from the Department of Psychology, to develop better treatment options for adult patients with severe dental anxiety. Professionals from the Public Dental Service and Gothenburg University designed together an intervention for patients with severe dental anxiety based on systematic desensitization. The intervention was administered by a psychologist at the dental clinic. The psychological intervention, integrated in the dental care, showed very promising results and was further developed through rigorous evaluation and research. It finally became a part of the ordinary dental clinic assignment of the specialized hospital dental clinic/oral medicine unit in Gothenburg and was later turned into its own organizational unit entitled the Dental Anxiety/Phobia Research and Treatment Centre in Gothenburg (DAPRTC). A treatment manual is available in a 9th edition from 2020, while the first treatment manual was published in 1985.

The research and development carried out at this clinic has played a major part in the important health policy advances to include psychologists in dental care for better oral and general health in Sweden, as described below. Both the Swedish National Board of Health and Welfare and the regional guidelines are based on the clinical research and development carried out by DAPRTC and the evidence base provided in a health technology assessment (HTA) report.

— The Swedish National Board of Health and Welfare decided in 1999 to cover treatment costs according to strict criteria (including the requirement that dentists and psychologists with special competences collaborate during both assessment and treatment), to make effective treatment of severe dental anxiety available in all regions of Sweden at a reasonable cost to patients. Patients fulfilling the criteria for treatment pay a standard fee for public medical care (approx. EUR 10–30) per visit.

— In 2017, Region Västra Götaland adopted regional clinical guidelines for adult individuals with severe dental anxiety/phobia, which included the provision of specialized cognitive behaviour therapy (CBT), administered by psychologists working in interdisciplinary collaboration with dental personnel within dentistry, to patients in the region.

Psychological treatment for adults with severe dental anxiety/phobia has thus been made available in all regions in Sweden according to the Swedish National Board of Health and Welfare. The treatment is provided in dental care clinics.

Over time, in addition to treating patients with severe dental anxiety, psychologists in dental care have also been assigned the tasks of contributing to dental care in other clinical areas (such as temporomandibular dysfunction), teaching of students and colleagues, and collaboration in research and development.

22.6.4.2 Clinical Work

Severe Dental Anxiety/Phobia in Adults

The major task for a psychologist in dental care is the *assessment and treatment of adult patients with severe dental anxiety/dental phobia*. In Sweden, as well as internationally, the evidence-based treatment for specific phobias is CBT with the focus on exposure-based interventions. Psychological assessment and treatment are usually performed in specialized hospital dental clinics/oral medicine units and are available in all regions in Sweden to varying degrees. Patients seek treatment via referrals or self-referrals.

In the Public Dental Service in Region Västra Götaland, the treatment is part of the regular dental care at three specialized hospital dental clinics/oral medicine clinics and follows the model developed at DAPRTC. Psychological treatment is delivered by a CBT-competent clinical psychologist employed at the dental clinic. There are several reasons why the psychologist works in the dental clinic, and why close interdisciplinary collaboration between the patient's psychologist and dentist is mandatory:

(i)   Individuals with severe dental anxiety are referred to dentistry (specialized hospital dental clinics).

(ii) For the psychologist to deliver the evidence-based treatment (CBT with exposure), the setting must be a dental treatment room with access to anxiety-provoking stimuli and situations.

(iii) To complete the CBT treatment, the patient needs to participate in "behavioural experiments" in the form of undergoing dental treatment by the dental team.

(iv) Since most patients have a deteriorated oral status and also need dental treatment, the CBT and the dental treatment must be sensibly planned and integrated, with the primary goal to cure the patients' severe dental anxiety/phobia.

In addition to the assessment of patients and the provision of CBT to patients with severe dental anxiety/phobia, the psychologist's assessment of the patient's mental health problems adds to the case formulation and to the dentist's understanding of the patient and of how to choose among the treatment options. When indicated, the psychologist can refer the patient to other psychological or psychiatric clinics. The psychologist also addresses compliance issues with patients using motivational techniques. Moreover, psychologists give consultations and provide supervision of the dental team.

Other Clinical Areas

Psychologists in Sweden can contribute to dental care in other areas as well; for example, assessment and treatment of children and adolescents with severe dental anxiety/phobia and dental behaviour management problems, behaviour change interventions for patients with poor oral health (caries, periodontal disease), assessment and treatment of patients with temporomandibular dysfunction and orofacial pain and support to patients with severe oral diseases (such as oral cancer).

At the Institute of Odontology, Gothenburg University, there is ongoing clinical research to evaluate a modified Acceptance and Commitment Therapy (ACT) intervention, a modern form of CBT, for behaviour change and better oral health in young adults with poor oral health. The brief, manualized ACT intervention is provided by a clinical psychologist working in general dental clinics within the Public Dental Service. The first evaluation showed promising results on oral health behaviour and oral health and has been well accepted by patients and the dental staff in the clinics.

22.6.4.3 Professional Development, Research, and Innovation

Psychologists in dental care are often engaged to supervise dental teams and provide teaching of basic psychological principles, communication, diagnostic, treatment issues, etc. This may take the form of *in-service training* for dental teams as well as *teaching at University clinics* with curricula for dentists and dental hygienists.

In many places, psychologists working in dental care take an active part in *clinical research and development* to develop diagnostic and treatment options for different groups of patients in dentistry, and in the planning, performance, analysis and reporting of clinical research and development projects.

References

Engel GL. The clinical application of the biopsychosocial model. Am J Psychiatry. 1980 May;137(5):535–44. https://doi.org/10.1176/ajp.137.5.535. PMID: 7369396. L G Ost Age of onset in different phobias J Abnorm Psychol. 1987;96(3):223–9. https://doi.org/10.1037//0021-843x.96.3.223. PMID: 3680761.

Newton JT. Interdisciplinary health promotion: a call for theory-based interventions drawing on the skills of multiple disciplines. Community Dent Oral Epidemiol. 2012;40(Suppl 2):49–54.

Kisely S. No mental health without oral health. Can J Psychiatr. 2016;61(5):277–82.

Öst LG. Age of onset in different phobias. J Abnorm Psychol. 1987;96:223–9.

Peres MA, Macpherson LMD, Weyant RJ, Daly B, Venturelli R, Mathur MR, Listl S, Celeste RK, Guarnizo-Herreño CC, Kearns C, Benzian H, Allison P, Watt RG. Oral diseases: a global public health challenge. Lancet. 2019;394(10194):249–60.

Widström E, Eaton KA. Oral healthcare systems in the extended European union. Oral Health Prev Dent. 2004;2:155–94.

Ford K, Brocklehurst P, Hughes K, Sharp CA, Bellis MA. Understanding the association between self-reported poor oral health and exposure to adverse childhood experiences: a retrospective study. BMC Oral Health. 2020;20(1):51.

de Jong-Lenters M, van Bussel J, Polak E, L'Hoir M, Duijster D. Toepasbaarheid van de 'Uitblinkers-interventie' om tandenpoetsen bij kinderen te verbeteren: een pilotonderzoek [Feasibility of the 'Uitblinkers' intervention to improve toothbrushing among children: a pilot study]. Ned Tijdschr Tandheelkd. 2020;127(3):189–98.

Lena Myran
Specialist in Clinical Psychology. Author and editor of textbook. Doing research related to dental anxiety, adverse childhood experience and oral health. Lecturer in psychology. Producer of psychological methods and tools (apps, handbooks, instructional videos and VR).

Jostein Paul Årøen Lein
Specialist in clinical psychology. Author and editor of textbook. Several years of experience in the treatment of dental anxiety in adults.

Margrethe Elin Vika
Psychologist/RN/PhD. Special interest in the treatment and research regarding dental anxiety in children and adults.

Ulla Wide
Professor Psychology (GU). Clinical psychologist treating patients with dental phobia, in dental care. Doing research and teaching students. Special interest in the evidence-based behavioural interventions.

Wendy Knibbe
Health care psychologist treating patients with orofacial pain and dysfunction, and maxillofacial prosthetics (adaptation, coping, and treating excessive gagging reflex). Also involved in research and teaching students.

Supplementary Information

Index